The Nursing Profession

The Nursing Profession

Views Through the Mist

Edited by
NORMA L. CHASKA, R.N., Ph. D.
Research Associate
Health Care Research Unit
Mayo Clinic and Mayo Foundation
Rochester, Minnesota

McGraw-Hill Book Company

A Blakiston Publication

New York   St. Louis   San Francisco   Auckland   Bogotá   Düsseldorf
Johannesburg   London   Madrid   Mexico   Montreal   New Delhi   Panama
Paris   São Paulo   Singapore   Sydney   Tokyo   Toronto

The Nursing Profession: Views Through the Mist

234567890   K P K P   78321098

This book was set in Press Roman by Allen Wayne Technical Corp.
The editor was Sally J. Barhydt; the cover was designed by Toni Goldmark;
the production supervisor was Jeanne Selzam.
Kingsport Press, Inc., was printer and binder.

Library of Congress Cataloging in Publication Data

Main entry under title:

The nursing profession

   "A Blakiston publication."
   Bibliography: p.
   Includes index.
   1. Nursing. 2. Nursing—United States. I. Chaska, Norma L.
[DNLM: 1. Nursing. WY100 N9784]
RT82.N87 610.73'0692 77-12025
ISBN 0-07-010695-9

TO
J. C.
L. E. T.
and my deceased parents
James and Edna
great teachers of growth
through living in the mist

Contents

Foreword

Teachers, researchers, clinicians, administrators, and consumers are witnessing considerable ferment and turbulence in the health field. The overall system may be visualized as a complex and dynamic mosaic constrained and influenced by a diverse group of dominant actors and interest groups. We strive to chart and understand the various forces and developments and hope to shape and influence them in order to achieve a more humane, equitable, and effective health system. But it is often difficult to keep up with the various developments or to stay abreast of the burgeoning and diffuse literature in the field.

The present volume is thus a welcome addition to the literature, for it contains a comprehensive and enlightening treatment of the nursing profession. It is impossible to conceive of the health delivery system of the future without contemplating the problems, deliberations, and changes in the nursing profession. A distinctive feature of the book is that twenty-nine of its contributors are nurse-sociologists who are unusually well equipped to enhance our knowledge and understanding of the profession of nursing. These contributors touch on a wide variety of subjects from different and stimulating perspectives. The authors also contribute to the more general area of sociology of the professions and occupations.

Dr. Chaska's introductions to the various sections of the book, the questions she raises after each of the chapters, and her final summary chapter should help make the book a useful teaching resource. The book should be helpful to nursing students, professional nurses who are taking continuing education courses, and students of the health professions in general. Dr. Chaska and her contributors are to be commended for producing this useful and timely volume.

Sol Levine, Ph.D.

University Professor of Sociology and Community Medicine
Chairperson, Department of Sociology, Boston University

Preface

Vague and nebulous is the beginning of all things,
but not their end,
And I fain would have you remember me as a beginning.
Life, and all that lives, is conceived in the mist and
not in the crystal.
And who knows but a crystal is mist in decay?*

Kahlil Gibran

Gibran presents a positive way of looking at change and uncertainty, which are inevitable in life. What he says might be applied to the professions, and specifically to the nursing profession. The beginning of nursing as a profession was clouded with doubt, and many questions arose about the directions nursing should take. As a pilgrim profession with no specific path to follow, nursing developed by taking a step at a time through the mist of uncertainty and change.

Seldom do we perceive anything as being crystal clear. Even when we do, our perception, like a crystal-clear sky, is temporary. For air, as well as life, is constantly moving. The time of mist in a profession is a time to reflect, question, plan, and reorganize. It is indicative of change. Visibility is reduced, but a luminosity still exists amidst the obscurity.

Mist provides moisture, which is needed for growth and life. Likewise, in nursing, diversity is the mist that nurtures the profession. This is not a time for absolutes. Professionals who ignore differing perspectives may limit their growth. As caring professionals, we need to identify the salient questions even though the answers may not be readily available. We must strive not for just any answer but for the best answer to each situation and problem that arises in the profession.

*Gibran, Kahlil. Reprinted from *The Prophet,* pocket edition, 1975, p. 100, with permission of the publisher, Alfred A. Knopf, Inc. Copyright 1923 by Kahlil Gibran; renewal copyright 1951 by Administrators C.T.A. of Kahlil Gibran Estate, and Mary G. Gibran.

A profession can seek answers in many ways. As different paths are explored or taken, the overall direction of nursing may become clearer. Inevitably, many different avenues will have to be explored in order to achieve the purposes of nursing. The answers may lie in finding the means to accept and take advantage of the diversity that exists.

Mist is a time to listen to many different voices, to identify options, and to take a step forward. In the time of mist, each one's "truth" needs to be questioned and tested in an open forum against the truth of others. This volume is a compilation of the knowledge of responsible professionals searching for answers in the profession of nursing. Most of the contributors are nurse-sociologists or recognized leaders in other branches of nursing. The perspective of sociology, and of other professions, may offer important contributions to nursing. We need to appreciate diversity: a member of a single profession cannot find truth alone.

Thus the purpose of this book is to provide a basis for reflecting on the present status of nursing as a profession and for dialogue in planning the future. A comprehensive presentation of nursing is needed at this time because of the ever-increasing rate of change in our society and in the nursing profession. Rather than reacting abruptly and haphazardly to changing forces, we must find an organized approach. This volume may provide the catalyst for perceptive planned change in the profession of nursing.

The book is divided into eight parts; the first seven parts contain chapters dealing with critical aspects of nursing as a profession: professionalization, nursing education, nursing research, nursing theory, nursing practice, interdisciplinary professional relationships, and the future of nursing. To facilitate the process of dialogue, questions for discussion are raised by the editor at the end of each chapter. Part Eight summarizes the current state of the profession, presents some conclusions, and raises further questions.

The questions that are posed throughout the volume may be helpful in a number of ways. Agencies or institutions employing nurses may use them in planning and establishing long-range goals. The questions may help identify and solve problems in organizations. It is hoped that they will greatly assist nursing educators at all levels in conducting discussion seminars for nursing students and, in addition, serve as the basis for specific course content. The questions should be of value to those interested in continuing education, whether they are instructors, practicing nurses, or nonpracticing nurses returning to practice. By reading the volume, reflecting on the questions, and positing possible answers, the reader should be able to gain a comprehensive perspective of the profession. The volume should help the reader to develop his or her own global view of the profession and to build a foundation for assessing possible future changes.

ACKNOWLEDGMENTS

This volume owes its existence to a happy association of interest in and concern for nursing on the part of the contributors, who had the difficult task of reviewing broad areas of nursing within the confines of a few pages. Their patience and good will in responding to stringent deadlines are gratefully appreciated.

I am much indebted to Mr. Norbert J. Gernes, whose volume *A View from the Mist**, suggested the title and theme of this book, and to the Alfred Knopf Publishing Company for permission to use a portion of a poem by Kahlil Gibran, from which the title originally developed. I am equally indebted to Sister M. Gretchen Berg, O.S.F., Ph.D., Sister Mary Brigh Cassidy, O.S.F., Consultant to Administration, Saint Mary's Hospital, Rochester, Minnesota, and Sister M. Kateri Heckathorn, O.S.F., Chairman of Intensive Care Nursing Services, Massachusetts General Hospital, for discussions about the theme of this volume and about the titles for the summary chapter and the book. Mr. Blaine Amann, National Weather Service Officer, Rochester, Minnesota, was helpful in defining the scientific concept of mist for its application in this volume.

My particular thanks are due to Miss Helen Jameson, Assistant Administrator of Patient Care Services, Rochester Methodist Hospital, Rochester, Minnesota, for discussions concerning the content of the book, and to Mrs. Sharon Tennis, Associate Director of Nursing, Rochester Methodist Hospital, Sister Gretta Monnig, O.S.F., Chairperson, Department of Nursing, College of St. Teresa, Winona, Minnesota, and Mrs. Mabelle J. Roberts Markee, Nurse Director (retired), Public Health Service, DHEW, for their discussions, suggestions, and review of the volume.

The encouragement, suggestions, and review of the summary chapter by Richard H. Hall, Ph.D., Professor of Sociology, State University of New York at Albany, were gratefully appreciated. I also want to thank John B. McKinlay, Ph.D., Department of Sociology, Boston University, for initially encouraging me to edit this volume.

I am indebted to Mrs. Verna Houlton for skillful secretarial services and to Mrs. Patricia Meyers for faithful and proficient secretarial assistance during the irregular hours required for the preparation of the manuscript.

Finally, I am greatly indebted to my family, friends, and colleagues of the Health Care Research Unit for their sustained support, encouragement, and interest; without them the development of this volume would not have been possible. This volume does not necessarily reflect the views or opinions of the Mayo Clinic.

I wish to extend special appreciation to the publisher and to Sally J. Barhydt at McGraw-Hill Book Company for their interest, counsel, and continued support in the production of this volume.

Norma L. Chaska

*Norbert J. Gernes, *A View from the Mist,* Vantage Press, New York, 1975.

Introduction

All professional nurses need this book. Nursing students, whether undergraduate or graduate, who are seeking to understand nursing's past, its present diversity, and its future potential, will find the contents challenging and will welcome the clear organization. Nursing faculty, whose aspirations for excellence are not always compatible with realistic time constraints, will bless the editor, the contributors, and the publisher—everyone who made this tremendous resource book possible. *The Nursing Profession: Views Through the Mist* should become a ready reference not only for nurses and medical sociologists but for our whole fraternity of interdisciplinary colleagues. The latter, although increasingly respectful, impressed—even downright fascinated—with nursing's contributions and potential, still admit to some confusion.

A text and resource book such as this is overdue. Its theme and organizational framework succeed in striking an appropriate tone—no small accomplishment considering the different publics which exist within nursing today. For instance, one chapter refers to three major criteria of a profession: a long period of specialization, a service orientation, and autonomy. These terms, as well as many others throughout the chapters, may seem controversial to some and will have different meanings to nurse readers. Yet interpretations of various aspects of professionalism are handled skillfully and sensitively by the authors throughout the text. The practical, service-oriented aspects of professionalism in nursing are not neglected even though this elite group of authors also demonstrates the capacity to ascend to the heights of philosophical thinking. The chapters that comprise this volume present many facets of the nursing profession and of the conditions that affect it. Each is distinctive in form and content; there is no pressure to mold the reader's mind to this or that formula.

In the final section dealing with the future, one author cites Florence Nightingale's vision of nursing as "... work designed to keep people well, to help them avoid disease and to restore them to their highest possible levels of health. She identified the need to discover knowledge that could be structured as the science of health. She knew that nursing one day would become a learned profession."[1] But even the forceful Miss Nightingale's design for nursing became enshrouded in mist and, as we are aware, its extrication after pressures from cultural, social and educational forces has been painfully slow. Mary Roberts' *American Nursing*[2] portrayed the misty origins of professional nursing in the United States by pointing out that in nineteenth-century America, as soon as the earliest hospital schools of nursing opened their doors, the term *professional* was applied to graduates—even though secondary school education was not required for admission!

The editor has defined *mist* as necessary for growth and life. Perhaps the very mist that has slowed our professional development has at the same time nourished and sustained Nightingale's vision. This tremendous volume testifies that many nurses have utilized "the time of mist" for thinking and doing—for developing into responsible professionals. I am not troubled that nursing does not yet have all the answers. I believe that the advent of the nursing profession's "clear day" will be related to continued effort on the part of the nurses themselves—efforts that are demonstrated so well in this remarkable volume.

Marion I. Murphy, R.N., Ph.D., L.H.D.
Dean and Professor, School of Nursing
University of Maryland, Baltimore

[1] Rozella M. Schlotfeldt, Chapter 39, p. 408.
[2] Mary M. Roberts, *American Nursing,* MacMillan, New York, 1954, p. 48.

Part One

Professionalization

The first section of this volume is concerned with the efforts of nursing to transcend the characteristics of an occupation and assume the status of a profession. Within that process we are interested in how members of an occupational group become socialized as professionals. The legitimation of nursing as a profession, which is treated in Part One, is the starting point for all the subsequent sections in this volume. To understand the challenges that face nursing today and to find appropriate ways to meet them, we need to examine nursing as a profession.

The contributions to this part stress the issues related to nursing as a profession and portray the values and behavior patterns of the contemporary professional nurse. Most often the term *profession* is conceptualized as an abstract ideal category, and specific occupations are located on a continuum in accordance with the degree to which each possesses characteristics defined as *professional*. The goal is to increase the number of professional attributes of nursing, in order to improve the quality of nursing and to achieve professional status. Throughout the ensuing pages, many characteristics of a true profession are shown to be present in nursing.

Chapter 1

Toward a Philosophy of Nursing

Juanita F. Murphy, R.N., Ph.D.
Dean, College of Nursing
Arizona State University, Tempe

It is appropriate that Murphy's article is the first contribution in this part because it provides a descriptive analysis of contemporary professional nursing. Murphy examines the philosophical positions of three nurse leaders—Dorothy Johnson, Martha Rogers, and Rozella Schlotfeldt—on the nature and scope of professional nursing, and outlines the perspective of each on the mission, knowledge base, and activities of the professional nurse. She concludes that these aspects of nursing are not the same for the professional nurse as for the technical nurse. The lack of recognition of these differences is a major dilemma for the nurse today.

Contemporary nurses are for the most part aware of their rich heritage, which has been accumulated through nurses collectively and enhanced through the momentous efforts of outstanding individuals. Historically, nurses have been concerned about the meaning, perceptions, and impact of their professional behavior. But in the present era of dramatic social change, some nurses are more concerned about the future of nursing as a profession. Where are we going? Should we build on the past? Can we define the essential mission of professional nursing in the past and use this definition as a stepping stone for the future? The uncertainties regarding nursing's mission and the responsibilities, roles, and accountability of those who practice nursing are profound indeed.

Helping people has been the major concern of nursing for more than a century. Nightingale, who was recognized as the visionary founder of professional, scientific nursing, indicated that the art of maintaining health as well as the art of nursing the

sick was the explicit prerogative of nurses. Included in Nightingale's list of future activities for nurses was maintaining the health and improving the health potential of all mankind. It is important to note that for more than a hundred years there has been an emphasis on health and illness behavior. Nightingale recognized the meager state of knowledge regarding nursing practice during her time, but envisioned the accumulation of inordinate amounts of knowledge by nurses in the future, which would increase the well-being of humanity and relieve human suffering.

Nevertheless, contemporary nursing is described generally as being impersonal, routine, and standardized. This is partly because it is not clear whether nurses are the handmaidens of physicians and/or of hospital administrators. Little evidence exists to show that nursing care has made a significant impact on the general welfare and well-being of society. Moreover, there is little agreement concerning the nature and scope of nursing knowledge, and this at a time when a knowledge explosion is occurring in many other fields. Technological advances have increased the responsibility of nurses for the technical management of various aspects of medical care, leaving them with little time to give personal services to patients. As a result, ancillary personnel have been employed in large measure to give personal services to patients under the supervision of professional nurses. In most modern, complex hospitals professional nurses have thus become only indirect providers of patient care. This means that nursing care as an art and science is not generally being offered by those who are best prepared educationally to provide it. Nursing as a field of scientific inquiry has been arrested in its growth. Many nursing methods and practices have not changed for years, and nursing practice has become static.

This kind of analysis of contemporary professional nursing has led nurses and others interested in the delivery of health care to question the status of nurses as professionals. Under particular scrutiny have been the service-oriented activities of nurses, the body of scientific knowledge that provides the rationale for nursing practice, and the ability of nurses to judiciously apply knowledge in an autonomous manner. The service orientation of nurses seems to have shifted from the welfare of patients to the welfare of the employing institution; documentation of the scientific basis for nursing practice is fragmentary; and the autonomy of professional nurses is continually challenged, since the knowledge base of nursing has been derived intuitively and experientially. Moreover, some professional nurses have been reluctant to assume the accountability for their profession, which is essential for professional autonomy.

What is the future for professional nursing? What changes can be made in the future that would not only ensure survival, but also enhance the development of professional nursing? Are there prescriptive recommendations? If so, can they be implemented?

Most of these questions have been given serious attention by nurse leaders who are concerned about the future of professional nursing. In this chapter selected philosophical positions of three contemporary nurse leaders (Johnson, Rogers, and Schlotfeldt) are examined with a view to pointing out their differences and similarities. Specifically, the assumptions of each nurse-philosopher regarding the *mission* and *knowledge base* of professional nursing, and the *activities* of professional nurses, are analyzed, as well as their recommendations for the future.*

MISSION

Occupational groups survive and are given recognition by society if they fulfill defined societal needs. Because the nature and scope of these needs changes over a period of time, the mission of these groups also changes. For example, Johnson points out that "patient care as a significant aspect of nursing practice has steadily lost ground in the last fifty years or more."[1] According to Johnson, patients need care by the professional nurse, but the nurse's time is consumed in monitoring medical activities delegated by the physician and managing the auxiliary personnel on the ward. For professional nurses to carry out their mission of patient care, they must be socialized as scholars in institutions of higher education, where they would develop a commitment to inquiry and "skill in the use of knowledge as applicable to the solution of the practical problems of man."[2] Thus, Johnson particularizes the mission of professional nursing by pointing out that professional nurses of the future must develop skill in the use of knowledge from the sciences and humanities in caring for patients.

Schlotfeldt maintains that the mission of professional nursing is "the promotion of health of all people."[3] She notes that this mission was clearly explicated by Florence Nightingale over a hundred

*It should be noted that the publications selected for this analysis were not written for the specific purposes for which the author has elected to use them. If, for this reason, erroneous references are drawn, this is certainly not intended by the author.

years ago and is still endorsed by nursing's leaders. However, until recently, this mission could not be fulfilled because our society placed limited importance on services for maintaining health. People tended to seek the services of health providers only in cases of illnesses. But in the future, with the growing recognition of the value of maintaining health as a personal and national asset, professional nurses will be the prime providers of services for the prevention of disease and the promotion and maintenance of health. Schlotfeldt evokes an image of nursing in the future as "the profession whose practitioners are responsible for and willing to be held accountable for assessing and promoting the health status, assets and potential of all human beings."[4] In her visionary plans for the "dramatic renewal" of nursing, educational approaches would focus "on providing students with opportunities to develop judgment in decision making and in the execution of the gamut of skills essential to the practice of professional nursing."[5] It is her expectation that nursing will become a recognized, learned profession and that nurses will provide essential services that will enhance the health and well-being of our society.

Rogers forthrightly states that "the purpose of nursing is to help people achieve their maximum health potential."[6] She adds that "nursing's first line of defense is promotion of health and prevention of illness. Care of the sick is resorted to when our first line of defense fails."[7]

The welfare of the whole person is seen as the focus of nursing and the practice of nursing should be directed toward dealing with human beings in every stage of the life process. Rogers maintains that the predictable health needs of our society demand that nurses as primarily "doers" be replaced by nurses who are proficient in using a core of knowledge both for nursing diagnosis and for interventions directed toward rationally formulated goals.

The similarities in these definitions of the mission of professional nursing are apparent. But, while Johnson tends to emphasize the care of the sick, Schlotfeldt and Rogers are firm in their convictions that health promotion and health maintenance, coupled with prevention of disease, are the prime concern of professional nursing. Nurses should be responsible and accountable to society for carrying out this essential mission.

BODY OF KNOWLEDGE

If nurses are to carry out the missions described above as *professionals*, they must be inculcated with a body of knowledge on which to base their practice. The apprentice-type education obtained in hospital schools of nursing during the first half of this century drew on a body of knowledge that was rather simple to extrapolate and identify. For the most part, this body of knowledge was derived intuitively and was taught primarily by physicians. Those methods and procedures which "worked" became a part of the traditional package of nursing knowledge. It was not important to understand why or how they worked, but rather to carry out the established procedures in an effective and efficient manner. The efficacy of such procedures and their impact on the well-being of patients were rarely questioned.

The content and the methods of teaching did not change measurably as nursing education programs shifted from hospitals to institutions of higher education. A series of general education courses was established as a prerequisite to the nursing major courses, but the applicability of the prerequisite courses to the practice of nursing was not always clear. Questions still arise as to what general education courses students should be required to complete before taking nursing courses, and on the relationship of general education to the practice of nursing. The three nurse-philosophers are quite explicit about general education requirements, the relationship of these courses to nursing practice, and the relationship of advanced general education courses to postbaccalaureate educational programs in nursing. All three agree that the education of professional nurses must be carried out in institutions of higher education.

Rogers is noted particularly for her stand on doctoral education in nursing. Perhaps less understood is her forthright stance on the education of professional nurses generally and the logical relationships she sees between baccalaureate education programs, master's education programs, and doctoral education for nurses.

Rogers' comments on the theoretical basis of nursing practice published in 1963 have not been modified to a perceptible degree.

> The theoretical base of nursing practice is nursing science. Nursing science is a body of scientific knowledge characterized by descriptive, explanatory and predictive principles about the life process in man. These principles rest on the views that man is a unified "bio-physical-psycho-social" phenomenon in constant interaction with all parts of the environment. This body of knowledge developed through synthesis and re-synthesis of selected knowledges from the humanities and the biological, physical and social sciences for new concepts and understanding about man and his environment (the hypothetical generalizations in scientific principles of nursing). It assumes its own "unique scientific mix" through selection and patterning of these knowledges.[8]

In another article published during the same year, Rogers adds that "the explanatory and predictive principles of nursing make possible nursing diagnoses and knowledgeable interventions toward predictable goals."[9] She continues in the same article by specifying the knowledge that students majoring in nursing must be familiar with.[10] Among these are knowledge of English, history, logic and philosophy, foreign languages, mathematics, biology, chemistry, sociology, physics, literature, anthropology, psychology, political science, and economics. Rogers infers that, based on this strong foundation in sciences and humanities at both the lower and upper college levels, an aggregate of theories has developed which represents the core of nursing knowledge. There is an explicit emphasis on the synthesis and resynthesis of this aggre-gate knowledge for the development and emergence of nursing principles. Rogers notes that nursing science is not additive, but creative. She states further that specialization in nursing should begin at the postbaccalaureate level, and maintains that traditional areas of specialization such as medical-surgical nursing do not form a rational basis for the development of nursing knowledge that could be logically related to nursing practice.

Further, Rogers maintains that doctoral students in nursing must gain knowledge of research tools and methodology. They must have cognate courses at the graduate level selected from the natural and social sciences and from the humanities. Doctoral students in nursing need courses in philosophy, in modern logic, and in advanced mathematics. There must be advanced study in nursing in the doctoral programs in which nursing is the major, since majoring in other subject areas does not provide the necessary knowledge base. Courses in other areas are selected (for the process of synthesis and resynthesis) for their applicability to the development of nursing principles.

Johnson proposes that knowledge in the basic sciences should be "substantial enough" at the baccalaureate level to provide a basis for either graduate study or a research career.[11] She decries the lack of knowledge in the humanities, since the development of leadership qualities is dependent upon a firm understanding of the humanities. Contrary to Rogers, Johnson believes that "nursing science and the content of nursing science courses may evolve more easily through the identification of common, but major, problems of patients that are of direct concern to nursing."[12] From this identification of common, major problems of patients, the content of nursing courses is derived inductively. Johnson questions the overemphasis on the application of skills and calls for an emphasis on skill in the use of knowledge. Her views on teaching strategies are logically related to her emphasis on skill and the use of knowledge. She challenges nursing educators' traditional methods of assigning students to patients on the basis of particular disease entity, and suggests that it would be more viable to assign students to the appropriate nursing care of the "whole person."

Johnson's view of levels of competence in research are noteworthy. She maintains that, at the baccalaureate level, students should learn to understand the gaps in scientific knowledge and the means by which knowledge can be increased; graduate programs should prepare nursing students in research competency. At all levels, students should be trained to think logically, analytically, and creatively. Curricula in nursing programs should not be standardized, but renewed attention should be given to the meaning of the application of knowledge.

It should be mentioned that Johnson has proposed an imaginative typology for the classification of knowledge required for the practice of nursing.[13] Included in her classificatory system are three types of knowledge: knowledge of order, knowledge of disorder, and knowledge of control. Concerted efforts by nursing researchers in the future should be placed on knowledge of disorder and knowledge of control. This typology of knowledge proposed by Johnson holds much promise for future scientific inquiry into nursing.

Schlotfeldt maintains that nursing theories are derived from systematic observation, and that the observations are guided by theory.[14] She begins with the premise that events do not occur by chance, and the development of nursing knowledge is dependent upon the abilities of nurses to search for "antecedent-consequent relationships between facts and phenomena."[15] Theoretical postulates are inductively arrived at when plausible explanations for associations can be formulated. Repeated tests are needed to ascertain the validity of a relationship so that predictions can be accurate.

Schlotfeldt indicates that the content to be mastered by students in programs of professional nursing is essentially the "theoretical and scientific concepts related to nursing . . . the study of man as a biosocial, psychological, value being and . . . the health-seeking mechanism available to man in differing environments and under varied circumstances affecting his health status and potential."[16] Students should be afforded a variety of opportunities to develop judgment and to make decisions as independent, primary care practitioners. Schlotfeldt proposes the operation of health assessment/health promotion clinics by schools of nursing for the development of these skills. It is essential nursing faculty supply good role models of professional nurses if students are to develop concern for high quality and standards.

Schlotfeldt foresees the rapid development of programs leading to professional doctorates in nursing (an N.D. degree) during the next 10 years. She also predicts that professional doctorates in nursing will be required for nurses entering practice. Additionally, in order to develop the scholars and researchers needed in the future, Schlotfeldt envisions the opportunity for the N.D. students to earn a Ph.D. degree simultaneously. She urges the recruitment of scholars from the biological and social-behavioral sciences into nursing to earn the N.D. degree.

A solid foundation in general education is thought essential by all three nurse-philosophers. Knowledge from other scientific disciplines can guide the observations of the nursing practitioner. The unique character of nursing knowledge is derived from the process of synthesis and resynthesis, as health-related phenomena are examined in the light of concepts and theories from other subject areas.

ACTIVITIES

There is general agreement among the three nurse-philosophers that the professional nurse of the future will be a practitioner able to use the scientific method for the analysis and resolution of health care problems. He or she will be expected to share findings and concerns with professional nurse colleagues. Direct involvement in all aspects of the health care of mankind must be the broad goal. In the process of direct involvement with patients, observations must be recorded routinely and systematically, and generalizing questions must be asked which derive from these clinical data. If professional nursing is to realize its true mission and to fulfill its potential, there must be a renewed commitment to use knowledge for the practical solution of problems of humanity.

RECOMMENDATIONS AND SUMMARY

Technical nursing must be separated both educationally and functionally from professional nursing. Both aspects of nursing are needed and should be supported. But the failure to recognize that the goals, body of knowledge, and expected activities of each aspect are different only perpetuates the many dilemmas of the contemporary nurse.

Nurses who are technically oriented should continue to be concerned with the routine prescribed management of patients. Their actions should be judged from the perspective of efficient and effective management of procedures. Nurses who are professionally oriented should develop the understanding and ability to use the scientific method as a basis for the nursing process. Some nurses may be proficient in both areas, but unless there is a renewed commitment to a broad knowledge base to serve as a rationale for implementing and evaluating health and illness care, nursing as a profession is in jeopardy.

In this era of increasing accountability, professional nurses must develop the courage and tenacity needed to meet the health care needs of society. Risk taking can be challenging and exciting, and unless we are willing to take risks our mission will go unfulfilled. Our rich heritage demands a renewed commitment to the ideals and standards of quality nursing care by qualified professional nurses.

NOTES

1 D. E. Johnson, "Nursing and Health Education," *International Journal of Nursing Studies*, 1:219, 1964.
2 Ibid., p. 222.
3 R. N. Schlotfeldt, "Can We Bring Order Out of the Chaos of Nursing Education?" *American Journal of Nursing*, 76:105, January 1976.
4 Ibid., p. 106.
5 Ibid.
6 M. E. Rogers, "Doctoral Education in Nursing," *Nursing Forum*, 5:77, 1966.
7 Ibid.
8 M. E. Rogers, "Some Comments on the Theoretical Basis of Nursing Practice," *Nursing Science*, 1:11, April 1963.
9 M. E. Rogers, "Building a Strong Educational Foundation," *American Journal of Nursing*, 63:94, June 1963.
10 Ibid., p. 95.
11 D. E. Johnson, "Patterns in Professional Nursing Education," *Nursing Outlook*, 9:608, October 1961.
12 Ibid., p. 609.
13 D. E. Johnson, "Theory in Nursing: Borrowed and Unique," *Nursing Research*, 17:206–209, May–June 1968.
14 R. N. Schlotfeldt, "Reflections on Nursing Research," *American Journal of Nursing*, 60(4):492–494, April 1960.
15 Ibid., p. 494.
16 R. N. Schlotfeldt, "Can We Bring Order Out of the Chaos of Nursing Education?" op. cit., 106.

EDITOR'S QUESTIONS FOR DISCUSSION

In the definition of the mission of the professional nurse, what has brought about the change in emphasis from the care of the sick to the promotion and maintenance of health? Currently, is the mission defined differently in the educational programs for the technical and the professional nurse? What changes in the health care delivery system and in educational programs are essential if the future professional nurse is to be the main provider of services for the prevention of disease? If the role of the professional nurse will be concerned primarily with prevention of disease, who will fulfill the role of caring for the ill? What type of knowledge and skills will be needed to prepare nurses for the roles of health maintenance and caring for the ill?

How can the application of a scientific knowledge base for nursing practice be instilled as a value? To what extent does the setting for nursing practice either inhibit or encourage the application of knowledge? Does the application of a scientific knowledge base for nursing make a difference in the outcome of patient care?

If professional doctorates in nursing (N.D.) were to be required for nurses entering practice, what type of service would such nurses provide? How would the role of a nurse who has a professional doctorate in nursing be legitimated? How could the need for a nurse who has a doctorate in nursing be justified economically, functionally, and educationally?

Chapter 2

Professional Socialization of Nurses

Ada Jacox, R.N., Ph.D.
Associate Dean for Research, Professor of Nursing
School of Nursing, University of Colorado, Denver

Jacox discusses the process by which the nurse acquires the identity characteristics of a professional in terms of three criteria for professionalism: specialized education, service orientation, and autonomy. Attributes the nurse may have acquired previously, such as obedience, are now deemphasized. Autonomy, which means that members of a profession are self-regulating and have control of their functions in the work setting, has become increasingly valued. Jacox emphasizes the importance of autonomous role models in the clinical setting as part of the socialization process. In the past, primary emphasis in this process was on education; today, service and practice are recognized as important factors in the development of professionalism.

Our interest today is to consider professional socialization, particularly with respect to how basic nursing education should and can contribute to the socialization of nursing students. Professional socialization is the process by which a person acquires the knowledge, skills, and sense of occupational identity characteristic of a professional (12). The process involves the internalization of the values and norms of a professional group into one's own behavior and self-conception. It is important to recognize that professional socialization does not begin with entry into a professional school, but has its roots in the earlier experiences of the person which result in the decision to join a particular occupational group. Before discussing professional socialization further, I'd like to consider briefly the sociological concept of professions, and comment on how sociologists have generally tended to view nursing.

The two major criteria for a profession are a long period of specialized education and a service orientation. A third characteristic, which is derived from these two, is autonomy. That is, members of the profession are self-regulating and have control of their functions in the work situation. Autonomy is granted a profession when society is confident that members of that occupation possess specialized knowledge and place service or community interests above self-interests. Because of the esoteric nature of the knowledge, only members of the profession are recognized as competent to define what tasks and practices are necessary and safe (17).

Occupations are not commonly divided into those which are and those which are not professions. Rather, they can be arranged along a continuum of professionalism according to the degree to which they are characterized by the above combination of attributes (4). The notion of degrees of professionalism gives rise to such terms

This article was originally published in *The Journal of the New York State Nurses Association*, 4(4):6–15, November 1973.

as "emerging profession," "marginal profession," "semi-profession," "professionalizing occupation," and so forth, all of which labels have been applied to nursing at one time or another. The points along the continuum are not clearly defined. To do so would be difficult, since the three major criteria—education, service, and autonomy—must be considered simultaneously, and there are many variations possible for each criterion. Etzioni (8) differentiates between "full-fledged" and "semi-professional" by placing those with five years or more of professional training into the full-fledged group and those with less education into the semi-professional group. Education, however, is only one of the ways in which he differentiates levels of professionalism.

Etzioni and other sociologists gave particular attention to three occupations—nursing, social work, and teaching—in a book entitled *The Semi-Professions and their Organization*. Etzioni asserts that semi-professions are distinguished from full professions by several characteristics. One, their training is shorter; two, their status is less legitimated; three, the right to privileged communication is less established; four, there is less of a specialized body of knowledge; and five, they have less autonomy from supervision or societal control than do the full-fledged professions (8). A common characteristic of the three semi-professions selected for study is that a majority of their members are women. This fact has major implications for how these occupations have developed, and is a point to which special emphasis will be given in this paper.

Simpson and Simpson observe that teaching, social work, and nursing are organized more along bureaucratic lines than they are professional collegial lines. They claim that this happens because semi-professionals lack the degree of specialized knowledge around which professionals build collegial authority patterns. These authors suggest that the fact that most semi-professionals are women seems to increase the tendency for these occupations to be organized along bureaucratic lines.

> The public is less willing to grant professional autonomy to women then to men, and . . . women are less likely than men to develop attitudes favorable to professionalism, because

most of them are oriented more toward family roles than toward work roles. So long as our family system and the prevailing attitudes of men and women about feminine sex roles remain essentially as they now are, this basic situation seems unlikely to change (15).

So far in the discussion, we have considered the concept of profession in terms of its three major characteristics and have seen that occupations are considered more or less professional according to the degree to which they possess these attributes. An analysis of nursing by sociologists suggested that the public's attitude toward women and women's notions about their own roles serve to define nursing as a semi-profession. Let us now look more closely at professional socialization into nursing.

As mentioned earlier, although the formal beginning of professional socialization is admission to a professional school, a person's expectations of and ideas about a profession—in this case nursing—actually begin to develop at a much earlier time. Many who decide to become nurses make this decision at a very young age. Nursing has been one of the few occupations that are commonly recognized as appropriate for girls to enter. One of the traditional gifts for little girls is a nurse's kit, by which they learn some of the activities and functions that presumably are associated with being a nurse. Favorite reading for many little girls was the Cherry Ames series, which described the adventures of a girl who became a nurse. Nurses are portrayed on television, in the movies, and other media, so that girls and boys who aspire to be nurses have a great deal of exposure to the role of the nurse as it has been defined in these varied sources. Considering those books, games, and so forth which propose to inform children about what it is to be a nurse, the characteristics portrayed usually are interest in people, warmth, and obedience of the doctor and of "superior" nurses. Movies and television programs often picture the nurse in much the same way with particular emphasis on obedience. Another common portrayal of the nurse for adult audiences is as a sex symbol.

It is a rare movie, TV program or book which characterizes the nurse as an intelligent, independent person who is making important decisions about the care of the patient.

School counselors reinforce the stereotype of the nurse. Preparation in nursing has long been considered to be particularly useful to girls from the lower and middle social classes since it not only prepared them to be "good" wives and mothers, but also gave them some training to fall back on in case they needed to contribute financially to the support of the family. In addition to these more vicarious contacts with nurses, many girls and boys have relatives or acquaintances who are nurses. Since most nurses work in hospital settings, the stereotype of the nurse as one who cares for acutely ill patients is reinforced.

An important point to remember in the usual portrayal of the nurse is the heavy emphasis on obedience. I'd like to refer to a few writings early in nursing's history which emphasize the importance of the nurse being obedient. The first is taken from a paper given by Lavinia Dock in 1893. An excerpt from this paper states:

> Absolute and unquestioning obedience must be the foundation of the nurse's work, and to this end complete subordination of the individual to the work as a whole is as necessary for her as for the soldier. This can only be obtained by a systematic grading of rank, a clear, definite chain of responsibility, and one sole source of authority . . . concentrated in the head of the school as their representative and delegate. . . . On one field only does the school properly come under the command of the medical profession, and that is in the direct care of the sick. Here indeed the command is absolute. The whole purpose of the school centers around this point, and the pride of the well-drilled nurse is to make this service perfect. Now for the first time in history of medical science can its orders be carried out faithfully, fully and at all hours (7).

Another excerpt from a document in 1887 outlined several directives for floor nurses. These included:

> In addition to caring for your 50 patients, each nurse will follow these regulations: . . . Daily sweep and mop the floors of your ward, dust the patient's furniture and window sills. . . . The nurse's notes are important in aiding the physician's work. Make your pens carefully; you may whittle nibs to your individual taste . . . . Graduate nurses in good standing with the director of nurses will be given an evening off each week for courting purposes or two evenings a week if you go regularly to church . . . . Any nurse who smokes, uses liquor in any form, gets her hair done at a beauty shop, or frequents dance halls will give the director of nurses good reason to suspect her worth, intentions and integrity (18).

The fact was that many nursing programs were developed in the context of religious orders and the military served to reinforce the obedience and authoritarianism that prevailed in nursing schools and programs. While nursing certainly has moved away from such absolute obedience as was stressed some hundred years ago, we have not moved far enough away. Obedience is still seen as a major virtue for young people who are interested in becoming nurses. The selection of students into some nursing programs reflects this emphasis on obedience as an important characteristic for nurses. Student nurses commonly rank high on obedience scores on personality tests when compared with students in other programs.

This discussion of how nursing is popularly portrayed, particularly in regard to the characteristic of obedience, is meant to emphasize the fact that the new recruit to nursing who appears for the first day in class already has more or less well-established notions of what it means to be a nurse. These attitudes and expectations necessarily influence how the student receives and responds to that which is encountered after entering the school. For example, during the past decade or so, there has been an attempt made in many nursing programs to emphasize health as well as illness. This often takes the form of introducing the student first to a healthy group of people before going into the acute care setting. The idea is to try to establish early in the student's mind the notions that nurses are concerned with health by focusing first on health. Those of you who have taught in such programs know that a common response of many of the beginning students is "when will we finish this part and get to the *real* nursing in the hospitals?" Because they have been taught to believe that real nursing is what takes place in acute care settings, this is what many come to school expecting to learn. And, they feel disillusioned or somehow cheated at not being able to get right on with this. If a program is successful of course, the student begins to change her view of nursing and to internalize some aspects of this new role—that is, nursing the healthy as well as the sick. Nurses entering associate degree programs, diploma programs, or baccalaureate programs all have some of the same expectations regarding the kinds of experiences they will encounter and the kinds of identities that they will develop as they become nurses. A common notion of the nurse is an obedient person who cares for acutely ill people.

Having brought the student to the door of the school, whether community college, hospital, or university, let us now consider some of the factors that contribute to the socialization of the student. These are many and varied, and they include the faculty, the clinical settings in which the student works, the patients, other students, members of other disciplines, and the larger community of which the school is a part. In the discussion to follow, we will consider two of these—the faculty and the clinical settings. These two factors will be considered in terms of the extent to which they provide experiences that reflect the three core characteristics of professionalism—education, service, and autonomy.

How successful faculty are in helping the student to develop a professional identity is partially dependent on how well faculty themselves have internalized the values of a professional. Many faculty reflect a good bit of ambivalence about what constitutes professionalism, particularly in regard to education and autonomy. Let us deal first with the criterion on which there is most

consensus, the one which specifies that professionals perform a service and act in the best interests of the client in performing that service. Nurses, including nurse educators, have a strong commitment to service. Nursing's origins in religious orders emphasized the importance of performing a service, and this emphasis has been largely retained. In recent years faculty have been self-critical and have been criticized by others for not being more involved in giving direct service themselves. This problem was addressed by the 1972 ANA House of Delegates, which passed a resolution urging that "faculty avail themselves of the opportunities for active involvement in providing nursing care. . . ." There does seem to be a strong effort by nurse faculty to identify and develop ways to engage in practice, confirming the service orientation that they share with other nurses.

A criterion upon which there is less agreement is that of education. The literature generally says something like "a long period of formal preparation" or "an extended period of training," leaving the interpretation of length of time open. Among the conflicts that arise within an occupation in the process of becoming a profession is one between those who are urging the upgrading of educational standards and those who do not want to be left behind or defined as less than professional. This conflict is reflected in the bitter controversies among nurses following the publication of two documents—the ANA's 1965 position paper on education (2) and the ANA Board of Directors' recent statement on graduates of diploma programs (1). The first document placed primary emphasis on education as a criterion for professionalism. The second stressed the importance of the service contributed by nurses, in this case graduates of diploma schools. The two statements have been interpreted in many ways, with some viewing them as contradictory. Rather than being contradictory, they seem to be emphasizing different criteria of professionalism, neither one of which is more important than the other. Performing a needed service for society and attaining specialized knowledge through a long period of education are both important attributes of a profession.

In any case, there has been and will very likely continue to be ambivalence and controversy among nurses as the move to upgrade educational standards and to locate all formal nursing education programs within the system of higher education progresses. This ambivalence will be reflected in nurse faculty as well as in other nurses, and will be an influence in the socialization of student nurses for some time to come.

Moving now to the third characteristic of a profession—that of autonomy—we come to the one on which nursing has made the least progress. For this reason, I would like to spend more time discussing this than was spent on education and service.

You recall that autonomy means that professionals have control over their own functions in the work setting. This notion is in direct opposition to the high value that nursing has traditionally placed on obedience. Nurses for years have been taught that obedience is a prime virtue, with students and graduate nurses alike expected to follow unquestioningly the orders of doctors and their "superiors" in nursing. In nursing service departments, authority was, and still is for the most part, vested in administrative position, rather than deriving from the expert knowledge of the professional. The model in which the top administrator and a few assistants unilaterally make all major decisions was carried over into schools of nursing, where it continues in far too many places.

In long established academic settings, there has been a strong tradition of faculty participation in matters of general educational policy and faculty status. Faculty determine curriculum, admission standards, and similar educational matters, and also evaluate the performance of each other in a system of peer review. Nurse faculties have not yet generally developed this kind of autonomy, especially in regard to decisions about faculty status. In many schools of nursing, decisions concerning initial appointments, promotions, and tenure are made solely by administrators, rather than through peer evaluation. Even in areas of educational policy, administrators have made unilateral deci-

sions, sometimes with little resistance from faculty. The model in which all authority resides in administrative position is contrary to the model of professionalism, in which authority derives from the knowledge of the profession.

In two separate articles in recent years, Marjorie Batey (5) and Janet Williamson (19) described very well the conflict experienced by university nurse faculty members who have completed doctoral programs and internalized the value of professional autonomy. On return to a nursing faculty, these persons often find it difficult to practice in accordance with their newly acquired values. Williamson describes the dilemma of the doctoral prepared nurse who has learned to expect that faculty will be able to exercise a great deal of control over how they teach. The role of administrator in such departments or institutions is as coordinator or consultant to other faculty members. Williamson states that:

> Many nurse-faculty members find it difficult to consult and coordinate. They are much more secure with the issuance and acceptance of commands or directives. These faculty members accept the mother surrogate role and oversee all aspects of student life, thus transmitting to the student an acceptance of the norms of the institutional system, or at least reducing the strength of the professional orientation (19).

While nursing faculties in some settings are making progress toward a professional model of academic decision making, many still have a long way to go. This is a problem which should concern us greatly in our attempts to help students develop professional identities, for we cannot transmit values that we ourselves do not believe in or exemplify.

Moving from faculty as an influence in the socialization of nursing students to another major influence—that of the clinical setting—some of the same problems become evident. In keeping with the major focus of this paper, I will deal primarily with the lack of autonomy of nurses in practice settings.

In most contemporary health agencies, there is a rather rigidly organized bureaucracy, with an emphasis on obedience rather than on autonomous behavior by nurses. Nurses' actions are so greatly determined by prescribed routines, policies, administrative directives, and physicians' orders that there is little freedom left for the exercise of professional judgment. The frustrations of new graduates in trying to act independently and creatively have been well described by Marlene Kramer (9) in her studies of professional-bureaucratic role conflict. Kramer has described the exodus of baccalaureate graduates from nursing as a result of their not being able to use the knowledge that they gained while in their education programs. Feeling frustrated and thwarted in their attempts to improve patient care, 20 percent of these nurses drop out of nursing completely. Others move from job to job looking for some place where they can behave somewhat independently with regard to patient care. It is unreasonable to expect students to develop a sense of autonomy when they see so few practicing nurses exercising autonomy. Faculty who value the development of professional judgment in nursing students and who seek opportunities to help students develop such judgment often find it frustrating to work within the bureaucratic practice systems. While nurses working regularly on patient units have little or no autonomy, faculty have even less in determining how care will be given. Clinical faculty are well-acquainted with the games that faculty play to maintain their status on the units. These include discouraging students from openly voicing complaints lest it jeopardize the status of other students on the setting, ignoring staff nurses who are insensitive in their remarks to patients or careless in their practice, and so forth.

It is encouraging to note that nurses are moving out of such settings to establish roles as more independent, autonomous practitioners. One of the most encouraging articles to appear in the past several years was the recent one by Barbara Schutt in which she described the efforts of nurses around the country to expand their roles and to develop as more independent practitioners (14). Some nurses also are trying to develop organizational models that will permit more autonomy and exercise of professional judgment by nurses within hospitals and other health agencies. As mentioned previously, the faculty and clinical settings are only two of the major influences in the professional socialization of nursing students. I would like to move now to another kind of influence, one that is interwoven with many of the other factors which contribute to the socialization of nurses.

Reference was made earlier to the identification of nursing as a "semi-profession" and the suggestion by some that it is not likely to obtain full professional status, partly because of the predominance of women in the ranks. The influence on nursing of this fact cannot be overestimated. Virginia Cleland addressed herself to this issue when she identified sex discrimination as nursing's most pervasive problem (6). Many of the characteristics associated with being a "good nurse"—that is, warmth, obedience, willingness to serve others, passivity, and so forth—are also attributes of "good women." A few minutes ago I spoke of the games that faculty members play in attempting to maintain their status as clinical instructors on units where they have no authority to control practice. Leonard Stein has described the doctor-nurse game that is commonly played (16). He observes that "the physician traditionally and appropriately has total responsibility for making the decisions regarding the management of his patient's treatment." In making these decisions it is necessary for him to obtain information and sometimes recommendations from nurses. How the nurse makes these recommendations and how the physician accepts them is the focus of Stein's analysis.

The object of the game is as follows: The nurse is to be bold, have initiative, and be responsible for making significant recommendations, while at the same time she must appear passive. This must be done in such a manner as though to make her recommendations appear to be initiated by the physician. . . . The cardinal rule of the game is that open disagreement between the players must be avoided at all cost. Thus, the nurse must communicate her recommendations without appearing to be making a recommendation statement. The physician, in requesting a recommendation from the nurse, must do so without appearing to be asking for it. . . . The nurse who . . . see(s) herself as a consultant, but refuses to follow the rules of the game in making her recommendations, has hell to pay. The outspoken nurse is labeled a "bitch" by the surgeon. The psychiatrist describes her as unconsciously suffering from penis envy and her behavior as the acting out of her hostility toward men. Loosely translated, the psychiatrist is saying she is a bitch. The employment of the unbright, outspoken nurse is soon terminated. The outspoken bright nurse whose recommendations are worthwhile remains employed. She is, however, constantly reminded in a hundred ways that she is not loved. . . . To understand how the game evolved, we must comprehend the nature of the doctors' and nurses' training which shaped the attitudes necessary for the game . . . the nursing student begins to learn to play the game early in her training. Throughout her education she is trained to play the doctor-nurse game (16).

Stein analyzes some of the factors that preserve this game. One of these is the sexual roles. "Doctors are predominantly men and nurses are almost exclusively women. There are elements of the game which reinforce the stereotype roles of male dominance and female passivity. Some nursing instructors explicitly tell their students that their femininity is an important asset to be used when relating to physicians" (16).

Another analysis of the sex roles acted out between physician and nurse is one by Hans Mauksch.

We are tempted to compare the physician to the traditional male, the master of the home who earns the wherewithal (in this case, by bringing in patients) and who comes home to obtain services, to inspect, to order, to reward, and to punish. The managerial functions of the nurse arise not only from her structural position, as the one who is located and assigned permanently to the patient care unit, but they are also compatible with the traditional female functions of homemaker and with other aspects of the mother role which are managerial in nature. This analogy suggests a distinction between manager and master which sheds light on the peculiar combination of managerial and deferential behavior, characteristic of nurses (10).

It has been recognized for some time that nursing has been at a disadvantage in moving to obtain professional status because of the number of women in nursing. One solution which has been frequently proposed in past years is to recruit more men into nursing. As a matter of fact, figures for entry into nursing programs in 1972 showed that roughly six percent of the people coming into nursing are men, which is a considerable increase over previous years (13). While it is possible that increasing the percentage of men in nursing would hasten the process of professionalization, such a proposition only reinforces and implicitly accepts traditional sexual stereotypes. Another suggestion for trying to make nursing a more independent occupation is to change the role of women in contemporary American society. During the past few years there have been tremendous gains made in this area and nursing is sure to benefit from them. The sex of its practitioners should be an irrelevant consideration in terms of how autonomous nurses can be. The nature of the service provided and the amount of specialized knowledge necessary to provide that service are what should be the primary determinants of autonomy.

So far in the discussion we have considered factors which influence the socialization of the nurse prior to admission to a professional school and during the program of formal education. Professional socialization continues beyond graduation from the basic nursing program, of course. This phase of the process will not be analyzed here, except to point out that the conflicts and ambivalence described on the practicing nurse.

For the remainder of this paper, I will address the issue of what basic nursing education should and can contribute to the professional socialization of nursing students. The obvious response to such a question is that it should help them to internalize the values of professionalism, which in these comments have been defined as specialized education, a service orientation, and autonomy. The first value that we must help students to internalize is a strong commitment to acting in the best interests of the patient. Nursing has an important service to contribute to society, and we must do whatever we can to assure that nurses will be spending a major part of their time and energy doing that which they are prepared to do—giving nursing care. It is unfortunate that in so many settings the majority of patient care is given by nursing personnel with little or no formal preparation. It is important that we continue to emphasize the view that the nurse's most important contribution is nursing care, rather than as a coordinator of the work of others.

The second professional characteristic to which students must be socialized is a strong commitment to education. This education should be related to the role that nurses are expected to be able to carry out at a particular stage in nursing's development. At the present time, for example, nurses are increasingly having opportunities for and being expected to practice such skills as physical assessment and diagnosis, health teaching, and counseling. We must continually examine and change our curricula to reflect society's changing nursing needs, and where possible, to anticipate what tomorrow's needs and nursing roles will be. The educational attributes of a profession go beyond simply requiring a student professional to spend X number of years in a prescribed course of study. Involved also is the notion that the professional will keep his knowledge of the specialty up to date by continuing to learn new knowledge as it is developed. In recent years, nursing has explicitly recognized this responsibility, and is making many opportunities available for nurses to update their knowledge. Students should be encouraged to view their basic nursing program as just the first major step in a learning process that will extend throughout their professional careers.

Another dimension of the education criterion is that a profession develops and tests its body of specialized knowledge. That is, new knowledge is created through research. Although nursing education has made considerable progress in incorporating research concepts into professional education, we have not gone nearly far enough in these efforts. Many nursing students still complete their basic nursing programs without having been exposed to research concepts and without developing a questioning attitude toward their practice and the knowledge on which it is based. We have tremendous gaps in our knowledge about basic nursing concepts and interventions. How well have nurses systematically studied such problems as increasing the quality and quantity of patients' sleep, alleviating patients' pain, facilitating patients' understanding of their illness, reducing the stresses associated with illness and hospitalization, and so forth? Such knowledge should constitute a major share of what nurses learn, yet little new knowledge has been systematically developed and tested by nurses. We must help students to understand that being a professional does not mean only that one learns already established facts, but that it means a commitment to expanding the specialized knowledge of the profession. I am not suggesting that every nurse should become a researcher, although there is certainly great need for many more nurse researchers. I am suggesting that all nurses must develop in their basic nursing programs a questioning, critical, research orientation toward nursing knowledge and practice.

The third professional attribute which basic nursing students should internalize is that of autonomy. This may be the most difficult to achieve with the positive value that nursing has traditionally placed on obedience. In my opinion, however, at this particular time in nursing's history, autonomy is the characteristic on which we should be placing the greatest attention. What use is it to patients if nurses have an important service to contribute and are knowledgeable about how to perform that service, if nurses do not have the ability to assure that such service will be delivered safely and effectively? So far, nursing has not been able to exercise enough strength to assure the delivery of safe and effective nursing. We have been too concerned with coordinating the work of others and with carrying out physicians' orders to attend to the provision of excellent nursing care. I am not suggesting that nurses do not need to work cooperatively with others, or that carrying out physicians' orders is not an important part of nurses' work. What I am suggesting is that we must be more aggressive in the promotion of nursing care, and in developing the ability for independent behavior in nurses. To this end, we must begin very early in a student's career to encourage the development of such characteristics and abilities as curiosity, critical appraisal of situations, a questioning reflective approach to practice, independence, and a willingness to take some risks.

Ingeborg Mauksch has identified several experiences for basic nursing students that will enhance their ability to be autonomous and self-directive (11). These include informal participation in determining the direction of the curriculum, sharing in the selection of clinical experience, learning leadership behaviors, pursuing some self-selected learning interests of their own, and participating with other health professional students to meet citizen responsibilities by volunteering their professional expertise in community clinics, day care centers, and so forth.

Another kind of knowledge and experience that would be useful for students in terms of developing the ability to function autonomously is how to operate effectively as professionals in organizations and the larger community. Students must be helped to gain a much broader understanding of how organizations operate and how to bring about change in such organizations. They need to be encouraged to act individually and collectively to bring about needed professional reforms. Students are currently seeing some excellent examples of

this by nurses in New York, Massachusetts, and other places. I am referring to the actions taken by many of you in your attempts to change the definition of nursing in the Nurse Practice Act, and to the successful organized effort of Massachusetts nurses to block changes in their licensing board which would have all but eliminated nursing's control over the licensing of professional nurses. As nurses increasingly take such actions, students should be able to identify with them and be encouraged to involve themselves in similar ways.

A service orientation and specialized education are only two of the major attributes of a professional. The third, and possibly at this time most crucial characteristic, is autonomy. We must not become sidetracked over the issue of whether a professional is one who has three or four years of education, using our precious energies and time to continue this bitter controversy. A good part of our collective energy ought now to be directed toward making nursing more autonomous.

Periodically throughout this discussion I have commented on how the fact that most nurses are women has influenced the development of nursing as an occupation and the kinds of values that nurses have been expected to internalize. In the past few years great progress has been made in challenging some of society's ideas about how women, including women professionals, should behave. Work options for both women and men are expanding. The desires of women to have professional careers, and to combine careers with families, are becoming more acceptable.

However, there is still a great deal of frustration involved for women who try to deal with the conflicting demands of the two roles. We should be doing more in our basic nursing programs to prepare young women for the fact that they will be encountering these kinds of conflicts. We should begin to help them think through how to deal with them or how to prevent some of them. Virginia Cleland currently is studying nurses who have married and begun to raise families soon after graduation from their basic programs. She is trying to identify the characteristics of those nurses who are successfully able to combine both roles. Her findings agree with other studies of working professional women, that one of the major factors that determines how well women are able to integrate the two roles is the husband's attitude toward egalitarianism. That is, those men who do not believe that the division of labor is rigidly classified by sex are able to be more supportive toward their wives in their careers as working women. While it may be neither possible nor desirable for us to encourage students to marry egalitarian men, we should certainly be discussing with them the consequences of marrying men whose expectations and values in this area differ from their own.

I have commented on some of the factors that influence the professional socialization of nurses and have argued that we must consider the several core attributes of a profession in determining the kinds of values that we encourage students to internalize. We have legitimately given a great deal of attention in nursing to upgrading educational standards and to developing a strong commitment to service. If nurses are to be able to use their knowledge in the interest of patients, they must have a significant influence on defining and controlling the kind of nursing care received by patients. For this reason, we must encourage nurses to be more aggressive, individually and collectively, in taking those actions necessary for nurses to become more autonomous and self-directive.

REFERENCES

1 American Nurses' Association, Board of Directors. "Statement on Diploma Nurse Education." *The American Nurse*, Vol. 5:6, June 1973, p. 5.

2 American Nurses' Association, Committee on Education. *Educational Preparation for Nurse Practitioners and Assistants to Nurses: A Position Paper*. New York: American Nurses' Association, 1965.

3 American Nurses' Association, House of Delegates, Resolution, ANA 1972. *American Journal of Nursing*. June (Vol. 72:6) 1972, p. 1105.

4 Barber, Bernard. "Some Problems in the Sociology of the Professions." *Daedalus*. Fall 1963, pp. 669–688.

5 Batey, Marjorie. "The Two Normative Worlds of the University Nursing Faculty." *Nursing Forum*. Vol. VIII:1, 1969, pp. 5–16.

6 Cleland, Virginia. "Sex Discrimination: Nursing's Most Pervasive Problem." *American Journal of Nursing*, Vol. 71:8, August 1971, pp. 1542–1547.

7 Dock, Lavinia. "Nurses Should be Obedient," in *Issues in Nursing*, Bonnie Bullough and Vern Bullough (editors). New York: Springer Publishing Co., 1966, pp. 96–97.

8 Etzioni, Amitai. (Editor) *The Semi-Professions and their Organization*. New York: The Free Press, 1969.

9 Kramer, Marlene and Constance Baker. "The Exodus: Can We Prevent It?" *Journal of Nursing Administration*, May–June, 1971, pp. 15–30.

10 Mauksch, Hans O. "The Organizational Context of Nursing Practice," in *The Nursing Profession: Five Sociological Essays*, Fred Davis (editor). New York: John Wiley and Sons, 1966, pp. 109–137.

11 Mauksch, Ingeborg. "Let's Listen to the Students." *Nursing Outlook*, Vol. 20:2, February 1972, pp. 103–107.

12 Moore, Wilbert E. *The Professions: Roles and Rules*. New York: Russell Sage Foundation, 1970, p. 71.

13 National League for Nursing. "Educational Preparation for Nursing — 1972." *Nursing Outlook*, Vol. 21:9, September 1973, pp. 186–593.

14 Schutt, Barbara. "Spot Check on Primary Care Nursing." *American Journal of Nursing*, Vol. 72:11, November 1972, pp. 1996–2003.

15 Simpson, Richard L. and Ida Harper Simpson. "Women and Bureaucracy in the Semi-Professions," in *The Semi-Professions and Their Organization*, Amitai Etzioni (editor). New York: The Free Press, 1969.

16 Stein, Leonard I. "The Doctor-Nurse Game," in *New Directions for Nurses*, Bonnie Bullough and Vern Bullough (editors). New

York: Springer Publishing Co., 1971, pp. 129–137.

17 Sussman, Marvin B. "Occupational Sociology and Rehabilitation," in *Sociology and Rehabilitation*, Marvin B. Sussman (editor). New York: American Sociological Association, 1966, pp. 179–237.

18 "The Role of a Nurse in 1887." *Nursing Forum*, Vol. X:1, 1971, p. 31.

19 Williamson, Janet A. "The Conflict-Producing Role of the Professionally Socialized Nurse-Faculty Member." *Nursing Forum*, Vol. XI:4, 1972, pp. 356–366.

EDITOR'S QUESTIONS FOR DISCUSSION

To what extent is it desirable for a nurse to have autonomy in a practice setting? What are the organizational and professional constraints that prevent the development of an autonomous role? How might students be socialized into autonomous roles? Is there a conflict between being autonomous and developing collegial relationships in a clinical setting?

Chapter 3

The Emerging Graduate

Rita F. Stein, R.N., Ph.D.
Professor and Director of Research
Indiana University School of Nursing, Indianapolis

Stein examines the socialization process that takes place as the student nurse develops into a professional. The findings of a 3-year longitudinal study of two classes of nursing students reveal the transformation of the attitudes and values of students progressing from the sophomore year through the senior year of their education. Stein is primarily concerned with role perception. She outlines the dominant personal attributes and values and the ways in which they change during the students' academic and clinical experience. The frustrations and conflicts of students are also discussed. Stein points out that the discrepancy between the real professional image and the ideal image of the nurse was a cause of constant concern. The majority of sophomores saw themselves as physician's helpers and emphasized various aspects of nurturance. As seniors, the students saw themselves as more autonomous and began to perceive the nurse as a potential teacher and leader in the profession. For all the students, the best experience in nursing was nursing practice itself.

INTRODUCTION

This is a study about the emerging professional nurse. It talks about young women who received baccalaureate degrees in nursing. The account deals with the confrontation between students and faculty in an institutional setting where ideals and idealogies must be upheld, yet need to change with changes in students, their needs, roles, conflicts, and demands. The kinds of change involve moving from adolescence to emerging adulthood, from lay to professional philosophies, and, in general, the process of professional socialization.

This is also a report of a study of continuities and discontinuities in nursing education in a large Midwestern university. The students enroll in a university school of nursing with certain needs and aptitudes, only to discover that the school of nursing prescribes status and roles, offering professional role models among the faculty to help the student shape herself into a nurse.

In assuming new roles the students adopt new attitudes and change old patterns. By stressing ideals, the instructors hope to teach good nursing that will endure throughout the students' careers. In this way, university schools of nursing behave as value guardians for the practice of good nursing.

Student expectations either fuse or conflict with the nursing school expectations. We might well ask, "How and when does a student change her self-image in emerging to professional status? Can we constructively evaluate the program from the eyes of the students?"

The Problem

The school of nursing helps the student to become increasingly self-directive and autonomous as he or she comes nearer to the goal of graduation. Students' feelings, opinions, and beliefs about professional performance reflect reality orientations in dissidence and consonance. Values instigate behavior, which can then be judged against the desirable standards of graduate professional performance. A study of student definitions of the situation enables a school to make a more reliable study of its curriculum and goals. This process keeps the school close to student needs and helps students to keep abreast of nursing requirements in the larger society.

The study reported here is a 3-year longitudinal study of two classes of nursing students. It attempts to determine transformations in the attitudes and values of the students as they progressed from the sophomore year to the senior year of schooling. It is concerned with role perceptions as they were related to each year of nursing education. Answers to the following questions were sought: (1) What are outstanding personal attributes of the student nurses in each year of schooling? How and when do these attributes change? (2) What are the dominant values of the senior-year students and how do these values change from the sophomore to the senior year? (3) What are the students' stressful academic and clinical experiences?

The vignette of the entering student is that of a naive young lady or young man arriving at the school to be fed knowledge and skills for nursing. Until now she has not thought of herself as a professional person. She becomes immersed in the profession mainly by conversing with faculty members and other peers with the same interests.

It is important to realize that the young people who take the student role do shape the role and take an active part in their own education. They are constantly choosing to work out situations for their own comfort among a range of possible alternatives. There is a borrowing of values, ideas, and ways of behaving, both from older students and from faculty. The ability to place their role in perspective is an important characteristic of student professionals that separates these students from the world of laymen. This and other such distinguishing characteristics need to be investigated, and this study attempts to accomplish at least a partial explanation of their development.

The following exploratory premises were developed:

1 Basic nursing students in the baccalaureate program reflect professional values oriented to achievement in nursing with emphasis on academic interests and achievement. These values and the images that derive from them develop in the course of 3 years of schooling in a professional school. Students' perceptions of their role as a nurse develop from a vague sense of nurturance and care of the less fortunate to the self-image of a teacher and leader in the nursing profession.

2 As a result of this developing self-image, the nursing students experience conflict between the ideal professional image as inculcated in the school and the imperfect nursing reality found in the hospital and community health agencies. Students react to the conflict between ideal conditions and actual clinical conditions.

The focal question becomes: "How do the students accommodate and integrate multiple facets of roles and selves?" With this question in mind, the author began the 3-year study of the world of student nurses.

Other Studies

The literature on personal need attributes describes nursing students from various theoretical frames of reference. Studies have been done in different geographical areas and in different kinds of nursing schools, such as diploma, associate arts, and baccalaureate settings. Freshmen nurses have been most often studied and compared with the college normative woman. The instrument most often used was the Edwards Personal Preference Schedule (Caputo, 1965; Gynther, 1962; Levitt, 1962; Mauksch, 1960; Navran, 1958; Schultz, 1963; Stauffacher, 1968).

Using the Edwards Personal Preference Schedule, Levitt (1962) found that sophomore nursing students were low on dominance, autonomy, and aggression. The less assertive needs of succorance, abasement, and nurturance predominated.

Gertz and Gynther (1962) found that hospital diploma students were significantly low in exhibition, autonomy, dominance, and need for change. They described nurses as women who learned to develop restraint and control and avoided blame and harmful situations.

In contrast to the above studies, which placed nurses in various feminine or dependent role positions, Caputo and Hanf (1965), in examining the difference between graduate nurses, freshmen nursing students, and senior nursing students, found no exclusive need patterns differentiating the three groups.

Comparative analyses between psychiatric and general medical nurses on graduate practicing levels indicated that nurses in general were higher in the need for order, deference, and endurance than college women. Navran and Stauffacher (1957) stated that general medical nurses were significantly more orderly and deferent in contrast to psychiatric nurses, who scored higher on the dominance variable.

Mauksch (1960) discussed the maternal instinct in nursing. He cited the nurse as one who was restrained and needed controls for her behavior. However, this description could also be applied to a nurse who has developed a professional attitude, which is characterized by cool appraisal and objectivity. This kind of objectivity could also be considered a defense against many traumatic stimuli found in hospital situations.

Although some consistency has been found by various investigators using the Edwards Personal Preference Schedule, there have also been inconsistencies in measuring attitudes of nurses. Furthermore, these studies date several years in the past. It has been the experience of the author that today's students have more outgoing personality traits.

METHODOLOGY

The Edwards Personal Preference Schedule, an interview, and a questionnaire were used in the investigation.

The Edwards Personal Preference Schedule (EPPS) (1954)

The purpose of the schedule is to measure a number of relatively independent personality variables.

Personal attributes as measured by the Edwards Personal Preference Schedule were analyzed for each class being studied (the classes of 1970 and 1971) from the sophomore to the senior levels. The exploratory premises were that alterations and patterns of personality traits would be consistent with redefinitions of professional roles and maturing female roles.

Edwards and Associates purport to scale values on a psychological continuum out of which two statements equal in social desirability value are taken. Therefore, it can be argued that if a subject is asked to choose the statement in the pair that is more characteristic of himself, social desirability will be of little importance in determining the response.

The testing procedure has been validated with different groups over a period of time (Edwards, 1954). Normative scores are available for comparative purposes (Edwards, 1954 and Klett, 1957).

The Questionnaire

It can be said that if a student believes and perceives that a situation is real, then the situation, for all practical purposes, is real. The frame of reference by which a student interprets an act is the important definition of the situation. This is the practical working situation in psychotherapy, for it is the condition that motivates feelings and behavior.

The questionnaire was constructed to test student attitudes toward academic personal, and clinical concerns. Questions were developed in each of the following areas: expectations in nursing, professional image, and conflicts during the course of nursing education. The items were multiple choice and free answer, coded by themes. All of the subjects tested were coded to prevent identification, and written comments were encouraged.

Validity and Plausibility

Junior students were pretested on the questionnaire and were asked to criticize the questions. They helped to revise, add, and delete questions for clarity, suitability, and accuracy.

The questionnaire was given to senior nursing students, which made it necessary for them to reflect on their sophomore year. At the same time the sophomores were given the questionnaire, and it was found that senior retrospection and sophomore answers correlated. The free-answer sections in the questionnaire were coded by theme, and coder agreement was accomplished by two pairs of independent observers. One pair (nurse-nonnurse) achieved 80 percent agreement. The second pair (researcher–faculty member) achieved 90 percent agreement.

The questionnaire did differentiate between religious, socioeconomic, and national groups in the areas of nursing practice, conflicts, and role image. Thus, the questionnaire was sensitive to subcultures in which certain common personal needs were manifested. The questionnaire helped to clarify the three psychological instruments and to point out the various positive and negative experiences and reactions by sophomore, junior, and senior students.

The Interview

Following the administration of the instruments (the questionnaire and the EPPS), interviews were conducted with a random sample of forty-eight students in each class. They were seen in groups of six students, and eight groups were interviewed in each class. The questionnaire was used as a basis for interviewing: the students were asked to amplify their answers with further explanations of meaning and substance. Amplification was made in the following categories: professional image, conflicts, changes in outlook, personal tensions,

and crises. The students were not identified and were not known personally by the interviewer.

Sampling

Data was collected by testing students consecutively during the spring semesters of the sophomore, junior, and senior years. We concentrated our efforts on two select classes (the classes of 1970 and 1971) preferring the intensity of this approach to the broader coverage that would be afforded by giving attention to all of the classes in the school at any one time. Such intensity seemed the most appropriate way to find answers to the questions we were asking about the process of student socialization. This approach allowed us to develop a composite picture of the students as they progressed from one year to the next. In the class of 1970, 125 of 130 students participated during the sophomore year. Five students failed to show for the testing. In the junior year 110 students were tested: 15 students were counted as dropouts. In the senior year 95 students were tested. Five students failed to appear for testing, and 10 students were counted in attrition. In the class of 1971, 130 students were tested, which represented all but 6 students who failed to show. In the junior year 120 students were tested and 10 students dropped out of school. In the senior year, 110 students were tested and 5 failed to show. Five students were counted as in attrition. Reasons for dropout included marriage, pregnancy, illness, and academic failure. When comparisons were made between those who took senior testing and those who did not there was no difference in mean Edward Personal Preference Scores between junior and senior years other than what is noted in Table 3-4. The answers of those who dropped out in their junior year and those who continued in the program revealed no differences between the groups in the junior year.

ANALYSIS AND INTERPRETATION

Description of Sample

The majority of the women in both classes of sophomore students were 18 to 19 years old. One male was present and was eliminated from the sample to preserve consistency in the pattern. The majority of students were fourth or fifth generation and came from Protestant, middle-class backgrounds; their parents' occupations were chiefly managerial or educational. In the class of 1970, 15 percent of the respondents belonged to the lowest social class (unskilled labor).

Nearly all the students stated that they and their parents regarded it important to have "a profession to earn a living" and had "concern with educational scholarship." Forty percent of them had gained some experience by working as hospital volunteers or by participating in the Red Cross.

Layman's View of Nursing

Although in time students accepted nursing practice as attending to emotional as well as physical needs, the sophomore students did not realize this overall objective in the beginning. Following orientation in the School of Nursing, they found out that nursing practice differed from their expectations; but they still had a layman's image that did not include the idea of becoming a leader in nursing. The majority of sophomores saw themselves as physician's helpers. They emphasized various aspects of nurturance and "helping humanity" until well into their sophomore year. It wasn't until then that they realized there was much emphasis in the school on developing clinical and team leadership. By graduation, the majority of students were emphasizing well-patient care and community health rather than the more limited freshmen concept of nurturance in sickness events.

As juniors and seniors the students saw, in retrospect, that the sophomore year was the most difficult. It was in this year that they came to realize the broader scope of nursing. They had to adjust to a heavy academic program with many science requirements, and they had to adjust to new roles as nursing clinicians on hospital wards. At this time they came to realize that the ideal forms of clinical nursing taught within the confines of the school were not always carried out in more realistic hospital practice.

During the sophomore year, the majority of

students endured personal tensions and expressed feelings of loneliness, restlessness, and depression. In spite of this, most missed only one to two days a month because of illness. With their friends and upper classmen they were able to discuss and ventilate personal issues. One of their greatest problems was the necessity of assuming more self-directed responsibility in academic and clinical nursing studies. Fifty percent of them felt they needed to learn how to deal with emotionally disturbed patients. They felt driven to assume poses of self-confidence even though they actually felt little confidence in working with patients.

They felt that by far the best experience in nursing was nursing practice itself. Clinical conferences were also considered beneficial for patient care. The students felt that one-fourth of their experience should be on night duty where a variety of experiences in 24-hour patient care added to the richness of nursing experience. Most

Table 3-1 Student Difficulties and Conflicts in Sophomore Year 1970–1971

	Question	Percent
1	Impersonality of patient care	83.0
2	Making mistakes in nursing practice	96.6
3	Caring for certain type patients	61.4
4	Combining career with marriage	29.5
5	Keeping mind on work	22.7
6	Concern with patients after I leave	59.1
7	Seeing patient as person not disease	42.0
8	Dealing with patients' families	64.8
9	Conflict between conducting a purposeful interview and socializing as a friend	64.4
10	Conflict between self-help patient and nurse dependency	58.0
11	Inability to adjust to those of different classes from own	33.3
12	Caring for patient who won't accept teaching	92.0
13	How to answer patient when there's no cure	97.7
14	Dealing with anxious patient	84.1
15	Frustrations about not being able to do more for patient	92.0
16	Hard to be objective about patients I don't like	51.1
		$N = 255$

of the sophomore students felt they required 15 to 20 hours a week of nursing practice for maximal benefits from clinical experiences.

The students in both sophomore classes expressed several areas of concern regarding nursing practice. The majority of the students felt that patient care was impersonal and therefore not conducive to helping patients cope with illness. They were afraid of making mistakes, especially in administering medications, hypodermic injections, and other technical procedures. They were concerned about their patients long after they left the wards and were frustrated about not being able to do more for them. The students were concerned about patients who did not accept their teaching. They felt inadequate in trying to answer patients' questions, especially when there were poor prognoses. They expressed lack of confidence in dealing with families and with anxious patients. They soon became troubled with the difficulty of trying to be objective with patients they disliked on a personal level.

The sophomore students saw themselves as moving quickly through the 3 years of education. During their sophomore year they were already concerned with the conflict between the idealism in school and the realism in hospital practice. The teachers regarded the students as learners of ideal situations, whereas the hospital nurses thought of them as helpers and as extra hands to get the work done. Their personal values meshed with beginning professional values, and consequently they experienced a difficult year of adjustments between self, school, and hospital.

Transition in the Nursing World

We now come to an analysis of the part played by junior and senior students as they progressed from sophomore-level neophytes to upperclassmen. Although these students could be thought of as legitimizers of the study (Whittaker and Olesen, 1968) conflicts can become keener in the upperlevel nursing courses, and the retrospection of these students can be revealing.

In the junior year, 55 percent of the students complained of nervousness, depression, and loneliness. In the senior year the symptoms were alleviated so that they occurred seldom or not at all. Sixty percent of the students now saw themselves as reliable and self-confident practitioners. From the grandiose desire to "help people" in the sophomore year they now said, "You do best you can—you must accept the inevitable in death and dying." Idealism was now beginning to dissolve into a view of nursing marked by realism. The older students felt that they could not control all phenomena in patient care and realized that they could not cure all patients. They turned their interest to prevention of disease and to care of the well. They aligned themselves with health teachers and saw themselves as physician's associates.

A sense of alienation in the sophomore year gave way to a painful process of identity shaping. It can be safely said that progression through the school was marked by a series of identity crises. Without being aware of it, the students approached their crises with attempts to form themselves into nurses. The tasks were infinitely more difficult than they imagined, and the psychological investment was more demanding than they had foreseen.

The students claimed that they were exposed to a whole kaleidoscope of human experiences in which distressful sights and sounds were predominant. The emerging nurses acquired new information and had more confidence about things that previously caused anxiety. By the senior year they had defined and formalized conflicts in nursing. As they looked forward to graduation, they began complaining about poor salaries and working conditions.

Both juniors and seniors felt that the care of critically ill patients was most educational for them. They also felt that multiple patient assignments with frequent rotation of patients helped hasten the learning process. The most favored method for evaluating patient needs was to have interactions with other personnel on wards. Clinical rounds and health team conferences were equally popular choices.

Table 3-2 Conflicts in Nursing Practice of Juniors and Seniors

	No concern		Concern	
Statement	1971 % Jr.	1972 % Sr.	1972 % Jr.	1973 % Sr.
1 Difficulty in accepting difference between expected and real nursing	42	55	58	45
2 Difficulty in correlating nursing theory with nursing practice	10	10	90	90
3 Conflicts in my role compared to other auxiliary nursing help	33	43	67	57
4 Not enough communication with physicians about patients welfare	3	5	96	95
5 Too much authority by physicians and little respect for nursing report judgments	5	3	95	97
6 Conditions of short help, poor salary, and poor working conditions lower morale	3	5	96	95
7 Am too busy to give good nursing care	6	5	94	95
8 Not enough ward administration experience for team management	13	18	87	83
9 Too much impersonality of patient care and neglect of emotional needs	6	8	93	92
10 Carrying out painful procedures on patients	5	5	95	95
11 Making mistakes in nursing practice	0	2	100	98
12 Dealing with death of patient	5	2	95	98
13 Caring for certain kinds of patients	15	20	85	80
14 Combining career with marriage	41	50	59	50
15 Keeping mind on work	49	52	51	48
16 Seeing patient as person and not as disease	38	45	62	55
17 Conflicts between interviewing and socializing	18	22	72	78
18 Conflicts between self-help and dependency	28	50	72	50
19 Conflicts between encouraging self-help and patient's reluctance to give up dependency	14	18	86	78
20 Inability to work with different socioeconomic class	39	50	61	50
21 Caring for a patient who will not accept my teaching	8	15	92	85
22 How to answer patients' questions when there is no cure	3	5	97	95
23 Dealing with anxious patients and those with emotional outbursts	4	15	96	85
24 Feeling frustrated that I can't make patients more comfortable	4	0	96	100
25 Find it hard to be objective with some patients	9	22	91	78
26 Not getting enough practice in nursing techniques	4	10	96	90
27 Dealing with patients' families	12		89	
28 Other	0	0	0	98
	$N = 110$	$N = 95$	$N = 120$	$N = 110$

Table 3-2 illustrates the conflicts which juniors and seniors felt needed resolution. This table shows that many of the conflicts in class of 1971 are unresolved from the sophomore year. In addition, upperclassmen felt that there was not enough communication with physicians, who had little respect for nursing judgments and reports. They felt that too much authority was exerted by physicians. They were concerned with conditions such as poor salary, short help, and lowered morale. They felt they had insufficient ward administration experience. These students also had more difficulty in understanding the professional nurse's role as it compares with other types of auxiliary health roles.

On a more personal level, these students were still concerned about coping with the death of patients. Still carried over from the sophomore year was their difficulty in accepting the differences between the expectations of the school and those of the hospital.

They had qualms about not doing enough for patients. Some felt like waitresses and others felt helpless and insignificant. The summer vacation proved to be an excellent opportunity for testing the self by working for pay. This also gave them the opportunity to broaden their experiences and increase their skills. Although the seniors had many of the same conflicts about hospital nursing as sophomores, they were able to stand aside and reflect more objectively, accepting those they could do nothing about and trying to resolve the others.

In summary, then, as the student progressed through school, she was still voicing doubts about the real professional image compared to her ideal image, but she no longer contemplated withdrawing. As the senior year approached there was a general desire for change, marked by plans for marriage, for joining the peace corps or the military, or for gaining clinical experience in new places. At the end of the senior year the students were legitimized as graduate nurses and as adults, although they carried their conflicts with them into the working situation.

Results of the EPPS

By means of the Edwards Personal Preference Schedule, the traits for each nursing class were examined and compared with the traits of the previous and subsequent classes. Efforts were made to determine whether these traits changed as students progressed from the sophomore to the junior and senior years and whether certain traits remained relatively constant. These traits were then compared to the college and high school normative samples.

Since data were nonscaler, the chi-square test of independence was used. Differences in means between the sophomore, junior, and senior groups of EPPS results were compared by t distributions.

If patterns of behavior are found in a single personality, patterns of behavior may be found among personalities within a culture. A group of individuals may possess more of one trait than another trait. This becomes a matter of relative dominance of a group's traits in another group. Enduring traits of personality are therefore ordered into interlocking networks of dominance and emphasis.

This study assumes that the adolescent ego is a directive power that develops from a particular social status before a school of nursing is entered. Upon being assimilated into a given culture, such as that of a school of nursing, the student has experiences that mold adjustment in the present and anticipate future goals so that certain character traits will become more or less dominant as the student proceeds through that particular culture.

The sophomores of 1970 and 1971 were compared to the class of 1965. The data for the latter was obtained by Eugene Levitt, Chief Psychologist at Indiana University–Purdue University at Indianapolis. He found high order, deference for authority, and low dominance in the 1965 class of sophomores. It appears that in the 1970s there was a different kind of entering student. The 1970 and 1971 classes of sophomores were higher in exhibitionism, autonomy, and heterosexuality. These students showed lower scores in deference for authority than the 1965 students. Interpretation

Table 3-3 Edwards Personal Preference Schedule Characteristics—Sophomore Classes

Traits	a Sophomores 1965		b Sophomores 1970		c Sophomores 1971		$\dfrac{t}{a-b}p$	$b-c$
	$\bar{x}$	S.D.*	$\bar{x}$	S.D.*	$\bar{x}$	S.D.*		
Achievement	12.05	4.09	12.29	4.092	12.13	3.77	NS	NS
Deference	12.15	3.25	10.91	3.25	9.99	3.95	2.66 $p < .01$	2.05 $p < .05$
Order	10.01	4.50	10.14	4.36	9.52	4.60	NS	NS $p < .05$
Exhibitionism	13.86	3.50	15.00	3.66	14.60	4.60	2.43 $p < .02$	NS
Autonomy	10.62	4.01	13.10	4.11	12.53	4.57	2.71 $p < .01$	NS
Affiliation	16.10	4.00	16.80	4.10	17.18	4.70	NS	NS
Intraception	17.72	4.50	17.32	4.83	17.22	4.70	NS	NS
Succorance	15.06	4.75	14.08	4.19	14.30	5.06	NS	NS
Dominance	11.88	3.89	12.33	4.49	12.41	4.74	NS	NS
Abasement	15.90	4.03	16.55	4.85	16.92	4.32	NS	NS
Nurturance	17.50	3.66	17.82	4.19	18.48	4.15	NS	NS
Change	16.50	4.09	17.26	4.25	16.87	4.99	NS	NS
Endurance	12.85	4.13	12.23	4.78	11.32	4.95	NS	NS
Heterosexuality	15.55	4.93	17.09	5.98	16.51	5.68	2.15 $p < .05$	NS
Aggression	9.71	3.98	10.60	4.34	11.28	4.42	NS	NS
	$N = 120$		$N = 125$		$N = 130$			

*S.D. = standard deviation

of these findings suggest that the sophomores of 1970 and 1971 desired to be independent of others while at the same time they tried to stay witty and clever, talk about personal adventures and experiences, and have others note and comment about their appearance. They appeared to be more vocal and exhibitionistic, and they engaged in social activities with the opposite sex more than the class of 1965 did. This is corroborated by the observation that the students in later classes have had a voice in school and curriculum affairs. They felt more free to question authority and combined intraception[1] with independence in working toward achievement goals.

[1] "Intraception" is defined by the EPPS manual as follows: "To analyze one's motives and feelings, to observe others, to understand how others feel about problems, to put one's self in another's place...."

The scores of both sophomore classes showed that heterosexual orientation was higher than it was for the normative college and high school groups. This may have been because several of the nursing students were either engaged or married.

Both sophomore classes, when compared to the high school samples, had higher achievement orientations, intraceptive abilities, and heterosexual demands. They were lower than the high school normative group sample in deference to authority, the need for affiliation with peers, abasement or self-consciousness, and aggression. This indicates a beginning maturity as well as serious academic orientation toward study and preparation for future goals.

When compared to the college students, the sophomore nursing students were higher in abasement scores. They were on the same level with col-

Table 3-4 EPPS Scores All Classes Compared with Normative Scores

Traits	a Sophomore 1970–1971 $\bar{x}$	S.D.*	b Juniors 1971–1972 $\bar{x}$	S.D.*	c Seniors 1972–1973 $\bar{x}$	S.D.*	$\dfrac{t}{p}$	d College norm $\bar{x}$	S.D.*	e High school norm $\bar{x}$	S.D.*	a/e $\dfrac{t}{p}$	a/d $\dfrac{t}{p}$	b/d $\dfrac{t}{p}$
Achievement	12.29	4.09	11.92	4.17	12.55	4.33		13.08	4.19	11.13	4.06	2.67 p<.01		
Deference	10.91	3.25	10.23	3.62	10.00	3.62	2.85 p<.01	12.40	3.72	11.81	3.55	2.81 p<.01	5.21 p<.001	5.75 p<.001
Order	10.14	4.36	9.85	4.50	10.55	4.90		10.24	4.37	10.68	4.14			
Exhibitionism	14.12	3.66	14.50	3.82	15.02	3.99		14.28	3.65	14.93	3.38			
Autonomy	13.10	4.11	12.78	4.35	12.47	4.74		12.29	4.34	11.89	4.20			
Affiliation	16.80	4.10	17.03	4.20	17.05	4.13		17.40	4.07	17.94	3.80	2.95 p<.01		2.90 p<.01
Intraception	17.32	4.83	17.75	4.54	17.00	5.19		17.32	4.70	15.87	4.27	2.85 p<.01		
Succorance	14.08	4.19	14.39	4.43	14.85	3.71	2.69 p<.01	12.53	4.42	12.70	4.50			3.42
Dominance	12.33	4.49	11.39	4.44	12.60	5.40	1.56 p<.20	14.18	4.60	11.99	4.39		3.66 p<.001	
Abasement	16.55	4.85	15.05	4.63	14.75	5.19		15.11	4.94	17.66	4.61	2.35	3.24	
Nurturance	17.82	4.19	18.47	4.38	16.70	4.61		16.42	4.41	17.35	4.30			
Change	17.26	4.25	16.26	4.71	15.72	4.47	1.57 p<.20	17.20	4.87	18.09	4.15			
Endurance	12.23	4.78	11.28	5.00	11.80	4.69		12.63	5.19	11.96	5.10			
Heterosexuality	17.09	5.98	19.53	4.77	19.10	4.83	4.85 p<.001	14.34	5.39	14.96	6.98	3.72 p<.001	5.34 p<.001	8.31 p<.001
Aggression	10.60	4.34	10.97	3.76	9.82	3.61		10.59	4.61	11.43	4.19	3.84 p<.01		
	N = 255		N = 230		N = 205			N = 749		N = 799				

Note: Answers to questions on the EPPS and the questionnaire revealed no differences between those who dropped out of school and those who did not in junior and senior years. Dropout reasons were illnesses, marriage, pregnancy, and academic failure.

*S.D. = standard deviation

lege students in intraceptive needs and achievement needs, but below the college level in deference to authority and dominance. They apparently maintained their autonomy on a par with college students. Although their scores in deference to authority were lower than college scores, in a situation of autonomy or independence this would be tempered by the high tendency toward abasement or self-conscious timidity when faced with life's problems. In other words, the student nurse has the capability to feel guilty and to accept blame.

Nurturance is considered very important in the personality of a nurse. It is the need to help people in trouble, assist those less fortunate, and treat others with kindness and sympathy. Contrary to Levitt's finding (1962), our tests showed that this trait remains up through 3 years of professional school. Although the scores during the senior year were lower than those of the previous two years, this is statistically not significant. In this trait the student nurses' scores were similar to those of the college normative group. Compared with the college group, the student nurses showed a greater need for succorance, which is the need to receive affection from others and to have others act kindly towards oneself. It would seem that these traits are related to the high heterosexual orientation since both traits, succorance and nurturance, serve in the give and take of interpersonal relations.

When nurturance was cross-tabulated with frustration in not being able to do more for patients and in thinking of them after leaving the clinical area, it was found that the majority of the high-nurturance students were most concerned about doing more for a patient (x^2 = 11.07, df = 4, $p < .05$). The majority of the low-nurturance students were concerned least of all.

In addition to frustration in patient care, high-nurturance individuals were afraid of making mistakes in nursing practice. This is a commonsense observation, since a person who feels the need to be kind and to assist others would also feel intense guilt upon making a mistake in nursing practice and abasement and humility in the performance of clinical skills.

When nurturance was cross-tabulated with the conflict between desiring patient dependence and encouraging patient self-help, 92 percent of high-nurturance student nurses had no conflict in these factors (x^2 = 9.82, df = 1, $p < .001$). These students encouraged self-help for patients under their care.

Most high-aggressive students were little concerned with being head nurse on a hospital ward, feeling that they could cope with the increased responsibility (x^2 = 13.57, df = 4, $p < .01$). Most low-aggressive students were very concerned about ward administration. Aggression may be a useful trait in determining administrative ability since planning for patient care and dealing with ward activities and personnel requires that a person be able to attack a wide range of problems.

When achievement orientation was analyzed with regard to anxiety in making mistakes in nursing practice, it was found that the high-achievement students were most concerned with making mistakes. The high-achievement students were also the most concerned with seeing the patient as a person who has various needs and feelings, rather than as a "disease."

In summary it may be said that student nurses have changed in the past few years with regard to the personality traits they bring with them as sophomores. They arrive with traits of autonomy, exhibitionism, and heterosexuality. Sophomore nursing students exhibit traits similar to those of college students. A few years ago they exhibited nurturance and deference to authority in excess of college normative values. They were different from college students in that they didn't show dominance, autonomy, and aggression in their lifestyle. Today we have a sophomore student nurse who is ready to question issues and practices in her school affairs and who is active in self-government. She shows more independence and autonomy in her thinking and in her relationships with faculty members as she steers a course between hospital and school in gaining nursing experience.

THE EMERGING NURSE

Amplification from the interviews led to the following summary of the student nurse's world of experience.

The student showed many starts and stops, as well as backsliding and regression, as her new, professional self began slowly to emerge. During the sophomore year, most nurses were aware of their academic and personal adjustment difficulties. They attempted to draw their nursing image out of a confusing student world in order to emerge with a sense of wholeness into the professional world.

Looming large was the student's feeling of ambiguity between the real world of the hospital and the ideal world of the school of nursing.

Early in her career the student appeared on the wards to carry out assignments and to occupy the position of student nurse. She was expected to take care of patients and to communicate with them regarding their problems. Inevitably she was burdened by a sense of her own lack of knowledge and competence. She was afraid of making mistakes and of giving the patients inadequate care, thereby losing the patients' confidence. She was not sure of herself when a patient asked her to do something requiring manual or psychological skill. Often the fledgling nurse was in the uncomfortable position of not having the answer to a patient's question or of making only a feeble attempt to answer. She would project her ambiguities upon the faculty, who she felt were not preparing her adequately to meet her experiences in the clinical area. It is realistic to assume that the student felt disillusioned, regretful, depressed, and anxious. She would often voice these anxieties in the form of headaches and feelings of nervousness. As she moved through the years of student nursing she engaged in self-scrutiny regarding her own suitability to nursing and her worthiness for the role. She endured growing convictions that there were incompatibilities between an ideal world of nursing presented in the school and the real world of nursing that she found in the clinic and hospital.

Although, as the student progressed through the years of education, she was still voicing her doubts about her real professional image compared to her ideal image, she no longer seriously contemplated withdrawing. As the years of study drew to a close and the senior year arrived there was a general desire for change, as evidenced in the students of the senior class who decided to marry, join the peace corps, join the military forces, or gain new clinical experiences in other places.

The student nurse came to see the clinical ward with certain realizations. The world of her chosen occupation was more complicated than she had imagined. The tasks were more socially oriented and were manually difficult. Her original, glorified idea of nursing was rather remote and even nonexistent after the sophomore year. Her image changed from one of God's helper in illness to one of practitioner-teacher, associate in wellness and in illness.

The sophomore classes today have more autonomous and independent students who have traits of intraception, aggression, and achievement orientation. However, as predicaments arise coincidently from the rhythms of hospital and student life, there was an unforeseen cycling of everyday experiences. The student was forced to identify herself with the student role if she was to survive in a school of nursing. She was forced to view herself in different ways. She moved through periods of confusion and feelings of inadequacy and self-righteousness. By the end of her time in student education she was forced to develop a professional image in which she rationalized that she can only do the best she can and that patients would die in spite of her care. She developed a professional poise which she considered to be composed of objectivity and a certain measure of cynicism.

She developed many conflicts regarding patient care in the hospital ward situations and in community health care. She felt that doctors were too authoritarian, did not listen to her, and did not communicate with her. She was afraid of making mistakes and felt inadequate in trying to answer patient's questions. She had feelings of frustration in caring for patients who did not accept her teaching, and she found it hard to be objective. Most of all the student was intent on collecting and mastering as many experiences and procedures as the instructors and curriculum permitted. She learned to carry as heavy a load of patients as she could safely handle and complained about an inadequate amount of time on the wards.

Working for pay as a student nurse provided her with an excellent opportunity for testing herself in realistic situations. In this way she helped to reconcile her inner world of nursing concepts with the realities she experienced in the outside world. The ability to work for pay and to deal with real problems indicates successful integration of nurse and student. Parts of her former self became altered so that the image of the professional nurse could emerge.

The students in the school of nursing held images of themselves as intelligent university students. During the junior and senior years, they complained about the ideology of the school and about insufficient procedural practice on hospital wards. Their conflicts were unresolved, but their role was legitimized on graduation.

Group dynamic conferences and team conferences on the ward encouraged self-awareness and provided the time and place for ventilating conflicts. Self-awareness was also heightened by courses in the social sciences that could be applied to patient care. All of these encounters served to make the students alter in minute ways the role that they had envisioned earlier as workable and viable.

With respect to their roles as adult women and their roles as nurses, the students were concerned about how they could marry and raise families and continue in nursing. The dominant outlook on graduation was a very practical one that is evident in the lifestyles of many women in our society: nursing work, withdrawal to marry and raise a family, and then a return to work. This is an example of a conflict that nursing students have in common with many American women who try to fulfill family responsibilities and work commitments at the same time. In the everyday experiences of the nursing students, the small details exemplifying bits of progress and of backsliding suggested that letting go of the traditional role was difficult; the new role was grasped tenaciously but timidly.

It is hoped that the student can not only be taught nursing but also that she or he can be given the motivation to live fully and deal with life's problems, tribulations, and happy events. The professional role is not enough. We need the insightful candidate who can realistically adapt to change and establish her own talent for originality and creativity. Just as patient care includes social and emotional considerations, so too must the teaching of nursing students. The student must be prepared socially and emotionally as well as academically if she is to meet her professional challenges.

BIBLIOGRAPHY

Bales, F. L.: "Position, Role and Status: A Reformulation of Concepts," *Social Forces*, **34**: 313–321, May 1956.

Becker, Howard S., Blanche Geer, Everett Hughes, and Anselm Strauss: *Boys in White: Student Culture in Medical School*, University of Chicago Press, Chicago, 1961.

Benne, Kenneth D., and Warren Bennis: "Role Confusion and Conflict in Nursing, Part I," *American Journal of Nursing,* **59**:196–198, February 1959.

——, and ——: "Role Confusion and Conflict in Nursing, Part II," *American Journal of Nursing,* **59**:380–383, March 1959.

Caputo, Daniel V., and Constance Hanf: "EPPS Pattern and the 'Nursing Personality,' " *Educational and Psychological Measurement*, **25**: 421–435, 1965.

Casella, Carmine: "Need Hierarchies among Nursing and Non-nursing College Students," *Nursing Research*, **17**(3):273–274, May–June 1968.

Davis, Fred: *The Nursing Profession: Five Sociological Essays,* John Wiley and Sons, New York, 1966.

Edwards, Allen: *Personal Preference Schedule. A Manual*, Psychological Corporation, New York, 1954.

Fox, David, and Lorraine K. Diamond: *Satisfying and Stressful Situations in Basic Programs in Nursing Education*, Bureau of Public Teachers College, Columbia University, New York, 1964.

Fox, Renee C.: "Training for Uncertainty," in R. K. Merton, G. Reader, and P. Kendall (eds.), *The Student-Physician*, Harvard University Press, Cambridge, 1957, pp. 207–243.

George, Janet A., and Margo Stephens: "Personality Traits of Public Health Nurses and Psychiatric Nurses," *Nursing Research*, **17**(2):168–170, March–April 1968.

Gynther, M. D., and B. Gertz: "Personality Characteristics of Student Nurses in South Carolina," *Journal of Social Psychology*, **56**:227–284, 1962.

Klett, C. James: "Performance of High School Students on the Edwards Personal Preference Schedule," *Journal of Consulting Psychology*, **21**(1):68–72, 1957.

Kramer, Marlene: "Role Models, Role Conceptions and Role Deprivation," *Nursing Research*, **17** (2):115–120, March-April 1968.

Levitt, Eugene E.: "The Two Faces of Eve: The Development of the Personality of the Nurse," an address to the Indiana League for Nursing, Nov. 8, 1962.

——, Bernard Lubin, and Marvin Zuckerman: "The Student Nurse, the College Woman, and the Graduate Nurse: A Comparative Study," *Nursing Research,* **11**(2):30–32, Spring 1962.

Linton, Ralph: "Concepts of Role and Status," in T. Newcomb and E. L. Hartley (eds.), *Readings in Social Psychology*, Henry Holt, New York, 1947, pp. 367–370.

Mauksch, Hans: "The Nurse: A Study in Role Perception," unpublished dissertation, University of Chicago, 1960.

Merton, Robert K.: "The Student-Physician," *The Cornell Program*, Harvard University Press, Cambridge, 1957.

Navran, Leslie, and James C. Stauffacher: "A Comparative Analysis of the Personality Structure of Psychiatric and Non-Psychiatric Nurses," *Nursing Research*, 7(2):64–66, June 1958.

——, and ——: "The Personality Structure of Psychiatric Nurses," *Nursing Research*, 5:109–114, February 1957.

Olesen, Virginia L., and Elvie W. Whittaker: *The Silent Dialogue*, Jossey-Bass, San Francisco, 1968.

Schultz, Esther D.: "Desirable Personality Patterns for the Nursing Student: A Longitudinal Comparative Study," unpublished doctoral dissertation, Indiana University, 1963.

Smith, Jeanne E.: "Personality Structure in Beginning Nursing Students: A Factor Analytic Study," *Nursing Research*, 17(2):140–145, March-April 1968.

Stauffacher, James C., and Leslie Navran: "The Prediction of Subsequent Professional Activity of Nursing Students by the Edwards Personal Preference Schedule," *Nursing Research*, 17(3): 256–260, May-June 1968.

Stein, Rita: "The Student Nurse, Part I," *Nursing Research*, 18(4):308–315, July–August 1969.

——: "The Student Nurse, Part II," *Nursing Research*, 18(5):433–440, September–October 1969.

Taves, M. J., Ronald Corwin, and Eugene Haas: "Professional Disillusionment," *Nursing Research*, 10(3):141–144, 1961.

Williams, T. R., and M. M. Williams: "The Socialization of the Student Nurse," *Nursing Research*, 8(1):18–25, 1959.

EDITOR'S QUESTIONS FOR DISCUSSION

Besides applying the current proposals of Kramer and others, how might students learn, while they are in a nursing program, to resolve the conflict between the ideal professional image that is developed in school and the realism with which they are confronted in nursing practice? What factors inhibit the resolution of this conflict? What is the importance of the ideal professional image in the development of professional roles? If conflicts of nursing students remain unresolved, what effects might be reflected in nursing practice after graduation? How might the Women's Movement influence the values of nursing students? What might account for the change in the nursing students' need for nurturance as they moved from the sophomore to the senior year?

Chapter 4

Professionalism of Nurses and Physicians

Sister Gretta Monnig, O.S.F., R.N., Ph.D.
Chairperson, Department of Nursing
College of St. Teresa, Winona, Minnesota

In the process of professionalization, it is helpful to investigate the degree to which members of a particular field possess professional characteristics. Monnig examines the professional model in the context of the degree of professionalism possessed by a random sample of nurses and physicians in Minnesota. For her study, Monnig used Hall's Professional Inventory Scale, which measures five attitudinal components of professionalism: use of a professional organization as a major referent, belief in public service, belief in self-regulation, sense of calling to the field, and feeling of autonomy. Nurses with master's degrees demonstrated a higher degree of professionalism in only one area—the use of professional organizations. Diploma nurses had the greatest sense of calling to the field, whereas nurses with master's degrees had the least sense of calling. Diploma nurses ranked higher in all dimensions of the professionalism scale than did the baccalaureate nurses, except for autonomy. There were few significant differences among physicians. However, when compared with nurses, physicians expressed a higher degree of professionalism on all of the scales except belief in public service.

Over the years the debate about the status of nursing as a profession has become more and more intense. The important question, "Who is the professional nurse?" is being asked. On the other hand, medicine has traditionally been accepted as a profession, and each physician as a professional person. The intent of this paper is to examine the professional model in the context of attitudes of nurses and physicians. The data used in this analysis are from a random sample of nurses and physicians in Minnesota.

BACKGROUND

The diverse ways in which the concept of profession has been defined and used provide various avenues for viewing the professional model. For the purposes of clarity and in order to separate certain identifiable aspects of a professional model, the concepts of profession, professionalization, and professionalism are differentiated in this discussion.

Profession

The term *profession* as an ideal type of occupational institution has been applied traditionally to medicine, law, and the ministry. However, profession as a title of distinction has been used by many other occupational groups, including nurses. Therefore, certain authors have formulated criteria for distinguishing a profession from other kinds of work (Flexner, 1915; Greenwood, 1957; Goode,

1957; and Becker, 1962). Flexner (1915) set forth six characteristics describing professional activity: (1) it is basically intellectual, carrying with it great personal responsibility; (2) it is learned, because it is based on a body of knowledge; (3) it is practical rather than theoretical; (4) its technique can be taught; (5) it is strongly organized internally; and (6) it is motivated by altruism (pp. 578–581). Since then, other authors have attempted to refine differentiating criteria that remain fairly similar to Flexner's original statements. These authors differ in their orientation toward various attributes, but all agree that there is something special about a profession and the way in which its members perform their activities.

After a lengthy review of the literature, Cogan (1953) concluded that "no broad acceptance of any 'authoritative' definition [of profession] has been observed" (p. 49). This statement remains true today, but for the purpose of this study the following definition of profession seems most pertinent. Profession, according to Moore (1970), is "an occupation whose incumbents create and explicitly utilize systematically accumulated general knowledge in the solution of problems posed by clientele, either individuals or collectivities" (pp. 53–54). Such a definition implies that a profession has a base of scientific knowledge that must be applied wisely and judiciously in the service to others.

Professionalization

Vollmer and Mills (1966) distinguished between the concepts of profession and professionalization. The term *profession* was applied only to the abstract model of occupational characteristics, and the concept of *professionalization* was used to refer to a "dynamic process whereby many occupations can be observed to change certain crucial characteristics in the direction of 'profession'" (pp. vii, viii). A. M. Carr-Saunder (1928), Caplow (1954), and Wilensky (1964) recognized a sequence of steps in professionalization. The established professions have followed a typical series of events in their development: (1) doing full-time work, (2) determining standards of work and establishing training schools, (3) promoting effective occupational organizations, (4) gaining legal protection for their skills, and (5) establishing a code of ethics.

Professionalism

Vollmer and Mills (1966) further separated professionalism and professionalization; they used *professionalism* to "refer to an ideology and associated activities that can be found in many and diverse occupational groups whose members aspire to professional status" (p. viii). Thus, over the years, different persons have identified and emphasized different facets of behavior as professional. Strauss (1963) delineated four traits associated with professionalism: expertise, autonomy, commitment, and responsibility. Moore (1970) suggested that professionalism should be properly regarded as a scale on which commonly noted attributes have differing values. Such a scale would provide order in arranging a hierarchy of the occupations and clarify the process of achieving professional status.

Recently, Richard Hall (1967, 1968, 1969) developed an attitude scale to measure the degree of professionalism among persons of different occupations. His Professional Inventory measured five attitudinal components of professionalism: use of the professional organization as a major referent, belief in public service, belief in self-regulation, a sense of calling to the field, and a feeling of autonomy. His scale was based on the premise that the attitudes and ideology held by its practitioners demonstrate the degree of professionalism characteristic of an occupation.

Profession of Nursing

In the literature of the past decades, the status of nursing as a profession has been debated (Goode, 1957; Corwin, 1961). Katz (1969) considered nursing a semiprofession because of the castelike relation of nurses to physicians and the lack of a particular body of knowledge in nursing. However, the earmarks of a profession as listed by Blauch

(1955)—specialized skill requiring training, success measured by quality of service, organization of professional association to maintain and improve service, and a code of ethics—are found in nursing.

Regardless of the status of nursing as a profession, the concept of professionalization can be useful in determining the place of nursing on a scale measuring the ideal-type professions. Nursing has passed through a sequence of steps in professionalization as documented by historical events. Modern nursing was initiated by Florence Nightingale during the Crimean War (1854–1856). In the late nineteenth century, training schools for nurses were opened, which led to the organization of the American Nurses' Association. Licensure laws were passed in several states as early as 1905 and are in effect to the present day. A code of ethics was formulated in 1950, and *Standards of Nursing Practice* was published by the American Nurses Association in 1973. Nursing theories are being refined, and the scientific bases for nursing practice are being developed (Spalding and Notter, 1970).

Despite the progress of nursing, Kleingartner (1967) recognized the existence of certain barriers to full professionalization. Resistance to professionalization developed both from within and without the nursing field. An example of controversy from within is the question of the legal status of nurses functioning in an expanded role. An example of resistance from the outside is the maintenance of a lack of autonomy in nursing; the majority of nurses work in hospitals or for organizations in which the client is not precisely defined. Autonomy and colleague authority are weakened in favor of the employing organization's bureaucracy. The degree to which nursing is professionalized depends upon the setting in which it is practiced, the manner in which the practitioner's performance is controlled, and the degree of expert judgment needed.

Goode (1970) sees the efforts of a profession to raise or maintain its position as a source of social change. The change occurs through research, alterations in education, legislation to protect the profession against new threats or to consolidate an emerging profession in its new privileges, and in distribution of the workforce. The efforts of the members to increase various rewards they obtain from society, to gain recognition, or to protect their privileged position from other aspiring occupations instigate the change. As a result, professionalism of the individual assumes a greater importance. Changing the social system and increasing the degree of professionalism of its members becomes a broader goal of the profession, and consequently the corresponding behavior receives high positive regard. The professional goal of status tends to overshadow the striving for professional expertise. According to French (1967):

> Nursing in America faces the alternatives of confining itself within well-defined areas where its technical knowledge and skill are well-established and respected, or of varying its single standard of preparation and extending its efforts to new problems over which it has special concern and commitment, but where it can't at this moment assert superior knowledge and skill. (p. 16)

The expanding role of the nurse, which demands greater cooperation between nurses and physicians, has presented just such a challenge to the nursing profession. A true partnership between nurses and physicians requires that nurses maintain the same degree of professionalism expected of physicians.

Profession of Medicine

Although medicine has traditionally been accepted as a profession, certain phenomena have affected its accepted status. Becker (1962), in his discussion of the nature of a profession, even challenges the right of law or medicine to serve as the prototype of a true profession since neither law nor medicine actually holds a monopoly over its esoteric knowledge and functions. Not all members of the profession are equally competent to supply basic service, nor are they completely autonomous; and the relationships between clients and professionals vary. In another study, Hall (1968) found that there is generally an inverse relationship between professionalization and bureaucratization even in the established professions. Work is becoming increasingly based on the organization, and this has had an affect on the professionalization process.

DESIGN OF THE STUDY

The present study was designed to test the attitudinal attributes of the professional model. Basically a professional model consists of a series of attributes, both structural and attitudinal, that distinguish professions from other occupations. Since the characteristics that are part of the structure of the occupation, such as formal educational and entrance requirements, are widely dissimilar, the structural attributes were not studied. The beginning practice in nursing is based on undergraduate education, whereas medical education usually begins after completion of the bachelor degree. However, attitudes of health professionals do reflect the degree of professionalization found in a particular profession. Studies on attitudes have shown a high correspondence between the attitudes measured and the behavior of the respondents.

Hall (1967) considered the following attributes important attitudinal constituents necessary to the professionalization process:

1 The use of professional organizations as major referents. This, according to Hall, includes the use of both the formal professional organization and the informal professional peer group as the major sources of ideas and for judgment of the professional's work.

2 A belief in service to the public. The conviction that the profession is indispensable and absolutely essential to society.

3 A belief in self-regulation. The opinion that only the peer group can judge performance.

4 A sense of calling to the field, reflecting the professional's dedication to the work and to serving society, above all other factors.

5 A sense of personal autonomy. The belief that the professional should have maximum freedom to act without constraints imposed by non-professionals or employing organizations.

Hall also noted that the professional model varies intraoccupationally: some members of the profession subscribe to professional ideas to a higher degree than do their colleagues.

The general hypothesis being tested was that differences exist in the degree of professionalism of physicians and nurses. Hall (1967) studied the dimensions of professionalism by constructing Likert scales to measure the five attitudinal components of professionalism: use of professional organization as the major referent, belief in public service, belief in self-regulation, sense of calling to the field, and a feeling of autonomy. Permission to use Hall's Professional Inventory Scale was obtained for this study (see Fig. 4-1).

Data was collected by means of a survey of nurses and physicians who were licensed and practicing in Minnesota. Questionnaires were mailed to a random sample of 300 nurses and 300 physicians. Completed questionnaires were returned by 257 nurses and 230 physicians.

Descriptive statistics were employed to summarize data, and inferential statistics were used to test for significant differences between study groups.

RESULTS

The general hypothesis that nurses and physicians differ in degree of professionalism was tested using the attitudes expressed on the Professional Inventory Scale. Secondary hypotheses were made concerning the relationship of professionalism to certain demographic factors. The hypotheses, the expected nature of their relationship to the variables, and the actual findings are specified in the sections that follow.

Attitudes of Nurses

Hypothesis 1 Nurses will differ in their level of professionalism when these nurses are grouped according to:

1 Using Professional Organization as Major Referent

    1 I systematically read the professional journals.
    2 I regularly attend professional meetings at the local level.
    3 I believe that the professional organization(s) should be supported.
    4 The professional organization doesn't really do much for the average member.
    5 Although I would prefer to, I really don't read the journals too often.

2 Belief in Public Service

    1 Other professions are actually more vital to society than mine.
    2 I think that my profession, more than any other, is essential for society.
    3 The importance of my profession is sometimes overstressed.
    4 Some other occupations are actually more important to society than mine.
    5 If ever an occupation is indispensable, it is this one.

3 Belief in Self-Regulation

    1 My fellow professionals have a pretty good idea about each other's competence.
    2 A problem in this profession is that no one really knows what his colleagues are doing.
    3 We really have no way of judging each other's competence.
    4 There is not much opportunity to judge how another person does his work.
    5 There are very few people who don't really believe in their work.

4 Sense of Calling to the Field

    1 People in this profession have a real "calling" for their work.
    2 The dedication of people in this field is most gratifying.
    3 It is encouraging to see the high level of idealism which is maintained by people in the field.
    4 Most people stay in the profession even if their incomes are reduced.
    5 My colleagues pretty well know how well we all do our work.

5 Feeling of Autonomy

    1 I make my own decisions in regard to what is done in my work.
    2 I don't have much opportunity to exercise my own judgment.
    3 My own decisions are subject to review.
    4 I am my own boss in almost every work-related situation.
    5 Most of my decisions are reviewed by other people.

Figure 4-1 Hall's Professional Inventory. *(Developed by Richard H. Hall, State University of New York—Albany.)*

1 Number of years actively engaged in nursing practice
  2 Highest degree related to nursing career
  3 Field of nursing practice
  4 Size of city of nursing practice
  5 Type of health care setting
  6 Degree of satisfaction with choice of nursing career

The researcher expected that nurses would differ in these ways:

1 Older nurses would have a higher degree of professionalism than younger nurses.
2 Nurses with higher degrees would have a greater degree of professionalism than other nurses.

Table 4-1 Comparison of Professionalism Scale Measures for Nurses Grouped According to Years Actively Engaged in Nursing Practice

Professional inventory scales	Mean scores				F-ratio	Significant pairs*
	Group 1 0–5 Yr (N = 70)	Group 2 6–10 Yr (N = 78)	Group 3 11–20 Yr (N = 60)	Group 4 Over 20 Yr (N = 49)		
Use of professional organization	3.01	3.37	3.56	3.38	14.43	Group 1 vs. 3 1 vs. 4 1 vs. 2
Belief in public service	3.56	3.62	3.59	3.67	0.59	None
Belief in self-regulation	3.65	3.79	3.72	3.70	1.22	None
Sense of calling to the field	3.35	3.36	3.46	3.55	2.18	None
Autonomy	3.22	3.41	3.44	3.40	3.70	None

*Newman Keuls Test

3 Nurses in medical-surgical nursing would have less professionalism.

4 Nurses in large cities would have a higher degree of professionalism.

5 Nurses in hospitals would have less professionalism.

6 Satisfied nurses would have a higher degree of professionalism.

Years in Nursing Practice The comparison of professional scale measures for nurses grouped according to years actively engaged in nursing practice is shown in Table 4-1. Older nurses were expected to have a higher degree of professionalism than younger nurses. It was thought that older nurses would be more active in professional organizations, have greater dedication, and be more accustomed to service. Nurses actively engaged in nursing practice for less than 5 years were significantly lower in the use of professional organizations than nurses who had been in practice for more than 5 years. The finding is consistent with the lack of membership in professional organizations by younger nurses. No differences were found on the other four scales: belief in public service, sense of calling to the field, belief in self-regulation, and a sense of autonomy. Apparently older nurses do not have a greater sense of dedication to nursing or a greater feeling of autonomy.

Highest Degree Professionalism scale measures for nurses grouped according to their highest degree related to a career in nursing are recorded in Table 4-2. Nurses with higher degrees were expected to have a greater degree of professionalism than other nurses. Nurses who have master's degrees should have more knowledge of the profession, a stronger sense of autonomy, greater ability to make decisions, and a deeper interest in the field of nursing, because they are expected to be the leaders in the field.

Nurses with master's degrees demonstrated a higher degree of professionalism only in one area: the use of professional organizations. Diploma nurses had a greater sense of calling to the field, whereas nurses with master's degrees had the least sense of calling to the field. This finding is probably consistent with the degree of dedication that has been cited in past literature as characteristic of diploma nurses.

Table 4-2 Comparison of Professionalism Scale Measures for Nurses Grouped According to Highest Degree Related to Career in Nursing

Professional inventory scales	Mean scores				F-ratio	Significant pairs*
	Group 1 A.D. ($N = 29$)	Group 2 Diploma ($N = 176$)	Group 3 B.S.N. ($N = 39$)	Group 4 M.S. ($N = 6$)		
Use of professional organization	3.05	3.33	3.27	3.88	7.87	Group 4 vs. 1 4 vs. 3 4 vs. 2
Belief in public service	3.57	3.64	3.54	3.36	2.33	None
Belief in self-regulation	3.72	3.76	3.60	3.41	3.98	None
Sense of calling to the field	3.24	3.50	3.37	3.03	6.79	Group 2 vs. 4
Autonomy	3.39	3.32	3.36	3.62	2.14	None

*Newman Keuls Test

Different educational backgrounds made no specific impact on nurses in three areas of professionalism: belief in public service, belief in self-regulation, and autonomy.

Field of Nursing Nurses grouped according to field of nursing practice are presented in Table 4-3. Since nurses in medical-surgical nursing are under much influence from institutions, it was conjectured that nurses in this group would feel less professionalism. Using the Newman Keuls test for significant pairs, no differences were found among nurses in various fields of nursing practice except on the autonomy scale. Medical-surgical nurses were lower in autonomy than nurses in specialties and other areas. As expected, nurses in medical-surgical settings experience less freedom in making decisions.

Size of City Table 4-4 compares the professionalism scale measures for nurses grouped according to the size of the city in which they practice. Nurses in larger cities were expected to have a higher degree of professionalism because of number of activities available in larger cities. No

significant differences were found on four scales: autonomy, use of professional organizations, belief in self-regulation, and sense of calling to the field. Nurses in large cities (of population over 100,000) had the lowest degree of professionalism on belief in public service. Apparently, the importance of the nursing profession to society is less significant to nurses in large cities than it is to those in smaller cities. It is probably true that nurses receive greater recognition or prestige in smaller cities.

Health Care Setting The comparison of professional scale measures for nurses in various health care settings is found in Table 4-5. Nurses in hospitals were expected to have less professionalism than other nurses because of the institutional structure. However, nurses in hospitals did not differ significantly from other nurses in degree of professionalism. Nurses in the community felt a greater sense of calling to the field, whereas office or clinic nurses had the least sense of calling to the field. A possible explanation for this finding is the degree of flexibility and the amount of responsibility that exist in community nursing.

Table 4-3 Comparison of Professionalism Scale Measures for Nurses Grouped According to Field of Nursing

Professional inventory scales	Mean scores				F-ratio	Significant pairs*
	Group 1 Medical-surgical (N = 101)	Group 2 Psych geriatrics (N = 40)	Group 3 Specialties (N = 53)	Group 4 Other (N = 63)		
Use of professional organization	3.28	3.31	3.43	3.33	1.16	None
Belief in public service	3.60	3.58	3.51	3.73	2.80	None
Belief in self-regulation	3.73	3.64	3.66	3.82	1.96	None
Sense of calling to field	3.36	3.38	3.41	3.55	2.25	None
Autonomy	3.22	3.32	3.54	3.45	8.52	Group 1 vs. 3 1 vs. 4

*Newman Keuls Test

Table 4-4 Comparison of Professionalism Scale Measures for Nurses Grouped According to Size of City of Nursing Practice

Professional inventory scales	Mean scores				F-ratio	Significant pairs*
	Group 1 Less than 10,000 population (N = 50)	Group 2 10,000–25,000 population (N = 47)	Group 3 25,000–100,000 population (N = 62)	Group 4 Over 100,000 population (N = 98)		
Use of professional organization	3.36	3.18	3.45	3.32	2.187	None
Belief in public service	3.64	3.75	3.78	3.43	10.941	Group 4 vs. 3 4 vs. 2 4 vs. 1
Belief in self-regulation	3.73	3.78	3.77	3.66	1.311	None
Sense of calling to field	3.45.	3.40	3.58	3.31	23.683	None
Autonomy	3.39	3.30	3.39	3.38	0.452	None

*Newman Keuls Test

Table 4-5 Comparison of Professionalism Scale Measures for Nurses Grouped According to Health Care Setting

| Professional inventory scales | Mean scores | | | | F-ratio | Significant pairs* |
	Group 1 Hospital (N = 175)	Group 2 Community (N = 32)	Group 3 Office or clinic (N = 20)	Group 4 Other (N = 30)		
Use of professional organization	3.30	3.38	3.37	3.42	0.47	None
Belief in public service	3.61	3.70	3.43	3.48	2.90	None
Belief in self-regulation	3.74	3.74	3.52	3.83	2.85	None
Sense of calling to field	3.44	3.54	3.12	3.36	6.41	Group 2 vs. 3
Autonomy	3.33	3.41	3.47	3.39	1.07	None

*Newman Keuls Test

Table 4-6 Comparison of Professionalism Scale Measures for Nurses Grouped According to Degree of Satisfaction with Career

| Professional inventory scales | Mean scores | | | F-ratio | Significant pairs* |
	Group 1 Very satisfied (N = 143)	Group 2 Satisfied (N = 95)	Group 3 Dissatisfied (N = 18)		
Use of professional organization	3.41	3.23	3.20	2.61	None
Belief in public service	3.64	3.58	3.40	1.61	None
Belief in self-regulation	3.78	3.66	3.42	4.21	Group 1 vs. 3
Sense of calling to field	3.55	3.26	3.02	12.97	Group 1 vs. 3
Autonomy	3.42	3.27	3.38	2.42	None

*Newman Keuls Test

Satisfaction with Nursing Career In Table 4-6 nurses are grouped according to degree of satisfaction with the nursing career. The very satisfied nurses apparently have a greater belief in self-regulation and a greater sense of calling to the field than the dissatisfied nurses. Although very satisfied nurses were expected to have a greater degree of professionalism on all scales, no differences were found in use of professional organizations, belief in public service, and sense of autonomy.

The degree of satisfaction of nurses, therefore, is not related to participation in professional organizations, freedom to function, or the recognition of nursing by society.

Summary There were very few significant differences when nurses measured on the Professional Inventory were grouped according to demographic variables. Younger nurses use professional organizations less than nurses actively engaged in nursing practice for over 5 years. Nurses with master's degrees use professional organizations the most but have less sense of calling to the field. Diploma nurses feel the greatest sense of calling to the field or, in other words, have a stronger sense of dedication. Medical-surgical nurses feel less autonomy than specialists and other nurses. Nurses in large cities manifest less belief in public service, whereas community nurses experience a greater sense of calling to the field than office or clinic nurses. Very satisfied nurses demonstrate a greater belief in self-regulation and sense of calling to the field than dissatisfied nurses.

Attitudes of Physicians

Hypothesis 2 Physicians will differ in their level of professionalism when these physicians are grouped according to:

1 Number of years actively engaged in medical practice
2 Highest degree related to medical career
3 Field of medical practice
4 Size of city of medical practice
5 Type of medical practice

The researcher expected that physicians would differ in these ways:

1 Older physicians would have a higher degree of professionalism.
2 Physicians with higher degrees would have more understanding of the profession, and therefore a greater sense of professionalism.
3 Family practitioners, having less need for professionalism than specialists, would demonstrate a lower degree of professionalism.
4 Physicians in larger cities would have easier access to professional activities and would therefore claim a higher degree of professionalism.
5 Physicians in solo practice would have less contact with the medical profession and would therefore have less professionalism.

Since all physicians except two were satisfied with their choice of a medical career, this variable was deleted for physicians.

Years in Medical Practice The comparison of professionalism scale measures for physicians grouped according to number of years actively engaged in medical practice is recorded in Table 4-7. Older physicians were expected to have a higher degree of professionalism than younger physicians. Physicians actively engaged in medical practice over 20 years had greater use for professional organizations and a greater sense of calling to the field than the very young physicians (under 5 years). It can be inferred from the findings that younger physicians participate less actively in professional organizations and have less dedication than older physicians. There were no significant differences on the other three scales: belief in public service, belief in self-regulation, and autonomy.

Highest Degree Table 4-8 records the professionalism scale measures for physicians grouped according to highest degree. It was conjectured that the physicians with the highest degrees would have a higher level of professionalism. Contrary to expectations, there were no significant differences on four scales: belief in public service, belief in self-regulation, sense of calling to field, and autonomy. Physicians with Ph.D.s demonstrated a very high use of professional organizations as compared to the M.D.s. This can be interpreted to mean that physicians with higher degrees understand the profession more deeply, read professional journals more regularly, and participate in medical societies and other activities more than less educated physicians.

Table 4-7 Comparison of Professionalism Scale Measures for Physicians Grouped According to Years Actively Engaged in Medical Practice

Professional inventory scales	Mean scores				F-ratio	Significant pairs*
	Group 1 0–5 Yr (N = 19)	Group 2 6–10 Yr (N = 34)	Group 3 11–20 Yr (N = 79)	Group 4 Over 20 Yr (N = 98)		
Use of professional organization	3.64	3.76	3.91	4.01	6.14	Group 4 vs. 1
Belief in public service	3.30	3.35	3.37	3.43	0.37	None
Belief in self-regulation	3.79	3.84	3.72	3.96	2.15	None
Sense of calling to field	3.39	3.53	3.54	3.71	5.33	Group 4 vs. 1
Autonomy	3.52	3.67	3.76	3.74	2.06	None

*Newman Keuls Test

Table 4-8 Comparison of Professionalism Scale Measures for Physicians Grouped According to Highest Degree Related to Career in Medicine

Professional inventory scales	Mean scores				F-ratio	Significant pairs*
	Group 1 M.D. (N = 164)	Group 2 M.S. (N = 51)	Group 3 Ph.D. (N = 2)	Group 4 Other (N = 13)		
Use of professional organization	3.82	4.13	4.55	4.09	10.45	Group 3 vs. 1
Belief in public service	3.35	3.55	3.84	3.46	2.28	None
Belief in self-regulation	3.81	3.96	4.00	3.82	1.64	None
Sense of calling to field	3.55	3.76	3.80	3.56	3.75	None
Autonomy	3.70	3.79	4.15	3.59	2.36	None

*Newman Keuls Test

Field of Medical Practice Professionalism scale measures for physicians in various fields of medical practice are compared in Table 4-9. Although family practitioners were expected to have less professionalism than specialists, the findings demonstrated otherwise. There were no differences in the professional attitudes of physicians in various fields of medical practice. This implies there is no relationship between degree of professionalism and field of medical practice.

Size of City In Table 4-10 physicians grouped according to the size of the city in which they practice are compared on professionalism scale

Table 4-9   Comparison of Professionalism Scale Measures for Physicians Grouped According to Field of Medical Practice

| Professional inventory scales | Mean scores | | | | F-ratio | Significant pairs* |
	Group 1 Family practitioner (N = 47)	Group 2 Internist (N = 45)	Group 3 Specialist (N = 81)	Group 4 Other (N = 57)		
Use of professional organization	3.78	3.96	3.88	3.99	2.69	None
Belief in public service	3.42	3.39	3.35	3.36	0.22	None
Belief in self-regulation	3.88	3.86	3.85	3.79	0.48	None
Sense of calling to field	3.54	3.64	3.62	3.57	0.76	None
Autonomy	3.77	3.64	3.74	3.76	1.61	None

*Newman Keuls Test

Table 4-10   Comparison of Professionalism Scale Measures for Physicians Grouped According to Size of City of Medical Practice

| Professional inventory scales | Mean scores | | | | F-ratio | Significant pairs* |
	Group 1 Less than 10,000 population (N = 49)	Group 2 10,000– 25,000 population (N = 24)	Group 3 25,000– 100,000 population (N = 52)	Group 4 Over 100,000 population (N = 105)		
Use of professional organization	3.74	3.89	3.97	3.95	3.40	None
Belief in public service	3.42	3.29	3.43	3.37	0.57	None
Belief in self-regulation	3.94	3.79	3.87	3.80	1.49	None
Sense of calling to field	3.50	3.69	3.59	3.62	1.45	None
Autonomy	3.73	3.62	3.76	3.71	0.67	None

*Newman Keuls Test

measures. Physicians in larger cities have easier access to other professionals and were therefore expected to express a higher degree of profession- alism. However, no significant differences were found in expression of professionalism by these various groups. There is evidently no relationship

Table 4-11 Comparison of Professionalism Scale Measures for Physicians Grouped According to Type of Medical Practice

Professional inventory scales	Mean scores			F-ratio	Significant pairs*
	Group 1 Solo (N = 32)	Group 2 2–5 Physicians (N = 75)	Group 3 6 or more Physicians (N = 98)		
Use of professional organization	3.80	3.94	3.91	0.84	None
Belief in public service	3.43	3.45	3.33	1.09	None
Belief in self-regulation	3.88	3.97	3.76	3.23	None
Sense of calling to field	3.69	3.60	3.57	0.76	None
Autonomy	3.81	3.77	3.66	1.73	None

*Newman Keuls Test

Table 4-12 Comparison of Professionalism Scale Measures for Nurses and Physicians

Professional inventory scales	Nurses (N = 257)		Physicians (N = 230)		T-ratio
	Mean	S.D.	Mean	S.D.	
Use of professional organization	3.34	0.70	3.91	0.56	–11.09*
Belief in public service	3.60	0.58	3.38	0.64	4.32*
Belief in self-regulation	3.72	0.57	3.84	0.55	– 2.69*
Sense of calling to the field	3.42	0.60	3.59	0.53	– 3.80*
Autonomy	3.37	0.57	3.72	0.52	– 7.75*

*Significant differences, at .01 level

between the size of the city of medical practice and the degree of professionalism expressed by the physician.

Type of Medical Practice Professionalism scale measures for physicians grouped according to type of medical practice are shown in Table 4-11. Physicians in solo practice have fewer restrictions from institutional structures but also associate less with

other medical persons. They were therefore expected to be less professional. The findings showed no significant differences among physicians in various types of medical practice. Apparently the type of medical practice bears no relationship to the degree of professionalism expressed by physicians.

Summary There were very few significant differences among physicians when they were grouped according to demographic variables. Older physicians use professional organizations more and have a greater sense of calling to the field than the very young physicians. Physicians with Ph.D.s demonstrate a very high use of professional organizations as compared with the M.D.s. No significant differences were found on professional scale measures for physicians grouped according to field of medical practice, size of city, or type of medical practice. Physicians in these groups have similar feelings and behavior as measured by the Professional Inventory.

Comparison of Attitudes of Nurses and Physicians

Hypothesis 3 Nurses will differ from physicians in degree of professionalism as measured by the Professional Inventory. It is conjectured that physicians will express a higher degree of professionalism than nurses.

A comparison of professionalism scale measures for nurses and physicians is shown in Table 4-12. The independent T-ratio for all five scales was significant at the 0.01 level. Physicians expressed a higher degree of professionalism on four scales: use of professional organizations, belief in self-regulation, sense of calling to the field, and autonomy. Nurses expressed a higher degree of professionalism in belief in public service. It seems that nurses feel very strongly that their profession is vital to society, whereas physicians simply accept the fact that their profession is essential. This is probably because the medical profession has a much higher recognition as a profession than the nursing profession.

Discussion The results on the attitude scales reveal some interesting patterns. Hall (1967) found that nurses emerged as strongly professionalized on the attitudes of belief in service to the public and sense of calling to the field, both of which are related to a sense of dedication to the profession. However, in this study, physicians emerge as more strongly professionalized in their sense of calling to the field.

The findings in this study support the findings in past literature that medicine as an occupation is more highly professionalized than nursing. The data from both physicians and nurses also show that some members of each profession subscribe to professional ideals to a greater degree than do their colleagues. However, the demographic variables used in this study shed little light on the cause of these differences.

Frequently persons comment on the apparent age level of individuals who participate actively in professional associations. This study validated the observation that older physicians and nurses use the professional association as a major referent. Professionals who have been actively engaged in practice for some years more systematically read the professional journals, attend professional meetings, and support the professional organization. Also, the use of the professional organization as a major referent can be correlated with the educational level of the professional.

In my estimation, the degree of professionalism expressed by satisfied nurses on the attributes of belief in self-regulation and calling to the field warrants further study. Apparently the dissatisfied nurses have less understanding of the competence of colleagues, do not really believe in their work, and express less idealism; measures could be instituted to promote attitudinal change in these areas.

As nurses work more directly with *Standards of Nursing Practice* and peer review, the belief in self-regulation will increase. A repetition of this study a decade from now would probably reveal increased professionalization of nursing and a greater sense of professionalism in most nurses.

BIBLIOGRAPHY

Becker, Howard S.: "The Nature of a Profession," in *Education for the Professions*, National Society for the Study of Education, University of Chicago Press, 1962, pp. 27–46.

Blauch, L. E. (ed.): *Education for the Professions*, U.S. Department of Health, Education, and Welfare, Washington, 1955.

Caplow, T.: *The Sociology of Work*, University of Minnesota Press, Minneapolis, 1954.

Carr-Saunder, A. M.: *Professions: Their Organization and Place in Society*, The Herbert Spencer Lectures, Clarendon Press, Oxford, 1928.

Cogan, M. L.: "Toward a Definition of Profession," *Harvard Educational Review*, **23**:33–50, Winter 1953.

Corwin, R. G.: "The Professional Employee: A Study of Conflict in Nursing Roles," *American Journal of Sociology*, **66**:604–615, May 1961.

Flexner, A.: "Is Social Work a Profession?" in *Proceedings of the National Conference of Charities and Corrections*, Hildermann Printing Company, Chicago, 1915.

French, D.: *Objectives of Profession of Social Work*, United Nations Economic Commission for Asia and Far East, Bangkok, 1967.

Goode, W. J.: "The Librarian: From Occupation to Profession?" *American Sociological Review*, **22**:194–200, April 1957.

Greenwood, E.: "Attributes of a Profession," *Social Work*, **2**:44–45, July 1957.

Hall, R. H.: "Components of Professionalism," paper presented at the meeting of the American Sociological Association, San Francisco, August 28, 1967.

————: "Professionalism and Bureaucratization," *American Sociological Review*, **33**:92–104, February 1968.

————: *Occupations and the Social Structure*, Prentice Hall, Englewood Cliffs, N.J., 1969.

Katz, F.: "Nurses," in *The Semi-Professions and their Organizations*, The Free Press, New York, 1969.

Kleingartner, A.: *Professionalism and Salaried Workers Organization*, University of Wisconsin, Industrial Relations Research Institute, Madison, 1967.

Krause, E. A.: *The Sociology of Occupations*, Little, Brown, Boston, 1971.

Moore, W. E.: *The Professions: Roles and Rules*, Russell Sage Foundation, New York, 1970, pp. 53–54.

Spalding, E. K., and L. E. Notter: *Professional Nursing*, J. B. Lippincott, Philadelphia, 1970.

Standards of Nursing Practice, pamphlet published by the American Nurses Association, New York, 1973.

Strauss, G.: "Professionalism and Occupational Associations," *Industrial Relations*, **3**:8–9, May 1963.

Vollmer, H. M., and D. L. Mills: *Professionalization*, Prentice Hall, Englewood Cliffs, N.J., 1966.

Wilensky, H. L.: "The Professionalization of Everyone?" *The American Journal of Sociology*, **70**:138–146, September 1964.

EDITOR'S QUESTIONS FOR DISCUSSION

What are the implications of Monnig's findings concerning graduate education for nurses? How can one explain why nurses with higher degrees did not show a greater degree of professionalism in this study than other nurses? Would you assume that the findings of this study would be representative of other geographic areas? What significance does the finding that diploma nurses ranked higher than baccalaureate nurses in all but one of the dimensions of the professional scale have for nursing education programs?

Why does the emphasis on autonomy tend to increase with higher education? What are the implications of increased autonomy for nursing as a profession and as part of the health care system?

Chapter 5

Rhetoric and Behavior in Conflict Resolution: The Professional Employee

Rita Braito, R.N., Ph.D.
Associate Professor, Department of Sociology
University of Denver, Denver

Patricia Prescott, R.N., Ph.D.
Assistant Professor, School of Nursing
University of Colorado, Denver

The definition of normative behavior in certain situations, even for professionals, is ambiguous. Thus, it is helpful to understand the actual attitudes associated with professional behavior, particularly in situations that lead to protest behavior, which some might regard as deviant behavior for a professional. The study by Braito and Prescott explores the reasons for the protest behavior of organizationally employed professional nurses. Protest behavior is defined as the stated behavior one will engage in or has engaged in to achieve a particular goal. The respondents were asked to indicate what types of protest behavior would be acceptable to them in support of a position on two issues: salary and control over who gives what type of patient care. Absenteeism and striking ranked twelfth and thirteenth, respectively, as types of protest activities that would be endorsed in support of the salary issue. Only two hypotheses were supported: (1) the greater the perceived deprivation of one's salary when compared with the salaries of another group, the higher the salary demands; and (2) the greater the information about salaries of other groups, the greater the perceived deprivation at the zero-order level. When control variables were introduced, marital status and number of children particularly, as well as socioeconomic status of the husband, altered many of the zero-order relationships. Job dissatisfaction was unrelated to demands for increased control over who provides what type of patient care. The findings also suggest that salary satisfaction and salary demands are related only for a small portion of the population studied. In addition, the authors point out that although bargaining originally may be used because of discontent with salaries, it can become established as a source of power for the bargaining representatives even

This is a revision of a paper presented at the Midwest Sociological Association, Omaha, Nebraska, April 3-6, 1974, supported in part by the American Nurses Foundation, 1967, and the University of Washington.

when the conditions necessary for its establishment no longer exist. In large organizations where upward mobility may be limited, members may depend on institutional bargaining to obtain a salary increase, which would be interpreted as recognition of merit. Contrary to what is reflected in the literature, relative deprivation, job dissatisfaction, salary, amount of knowledge, and reference group support did not explain the attitudes of the population studied concerning salary demands and increased control over who gives what type of care.

The professional and the blue-collar occupations have been viewed as polar types. Each type has had its own problems and tensions that have led to institutionalized solutions. However, circumstances frequently have arisen that have led to pressure by blue-collar workers for professionalization, on the one hand, and the encounter of professionals with blue-collar-like conditions on the other. In these situations each occupational type has confronted problems for which there are no institutionalized solutions. The problems of concern in this research are of this transitional type. They may be approached most efficiently by way of a review of the typical problems of professionals and blue-collar workers.

THE PROFESSIONAL

The traditional model of a profession has been based upon the individual practitioner, with the medical doctor, the lawyer, and the dentist as prototypes. The criteria for professionalization, which have been identified by authors with varying degrees of emphasis, are "the unstandardized product, degree of personality involvement of the professional, wide knowledge of a specialized technique, sense of group identity and significance of the occupational service to society" (Gross, 1958, p. 7; see also Vollmer and Mills, 1966; Moore, 1970; Pavalko, 1972).

The problems faced by ideal-type professionals derive from the characteristics of professional occupations. They include:

1 Problems related to autonomy or the right to independent decision making

2 Problems related to personal commitment or

orientation to a career and the high degree of time and energy involved in career pursuits

3 Problems related to professionalization, relations with associations and colleague groups, and definitions of standards of practice

4 Problems related to honor, prestige, and extrinsic and intrinsic rewards

BLUE-COLLAR WORKERS

It is interesting to note that there appears to be no composite description identifying the characteristics of blue-collar workers such as there is for the professional. However, as a polar opposite of the professional, the blue-collar worker tends to be characterized by little autonomy, the absence of a theoretically based body of knowledge, the absence of career commitment, and a reward system based on remuneration rather than prestige and honor.

Problems of blue-collar workers may also be defined in terms of the nature of their occupations. These workers are likely to have problems in finding meaning in the tasks they perform and problems related to increasing control or influence over conditions associated with work, job security, profit sharing, and fringe benefits.

THE PROFESSIONAL AS AN EMPLOYEE

Several persistent trends in the nature and organization of professions are apparent. First, occupational census data indicate that "professionals represent the most rapidly growing occupational category in highly-developed, modern economies, and the end is nowhere in sight" (Moore, 1970, p. 3). Second, professionals are increasingly employed by organizations. In 1960, four-fifths of males categorized as professional or kindred workers were not self-employed (Moore, 1970, pp. 187–188).

Much of the research on the professional employee has been concerned with conflict as it relates to the bureaucratic role versus the professional role or to a local versus a cosmopolitan orientation (Kornhauser, 1962; Corwin, 1961; Wilensky, 1964; Becker, 1958; Pearlin, 1962; Freidson and Buford, 1965; Strauss and Rainwater, 1962; Perrucci and Gerstl, 1969; Habenstein and Christ, 1963; Goldner, 1957, 1958; Miller, 1966; Ben-David, 1958).

Despite the large body of literature addressing the problems of professional autonomy and role conflict experienced by professional employees of organizations, there has been relatively little research on the issue of remuneration or on other issues generally considered to be problems of organizational employees. For example, much has been written about unionization of blue-collar workers, but comparatively little is available on the professional equivalent of the union, the professional association, as it relates to the welfare of the professional worker who is also an organizational employee.

NURSING

Nursing is a profession that is most frequently practiced in organizational settings. Consquently, nurses demonstrate many of the occupational characteristics of both the professional and the blue-collar worker. For example, they are concerned with professional issues such as quality of care, but they are also concerned with issues of interest to blue-collar employees, such as salary and working conditions. They have two sets of contrasting values—those of the employee and those of the professional. The ways in which workers have attempted to control their working conditions have centered on the strike, the boycott, and the demonstration; the ways in which the classical professionals have attempted to con-

trol their conditions have centered on the professional organization and the political pressure group.

Forms of Protest

Forms of protest taken by different groups have varied from strike behavior to slowdown. Such actions are a deliberate transfer of attention from the goal ends of the organization to the means (Muskow, 1966; Dubin, 1960; Sheppard, 1954; Schneider, 1964). Two broad types of factors or conditions have been identified as contributing to such protest behavior: (a) conditions external to the occupation, such as a change in the social distribution of rewards or wages, alterations in the opportunity structure, and wider dispersion of knowledge, or mass acculturation (National Manpower Council, 1958; Wilensky, 1964) and (b) conditions internal to the occupation or work situation, such as a decrease in job satisfaction due to alterations in tasks, an alteration in the reward system, and decreased opportunity to exercise acquired skills (Palola and Larson, 1965; Georgopoulos and Mann, 1962; Blauner, 1964; Morse, 1953; Pearsall, 1963). In either type of condition there is an alteration in the extrinsic or intrinsic rewards associated with a given occupation.

Integral components of protest behavior are the issues or goals and their legitimation (Dubin, 1960; Barth and Johnson, 1959; Harbison and Coleman, 1951). The basis for the legitimation of an issue and its translation into advocacy is problematic (Blau, 1964; Kerr and Fisher, 1949; Blumer, 1951). The sources of legitimation are located in the important social groups of which one is a member. For example, the professional as a member of a professional group can utilize improvement of care to the client or increased recruitment in a field important to public welfare as justification for a present or proposed action of the professional group. Although professionalism can provide a basis for legitimation (Gross, 1960), paradoxically, it may inhibit particular types of protest behavior, such as strikes and mass demonstrations. Yet a no-strike orientation reduces the amount of power that protesting individuals can exert.

Another source of legitimation anchored in group membership is distributive justice. Aware of current norms, people in our society expect given rewards based upon given investments. When a discrepancy exists, it can be used as the basis for the legitimation of conflicts.

The power of any group and the strategy available to that group may be partially dependent upon the type of organization that is utilized for goal achievement. Unions can mobilize groups and be effective in bargaining situations because adherence to the agreed-upon course of action is insured by sanctions that may be enforced. Professional bargaining associations do not have such sanctioning power available to them. Even when sanctioning power is used, the compliance on the part of the membership is voluntary and may have little impact upon their employment by a given organization. An indirect measure of the potential power of a group of employees is the degree of consensus on issues, bases of legitimation, and forms of protest. Several factors may mediate the degree of consensus attained within a given group. Such factors include type and amount of professional education, tenure in the organization, proximity to retirement, position held in the organization, and membership in professional associations. These statuses are related to placement in the organization and may differentiate management from nonmanagement positions.

KEY CONCEPTS FOR A STUDY OF PROFESSIONAL TENSIONS

Conditions both external and internal to the occupation, such as societal distribution of rewards, an increase in knowledge about reward distribution, changes resulting in decreased job satisfaction, or alteration in the reward system, have consequences for individual behavior. The meaning and importance of these changes are influenced by the groups to which one belongs.

REFERENCE GROUP AND RELATIVE DEPRIVATION

The concept of reference group has been shown to have several meanings and can be used to serve a variety of functions. Some meanings have been suggested by Turner (1966). The very broad usage of the term has been dealt with in great detail by Merton (1957). However, the definition used in this study is that which was summarized by Secord and Backman:

> A reference group is a group taken as a frame of reference for self-evaluation and attitude formation. It may have two functions: a normative function and a comparison function. The normative function is that of setting and enforcing standards of conduct and beliefs. The comparison function is that of establishing it as a standard or a comparison point against which persons may compare themselves and others (1964, p. 212).

This study focuses on groups serving both normative and comparative functions. With regard to the normative function, a study was made of reference groups and loyalties in the outpatient department by Bennis, Berkowitz, Affinito, and Malone (1959). The reference groups defined as relevant were the nursing profession, the outpatient department, the hospital, the immediate work group, the medical field, and the hospital nursing service. In another study based on the same population, Benne and Bennis (1959) expressed regret that they did not include the school from which the nurse graduated because they felt that it was an important reference group. These groups or categories, the hospital nurses, the hospital administration, and an unidentified, highly respected person, as well as their own professional image, were selected as sources of social support for the nurses included in the sample of this study.

The second function of reference groups as suggested by Secord and Backman is a comparative function. They state:

> Basic to the phenomena of status is a process of comparison. Persons compare themselves and

others with respect to rewards received, costs incurred, and investments accumulated and they are in varying degrees satisfied or dissatisfied with the comparisons (1964, p. 297).

This process of social comparison has been discussed by Homans (1961, p. 73) and Merton (1957, p. 227). It involves two central concepts: distributive justice and status congruence. Homans says:

> Distributive justice is a matter of the relation between what a man gets in the way of a reward and what he incurs in the way of cost, here and now status congruence is a matter of the impression he makes on, the stimuli he presents to, other men, which may effect their future behavior toward him and, therefore, the future reward he gets from them. There is a difference between the two phenomena and so we have called them by different names, but of course the two may overlap (1961, p. 250).

Merton (1957) suggests the concept of relative deprivation refers to the results of the comparison process in which dissatisfaction, deprivation, or injustice are felt as a consequence of comparing one's situation with that of others. The comparison process may result in a feeling of relative deprivation or it may result in a feeling of violation of distributive justice. Distributive justice, however, refers explicitly to the relationship between cost or investment and reward, and, depending upon the individual's circumstances, will either give rise to a notion of being fairly treated or to the feeling that distributive justice has been violated. Deprivation, as suggested by Homans and Merton, may be an example of violation of distributive justice; however, the term distributive justice is used to refer to the basis of legitimation. It is important to note that both relative deprivation and violation of distributive justice derive from the same basic process of social comparison. The separation of the two terms in this research is for clarity in presentation rather than for theoretical clarification or elaboration.

JOB DISSATISFACTION

Conditions internal to the occupation or work situation, such as decreasing job satisfaction due to alteration in task, alteration in the reward system, or decreased opportunity to exercise acquired skills, may lead to protest behavior. Although job dissatisfaction is distinct from relative deprivation and distributive justice, it may arise from the same social comparison process. Job dissatisfaction may originate in the work situation because of changes that have occurred; it may also arise from failure of the work situation to meet expectations acquired in the socialization process.

There is an abundance of literature on job dissatisfaction (Friedman, 1961; Barton, 1961; Katzell, 1964; Taylor and Weiss, 1969; Graen, Dawis, and Weiss, 1968; Blauner, 1964; Stagner and Rosen, 1965; Tannenbaum, 1966; Morse, 1953). Much of the literature cited is concerned with job dissatisfaction as it is related to productivity, turnover, and ego needs.

Studies of job dissatisfaction in nursing have identified the following as related factors or possible sources:

1 Discrepancy between an ideal conception of nursing and the actual tasks performed (Katz, 1969; Corwin, 1961).

2 Discrepancy between an ideal conception of nursing and the criteria used by the organization for promotion; in other words, conflicts between clinical and administrative duties (Leonard, 1977; Benne and Bennis, 1959).

3 Conflict between physicians and nurses, particularly in the area of the nurses' discretionary freedom.

4 Consensus regarding definitions of role. Larsen (1968) has shown that consensus is directly related to job satisfaction, with low consensus related to high job dissatisfaction.

5 The relatively low social position of the nurse and the poorly defined professional hierarchy within the work setting (Devereax and Weiner, 1950).

6 Conflict between the behaviors rewarded and

the values held by nursing educators and nursing administrators (Smith, 1965).

7 High staff turnover rates and accompanying instability within the nursing group (Yett, 1965).

8 Knowledge about the wages, working conditions, job security, and fringe benefits of other work groups. Such knowledge may give rise to satisfaction with one's own form of remuneration, or it may cause dissatisfaction as a result of the process of social comparison and an ensuing sense of relative deprivation. Knowledge is viewed as an external source of potential job dissatisfaction in contrast to the conditions listed above, which are considered internal to the job.

It seems reasonable to infer that there is widespread knowledge about what various groups are earning, the types of fringe benefits they receive, and the nature of other work-related conditions. It is suggested that increased knowledge of this type, if it results in relative deprivation in the area of wage comparisons, will give rise to job dissatisfaction, salary demands, and forms of protest behavior.

Job dissatisfaction has multiple sources within the nursing occupation. In addition, it may have multiple consequences. For example, it could result in innovative changes within the organization, which might then bring about changes in the actual situation causing the dissatisfaction. It is also possible that a form of "goal displacement" would occur and that this would be reflected in traditional demands of the worker or the person of employee status. It is conceivable that job dissatisfaction could lead to a variety of demands similar or identical to those frequently made by anyone in an employee position. For the professional of employee status, job dissatisfaction could produce demands commonly made by the employee as well as demands in the professional domain. For example, such a professional might make demands for greater autonomy, whether or not the autonomy is actually at issue. Job dissatisfaction could also give rise to demands that would enhance the status of one's own field in relation to other fields.

The main point is that job dissatisfaction may have pervasive effects that have not yet been explored.

ISSUES AND LEGITIMATION

Integral components of protest behavior are issues or goals and their legitimation. Blau has suggested that:

> Serious social deprivations experienced in a collective situation create . . . a surplus of resources . . . this surplus is the resource that produces social legitimation. Rewards that are entirely insufficient to meet expectations of fairness and basic needs paradoxically also create a potential surplus, and if conditions are favorable for its realization this surplus becomes the resource that produces social opposition.
>
> Opposition is a regenerative force that introjects new vitality into a social structure and becomes the basis of social reorganization. It serves as a catalyst or a starting mechanism of social change, which is sometimes carried out in large part by others rather than those active in the opposition that stimulates it (1964, p. 301).

Social deprivation could be translated into issues that require legitimation. As collective bargaining has been institutionalized, it is necessary to look at those issues which in prior agreements have been relevant to nursing, at the issues in which the nursing association has participated, and at agreements between the association and the hospital council (Kerr and Fisher, 1949). The issues negotiated previously by the parties involved have related to hours of work and overtime, salary, premium pay, vacations, holidays, sick leave, leaves of absence, health programs, employment status, part-time nursing, equal employment opportunity, conference committees, grievance procedures, retention of benefits, and effective date and duration of the agreement. These are the traditional issues of concern to blue-collar workers, and the majority of the unions have focused on them. For analytical purposes, Dubin has defined two broad categories of collective bargaining:

> Fundamental issues are those not yet incorporated into collective bargaining. Control over the functions of defining such issues may be in the hands of either party exclusively or located at some other point in the social system. Conventional issues are defined as those which have been included in collective bargaining through past negotiations between the parties and incorporated in union contracts (1960, p. 509).

The issues cited above would be considered conventional issues. Fundamental issues would cause the greatest amount of conflict. However, within this formulation the amount and type of conflict over the issues would depend upon the power of the respective groups. In 1965 the hypothesis that equal power would give rise to greatest amount of conflict over fundamental issues was tested and supported (Dubin, 1965). Goldhammer and Shils suggest:

> The motivation for obedience and disobedience is instrumental to the extent that it is based on an anticipation of losses and gains, and noninstrumental to the extent that it is based on ethical or affective imperatives of conduct dictating obedience or disobedience to the command (1939, p. 173).

These authors have looked at fundamental and conventional issues in relation to attempted domination of one group by another and the amount and length of conflict involved. It seems equally appropriate to look at issues within the same context as well as the norms for conduct. Within this framework a fundamental or a conventional issue could be instrumental or noninstrumental. Bidwell and Vreeland (1963, p. 236) have suggested "solitary incentives centered upon professional values and commitments" as the principal means of control in client-serving organizations. They also suggest that these incentives would be related to professional values. Using this formulation, profes-

sionalism or distributive justice could serve as a basis for legitimation. An example of a conventional issue for teachers, nurses, and other groups would be salary. A fundamental issue would be one that a group defines as not in the area of negotiation. Examples of fundamental issues for registered nurses might be such things as increased control by nurses themselves over who will provide what type of care and increased control over the quantity and quality of care they provide. These issues have not come up for negotiation. Considering for a moment the teaching profession, it is important to note that, although the most important early issues did relate to salary and similar types of benefits, the issues currently under negotiation, while still of that type, have been broadened considerably to include other issues more related to the professional work of the teacher. If nursing follows a similar pattern it can be expected that such a transformation in the type and nature of issues will also occur. Therefore, the issues selected for this research include one of the conventional type (salary) and one that could at some later time become a fundamental issue (control over who provides what type of care). The two types of issues selected could also be dichotomized into instrumental and noninstrumental.

Bases of legitimation can be conceived of as strategies of action. Such strategies could derive from a variety of sources, such as service to God, service to humanity, service to the sick, and greater enhancement of personal development. It is likely that these strategies will develop out of the position the individual occupies in the social situation requiring action. The strategy of a professional employee is apt to stem from two bases: that of the worker and that of the professional. As a worker the nurse can draw upon the vocabularies of motives that have been used by other workers in the past, such as education, amount of work, responsibility, type of work, irregularity of the hours, or stress associated with such activities. As a professional, the nurse can draw upon service to the public, particular types of responsibilities, professional jurisdiction as acquired through the professional association, or protection of the public. Since nurses are not unionized it is necessary for them, through their vocabulary of motives, to gain the support of their group and at the same time avoid alienating the public whose support they need. The more effectively nurses mobilize and legitimate their behavior, the greater their power will be. Gross (1960) has suggested that power of professional groups is a result of their bargaining positions in the society, their social importance, and the criticalness of their service, as well as the law of supply and demand. Professional personnel, then, can be conceived of as occupying relative power positions. Yett has suggested:

> It is quite likely that as the shortage of nurses continues, or even grows, nurses will, more and more, come to realize that they are not taking full advantage of the collective power they could have to improve their salaries and other conditions of employment. The "monopsonistic" power of hospitals is too obvious to go unnoticed, and the same can be said for the potential "contravailing power" of organized nurses. Either the ANA and its affiliated state organizations will have to greatly improve and expand its "economic security" program or else it will gradually lose out to bona fide trade unions (1965, p. 102).

As nurses and hospitals become more equal in power or become more aware of the power they control it is possible that greater conflict, particularly over fundamental issues, may result. It also follows that leaders of the American Nurses Association, in order to maintain their position and strength and that of the organization and in order to prevent inroads by unions, will become more demanding and more militant. But as we mentioned earlier, professionalism, while providing a basis for legitimation, may also inhibit particular types of protest behavior such as strikes or mass demonstrations; and a no-strike orientation reduces the amount of power that protesting individuals can exert. The next important concept to examine, then, is protest behavior.

PROTEST BEHAVIOR

The types of collective action behavior a group uses to achieve its goals depend, in part, upon the organization of the group. A union, for example, is able to exert sanctions against members who violate measures that the group has decided to take against a given company or organization. In the professional organization, where the behavior is not subject to sanctioning, high group solidarity is important. In the state where the three hospital organizations and the population to be studied were selected, the nurses' association required 75 percent membership on the part of the registered nurses in a given hospital prior to serving as the negotiating agent. Such a large membership—75 percent as compared with the 51 percent required by law—at the time of negotiation indicates the power of the nursing group to the hospital board. Just as the vocabulary of motives grows out of the individual's position in the social structure, so the type of protest behavior considered appropriate grows out of one's position in the organization. Such things as slowdown and sabotage have not, therefore, been appropriate tactics in the achievement of group goals in nursing. In some states it is illegal for particular categories of personnel to strike. In these cases, alternatives that would have the same result might be utilized, such as mass resignations or calling in sick or absent. Both of these types of behavior would have the same consequences but would not violate a no-strike statute on the books. It is necessary to differentiate between legitimation as conceived in law and legitimation as related to right to protest, which may be restricted by law. Such a law might be considered illegitimate or not applicable in a given situation. If the members of a group view a law as "illegal," they might engage in strike behavior even though such behavior is defined as illegal. Striking or threatening to strike may also have consequences in areas other than collective bargaining. Such action may serve as a device for informing the public of the issues and the demands that are under negotiation. Depending upon the orientation of a given public, it may also serve to bring public pressure to bear on various groups. The ability to solidify around a given issue may also serve to strengthen a professional association, since the involvement in economic issues can lead to interest in other areas and activities. For example, the economic security program of the American Nurses Association has been evaluated positively by nurses and therefore may be a route by which individuals active in this program alone become involved in other aspects. The greater the numbers of the individuals who are willing to engage in behavior that would have the same consequences as a strike, the stronger the negotiating power of their representative becomes. It also seems likely that not only the type of behavior but the range of behavior in which individuals are willing to engage might tend to increase the power of their group, provided that they are able to legitimate their issues to the particular publics whose support they are seeking.

MARITAL STATUS AND ROLE OF THE FAMILY

The influence of the family on both the male and the female in their actual occupational behavior has received little attention in sociological research. An article by Kemper (1968) has shown that the influence of an individual's various roles on his or her organizational behavior is potentially great. The role of the family may have great significance for the issues and forms of protest and legitimation that an individual would consider. Although the economic and the occupational role of the husband has traditionally been the basis for establishing family orientation in terms of values and class-related behavior, family research has shown some variation with respect to the husband's influence. In husband-wife discussions of various issues, it has been shown that the husband's position on labor issues usually dominates. But there is evidence too, that the working wife exerts more influence than the nonworking wife, although this finding varied with the number of

children (Axelson, 1963; Heer, 1963; March, 1963; Blood, 1963). It might be argued that the nurse whose spouse is a blue-collar worker might be more prone to strike activities, since the strike is the activity that has been most effectively used by this group. It is equally plausible, however, since the nurse occupies a position of higher status and is regarded as a professional by the public, that the spouse would consider the nurse to be in the position to make the decision. The nurse whose spouse is professionally employed might agree on a particular issue, whether it be that of the employee or the professional. The spouse who is a private-practice professional might also agree on an issue related to the deprivations the nurse is experiencing and support any action undertaken. On the other hand, the spouse may be less willing to encourage such active protest behavior as striking, calling in ill, or participating in mass resignation. It would be possible to build up a plausible argument for whatever position one chose to take. Although it is expected that the marital role and the occupation of the spouse will have some consequences, there is insufficient information in this area to suggest specific consequences.

Figure 5-1 summarizes the relationships among the major concepts discussed in the preceeding sections. The hypotheses of this study are derived from these relationships.

HYPOTHESES OF THE STUDY

I The greater the relative deprivation of nurses the greater the salary demands.

II The greater the relative deprivation of nurses the more protest activities used to obtain a salary increase.

IIIa The greater the job dissatisfaction of nurses as measured by global indicators the greater the number of protest activities used to obtain a salary increase.

IIIb The greater the job dissatisfaction of nurses as measured by activities enjoyed the greater the number of protest activities used to obtain a salary increase.

IV The greater the job dissatisfaction of nurses

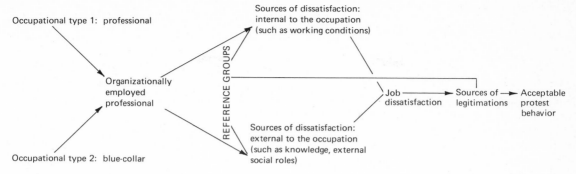

Figure 5-1   Relationships among major concepts

as measured by global indicators the greater the number of protest activities used to obtain increased control over who provides what type of patient care.

V   The greater the knowledge of nurses the greater the relative deprivation.

VI   The greater the knowledge of nurses the more protest activities used to obtain a salary increase.

VII   The greater the reference group support of nurses the greater the number of protest activities used for salary increases.

VIII   The greater the reference group support of nurses the greater the number of protest activities used to obtain increased control over who provides what type of patient care.

IX   There will be higher agreement among nurses on legitimation of the patient control issue than on the salary issue.

Family control variables were introduced to assess their impact on the hypothesized relationships under the null hypothesis; marital status, number of children, and socioeconomic status of the spouse will have no effect on the above hypotheses.

Organizational control variables were also introduced to assess their impact on the hypothesized relationships under the null hypothesis: organizational position, employment (full-time or part-time), education, and age will have no effect upon the aforementioned relationships.

METHODOLOGY

Sample and Statistic

Registered nurses, professional employees of three hospitals in the Northwest, met the condition of being workers as well as employed professionals and were selected for the study. The group was in negotiation with the representatives of the hospital association concerning a salary increase. Therefore, the research was relevant to the group's activities at the time. A questionnaire that had been pilot-tested was sent to all nurses from the three hospitals. A cover letter from the director of nursing at each hospital encouraging participation was sent with the researcher's cover letter, which assured anonymity and stressed the importance of the response. A postcard was enclosed for the nurse to sign and mail back at the same time the questionnaire was returned. The overall response rate was 64 percent and varied by hospital from 55 to 75 percent. The number of respondents was 467. Gamma was the statistic used in assessing the strength of the relationships proposed (Goodman and Kruskall, 1963; Costner, 1965). A gamma of .40 and above is considered strong support, a gamma of .30 to .39 as moderately supporting a given proposition, and a gamma of .20 to .29 as providing directional support. Percentage was also utilized (Anderson and Zelditch, 1968).

Operational Indicators

Issues Issues have been defined as the goals over which bargaining is or will be relevant (Dubin, 1960). These have been included under two classifications: conventional and fundamental.

Conventional Issue (Salary) Do you think nurses in _____ should have a salary increase at this time? _____ no; _____ yes; if yes, $_____ per month.

Fundamental and Professional Issue Do you think nurses should have increased control over who gives what type of patient care? _____ no; _____ yes.

Legitimation Rhetoric Eleven judges were asked to classify the issues according to whether they were professional issues or issues of distributive justice. (See Figure 5-2 for examples of each type of legitimation.) The respondents were asked whether they favored or opposed each issue. They were also asked to indicate the first and second reasons for their position.

Job satisfaction was defined as the discrepancy between what the individual wants and what is received in the occupational sphere including expressed enjoyment of a given activity (Morse, 1953). Two summary scores were obtained. One was based on general indicators; the other was based on specific tasks. The general measures reflected a possible range of 1 to 6, with 6 representing high satisfaction. The number of times 4, 5, and 6 were checked was totaled, and a summary score was obtained. The general indicators in question were: having a chance to do the things you do best, having a feeling of accomplishment from the work you are doing, having an opportunity to give the type and quality of nursing care which you are capable of giving, having the opportunity to give the type and quality of nursing care which you think should be given, having an opportunity to give the type and quality of supervision which you are capable of giving, feeling that what you are doing is important, feeling that you are an impor-

tant member of the health team, feeling that you are recognized as an important member of the health team, feeling that the people for whom you work are concerned about your welfare, feeling that learning experiences are provided for you within your job, and feeling that you have an opportunity for promotion.

The specific tasks related to enjoyment of activities in the work situation were as follows: talking with patients; talking with visitors; giving medications; giving treatments; charting; noting orders; collecting specimens; providing direct physical care to patients; socializing with other nurses or personnel in the area; working with interns, residents, and doctors; working with instruments and equipment; supervising others in the provision of patient care; teaching patients; providing patients with information. A total score was obtained by totaling the number of times a like score was checked.

Protest behavior was defined as the stated behavior one will engage in or has engaged in to achieve a particular goal. The respondents were asked to indicate what protest behaviors would be acceptable to them in support of a position. Eighteen different forms of protest behavior were presented on the salary issue and sixteen on the control issue. They could check as many as they wished. The activities presented were: striking; participation in mass resignations; participation in mass calling-in-absent; participation in writing a group letter of protest to the administration; talking directly to the hospital administration; writing a letter to the *Journal of Nursing*, newspaper, city council, etc.; being less accommodative to the administration's requests for overtime, float, unpleasant hours; attending meetings where this issue was being discussed and voting for it; complaining to physicians; attempting to enlist the support of physicians; discussing the matter with patients; discussing the matter with colleagues; changing to another area of nursing (office, private duty, etc.); resigning individually and going to another hospital. The total number of activities checked from the above list was obtained for each respondent and constituted a summary score. Other activities, such as keep it to myself and say nothing, or in the event of a strike keep on providing patient care, were not totaled.

Reference group was defined as relevant groups, significant others, or symbolic images utilized for social support or nonsupport of a particular position on selective issues. A summary score was developed based on the number of groups or significant persons out of the eight following categories that the respondents said would be in favor of a salary increase or increased control over patient care. The categories included: a person whose opinion you value highly, your spouse (for single nurses, imagine how your spouse would respond), the majority of nurses on your ward, the nurses in your hospital, your school of nursing, the professional image you hold, the nursing administration, the hospital administration.

Relative deprivation refers to the perceived deprivation in terms of one's salary when it is compared to the salaries of another group (Merton, 1957). A summary indicator was developed for each respondent based upon thirteen comparisons. The comparison groups were nurses in other areas of employment, directors of nursing, doctors, laboratory technicians, social workers, beauticians, clerks in department stores, elementary and junior and senior high school teachers, engineers, gardeners, firemen, policewomen, and plumbers. For each of these occupations the respondent was asked to indicate whether the nurses earned less, the same, or more than the particular category.

SALARY ISSUE

Professional Legitimation
> It would encourage more nurses to return to the field.
> It would improve quality of patient care.
> It would attract more young people into the field.

Distributive Justice Legitimation
> Nurses have subsidized patient care long enough.
> Nurses are underpaid for the education required.
> Nurses are underpaid for the amount of responsibility held.
> It would give recognition for the unique responsibility held.
> It would give recognition of worth—the more you earn the more important your work is evaluated.

INCREASED PATIENT CONTROL ISSUE

Professional Legitimation
> One can better utilize the auxiliary personnel.
> It would provide better nursing care.
> It is essential to protect the welfare of the patient.
> It would enable one to better coordinate the care or services that patients receive.
> This should be primarily the responsibility of professional nurses.

Distributive Justice Legitimation
> It would encourage more nurses to return to the field of nursing.
> People with our preparation are equipped to make such decisions because of our unique relationship with the patient.
> Displacement of professional nurses by practical nurses will occur otherwise.
> It would improve the public image of the professional nurse.
> Hospital administration has been making these decisions without consulting us.

Figure 5-2 Legitimation of issues.

They were also asked to state whether nurses *should* earn less, the same, or more than the category. A relative deprivation global score consisted of the total number of times a respondent indicated she should earn more but actually earned less than or the same as the other groups.

Knowledge was defined as the information about the salaries of other groups. The occupational categories mentioned above were used to assess the knowledge of the nurses who participated in this study. For each of the categories selected, respondents were asked to indicate their knowledge of the group's earnings today compared with two years ago—whether it was less, the same, or more. A global score was developed based on the number of times the respondents stated more.

Control variables were the socioeconomic status (SES) of husband and father based on Hollingshead's two-factor index, marital status, number of children, position in hospital (staff nurse, head nurse, assistant head nurse, supervisor, assistant director of nursing), and type or amount of education (2 years, 3 years, B.S., M.S., Ph.D.).

FINDINGS

Only two of the eight hypotheses were even weakly supported. They are: the greater the relative deprivation of nurses, the higher the salary demands; and the greater the increase in knowl-

Table 5-1 Zero-Order Measures of Association of Eight Hypotheses Concerned with Relative Deprivation, Salary Demands, Protest Activities, Job Dissatisfaction, Increased Knowledge, and Reference Group Support

Hypothesis number	Hypotheses	Gamma measure of association
I	The greater the relative deprivation of nurses the greater the salary demands	+.21
II	The greater the relative deprivation of nurses the more protest activities used	+.08
IIIa	The greater the job dissatisfaction of nurses as measured by global indicators the greater the number of protest activities used	+.09
IIIb	The greater the job dissatisfaction of nurses as measured by activities enjoyed the greater the number of protest activities used	+.005
IV	The greater the job dissatisfaction of nurses as measured by global indicators the greater the number of protest activities used to obtain increased control over who provides what type of patient care	-.04
V	The greater the increase in knowledge of nurses the greater the relative deprivation	+.25
VI	The greater the increase in knowledge of nurses the more protest activities used to obtain salary increase	+.15
VII	The greater the reference group support of nurses the greater the number of protest activities used for salary increase	+.001
VIII	The greater the reference group support of nurses the greater the number of protest activities used to obtain increased control over who provides what type of patient care	-.001

edge, the greater the relative deprivation. One of the assumptions that is generally accepted in the literature is that when a salary increase is asked for, the demand is based on relative deprivation. But the weak support found in this study suggests that, while this may be true, other factors must be operating as well. A further assumption made in most of the past literature and called into question by these results is that salary dissatisfaction is reflected in job dissatisfaction.

Another question that was asked about salary on a range of 1 to 6 was: "How satisfied are you with your salary?" The responses were as follows:

	Not at all					Very much
	1	2	3	4	5	6
Number	71	69	85	118	72	48
Percent	15.2	14.8	18.2	25.3	15.4	10.3

As can be seen, 50 percent checked 4 or higher. Yet when asked: "Do you think nurses in _____ should have a salary increase?" 450 out of 461, or 96 percent, said yes. When asked $_____ per month, 66, or 15.9 percent, wrote between $5.00 and $80.00, 315, or 75 percent, wrote in exactly $100.00, and 34, or 8.2 percent, answered from $120 to $250. Another way of looking at the results is presented in Table 5-2.

Of the 34 who had the highest salary demands, 77 percent checked 3 or below on the general measure of satisfaction with salary. Of the 66 who had the lowest salary demands, 67 percent checked 4 or above. Furthermore, when asked about a salary increase, of the 11 who had opposed a salary increase, all checked 4 and above. This suggests that salary satisfaction and salary demands are intimately related only for a small portion of the population studied. General satisfaction could not be used to predict with great precision how a person within the $100 category (where most fell) would rate his or her salary, since 53 percent checked 3 or below, and 48 percent checked 4 and above.

Kralewski (1969) suggested that nurses saw

Table 5-2 General Satisfaction with Salary by Salary Demands

General satisfaction with salary	Salary demands		
	$0–$80 (N = 66)	$100 (N = 313)	$101–$250 (N = 34)
	Percent	Percent	Percent
Very low			
1	6	17	24
2	8	17	26
3	20	19	27
4	23	27	15
5	26	14	6
6	18	7	3
Very high		Gamma: +.37	

bargaining as something quite apart from themselves and their work. If this is the case, the findings in this study and Kralewski's can be used in support of the following alternative explanation.

Bargaining may originally emerge out of conditions that create discontent with salary. However, once bargaining is institutionalized and contracts are routinely renegotiated, the expectation of increase in salary and other benefits is present even in the absence of dissatisfaction. These expectations are perhaps also fostered by the bargaining representatives such as union heads and representatives who bargain for professional organizations. For such representatives, bargaining is a base of power and may become an end in itself. In other words once established, bargaining has a life of its own, no longer requiring the preconditions necessary for its establishment. It is also important to consider that for employed professionals, and maybe nonprofessionals, when the opportunity for upward mobility is limited, the increase in salary becomes an alternative way of recognizing merit, particularly in the absence of promotion. In large organizations, there is only room for so many at the top, and this means that large numbers will depend upon institutional bargaining situations to obtain the salary increase that is interpreted as recognition of merit.

It is interesting to note that job dissatisfaction was unrelated to demands for increased control over who provides what type of patient care. The increased control issue was not a conventional issue. Perhaps, even though it was perceived as a desirable goal, it was not distressing enough to be considered detrimental to the types of services the nurses were providing, and therefore was not reflected in job dissatisfaction.

As can be seen from Tables 5-3 and 5-4, with the introduction of control variables reflecting society or family statuses, the relationships among the original variables altered considerably. Being single affected only the relationship between relative deprivation and salary demands, changing it from .21 to .40, and the relationship between job dissatisfaction and salary demands (for the latter the change is in the opposite direction from the prediction). The original zero-order relationship between job dissatisfaction and salary demands, which was +.005, became −.31. Being married introduced little change, but being separated,

widowed, and divorced affected the strength of the relationship for all but two of the eight hypotheses. Perhaps this group is more vulnerable and therefore more responsive to conditions in the environment. While it is true that single people are increasingly heads of homes, the probability of dependents for this group is not as great as it is for the separated, widowed, or divorced. The number of children made a difference depending upon the hypothesis. However, having four children consistently made a difference regardless of which hypothesis was under consideration.

The introduction of the SES of the spouse as a variable had differential effects depending upon the hypothesis. Working-class status and lower-class status had more pervasive effects than any of the others. The pattern is so variable that a synthesizing formulation is not apparent.

Control variables reflecting organizational employment plus age had little impact upon the original relationships. (See Tables 5-5 and 5-6.) As a person moves up in the hierarchy of positions, it

Table 5-3 Zero-Order Relationship as Measured by Gamma of Deprivation and Dissatisfaction Hypotheses by Partial Relationships of Family Variables: Marital Status, Number of Children, and Husband's SES

	Relative deprivation and salary demands	Relative deprivation protest for salary	Global job dissatisfaction and salary demands	Activity job dissatisfaction and salary demands	Global job dissatisfaction and increase control	Activity job dissatisfaction and increase control
Original relationships	+.21	+.08	+.09	+.005	−.02	−.04
Marital status						
Single	+.40	−.009	+.07	−.31	+.18	+.19
Married	+.07	+.08	+.08	+.17	−.12	−.17
S.W.D.	+.27	+.36	−.25	+.37	−.14	−.01
Number of children						
0	−.12	+.10	+.19	+.02	+.48	−.79
1	+.43	+.51	+.06	−.04	−.38	−.10
2–3	−.13	−.11	+.46	+.27	+.44	+.19
4+	+.36	+.20	−1.00	+.51	−.27	+.02
Husband's SES						
Upper	+.29	+.08	−.22	−.06	−.70	−.22
Upper-middle	+.24	−.14	+.41	+.35	+.55	+.06
Middle	+.15	+.30	−.15	−.25	−.08	−.44
Worker	−.67	+.15	+.63	+.67	−.33	+.39
Lower	−.67	−.50	−.33	—	−1.00	—

Table 5-4 Zero-Order Relationships as Measured by Gamma of Knowledge and Reference Group Support Hypotheses by Partial Relationships of Family Variables: Marital Status, Number of Children, and Husband's SES

	Knowledge and deprivation	Knowledge and protest for salary	Reference groups and protest for salary	Reference groups and protest for control
Original relationships	+.23	+.15	+.001	−.001
Marital status				
Single	+.14	+.12	−.07	+.02
Married	+.15	+.12	−.005	+.04
S.W.D.	+.74	+.21	+.14	−.20
Number of children				
0	+.20	+.13	−.38	+.37
1	+.31	+.18	−.05	−.14
2–3	+.27	+.05	+.18	−.33
4+	+.25	+.25	+.34	+.28
Husband's SES				
Upper	−.13	+.05	+.11	+.20
Upper-middle	+.48	+.39	+.00	+.14
Middle	−.03	+.001	+.12	−.11
Working	+.42	+.36	−.16	−.11
Lower	+.60	−.80	−.27	−.23

Table 5-5 Zero-Order Relationship as Measured by Gamma of Deprivation and Dissatisfaction Hypotheses by Partial Relationships of Organizational Variables: Position, Employment, Education, and Age

	Relative deprivation and salary demands	Relative deprivation protest for salary	Global job dissatisfaction and salary demands	Activity job dissatisfaction and salary demands	Global job dissatisfaction and increase control	Activity job dissatisfaction and increase control
Original relationships	+.21	+.08	+.09	+.005	−.02	−.04
Position:						
Staff	+.17	−.04	+.08	−.02	+.03	−.03
Assistant and head	+.44	+.56	−.01	+.17	−.15	−.23
Supervisor	+.32	−.17	+.50	−.43	−.44	+.44
Employment						
Part-time	+.01	+.06	+.10	+.11	+.30	+.11
Full-time	+.30	+.09	+.10	−.06	−.19	−.10
Education						
2–3 years	+.01	−.02	+.24	+.04	−.04	−.35
3 years+ B.A.	+1.0	+.58	−.33	−.06	−.32	−.07
B.A.+	+.47	+.06	−.10	−.07	+.21	+.55
Age						
20–25	+.25	−.18	+.17	+.25	+.005	−.19
26–35	+.29	−.17	.00	−.24	+.19	+.24
36–50	+.42	+.42	+.31	−.02	+.06	−.07
51+	−.00	+.40	−.27	−.09	−.26	−.17

Table 5-6 Zero-Order Relationships as Measured by Gamma of Knowledge and Reference Group Support Hypotheses by Partial Relationships of Organizational Variables: Position, Employment, Education, and Age

	Increased knowledge and relative deprivation	Knowledge and protest activities for salary	Reference groups and protest activities for salary	Reference groups and protest activities for control
Original relationships	+.23	+.15	+.001	−.001
Position				
Staff nurse	+.21	+.19	−.01	−.01
Assistant and				
head nurse	+.20	+.13	−.19	−.14
Supervisor	+.50	−.22	+.10	−.06
Employment				
Part-time	+.08	+.18	+.15	+.21
Full-time	+.27	+.12	−.11	−.10
Education:				
2–3 years	+.21	+.20	−.02	−.08
3 years+ B.A.	+.29	+.25	+.14	+.40
B.A.+	+.22	−.06	+.04	+.11
Age				
20–25	−.07	+.23	−.22	+.28
26–35	+.17	+.15	+.18	−.13
36–50	+.16	+.13	+.14	+.07
51+	+.61	+.12	−.10	−.13

appears that he or she is increasingly affected by conditions of work. It is possible that movement up the organizational ladder represents a greater career commitment on the part of the individual, who is also apt to be more highly educated and older. The type and amount of education made a difference. The other statuses had differential effect depending upon the specific hypothesis.

Concerning issue legitimation, the last hypothesis was that there would be higher agreement on legitimation for the patient control issue than for the salary issue. As can be seen from Table 5-7 the difference is always 30 percent or greater, supporting the suggestion that the issue influences the type of legitimation that will be utilized. The salary issue, since it can be defined either way with greater facility (as a professional or blue-collar concern), receives both types of endorsements, whereas the patient control issue is defined as strictly professional.

It is apparent that some of the accepted explanatory variables, which are an integral part of the literature, such as relative deprivation, job dissatisfaction, salary, knowledge, and reference group support have little explanatory power concerning the issues of salary demands and increased control over who gives what type of care. It may be that nurses as an occupational group are different, and therefore some of our "pet" variables do not explain the behavior. However, to the degree that the findings of this study may not be unique to nursing and to the degree that this is a test of many assumptions in the literature, there is a need to further explore, both conceptually and empirically, the reasons for protest behavior in organizationally employed professionals. Further, it is apparent, that the individual's status external to the organization needs to be considered if the behavior of people in the work situation is to be understood.

Table 5-7   Ranked Percentage Representation of Endorsement of Protest Activity in Support of Salary Issue by Percent of Single, Married, Separated, Widowed, and Divorced Registered Nurses Willing to Engage in Presented Activity

Activity	Rank	Percentage (N = 458)	Married status		
			Single (N = 155)	Married (N = 249)	Divorced (N = 54)
Attend meetings	1	73.58	80.65	71.49	62.96
Resign	2	70.74	72.26	73.09*	55.56
Attend meetings and vote	3	63.76	71.61	60.64	55.56
Discuss with colleagues	4	63.32	75.48	59.04	48.15
Attend meetings and voice opinion	5	60.70	62.58	59.44	61.33†
Group letter to administration	6	50.66	58.71	47.39	42.59
Talk to hospital administration	7	37.77	49.03	32.13	31.48
Provide patient care in the event of a strike	8	31.44	31.61	28.51	44.24‡
Letter to journal or newspaper, etc.	9	25.11	30.97	21.29	25.93†
Enlist support of physicians	10	22.93	34.19	18.07	12.96
Be less accommodative	11	19.43	29.68	14.06	14.81
Call in absent	12	17.69	15.48	20.80*	9.26
Strike	13	10.92	11.61	12.05*	3.70
Complain to physicians	14	6.77	12.26	4.42	1.85
Change to another area of nursing	15	4.80	4.52	5.22*	3.70
Resign and go to another hospital	16	4.59	9.68	2.01	1.85
Complain to patient	17	4.37	9.03	2.01	1.85
Keep to self and say nothing	18	1.53	.65	1.20	5.56‡

*Endorsement by married exceeds endorsement by single.
†Endorsement by divorced exceeds endorsement by married.
‡Endorsement by divorced exceeds endorsement by married and single.

BIBLIOGRAPHY

Anderson, Theodore A., and Morris Zelditch, Jr.: *A Basic Course in Statistics with Sociological Applications*, Holt, Rinehart and Winston, New York, 1968.

Barber, Bernard: "Some Problems in the Sociology of the Professions," in Kenneth S. Lynn et al. (eds.), *The Professions in America*, Houghton Mifflin, Boston, 1965.

Barth, E. T., and Stuart D. Johnson: "Community Power and a Typology of Social Issues," *Social Forces*, 38:29–32, October 1959.

Barton, Allen H.: *Organizational Measurement and Its Bearing on the Study of College Environment*, College Entrance Examination Board, Princeton, 1961.

Becker, Howard S.: "The Teacher in the Authority System of the Public Schools," *Human Relations*, 2:225–274, August 1958.

Ben-David, Joseph: "The Professional Role of the Physician in Bureaucratized Medicine: A Study of Role Conflict," *Human Relations*, 2:225–271, August 1958.

Benne, Kenneth D., and Warren Bennis: "Role Confusion and Conflict in Nursing: The Role of the Hospital Nurse," *American Journal of Nursing*, 59:196–198, February 1959.

Bennis, W. G., N. Berkowitz, M. Affinito, and M. Malone: "Reference Groups and Loyalties in the Out-Patient Department," *Administrative Service Quarterly*, 2(9):481–500, March 1959.

Bidwell, Charles E., and R. S. Vreeland: "Authority and Control in Client-Serving Organizations," *Sociological Quarterly*, 4:231–242, 1963.

Blau, Peter M.: *Exchange and Power in Social Life*, John Wiley, New York, 1964.

Blaunder, Robert: *Alienation and Freedom*, The University of Chicago Press, Chicago, 1964.

Blumer, Herbert: *Principles of Sociology*, 2d ed., Barnes and Noble, New York, 1951.

Caplow, Theodore: *The Sociology of Work*, University of Minnesota Press, Minneapolis, 1954.

Corwin, Ronald G.: "The Professional Employee: A Study of Conflict in Nursing Roles," *The American Journal of Sociology*, **66**:604–615, May 1961.

Costner, Herbert L.: "Criteria for Measures of Association," *American Sociological Review*, **30**:341–353, June 1965.

Devereux, George, and F. R. Weiner: "The Occupational Status of Nurses," *American Sociological Review*, **15**(5):628–634, October 1950.

Dubin, Robert: "A Theory of Conflict and Power in Union Management Relations," *Industrial and Labor Relations Review*, **13**:304–518, July 1960.

———: "Industrial Conflict: The Power of Prediction," *Industrial and Labor Relations Review*, **18**(3):352–363, April 1965.

Freidson, Eliot, and Rhea Buford: "Knowledge and Judgment in Professional Evaluations," *Administrative Science Quarterly*, **10**:107–124, June 1965.

Friedman, George: *The Anatomy of Work*, The Free Press, Glencoe, Ill., 1961.

Georgopoulos, Basil S., and Floyd C. Mann: *The Community General Hospital*, Macmillan, New York, 1962.

Goldhammer, Herbert, and E. A. Shils: "Types of Power and Status," *The American Journal of Sociology*, **45**:171–182, September 1939.

Goodman, Leo G., and William H. Kruskall: "Measures of Association for Cross Classification, III: Approximate Sampling Theory," *Journal of American Statistical Association* **58**:310–364, June 1963.

Gouldner, Alvin W.: "Cosmopolitans and Locals," *Administrative Science Quarterly*, **2**:281–306, December 1957; **2**:444–480, March 1958.

Graen, George B., R. U. Dawis, and D. J. Weiss: "Need, Type, and Job Satisfaction Among Industrial Research Scientists," *Journal of Applied Psychology*, **52**:4, 1968.

Gross, Edward: "Industrial Relations," in Robert E. L. Faris (ed.), *Handbook of Modern Sociology*, Rand-McNally, Chicago, 1964.

———: "Sociological Aspects of Professional Salaries in Education," *The Educational Record*, **41**:904–913, April 1960.

———: *Work and Society*, Thomas Y. Crowell, New York, 1958.

Habenstein, Robert W., and Edwin A. Christ: *Professionalizer, Traditionalizer and Utilizer*, University of Missouri, Columbia, 1963.

Harbison, Frederick H., and John R. Coleman: *Goals and Strategy in Collective Bargaining*, Harper Brothers, New York, 1951.

Heer, David M.: "Dominance and the Working Wife," in F. Evan Nye and Lois M. Hoffman (eds.), *The Employed Mother in America*, Rand-McNally, Chicago, 1963, pp. 251–262.

Homans, George C.: *Social Behavior: Its Elementary Form*, Harcourt Brace, and World, New York, 1961.

Katz, Fred E.: "Nurses," chapter 2 in Amitai Etzioni (ed.), *The Semi-Professions and Their Organization: Teachers, Nurses, Social Workers*, The Free Press, Glencoe, Ill., 1969, pp. 54–81.

Katzell, Raymond A.: "Personal Values, Job Satisfaction, and Job Behavior," in Henry Borow (ed.), *Man in a World of Work*, Houghton Mifflin, Boston, 1964, pp. 341–361.

Kemper, Thomas: "Third Party Penetration of Social Systems," *Sociometry*, **31**:1–27, March 1968.

Kerr, Clark, and Lloyd H. Fisher: "Multiple-Employer Bargaining: The San Francisco Experience," in Richard A. Lester and Joseph Shister (eds.), *Insights into Labor Issues*, Macmillan, New York, 1949, pp. 25–61.

Kornhauser, William: *Scientists in Industry: Conflict and Accommodation*, University of California Press, Berkeley, 1962.

Kralewski, John Edward: "The Professional Nurse in the Hospital Organization: A Study of Conflict Resolution," unpublished doctoral dissertation, University of Minnesota, August 1969.

Larsen, Donald E.: "A Study of Consensus on the

Role of the Psychiatric Nurse," Dissertation Abstracts, *Humanities and Social Sciences*, **38**: 10, April 1968.

Leonard, Robert C.: "The Impact of Social Trends on the Professionalization of Patient Care," in Jeanette R. Folta and Edith S. Beck (eds.), *A Sociological Framework for Patient Care*, John Wiley, New York, 1977, pp. 71–82.

March, James G.: "Political Issues and Husband Wife Interaction," in F. Evan Nye and Lois M. Hoffman (eds.), *The Employed Mother in America*, Rand-McNally, Chicago, 1963, pp. 201-207.

Merton, Robert K.: *Social Theory and Social Structure*, The Free Press, Glencoe, Ill., 1957.

Miller, George A.: "Professional in Bureaucracy: Role Orientations and Alienation Among Industrial Scientists and Engineers," unpublished Ph.D. dissertation, University of Washington, Seattle, 1966.

Moore, Wilbert E.: *The Professions: Roles and Rules*, Russell Sage Foundation, New York, 1970.

Morse, Nancy C.: *Satisfactions in the White-Collar Job*, University of Michigan, Survey Research Center, Ann Arbor, 1953.

Muskow, Michael H.: *Teachers and Unions*, University of Pennsylvania, Philadelphia, 1966.

National Manpower Council: *Work in the Lives of Married Women: Proceedings of a Conference on Women Power*, Columbia University Press, New York, 1958. (Conference held October 20-25.)

Palola, Ernest G., and William R. Larson: "Some Dimensions of Job Satisfaction Among Hospital Personnel," *Sociology and Social Research*, **49**: 203-213, January 1965.

Pavalko, Ronald M. (ed.): *Sociological Perspectives on Occupations*, F. E. Peacock Publishers, Itasca, Ill., 1972.

Pearlin, Leonard I.: "Alienation from Work: A Study of Nursing Personnel," *American Sociological Review*, **27**:314-326, June 1962.

Pearsall, Marion: *Medical Behavioral Science: A Selected Bibliography of Cultural Anthropology, Social Psychology, and Sociology in Medicine*, University of Kentucky Press, Lexington, 1963.

Perrucci, Robert, and Joel E. Gerstl: *The Engineers and the Social System,* John Wiley, New York, 1969.

Schneider, B. V. H.: "Collective Bargaining and the Federal Civil Service," *Industrial Relations*, 3(3):94-120, May 1964.

Secord, Paul F., and Carl W. Backman: *Social Psychology*, McGraw-Hill, New York, 1964.

Sheppard, Harold L.: "Approaches to Conflict in American Industrial Sociology," *The British Journal of Sociology*, **5**:324-341, December 1954.

Smith, Kathryn M.: "Discrepancies in the Role-Specific Values of Head Nurses and Nursing Educators," *Nursing Research*, **14**:196-202, Summer 1965.

Stagner, Ross, and H. J. Almar Rosen: *Psychology of Union-Management Relations*, Wadsworth Publishing, Belmont, Calif., 1965.

Strauss, Anselm, and Lee Rainwater: *The Professional Scientist: A Study of American Chemists,* Adline Publishing, Chicago, 1962.

Tannenbaum, Arnold S.: *Social Psychology of the Work Organization,* Behavioral Science in Industrial Series, Wadsworth Publishing, Belmont, Calif., 1966.

Taylor, Kenneth E., and D. J. Weiss: "Prediction of Individual Job Termination from Measured Job Satisfaction and Biographical Data," Research Report No. 30 Work Adjustment Project, University of Minnesota, Minneapolis, 1969.

Turner, Roland H.: "Role-Taking, Role-Standpoint, and Reference Group Behavior," *American Journal of Sociology*, **61**:316-328, 1956; rpt. in Bruce J. Biddle and Edwin J. Thomas (eds.), *Role Theory: Concepts and Research*, John Wiley, New York, 1966, pp. 151-159.

Vollmer, Howard M., and Donald L. Mills (eds.): *Professionalization*, Prentice-Hall, Englewood Cliffs, N.J., 1966.

Wilensky, Harold L.: "The Professionalization of Everyone?" *American Journal of Sociology*, **70**(2):137-158, September 1964.

Yett, Donald E.: "The Supply of Nurses: An Economist's View," *Hospital Progress*, **46**: 88-92, 94, 96-99, 102, February 1965.

EDITOR'S QUESTIONS FOR DISCUSSION

What explanations can you offer for the finding that salary satisfaction and salary demands were unrelated for most people in this study? What other variables might more adequately explain protest behavior? What relationship might exist between the professional's status external to the organization and the type of protest behavior he or she considers acceptable? Given the expected normative behavior of a professional (learned by nurses through the socialization process of their educational programs), what might a professional consider before engaging in any type of protest behavior? What are the implications for nursing as a profession in the finding that job dissatisfaction was unrelated to control over who provides what type of patient care? Do the findings relating marital status to the deprivation and dissatisfaction hypotheses offer suggestions about the type of professional commitment the respondents might have?

Chapter 6

Feminism and the Nursing Profession

Rosalee C. Yeaworth, R.N., Ph.D.
Assistant Dean, Graduate Programs in Nursing; Associate Professor of Nursing
College of Nursing and Health, University of Cincinnati, Ohio

Yeaworth's article focuses on the unique problem of a profession in which the majority of individuals are women. The problem is compounded by the fact that these women do not perceive this as a problem. Yeaworth specifies several factors that seem to limit nursing to an occupation and impede its progress toward becoming a profession. These include the traditional socialization process of women and the image of the nurse as nurturing, feminine, and self-sacrificing; the attitude of many nurses that nursing is a "job," often to supplement family income, rather than a career; the lack of recognition for the many independent, decision-making functions nurses have traditionally performed; nursing education programs that are not in accredited, degree-granting colleges or universities; the lack of sufficient research and theory-building skills among nurses; and nursing's lack of representation in administrative positions for planning of health care education and services.

Yeaworth relates the problem areas in nursing to the overall problem areas of women in our society. Besides suggesting means of supporting one another and of helping to validate the competency of nurses, she proposes that one solution would be for nurses to develop power by uniting within their professional organizations.

Since Florence Nightingale's efforts to establish modern nursing as a profession for women like law and medicine were for men, nursing has persisted as a woman's occupation. Elementary education and social work, the other so-called occupational ghettoes for women, now have increasing percentages of males in their ranks, but 98 percent of all nurses are women. Thus, we cannot speak of roles and statuses of nurses without realizing that they are a reflection of the roles and statuses of women. The most fundamental problems in nursing are: (1) that it is a woman's occupation, and (2) that the majority of nurses, like the larger society, do not perceive this as a problem at all. Usually efforts to solve a problem that is not perceived by most people as a problem are not only frustrating and ineffective, but are also likely to cause the would-be problem solvers to be viewed as a bit strange or even humorous.

WOMEN IN AMERICAN SOCIETY

Women in the United States may be educated for occupations or even for careers, but they are still effectively socialized to be wives and mothers despite the fact that improved household technology and reduced family size may mean that the wife-mother role fills only a small portion of a woman's life. There are very strong norms that stereotype certain household and childrearing chores as "women's work," and imply that the working wife and mother is neglecting her rightful duties and denying her femininity. These norms serve to force the working woman to add work responsibilities to homemaking and childrearing chores since she has no "wife" to do them.

The above comment about women lacking wives may sound like a joke, but only to those who have not stopped to analyze the supportive, socioemotional role placed by the wives of many successful career men. If an individual is interested in a career and advancement into management positions, there are typically reports, budgets, or manuscripts that get prepared at home after the usual working day. Wives serve as gatekeepers, protecting their husbands from the interruptions of children, telephone calls, and other demands. Often wives also serve as idea people, editors, and typists. A lack of this kind of support can prevent the accomplishment—or even the undertaking—of tasks that are necessary for career mobility.

Internal Factors

The socialization process develops self-image in regard to what it means to be male or female. From infancy both little boys and little girls learn that females are to be nurturing, empathizing, non-competitive responders who meet others' needs, while males are aggressive, competitive, analytic decision makers who initiate ideas, take risks, and lead others. Males are socialized for achievement, females for affiliation. Men gain status, power, and high salaries by moving up in an organization to occupy administrative positions and by being elected into high political offices. Women gain status and power by aligning themselves with and pleasing the right man, giving him support and ideas so that he can maintain his high-status position or advance even further.

If women aren't discouraged from undertaking

to gain high-power–high-status positions by attitudes, beliefs, indeed by the very identity that they've assumed during their socialization as women in our society, then they have to deal with the interpersonal influence of the expectations held and rewards given by both male and female associates. For example, women often are denied the informal signs of belonging and recognition once they do manage to get to higher-level positions. Some of the ways this is done include: failing to use titles in introductions (Ms. or Mrs. instead of Dr.); referring to the woman as "our attractive member" or the "representative of the fairer sex"; or having men greet her with a kiss when she walks into a formal meeting. Telephone operators make a thing of converting Dr. back to Ms. when it is attached to a woman's name or of assuming that the woman making the call must be the doctor's secretary or receptionist. These are all little things that, if they are mentioned, make the person calling attention to them sound like a status seeker; but day after day, they take a psychological toll and give women the silent message that regardless of their accomplishments or positions they don't quite measure up to the males, even the less accomplished ones.

External Arrangements

Society doesn't trust everything to these strong blocks that women build up within themselves or to the influence of other people. Social institutions and organizations seem to be carefully arranged to provide obstacles to women's efforts to reach higher-level positions. These arrangements include discrimination in educational opportunities and in hiring and promotion, nepotism, full-time work requirements, and the lack of child care facilities and maternity-paternity leaves. Affirmative action has helped to get women into organizations, but relationships and opportunities are structured to minimize their influence once they are part of an organization. A woman does not usually get on important committees and boards—the important policy-making bodies—or if she does, she is the token woman who would need to be something of a miracle worker to have real impact.

We have a society that provides access to status in the community and financial rewards through work. Self-worth becomes closely associated with the status and salary resulting from that work, and the definition of work does not include family and domestic roles or community volunteer roles; it includes only the occupational and career roles. Statistics may show that one-third of the labor force is made up of women, that 97 percent of all women spend some part of their life in marriage, and that families in which both husband and wife work are in the majority; but the norm persists that a "real man" should support his wife and family in such a fashion that the wife does not have to work. Our public laws and policies are set up to deal with families in which there is a head of the household, who is the breadwinner, and a dependent spouse. Generally, other cases are seen as deviations from the norm.

The tax structure effectively deprives the working wife of much of the reward for her labor. Some states require that persons who file their federal income taxes jointly at the federal level in order to take advantage of a lower rate must also file jointly at the state level. The state tax, with increasing percentages for higher incomes, makes little allowance for the fact that two incomes with accompanying expenses are involved in the joint husband-wife income. Allowances for money paid for homemaking help have been slow in coming and are now only allowed on federal taxes to women who have children under the age of 15 or a disabled individual living in the home. Thus, the message once again is that working women should be able to manage their own homemaking if they don't have young dependents, even though more liberal tax deductions might result in more jobs. Cleland (1970) showed how taxes and work-related expenses could reduce a salary of $12,000 to an actual increment of $4,787 in family income.*

*These figures were for Detroit, Michigan, in 1970.

WOMEN IN NURSING

The Nursing Image

Nursing has provided an occupation for large numbers of women and a career for a few. At the same time, nursing has been effective in maintaining the status quo and in remaining a predominantly female occupation. One of the first factors that accounts for this is the maintenance of the image of the nurse as the nurturing, feminine, self-sacrificing person who meets the needs of others. This image does not conflict with the feminine, wife-mother image. In fact, the very title of the occupation is enough to prevent many men from ever considering it as a serious career choice.

Nursing as a Job

Nursing includes a wide range of services that are usually available on a part- or full-time basis with rotating shifts, and that, until very recently, were much in demand. Nurses who were wives and mothers could usually find some kind of work that fit family schedules. They were often working to supplement family income, to keep their knowledge and skills as a contingency plan for emergencies, or as a diversionary interest. For some women, nursing filled the spot that hobbies, volunteer work, or bridge filled for others. These nurses usually did not have to be that concerned about the salary; for them nursing was an occupation not a career. Two-worker families or one-worker–one-career families are much less stressful than two-career families. If the demands of the work interfered with the wife-mother role, nurses could quit and retreat to the domestic, family role or find a less conflicting job. This has been a very positive and valuable feature of nursing for many women, but it has also forestalled their securing a wage commensurate with the preparation required and the work performed. It has weakened the bargaining power of career-oriented nurses.

The Nurse-Physician Relationship

Physicians have been granted very high status in our society. This status has been based on the importance of the physician's role in treating ill persons and facilitating their recovery and on the scientific knowledge and expertise gained through the medical education process. This status is functional in promoting compliance with physicians' orders, but it often prevents nurses from questioning orders or refusing to carry out an unsafe order (Hofling et al., 1966). The hospital social structure fosters a status schism between physicians and nurses (Seeman and Evans, 1962). This imbalance of power causes nurses to look to physicians for the validation of their self-worth and to emulate the physician's activities and knowledge. A recent advertisement for the Nurse's Book Society listed nineteen books, only three of which appeared to have been written by nurses. The list included such titles as *Primer of Clinical Radiology, The Principles and Practice of Medicine*, and *Functional Anatomy of the Newborn/Nonoperative Aspects of Pediatric Surgery*. The advent of the physician's assistant and ensuing pressure on nurses to accept orders from them as well as the expanding role of the nurse have further stimulated the emulation of physicians.

The innumerable, independent, decision-making functions of nurses have been carefully secreted. The physician is responsible for making the diagnosis and ordering medical treatment. The nurse may be the one who gathers the information or observes the symptoms that confirm the diagnosis, or she may even be the one who suggests the diagnosis, but this is not formally recognized. The nurse may suggest that a specific medication or treatment be tried, that an order calls for an incorrect amount of a drug, or that a treatment or medication be discontinued because of adverse reactions. She may even write the prescription over the physician's signature on the prescription blank. But legally the nurse only suggests; the physician alone prescribes. If the nurse wishes to carry out clinical research to find out whether one nursing procedure or approach is more effective than the other, she must ask the physician's permission, or at least inform him of her plan; and giving that information carries with it the under-

standing that if the physician does not consent, nothing can be done. If nursing care is required by a noninstitutionalized person, the nurse cannot provide it and bill for third-party payment. The physician can hire the nurse, pay her a salary, and bill for the services she gives to patients, but the nurse's license to operate as an independent practitioner in the health care system is hampered by society's formal norms.

Nursing's Educational Patterns

Nursing's educational patterns have severely hindered efforts to professionalize. Until all nursing education takes place in accredited, degree-granting colleges or universities, nurses will have the problem of being blocked from upward educational mobility. College courses taken in accredited colleges for credit hours have the legitimacy of being taught by qualified faculty and of having proper course content, evaluation, etc. Such courses also have the potential of being negotiable for a higher degree in nursing, for transfer to another discipline with a change of career plans, or for being seen as legitimate even after some time lag. Nurses themselves have created some of the biggest blocks to moving nursing education into colleges and universities. As diploma programs across the nation are beginning to phase out (primarily because of economic and social pressures), nursing educators are busy doing the same thing at a different level—creating nurse practitioner programs in which nurses may spend as much as a year or even two of study to earn, not a Master's degree, but a certificate.

For the nursing programs and faculty who make it to the university setting, there are specific problems. Many of nursing's best-educated persons are faculty members in university settings, but they are torn between the people-oriented values of nursing and the creativity-oriented values of research and publication. Promotions, memberships on university graduate faculties, and other opportunities for influence and recognition are closely tied to research and publication. Howe

(1975) states that overcommitment is a significant aspect of the lives of academic women. This is especially true of members of nursing faculties, who are caught between the demands of clinical courses with low credit-hour ratio for faculty time involvement and the need to keep their own clinical skills and judgments current, and who, in addition, are pressured by the usual classroom teaching expectations. Grants are the lifeblood of nursing's graduate education, but the time spent writing grant proposals and grant reports cuts heavily into time that could be spent in research and writing.

There is now a tightening of regulations concerning credentials at universities as budgets shrink and enrollments decrease. The latest HEW figures indicate that women are losing ground in universities at the higher rank and salary levels (National Center for Education Statistics, 1976). Barriers to women's admission to graduate schools have been lowered at a time when financial support to students is decreasing.

More nurses must gain the research and theory-building skills normally acquired in graduate education if nursing is to make greater progress toward professionalization. In defining professions, a major criterion has been the possession of a systematic body of theory (Vollmer and Mills, 1966). There is a pool of "pure" theory about humankind, with areas claimed by sociology, psychology, anthropology, medicine, and physiology; but these areas are also necessary to formulating a theory of nursing, of giving care, of promoting wellness, and of preventing illness. Nurses in specific leadership positions need theory from administration and education. Nurses need to draw from this pool of knowledge claimed by many disciplines and apply, test, and refine it to build nursing theory. Until adequate numbers of nurses are prepared at the doctoral level, doctoral programs in nursing will remain few in number. Sociologists, psychologists, and physiologists are much more comfortable with the idea of providing members of their discipline to do the research for nursing than with the idea of providing doc- toral preparation for nurses who then return to nursing to apply their knowledge.

Nursing's Lack of High-Status Positions

Changes in our system for delivering human services have resulted in more administrative positions and more upper-level positions in planning and research. This has attracted more men into the traditionally female occupations of social work and elementary school teaching, and men rise quickly to the upper-level positions. Nursing has been kept embedded in the administrative hierarchy of bureaucratic organizations, so that the top-level management positions have traditionally not been held by nurses, but by males with business and management training. The majority of nursing service directors do not control their own budgets (Cleland, 1971). Even collegiate schools of nursing are frequently set up administratively under colleges of medicine or education, rather than as autonomous colleges. The pattern is holding: males who enter nursing usually rise quite rapidly to the existing upper-level positions.

Blaming the Victim*

Nurses have been admonished for contributing to their own oppression and inhibiting nursing from achieving the status of a profession (Stein, 1972). Much energy and time has been wasted through intradisciplinary battles between nursing service and nursing education and over types of educational programs and levels of entry into practice. Nurses invalidate other nurses by bringing in "experts" from other disciplines to tell nurses how to do things that are already being done by nursing "experts." This blaming, self-flagellation, and infighting must be recognized by nurses as deriving from the more general social problems of women. And, like women generally, nurses must understand that they alone are not to blame for these problems.

*William Ryan, *Blaming the Victim*, Random House, New York, 1971.

APPROACHES TO SOLUTIONS

The Women's Movement has resulted in a general consciousness-raising and some budding feelings of sisterhood, but it will take carefully organized strategy to create real change. Cleland (1974, p. 563) has proposed that we "agitate, educate, legislate and negotiate." An example of agitation for changes in legislation is the complaint filed by the American Nurses Association in opposition to the practice of the Teachers Insurance Annuity Association paying retired female teachers less per month than male teachers with equal units of investment. Divisions of Women's Studies are offering college courses that can do much to educate some, and collective bargaining is proving to be a negotiating tool in academic and hospital settings.

Howe (1975) contends that the most talented women should not be encouraged to enter physics or law to spread a thin token population of women into the nontraditional areas, but that women's power should be developed in those areas where women are the most numerous. She suggests that by developing their power in nursing, social work, and teaching, women can change three of the most important service institutions in society. School teachers can play an especially important role through socialization of the young. Nurses and social workers can create change through their daily contacts with clients.

The School of Social Development at the Univeristy of Minnesota (Duluth) has developed a special training program for its students (Hooyman and Kaplan, 1976). The initial training focuses on the individual's values, goals, and attitudes. Using experiential tasks called "Life-script," "Life Line," "Internal Dialogue," "Life Planning," and "Skill Assessment," the school has helped women deal with issues of personal growth. Interpersonal skills that foster effective working relationships with both men and women are developed through such techniques as assertion training, values clarification, and the use of case situations to increase problem-solving and decision-making skills. Skills in conflict resolution, organization of others, and group leadership are taught through simulations and role playing.

Nursing is being threatened by institutional licensure and being squeezed by the paraprofessionals. Only by uniting behind their professional organization and presenting a united front can nurses move nursing toward greater professionalization and power. If this cannot be done, the talented, career-oriented women will be drawn to other professions with higher status and higher salaries.

Nurses and women in general need to be more active politically. Nurses who achieve position and status need to advise and groom other nurses. Nurses who are in lower-level positions need to give support to nurse leaders and help to validate other nurses' competencies. Nursing educational programs should teach nurses to write resumés or curriculum vitaes that present their education and experiences in the best light and to negotiate contracts, not just for salaries, but for fringe benefits and, even more important, for active participation in the decision-making process.

SUMMARY

Most of the identified problem areas in nursing reflect the problem areas of women in general. The first step in solving the problems lies in recognizing them as the wider social problems they are. Nurses have the power of numbers in health care organizations. Nursing educational programs and professional nursing organizations can be powerful forces for change. To create change will take energy. It will take a psychological toll; but in the process not only will nursing improve and women make gains, but health care will improve and men will make gains. Greater humanization and recognition of others as individuals will, in the long run, take from no one and benefit all.

BIBLIOGRAPHY

Cleland, Virginia: "Role Bargaining for Working Wives," *American Journal of Nursing*, **70**:1242–1246, June 1970.

———: "Sex Discrimination: Nursing's Most Pervasive Problem," *American Journal of Nursing*, **71**:1542–1547, August 1971.

————: "To End Sex Discrimination," *Nursing Clinics of North America,* **9**:563–571, September 1974.

Hofling, Charles K., Eveline Brotzman, Sarah Dalrymple, Nancy Groves, and Chester Pierce: "An Experimental Study in Nurse-Physician Relationships," *The Journal of Nervous and Mental Disease*, **143**(2):171–180, 1966.

Hooyman, Nancy R., and Judith S. Kaplan: "Increasing Women's Power: Skills for Change," paper delivered at the Pioneers for Century III Bicentennial Conference on Men and Women, Cincinnati, Ohio, April 1976.

Howe, Florence: *Women and the Power to Change*, McGraw-Hill, New York, 1975.

National Center for Education Statistics, Office of the Assistant Secretary for Education, Department of Health, Education and Welfare, January 1976.

Ryan, William: *Blaming the Victim*, Random House, New York, 1971.

Seeman, Melvin, and John W. Evans: "Apprenticeship and Attitude Change," *American Journal of Sociology*, **67**:376, January 1962.

Stein, Leonard I.: "Liberation Movement: Impact on Nursing," *AORN Journal*, **15**:75, April 1972.

Vollmer, Howard M., and Donald L. Mills: *Professionalization*, Prentice-Hall, Englewood Cliffs, N.J., 1966.

EDITOR'S QUESTIONS FOR DISCUSSION

What social factors inhibit women from changing their orientation toward nursing to view it as a "career" rather than a "job"? Is orientation toward nursing as a job incompatible with orientation toward nursing as a career? What obligations or responsibilities does the profession have to women who view and need nursing as a job? What obligations or responsibilities do these women have to the profession? What rights and expectations does the profession have in regard to members who are employed? What rights and expectations do members have in regard to the profession?

What effects might one anticipate from the Women's Movement in terms of a job or career orientation in nursing? Would one anticipate a decrease in values such as nurturance (as discussed in Stein's study), that would change the image of the nurse? What are the pros and cons for society, the family, the profession, the organization, and the individual for encouraging or discouraging the employment of part-time nurses?

If nurses continue to strive for professional status, what would be the ultimate advantages for nursing? Should nursing be content to be primarily an occupation? What societal functions does nursing serve as an occupation that might be threatened by increased professionalization?

Part Two

Nursing Education

Perhaps no area of nursing has evidenced so many changes as that of nursing education programs; in this regard, many questions have been raised but few answers provided. As nursing has assumed more of the attributes of a profession, the basic question has been, "How do we prepare our prospective members to be competent professionals?" Regardless of the type of program from which they graduate, nurses have been socialized to believe in their own professional competency. As a result, nurses find it difficult to accept the differences they encounter between the value of various education programs and the level of competency expected from them as graduates of such programs.

The concept of professionalism does not necessarily include a certain type of education, although occasionally this factor is implied. The challenge is not in determining who best qualifies for the label "professional" but rather in conceptualizing and defining the expected levels of competency in practice and in determining the educational requirements to prepare competent practitioners. The disparity between nursing education and nursing practice may have evolved because the primary focus has been on assumed educational needs rather than on needs determined by the actual practice setting. Thus, some students find it difficult to apply the knowledge they have acquired in the classroom and they may question the utility of applying such knowledge in actual practice situations. As more nursing faculties become models for the role of nursing practice, students may find it easier to assume role-making and role-taking responsibilities.

Chapter 7

Leaders Among Contemporary U.S. Nurses: An Oral History

Gwendolyn Safier, Ph.D., R.N.
Postdoctoral Fellow
Department of the History of Health Sciences
University of California, San Francisco

Through Gwendolyn Safier's contribution we glimpse the historical socialization process of the nurse; review commentaries on tasks, schedules, and expectations of the earliest nursing students; and view some of the historical events that were the foundation of nursing education. By means of her interviews with twelve nursing leaders we are able to reflect on the past and assess the progress nursing has made. Safier queries the nursing leaders on their perception of the current issues in nursing, nursing roles, and the future of nursing. These leaders concur that all nursing education programs should be located in college or university settings but dissent on such topics as establishing the role of the nurse practitioner and the future of nursing. Some issues cited as being relevant to nursing are: the lack of consensus as to the purpose of the profession, the tendency of nursing to react to change rather than to design change, and the rights of patients in clinical research.

Although nursing as a profession has undergone profound changes since World War II, neither the changes themselves nor the individuals instrumental in effecting them have received sufficient public recognition or scholarly attention. Many of these changes were brought about as the result of new directions taken by nursing leaders. Accordingly, this chapter is based on interviews with wartime and postwar nursing leaders selected by their professional peers as individuals who significantly altered the course of nursing in the United States. These interviews illuminate some of the principal areas of change and showcase the specific contributions of several especially notable leaders. In addition, this study aims to uncover information and perspectives heretofore largely absent from the historical record of American nursing. Finally, this study speculates on the viability of using the oral history approach for investigating neglected aspects of feminist studies.

This article is a revision of " 'I Sensed the Challenges,': Leaders Among Contemporary U.S. Nurses," *The Oral History Review*, New York, 1975, pp. 31–58; and selected parts from *Contemporary American Leaders in Nursing: An Oral History*, McGraw-Hill, New York, 1976. Permission to use the material from the above sources is acknowledged. I want to express my appreciation to Willa K. Baum, Director of the Regional Oral History Office, University of California, Berkeley, and Arthur A. Hansen, Director of the Oral History Program at California State University, Fullerton, for their help and encouragement; I am grateful to the American Nurses' Foundation for a grant award (1974) enabling me to interview identified nursing leaders throughout the United States.

METHODOLOGY

Oral history is a relatively new phenomenon in American historiography, and a brief note as to its development, purpose, and procedures will serve to put this article in perspective (Safier, 1976). *oral history* is defined as a developed technique of collecting information on recent events by interviewing knowledgeable people, recording the data on magnetic tape, and keeping it available for the use of researchers and scholars. An example of this is the oral history collection currently being done for the Nursing Archives at Boston University's Mugar Library. Another example of the scholarly use of oral history is Safier's (1975) work on nursing leaders. Her immediate objective was to document in the leaders' own words their careers and contributions since their recognized leadership had had a strong and innovative impact upon nursing. By interviewing women who were advancing in age (most were in their seventies), and thus obtaining their reflections upon their lives and their views about issues in nursing, Safier intended to improve the record available to future scholars. The oral history interviews are structured in question (interviewer) and answer (interviewee) form from pre-planned interview guides.

There has been oral history—an oral tradition—for centuries. Anthropologists, especially, have collected tales, legends, and folklore of different cultures. It was in 1948 that the term *oral history* as it is used today was used by Professor Allan Nevins, a historian at Columbia University, to refer to interviews he conducted systematically. He taped oral history interviews with people who had special knowledge, and these interviews were transcribed and then housed in the Columbia University library archives. Professor Nevins is acknowledged by oral historians to have been the pioneer in the collection of oral history with a scholarly orientation. As Benison (1967, pp. viii–ix) points out, however, oral history is misnamed; that is, the oral historian does gather oral material, but the transcript must be edited and sometimes very heavily

edited and/or revised before the final prepared transcript conveys what the subject wants it to say.

RATIONALE FOR THE USE OF ORAL HISTORY

The first and most obvious reason why oral history is available is that verbal responses can be obtained directly from living persons who have special knowledge about something. One is able to obtain information that might not be available later, especially in these modern, fast-paced times when the telephone is used a great deal and personal letters and diaries are rapidly vanishing. The material as mentioned earlier can be used to set the record straight or to improve upon the record for future scholars. An example of this is to interview a number of individuals who hold divergent views about some particular issue, and the resultant oral history materials can supplement manuscript collections already deposited in library archives. By enabling a subject to talk in his or her own words, one hopes to capture somewhat the personality and conversational style of that person. Also, one is able to probe and to elicit personal feelings, views, and thoughts about certain areas, such as the subject's backward glance at a lifelong pursuit of a career goal. One of the big advantages of oral history is that through the *process of interaction* between the interviewer and interviewee, a dialogue ensues that allows for an in-depth analysis of a reply.

LIMITATIONS OF ORAL HISTORY

There are certain limitations to the use of oral history. An obvious one is that the interviewee material may be too subjective, that is, the material may be overly biased or inconsistent. However, one can substantiate some oral materials with written documents. One also assumes that the person being interviewed will be honest. However, the person may desire that what she or he says remain confidential. In addition, there may be problems of memory recall and of some individuals being more articulate than others.

How reliable are the data? Some of the data are specific and unique to an individual, and you may have to accept on good faith that it is true. Some persons may not say what they really think or feel because they are afraid of lawsuits. Some of the oral history information may be checked later against secondary sources such as newspapers, published records, letters, or by interviewing someone else who may have been involved in the same situation. All the previous examples relate to the validity of the data.

A sample of nursing leaders was selected during the summer and fall of 1973 by the *reputational method*, a method permitting the determination by other nurses of "who is a leader and why." First, a letter outlining the project's research objectives was sent to all deans and directors of accredited nursing education programs, as well as to presidents, executive directors, and chairpersons of professional nursing organizations and national commissions, requesting their cooperation. Specifically, they were instructed to list the names of thirty living American nursing leaders presently in or near retirement, and to indicate the reasons governing their selection. Respondents were asked to be mindful of all areas of nursing, such as administration, research, education, and practice. To encourage candor, they were assured confidentiality for their choices. A strength of the reputational method was that it allowed respondents to indicate *why* they chose the individuals they did rather than imposing a strict set of criteria for their selections. A possible shortcoming of this approach was that respondents may have had a conscious or unconscious tendency to compromise their professional judgment by displaying inordinate consideration for friends.

Out of 432 letters sent, 345 were received. The thirty names most frequently cited were then compiled into an alphabetical list that was subsequently sent to 60 nurses selected at random from the original list of 432. Each respondent was asked to rank the top seventeen, a number chosen to accommodate time and funding limitations.

After the seventeen leaders were determined, the project director sent each a letter.[1] Therein she identified herself, informed them that they had been selected for a study, asked if she could meet with them to interview them in depth, and requested that they forward her a photograph and curriculum vitae to help her prepare specific interview questions.

General questions of a biographical nature were designed for all interviewees: What is your family background? What early childhood experiences were influential in your life and career? What type of education did you receive? Why did you enter nursing? How was your education financed? Did you ever desire to leave nursing and take up something else? Did you ever want to switch from nursing to medicine? What do you consider to be your unique contribution to nursing? What do you consider your failures? What obstacles, frustrations, and disappointments did you encounter? What help did you get along the way? What do you consider to be the most critical decisions you have made? What impact did these have? What social and personal conflicts did you have? How did you resolve them? What are your work habits? What is your lifestyle? What do you consider to be the biggest changes in nursing? Where do you think nursing is going? What, if anything, would you now do differently in your life if you had the opportunity? What was your first leadership position? How did you get it? Did you ever feel discriminated against? By whom? Why did you stay (or, if you left, leave)? If married, did you

[1] Before commencing any interviews, the author was required to submit fifteen copies of her entire research protocol and procedure for approval to the University of California, San Francisco, Committee of Human Subjects and Experimentation. The committee recommended that a provision be included whereby, if any subject became tired and desired to discontinue her participation in the project, she could. Upon inclusion of this provision, the research plan was approved September 12, 1973.

ever feel that your home life was neglected because of your career? If unmarried/never married, did you ever want to get married and have a family? Did you ever feel that you had to make a choice between marriage and a career?

Next a list of specific questions was prepared relative to each leader's career. These were formulated after scrutinizing the leader's curriculum vitae, doing preparatory reading about her and her activities, and engaging in informal conversations with various people who worked with or who knew her well. A list of general and specific questions was forwarded prior to the actual interview. Each interviewee was told the interviews would be taped and that interview time would run approximately one and a half to two hours in length. All were assured that interview material would be kept confidential, and that each interviewee would be sent a copy of the transcript for emendation and amplification. Should the leader desire, she could select one other person familiar with her career to read and comment upon the revised transcript. Fifteen of seventeen leaders ultimately agreed to be interviewed; one became to ill to participate, while another was out of the country and therefore unable to participate. The following are selected portions of the interviews with thirteen nursing leaders.

ORAL DOCUMENTATION

Early Days of Nursing Education

Almost all of the nursing education took place in hospital schools of nursing that were the 3-year diploma programs.

Marion Sheahan was the first Executive Director of the National Committee on the Improvement of Nursing Services and later of the Department of Nursing Services of the National League for Nursing. In her notes regarding diploma nursing education around 1913 she said:

> My class consisted of ten, all of us just from high school.

We had a very well equipped teaching class room, Susan, our doll, and all the gadgets needed. That was the era when nurses had to reduce a half grain tablet of morphine to an eighth or whatever strength was needed. On the floors the senior students mixed the solutions. We sterilized the equipment, etc. etc.

We were sent to the Teachers College in Albany, New York, for a course in nutrition for which we received some credit. . . . We had a massage instructor who came to our teaching lab to teach us massage. . . .

Our lectures outside our own teaching lab were largely from the chiefs of medical staff. Not too long ago when I broke up my parental home, I came across note books of "medical lectures." They are fine at a given period but for teaching students of my vintage they were a waste of time.

All in all I enjoyed my training. . . . We learned to really know our patients. . . .

We had the standard text books. I remember getting one assignment that prompted me to go to the State Medical Library to do some additional research.

We, as usual at that time, had to count the linen, order it, etc. We kept the unit around each bed (bedside stand, etc.) clean and I think the senior on the ward had to keep the medicine cabinet in order. At that period we did our own sterilizing of items like rectal tubes, hypos, etc. Dressings and big items were done in the autoclaves by operating room nurses. There was no central supply for packaged materials. (October 1974).

A distinguished educational nursing leader (Helen Nahm) tells about her nursing education:

> When I finished high school in Columbia, Missouri, I wanted very much to go to the University of Missouri, but I had no money. I obtained a job teaching in a country school for one year. I wasn't paid very much, but also it didn't cost very much to live either. And as I remember, I saved, in that year, two hundred dollars. That was enough to pay my tuition at the University of Missouri. . . . Tuition then was not high. . . . We paid thirty dollars a semester, and I had

money enough for books and other necessities (Safier, 1977, p. 257).

I started out in home economics with the idea I'd like to get into extension work. . . . During my freshman year, I became sick and was sent to the University hospital. I was so excited about that experience that I decided to go into nursing. . . .

I went over to see the Director of the School of Nursing, who was also director of Nursing Service. At that time, the hospital was a small university hospital. I told her I'd like to enter the School of Nursing. It was rather unusual then for girls who had had some college work to come into nursing. I was one of a class of eight to begin with, of which, five graduated three years later. I didn't get a degree. I received what was called a G.N., Graduate Nurse Degree that had been specially created because they didn't know quite what to do with us. I think I had a very wonderful experience. . . .

At the University of Missouri the nurse who came to be in charge of the school, Nance Taylor, had been the Superintendent of Nurses of the School of Nursing at St. Luke's Hospital at St. Louis, Missouri, prior to World War I. She was a very able and intelligent woman.

After World War I Miss Taylor, who was a very foresighted person, decided to go to Columbia, Missouri to start a University School of Nursing. . . . Miss Taylor planned a 3-year nursing course, but she developed the program in such a way that students could take all of their science courses right along with other students on the University campus.

In addition to that, they took courses in English and History in order to meet the Arts and Sciences requirements for Bachelor of Arts degree. Nearly everything we took counted for credit, with the exception of some of our nursing courses, toward the Bachelor of Arts degree. We had, as a result of this, continuous association with university students. This was relatively rare at that time. Though we lived in a nurses' residence, it was right on the campus, and there were many advantages in this. We felt that our work was just as important as that of any other student on the campus. . . .

We had, which was very unusual at that time, an 8-hour day, including classes. . . . We only had one half day off during the week and a half day on Sunday. . . .

I've always valued that our job was to care for patients and patients had a right to expect of nurses the best they could give.

The hospital was small; so we were sent to Kansas City, Missouri to Research Hospital for experience in maternity nursing and additional experience in medical nursing, and to Mercy Hospital in Kansas City for pediatric nursing. . . . We had good maternity nursing experience in Kansas City. . . . This was the first time we no longer had an 8-hour day. We worked very long hours. In fact, students provided all the care of patients. They served as head nurses at Research Hospital and at Mercy Hospital too. . . . It was difficult to give the kind of care I felt patients needed. The students at Research School of Nursing lived under very strict rules and regulations.

I began to sense what this did to students. I listened to the girls who were about ready to graduate, and they seemed to have no ambition or even to have any vision of what could be done except to be private duty nurses, because all the work in the hospital was done by students. Many of them were just waiting to graduate. They talked about finishing their nursing program. That was the chief thing. They also talked about what you would have to do to be a private duty nurse, the kind of gowns and negligees you had so you could sleep in the patient's room at night. Private duty nurses did 24-hour duty at that time (September 1973).

Following America's entry into World War I, the Army School of Nursing was organized in 1918.[2] There were 10,000 applicants for that school, and 2,000 were taken (Henderson, 1974).

[2] For a brief overview of this school, see Josephine A. Dolan, *Nursing in Society*, W. B. Saunders, Philadelphia, 1973, p. 268. There were 500 graduates in the first graduating class in 1921, a figure representing the largest class of nurses graduating at one time in the world's history.

Lulu K. Wolf Hassenplug, a graduate of the Army School of Nursing relates:

> I entered the program in the fall of 1921 straight from high school . . . we had a class of only 65, and there were about 4,000 patients at Walter Reed Hospital where all of the classes were then consolidated. . . . At Walter Reed we had about eight or nine months of classes and then my group went to Philadelphia General for Women and Children and then to Henry Street in New York for four months of public health and two months psychiatry at St. Elizabeth's. I think that the army school was the first of its kind that required psychiatric nursing and public health in the thirty-six month program, which was unusual in those days. . . .
>
> When we went to New York we lived in apartments, and at Philadelphia General we lived in the nurses' residence which we thought was pretty bad. . . . We had our classes and laboratory all in our eight hour day, and all the other nurses in the country were on a ten hour or longer day. When we showed up on any affiliation, they said, "Here comes the army. Give them the keys and let them do the work," and this is really what we did. . . . There were moments in my career when I really thought being in nursing was the worst thing I could ever have done. The hours were long; it was not stimulating . . . we did an awful lot of repetitive work. We did a lot of things that I could see no reason for intelligent women to do. I thought the emphasis on how to make a bed and all its tight corners were just crazy and we were thrown into responsibilities that we were not prepared for, and it got to be that you did things whether you knew how or not and then you pretended you hadn't done them . . . so it was a case of you're really trying to lie about things. . . . Some of our teachers were very good; some were quite pathetic. We stuck to text books . . . we had the discipline of the Army and on top of that we had the discipline that always goes through any nursing program (May 1974).

Although designed as a wartime measure, the Army School of Nursing continued into the post-war period and was discontinued in 1932 for economic reasons.

The "launching of the United States Nurse Cadet Corps occurred later due to the United States's further involvement in war. The formation and development of the United States Nurse Cadet Corps provides an illustration of the transformation nursing underwent during World War II. Emerging in response to an urgent need for more and better nurses to meet the wartime emergency situation, this unit was launched in 1943" (Safier, 1975, pp. 34–40). Designed, developed, and evaluated by Lucile Petry Leone, the Corps[3]—and Mrs. Leone's leadership role—deserves attention for its contribution to both nursing education and the public image of nursing. The Corps became a reality with the passage of the Bolton Act (1943). Between 1944 and 1946 the Corps oversaw the education of some 170,000 cadets, which comprised 90 percent of the total enrollment in nursing programs for those years, and nearly doubled the number of nursing students previously enrolled.

What was the achievement of the Cadet Corps relative to the development of nursing education and the public image of nursing? There had to be a program to tap the quantitative need for nursing personnel while maintaining and improving the system of nursing education. Clinical and educational resources were rapidly expanded; Congress financed it. Under the terms of the Bolton Act the Corps was granted a 60 million dollar appropriation to subsidize scholarships and subsistence grants to attract prospective cadets into the Corps. This measure can now be viewed as a landmark in the development of American nursing, for it marked the first time that federal money was allocated for nursing education. The infusion of federal monies, however, was hardly sufficient in itself to alleviate the shortage of nurses. While adequate financing was assuredly a step in the right direction, explains Mrs. Leone, there were other

---

[3] A detailed history of the Corps activities can be found in Lucile Petry, *The United States Cadet Nurse Corps*, Government Printing Office, Washington, 1950.

factors involved in the success of the Cadet Nurse Corps.

> It was the spirit that was important. I was always interested in making nursing meet people's needs. Public relations was important as an expression of how people work together in meeting needs. . . . One of my skills, then, was in getting people to work together, along with my interest in the vast, multi-interest complex and the interrelatedness of health, society, politics, and the war effort. It was a constant awareness of all the parts as they relate to one another.

> I was primarily interested in the people who would be *nursed*. What were the demands on nurses from people? What did rich and poor people need? What did people need to keep their families healthy? What did the very sick person need? What did the well person who might get sick need? All of these kinds of things are what makes nursing what it is. My main interest was in what did people need? . . . I wanted people to be able to express what they needed from nursing, and that is the consumer movement as it is known today. Consumerism and good public relations were to me in some respects synonymous (Safier, 1975, pp. 36–37).

In 1949 Mrs. Leone was appointed assistant surgeon general of the United States Public Health Service (USPHS). This appointment gave her a rank equivalent to rear admiral in the navy and brigadier general in the army, and marked her as the first woman to attain such high office in the USPHS. In this capacity she helped obtain federal funds for nursing education. Partially because of her efforts nursing became one of the first fields to receive federal subsidization for programs in nursing education, public health nursing, psychiatric nursing, and research. Truly an outstanding leader in her profession, she pioneered the role of the federal government in nursing both in the United States and abroad.

Just prior to Mrs. Leone's appointment as assistant surgeon general of the USPHS, there appeared an influential study of basic nursing programs. Entitled *Nursing for the Future* and commissioned by the National Nursing Council, it was written by Dr. Esther Lucile Brown (1948), a non-nurse anthropologist. She recommended that if society's future nursing needs were to be met, the profession would have to prepare two types of nurses: professional and vocational. This recommendation, along with the entire report, provoked a spirited controversy within nursing circles, but ultimately a national committee, the National Committee for the Improvement of Nursing Services, was established to implement the Brown plan. The committee agreed early that improvements in nursing services could not result without increasing the quality of nursing education.

Strong leadership was now required within the nursing profession. One individual ideally suited for the task at hand was Dr. Helen Nahm, who was completing a doctoral dissertation at the University of Minnesota on "An Evaluation of Selected Schools of Nursing with Respect to Certain Educational Objectives." Dr. Nahm firmly believed that the quality of nursing education had to be improved; otherwise, she cautioned, "nurses would be severely handicapped in their efforts to provide quality patient care." She believed that with scientific knowledge increasing and accelerating in pace, health care concepts and therapies were undergoing rapid changes. Accordingly, she agreed with Dr. Brown that there had to be different types of nurses, such as vocational or practical and professional nurses. She also believed that there had to be educational structures to prepare the different types of registered nurses as well as professional nurses for advanced positions in patient care and in teaching, supervision, administration, and research (Safier, 1975, p. 40).

When in 1949 the National Nursing Accreditation Service (NNAS) was instituted, Dr. Nahm was appointed its first director. The choice was an apt one: in addition to being one of the few nurses with a Ph.D. degree, she had also held teaching and administrative positions in Texas and Missouri. As one nurse-historian, Mary M. Roberts, had noted, "Miss Nahm with experience in both large and small schools was *temperamentally* as well as academically and professionally unusually well qualified for this *exacting* and influential position" (Safier, 1975, p. 40).

Her main concern as director was with accreditation.[4] Tackling the rigors associated with evaluating the array of nursing programs scattered throughout the United States was an imposing assignment but one that Dr. Nahm readily undertook. "Except for the job I had later at the University of California [Dean of the School of Nursing]," she later recounted, "it was by far the most challenging position that I have ever had" (Safier, 1975, p. 262).

At the time that the NNAS began its work, there were two types of undergraduate educational programs: the 3-year hospital diploma and a small number of college-university baccalaureate programs. In addition, programs for graduate nurses, most of which were also at a baccalaureate level, prepared nurses for public health nursing, teaching, administration, or supervision. The first task confronting the NNAS, then, was to formulate specific criteria for the evaluation of each type of program for accreditation.

It was agreed that a program of temporary accreditation should be developed for all programs not then fully accredited. Criteria for temporary accreditation were much less stringent than those for full accreditation. Of a total of 904 basic programs that applied for temporary accreditation during 1951–1952, 624 were approved for a period of five years and 276 were not approved. It was initially hoped that, at the end of a five-year period (1952–1957), the majority of temporarily accredited schools would have met criteria for full accreditation. However, this period of time was much too short, and it was not until 1962 that it was possible to discontinue listing, as a separate category, certain developing programs that were not

[4]For a judicious treatment of the entire question of accreditation, see William K. Selden, *Accreditation—A Struggle Over Standards in Higher Education*, Harper Brothers, New York, 1960.

yet ready for full accreditation (February 1974*b*).

After serving as Director of the NNAS for 2 years, Dr. Nahm was appointed the director of the Division of Nursing Education of the National League for Nursing. Since this organization assumed responsibility for accreditation in 1952, Dr. Nahm's tenure in the directorship (1953–1958) represented a continuation of her former duties.

There were problems concerning the emotional reaction to accreditation:

The most difficult problems were those associated with the hospital schools of nursing. From the time these schools were first established, students had been depended upon to furnish the bulk of hospital nursing service. To say that, to be accredited, a school should have a well-prepared faculty, a library, adequate physical facilities, and a budget, and that students should have time for study and recreation was looked upon by some schools as absolute heresy. Many collegiate schools of nursing were also very poor. College and university, as well as hospital administrators, did not relish being told their programs did not meet agreed-upon national criteria (February 1974*a*).

But in spite of this delicate situation, the accrediting program survived and continues as an established function of the National League for Nursing. In a paper Dr. Nahm delivered in 1974 on "The Accrediting Program in Nursing Education" at the American Nurses Association Convention, she unveiled a striking statistical portrait: "In 1950, there were approximately 1,170 basic programs of which 35 basic collegiate and 113 noncollegiate programs were accredited [total of 148]. In 1974, there are approximately 1,492 programs that prepared for licensing as registered nurses. Of these, 433 diploma, 207 associate degree and 234 baccalaureate degree programs are accredited [total of 874] (1974)." In great measure, this success story can be attributed to Dr. Nahm's skillful leadership.

It is perhaps instructive, therefore, to consider her formula for successful leadership.

One thing that is very important if you're working for a nursing organization is that you . . . try to state the issues as clearly as you can. . . . You try to state the strengths and weaknesses of what is proposed. . . . You (must) learn . . . to respect the human beings with whom you are dealing, whether you agree with them or not, to listen to people, to treat what they say as important, to avoid making them feel inadequate. . . . If decisions that are made are basically sound decisions, they can be defended. In the defense it is not necessary to antagonize or hurt people that initially do not agree. As a staff member you can listen and interpret and reinterpret. Gradually people themselves who have disagreed go through a process of change, and sooner or later you begin to get consensus (February 1974*a*).

In 1958 Helen Nahm was appointed Dean of the School of Nursing at the University of California, San Francisco. There, until her retirement in 1969, she again demonstrated her brilliance as an administrator, developing the University of California school into a leading institution of nursing education.

Other recognized nursing leaders were asked[5] what they perceived as current issues in nursing. Mary Kelly Mullane replied:

I think the biggest issue is how much unanimity of purpose we can hope for in a profession as diverse as our own. Internal warfare in the nursing profession is scandalous. Antagonism between the ANA [American Nurses Association] and the NLN [National League for Nursing] is one case in point. Another is continuing mutual criticism of nursing education and nursing service. A more recent one is the emerging chasm between nursing administrators

[5]Due to space limitations, the author's original questions are not included but instead a general passive voice is used. This represents a departure from the present recommended standard oral history format.

and nursing staff precipitated by Taft-Hartley revisions. Yet, even though these kinds of things come up from time to time, we tend to get them resolved. I'm confident that we shall continue to resolve them, that our professional leadership will be adequate to the task as it always had in the past.

I often wonder whether young nurses will be astute enough to understand the strength they have in organized nursing—that is, the state and national organizations—and to use that strength. . . . Another crucial issue is nursing's tendency to react to changes rather than help design them. If we have less internal dissension, we'd have a political clout, and in our society political clout is the name of the game. We're not yet in a position to play that game as national health insurance, quality controls, PSRO's [Professional Standard Review Organizations] and other major developments come tumbling out of Washington. If nursing could provide the public with a well-defined redefinition of the role of nursing in modern society— what it ought to be—we couldn't fail, given our large numbers. . . . I hope the next generation of professional nurses will demonstrate their expertise and dedicate their money and energies to speaking with one voice about future goals of Americans' health care. If they can, the public and nursing itself will be better for it (Safier, 1977, pp. 251–253).

Marion Sheahan comments on nursing education:

I think that nursing education belongs in both junior colleges and colleges, because there is a place for a level of nursing to work in relation to professional nursing, comparable to physicians' assistants with physicians. And I don't think it makes any difference whether the nursing profession . . . calls the person "nurse" or not . . . . Someone is going to be needed who fulfills the role of the prepared nurse (October 1974).

Martha Rogers addresses the issue of different careers in nursing:

If I were going to identify one single issue, then I would say differentiation of professional and technical careers in nursing, legally and openly and honestly, is the most critical issue that must be resolved. . . . Nursing *does* have professional and technical careers. . . . We cannot discuss fulfilling our responsibilities and accountability to society until we differentiate careers honestly. . . . Professional education does start with the baccalaureate degree. I can't imagine any of us wanting a dental hygienist to make decisions for dentistry, or a dental hygiene license as adequate for dentists. But this is precisely what we do. . . . The "ladder game" is nothing but setting up a second-rate citizenship and denying the right to respect and dignity to nursing technicians (Safier, 1977, pp. 328–329).

Virginia Henderson views the roles of the nurse at a macroscopic level:

I think that a national health service is coming and that it would provide health insurance for all citizens in the United States. . . . The only way that health care can be made universally available is to give nurses a much broader and more responsible role than they now have. . . . The role of nurses is going to be a more responsible one (Safier, 1977, p. 131).

Lucille E. Notter raises the issue of clinical research:

One issue is that of nurses interested in doing clinical research. . . . The issue of patients' rights complicate the picture and institutions are increasingly cautious about granting permission for research to be carried out using their patients. It is possible that nurses wanting to do patient care research will find themselves in competition with physicians for the available patients (Safier, 1977, pp. 279–281).

Florence Blake enlarges upon the issue of research, the role of faculty and graduate education:

One issue is that persons believe that all faculty should be involved in pure research. Personally, I can't believe that productivity grows from coercion or constant reminders that research is necessary for promotion. . . . I used to hypothesize that more research would be done if the energy dissipated in coercion would be diverted into study of how time for research could be made available to faculty members who had already identified problems worthy of and appropriate for controlled designs. Faculty who are interested in doing research should have support in doing it, but I can't see why every faculty member must be cast into the same mould. Is this really the best use of the varied, unique talents observable in faculty members?
. . .

I would like to see some of our best-prepared faculty become more involved in nursing service than they are today. Maybe then some of the stumbling blocks to our professional growth might vanish. . . . Teachers and nursing service personnel have a great deal to share with one another. . . . Progress could be made faster if we could all learn to work together.

I'm convinced that graduate students need tools and motivation for continued learning. . . . Pure clinical courses are being offered at the baccalaureate level. It seems even more important to have intensive clinical study at the graduate level, and not programs which focus primarily on research methodology (Safier, 1977, pp. 30-31).

Concerning perceptions of the nurse practitioner roles, Florence Blake replied:

I wish there weren't so many different categories of nurses. It's confusing, especially to lay people and others on health teams. I can't quite see why settings should determine the titles provided for nurses. I think educational experiences to help nurses learn to make thorough physical assessments of patients are an asset. . . . Nursing diagnosis and plans for care or for continued health supervision require it. We glossed over the area of preparation for planning patient care in the recent past, and I'm delighted to learn that more thorough preparation for making total health assessment is being provided. I just hope nursing practitioners are doing nursing and not just doing those procedures and routines delegated to them by doctors (Safier, 1977, p. 31).

Ruth Freeman discusses the expanded role of the nurse in terms of a primary health referent.

If nursing maintains a narrow approach it's going to become terribly expensive and pretty ineffective. We need some way in which we can get a primary health referent for every family in this country, and it's my opinion that it will not occur through the further development of the family physician. The family physician is overprepared for many things families need in health care. Another very real issue is what should be done with respect to the organization and management of the multidiscipline team. First, I think the hierarchical concept under which such teams are usually set up is no longer useful for the kind of services we're expected to render. Secondly, I think there are great difficulties in defining the responsibilities of the individual members so they feel content within some kind of reasonable framework, and at the same time allowing them to interchange responsibilities when that is necessary for purposes of economy or effectiveness in dealing with patient care situations. Another problem is . . . the organization of medical care in general. I feel that, if everyone is to have a primary health referent, someone to whom he can turn, this health referent has to be one of a large group of professionals, readily available psychologically as well as physically. . . . The public health nurse could be this referent. . . . The issue is: Who is going to take the leadership or maintain control of the health programs, as differentiated from medical care programs? (Safier, 1977, pp. 78–79).

Rozella Schlotfeldt demonstrates a pragmatic approach to the issue.

I don't know what the term "nurse practitioner" means. When anybody . . . [uses the term], I'll say, "do you mean a nurse?" That's my standard question. If you ask the question often enough, maybe you open up these people [stimulate some people to really define it] (Safier, 1977, p. 351).

The nursing leaders were also asked their concerns about the future of nursing. Rozella Schlotfeldt believes nursing is:

. . . at the crossroads. . . . I'm really quite worried about nursing at the present time. . . . I like to think that we will have a sufficient number of bright people that will act wisely and give the leadership that is needed. However, I see much "selling out" to the notion of nurses being a physician's assistant. They don't call themselves that, but rather a "nurse practitioner." However, some are actually in the position of being a physician's assistant. Therefore they will attain prestige, reward, money and forget nursing. . . . I think we have to stand up and be counted, that nursing is going to control its own destiny. But then try to give forthright leadership that's effective and if it is effective there will be recognition that nurses have a contribution to make (Safier, 1977, pp. 349–350).

Dorothy Smith predicts that:

If enough people can be found who are career-oriented, and really motivated toward patients rather than something outside nursing, then great things could happen in nursing. . . . The forces that operate against good nursing care are tremendously strong, . . . that includes a tremendous number of nurses, who really don't want things to change (Safier, 1977, pp. 349–350).

Florence Blake outlines future roles for nurses:

I'd like to see nurses expand their role to the limits of their capacity. They can do a great deal more in the prevention of all types of disease than they have in the past. There is plenty for all professional workers to do which isn't being done well enough now. Nurses can play a significant role in rehabilitation and in helping people learn how to protect themselves from disease and from further disability if they already have a chronic disease. People need so much more knowledge about their disabilities and the purposes of the treatment prescribed than they are being given. If they got it, they would be much better prepared to help themselves, and would value themselves more highly as a consequence (Safier, 1977, pp. 32–33).

ORAL HISTORY AND FEMINIST STUDIES

In addition to these specific examples, there are some general conclusions that emerge from interviewing this designated nursing elite that have implications for feminist studies. First, most of these women were not prepared for specific leadership, but instead had leadership roles thrust upon them as a result of circumstances. Second, most of the leaders were forced to choose between marriage and a career. Questionnaire responses reveal that of the sixteen, seven never married, four were married, and five married for the first time after the age of 40.

These conclusions raise questions that can profitably be pursued by others researching women in leadership positions outside the field of nursing. For example, how does the social climate differ today in creating opportunities for women? How and why do women enter the fields they do? What is their career trajectory? What are the social costs involved for those achieving leadership roles? What are the comparative opportunities for men and women who choose the same vocation?

Although answers may further expose the sexist basis of American life, the accompanying consciousness that such knowledge brings can serve as a starting point between bridging the gap between the *is* and the *ought* of American ideas and practices. Viewed in this sense, oral history can be seen as a tool of social reorientation, an instrument in forging a truly free and open American culture.

BIBLIOGRAPHY

Benison, Saul: *Tom Rivers: Reflections on a Life in Medicine and Science*, M.I.T. Press, Cambridge, Mass., 1967.

Hassenplug, Lulu K. Wolf: May 15, 1974, unpublished interview.

Nahm, Helen: September 11, 1973, unpublished interview.

_____: February 19, 1974*a*, unpublished interview with the author.

_____: February 19, 1974*b*, unpublished letter to author.

Safier, Gwendolyn: *Contemporary American Leaders in Nursing: An Oral History*, McGraw-Hill, New York, 1977.

_____: " 'I Sensed the Challenges': Leaders Among Contemporary U.S. Nurses," *The Oral History Review*, pp. 31–57, 1975, Published by the Oral History Association, New York.

_____: "What is Oral History?" Published under the Questions and Answers column in *Nursing Research*, 25(5):383–385, September-October 1976.

Sheahan, Marion: October 21, 1974, unpublished interview.

EDITOR'S QUESTIONS FOR DISCUSSION

What historical norms and values portrayed by the interviewers are present today in nursing? What issues of concern to nursing today have historical roots? How can leadership be developed in nursing? What instrumental factors in society and in the profession encourage or inhibit leadership development?

Chapter 8

Entry into Professional Practice: The New York Proposal

Margaret L. McClure, R.N., Ed.D., F.A.A.N.
Director of Nursing,
Maimonides Medical Center, Maimonides Hospital, Brooklyn, New York

Perhaps the most controversial issue within the nursing profession today concerns proposed legislation that by 1985 the baccalaureate degree in nursing be the requirement for licensure as a registered professional nurse. Margaret L. McClure clarifies some of the implications and issues of the proposed legislation. She illustrates that the division of labor between technical and professional tasks is not possible in nursing and proposes a third model for conceptualizing nursing practice. The issues of the lack of prepared leaders in nursing, the lack of opportunity for current registered nurses to obtain baccalaureate degrees, the quality of baccalaureate education, and the ratio of types of nurses needed are discussed.

At the 1974 New York State Nurses Association convention, a resolution was introduced and passed that, if enacted into law, will undoubtedly have far-reaching effects on the quality of nursing care that future patients in that state will receive. The resolution proposes, in essence, that the baccalaureate degree become the minimal educational preparation for entry into the profession by the year 1985 (Figure 8-1). The directors of nursing special interest group sponsored this action, a fact which both is appropriate and should be a source of pride to this group. Nursing service administrators are entrusted with the full responsibility for the quality of nursing care that patients receive, and for that reason they have a vested interest in ensuring that the nurses whom they hire and place in a variety of critical positions come to the employment setting with the best possible preparation. Unfortunately the present situation in which we find ourselves does not offer such insurance.

It would seem apparent that the majority of the problems we currently face came about as a direct result of the initiation and implementation of the so-called technical nursing education programs that were developed in the early 1950s.

The rationale for this level of preparation was built on an analysis of practice that would appear to be indisputable:

The functions of nursing can be said to be on a continuum or as having a spectrum-like range. At one extreme of the range of the spectrum are those activities which are very simple and which serve to give assistance to the nurse or

This article originally appeared in *The Journal of Nursing Administration*, vol. 6, no. 5, June 1976.

**Resolution on Entry
into Professional Practice**

Approved by the 1974
New York State Nurses Association
Voting Body

WHEREAS, The existence of multiple kinds of basic nursing education programs leading to licensure as a registered professional nurse creates immeasurable public and professional confusion, and

WHEREAS, It has also long been recognized that baccalaureate preparation is basic to professional nursing practice.

THEREFORE BE IT RESOLVED, That the New York State Nurses Association develop a plan for establishing by 1985 the baccalaureate degree in nursing as a requirement for licensure as a registered professional nurse, and be it further

RESOLVED, That this effort provide through grandfather clauses and/or other appropriate means, full protection of all practice privileges, titles and status of all individuals currently licensed or preparing for licensure as a registered professional nurse.

Figure 8-1

physician. . . . At the other extreme of the range of function are those which are extremely complex and require a high degree of skill and expertness acquired through long periods of training. . . . The main volume of nursing in hospitals, clinics, and other agencies giving nursing care lies somewhere between the two extremes just described. It occupies the middle of the spectrum range. The functions performed in this portion of the range may be described as semiprofessional or technical[1].

On the basis of this analysis, the community college program was developed. Since that time, directors of nursing have been chastised by themselves as well as by others for their failure to operationalize two distinct practices, one professional, the other technical. Yet despite these castigations, the two categories have never been differentiated,

and one must be forced at this point to ask why. Although it may be possible that part of the problem has been a lack of vision and creativity on the part of the directors, this factor certainly does not begin to account for the entire difficulty. All directors are not recalcitrant reactionaries; some are actually bright, innovative professional people who are anxious to see practice improved and to initiate programs designed to accomplish that goal. After almost 25 years of working with this problem, perhaps it is time that we reexamine the entire issue beginning with the fundamental concepts.

It would seem evident that the difficulties with the concept of technical practice begin to emerge at the point at which this practice touches on actual nurse-patient interaction. The patient is basically the root of the difficulty. He refuses to cooperate. He simply does not emit his needs in neat, carefully itemized packages that can be clearly labeled as belonging to either the technical or the professional realm. Instead, he gives them off in muddled, unsorted, and quite unpredictable bundles which confront and too often confound whatever level of practitioner happens to be present at the time. As an example, the changing of a colostomy dressing is in itself a technical task; indeed, if one could detach the task from the patient it would be totally technical in nature. This detachment is obviously not possible, however, and thus the individual dealing with the dressing must also deal with the total patient and all the needs he is expressing at that point in time. Obviously he needs someone who can cleanse the area adequately, note the condition of the stoma, provide appropriate skin care to the surrounding area, and apply the clean dressings in an effective and comfortable manner; however, he also needs someone to assist him in coping with his anxieties, dealing with his learning needs, interpreting his symbolic language (in Kubler-Ross terminology)[2], and planning for ways to manage the changes that such a physical impairment will impose on his entire way of life. In short, he needs a professional nurse. Much the

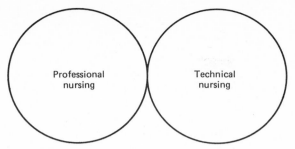

Figure 8-2

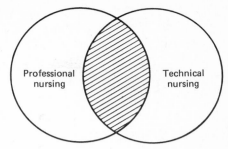

Figure 8-3

same case can be made for most technical nursing tasks that might be cited: as long as a human being is involved, the need will be for a professional nurse in the majority of situations.

This perhaps is an important clue for us. One of the professions that we have frequently been compared to is that of engineering. There apparently does exist a differentiation, both in education and in practice, between the professional and the technical engineer. Undoubtedly, the success of this pattern is due largely to the fact that engineers are dealing with inanimate objects that lend themselves to such a division of labor; the human being simply does not.

What this ultimately boils down to, then, is a basic difference in the conceptualization of nursing practice. A literal translation of Montag's work might be illustrated in Model 1 (Figure 8-2). In this model, professional and technical nursing are viewed as adjoining one another although carrying out separate, discrete, and easily identifiable functions. It would be expected that the educational components of the curriculums preparing the respective practitioners would be equally as separate, discrete, and easily identifiable.

Undoubtedly many nursing leaders (and perhaps Montag herself) would not agree entirely with the above interpretation. It is probably safe to say that their conceptualization would involve some degree of overlap in the functioning of the two levels, as diagrammed in Model 2 (Figure 8-3). Such an approach would indicate that there are some patient needs that fall within the purely professional realm, some that fall within the purely technical

realm, and some that fall within a gray area that can be met by either level of practitioner. It is obvious, however, that large portions of the practice of each of these nurses are still conceived to be separate, discrete, and easily identifiable, and one would expect that the curriculums would clearly reflect the differences between the two. In reality, such is not the case. On close examination, one finds very little of any substance that is unique to one or the other type of educational preparation and, in fact, a good deal of confusion exists between them.

If we return to the patient in the real world, it would seem that neither of these conceptual schemes is actually based on his needs, for each presupposes that these needs are easily separated into the respective domains of the professional and the technical nurse. Rather, a third model in which the technical aspects of care can be illustrated as a part of the professional nurse's realm would appear to be more appropriate, as illustrated in Model 3 (Figure 8-4). This interpretation indicates that although the professional nurse may delegate some of the technical aspects of care to another level, these aspects nonetheless remain an integral part of the professional nurse's total responsibility. Further it is not intended that the area designated in Figure 8-4 as "technical nursing" necessarily indicates such delegation; there may or may not be a lesser prepared individual involved, depending on the circumstances of the particular situation. The curriculum for preparing the professional nurse in this model would follow closely the classic educational philosophy of Alfred North Whitehead, who said:

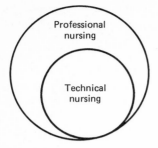

Figure 8-4

The antithesis between a technical and a liberal education is fallacious. There can be no adequate technical education which is not liberal, and no liberal education which is not technical: that is, no education which does not impart both technique and intellectual vision. In simpler language, education should turn out the pupil with something he knows well and something he can do well [3].

In keeping with this model, a second level of practitioner would be prepared to assist in carrying out selected components of care. The curriculum for that level would appear to be much like that of the better practical nurse programs extant throughout the nation today.

Again, there is a distinct possibility that the original intent for operationalizing technical nursing was a model 3 approach. However, licensing laws, the proportion of practitioners prepared at the two levels, and salary scales would tend to negate any attempt in this direction.

It is my contention that a large number of the problems that we have encountered and continue to encounter in our profession are a direct result of our attempt to impose either a model 1 or 2 concept on a model 3 world. Thus, when the technical nurse appears in the health care setting, she is called upon to do an enormous amount of work for which she is ill prepared. The practical consequences of this situation for nursing, and therefore for patients, have been serious.

The most obvious consequence of the technical program has been that it has placed large numbers of practitioners with only superficial knowledge in

situations where in-depth knowledge is required. The knowledge explosion has been very well documented and is a familiar, frightening phenomenon to all of us. A mastery of large amounts of content from both the physical and the social sciences is required in order for the practitioner to be safe and competent. More important, this nurse needs to be able to synthesize these diverse pieces of knowledge in such a way as to provide maximum benefit to the patient—a task that requires not only substantive coursework but also intensive study of practice within the framework of the academic program. In looking to the future, keeping in mind that the twenty-first century is almost around the corner, one can only anticipate that the knowledge base for nursing practice will continue to expand in staggering, geometric progression. Therefore, given the magnitude of the knowledge dimension, it is difficult to envision how the associate degree program can continue in its present form. What we end up with is an intellectual "blivett," which is essentially an effort to put 5 pounds of potatoes into a box designed to hold 3 pounds.

A second and obviously related consequence is the acute disappointment of patients and their families in the nursing care that is generally rendered. They do not understand (and what is more, they do not want to understand) the differences among the various educational preparations[4]. They do, however, understand very well that the quality of services received is far inferior to what it should be, given the cost of health care today. To say that the image of nursing has suffered as a result of this factor would be a tremendous understatement. Patients in particular and the public in general continue to view the nurse as a task-oriented handmaiden to the physician with little intellectual ability or expertise[5].

This brings us to the third consequence, namely, a lack of colleagueship with other health professional personnel. For a number of years we have endeavored to take our rightful place on the health care team—as a colleague of the physician, the social worker, the dietician, the physiotherapist. Yet we have met with extremely limited success.

There can be little question that the educational preparation of the majority of our practitioners is a factor that must be reckoned with in this regard. The technical nurse is not prepared on a peer level and, therefore, remains in a one-down position. In the past we have raised many a hue and cry about this issue, but one is tempted to question whether our continued support of community college education for registered nurses is not an unconscious desire to remain one-down: the poor, helpless female depending on the superior male to shoulder the bulk of the responsibility.

A final consequence for this discussion is the dearth of nurses prepared in graduate programs to provide leadership and scholarship for the profession. Approximately 85 percent of the registered nurses in this country hold the diploma or the associate degree as their highest credential. In light of the fact that many baccalaureate programs do not encourage these nurses to pursue further study, it is little wonder that the percentage of nurses holding advanced degrees is startlingly small. This has had disastrous results for all areas of nursing: education, service, and research. The general effect is again a one-down position. For example, in education, the baccalaureate and higher degree programs do not begin to have adequate numbers of teachers prepared at the doctoral level. This means that concessions must frequently be made in appointing individuals to nursing faculties in universities, and as a consequence the department does not measure up well against other departments in the college or university—a lightweight competing in the heavyweight's arena.

A lack of prepared leadership in both the clinical and the administrative service areas is also a critical problem. A well-qualified clinical specialist and a well-qualified director of nursing are both very scarce resources, and in some geographic areas they are both almost nonexistent. Because leadership positions, like nature, seem to abhor a vacuum, the positions do get filled; but when the individuals involved are not fully prepared, then the one-down syndrome appears again. An inadequate director of nursing will never be considered a colleague of such powerful individuals as the director of medicine or the director of surgery.

Undoubtedly the single area in which a lack of leadership is most evident is that of research. There are two problems in this regard. The first is our pitifully small number of individuals prepared to carry out research, because the technical aspects required to do this type of work are taught exclusively at the graduate level. As a result, most of our nursing practice is based on personal wisdom rather than on scientific investigation. Questions related to such fundamental nursing problems as the treatment of decubiti and the temperature for tube feedings are only now beginning to be addressed by nurse-researchers; the study of highly complex subjects such as the psychosocial factors related to senility and other aspects of care for the elderly is still in the distant future. At the present time many nurses have their own personal theories about these matters, but these theories have not been validated by rigorous testing. The second problem is that only a small proportion of our colleagues understand how to read a research report, and therefore even the few research findings that are generated are not put into practice [6]. Compared to other health professions, the practice of nursing is more an art and a skill than it is a science. One-down again.

Clarifying the above fundamental issues and problems only lays the groundwork for the major focus of our concerns today, namely, (1) what has been done and what is being planned in order to ensure that the Entry into Professional Practice resolution comes to fruition; and (2) what implications the resolution has for directors of nursing in New York as well as in other states. Since the 1974 New York State convention, work has progressed to the point where a proposal has been drafted for a revision to the Nurse Practice Act. The major ideas contained in the proposal are as follows:

1 The requirement of a baccalaureate degree in nursing for all registered nurses *entering* the profession, effective 1984

2 The requirement of an associate degree in nursing for all *entering* practical nurses, effective 1984

3 Transitional mechanisms designed to protect any nurse licensed in either of these two categories prior to the effective date

It is particularly important to note the future orientation of this proposal. No attempt is being made to force any change whatever on nurses currently in practice. Rather the entire emphasis is on ensuring adequate and appropriate educational preparation for future generations of practitioners.

The 1975 New York State Nurses Association convention voted its approval of the above proposal by an overwhelming majority, and plans are underway to introduce the bill in the state legislature in 1976.

Clearly these revisions to the Nurse Practice Act have been long in coming and should be viewed as evolutionary rather than revolutionary. They do carry with them, however, a number of implicit and important issues which we, as directors of nursing, must confront vigorously. One of these issues is the relative lack of opportunity for current RNs to obtain their baccalaureate degrees. Although this situation has improved slightly, it remains a serious problem and one which has caused bitterness and resentment among many nurses. We have a responsibility to press our colleagues in education for more and better opportunities for these RNs. It may even be possible for federal and state grants to be obtained for support during this limited, transitional period. Nurse educators should be encouraged to explore all possible avenues in this regard.

A second issue of paramount concern is improvement in the quality of baccalaureate education. Many directors of nursing have been disappointed in the practice skills demonstrated by beginning practitioners, and although this practice training varies considerably from school to school, it continues to present problems to both the neophyte nurse and his or her employing agency. In fact, a very fine editorial in *Nursing Outlook* addressed itself to this very issue[7]. The value of clinical practice is one that should not be underestimated. It offers the student an opportunity to try out classroom knowledge in a variety of situations, and it also begins the important process of socializing her into the role of "nurse" while she is still exposed to instructors who are, ideally, serving as role models.

We administrators, also, have an important responsibility in relation to the student's clinical experience. We have the obligation to provide a setting in which the student nurse's learning can take place and to work out smooth and harmonious relationships between the staff and the faculty and students. One of the serious handicaps that many baccalaureate programs face is a limitation in the availability of clinical facilities for their use, in spite of the fact that such facilities exist within the community. Obviously, if we want to obtain well-qualified graduate nurses, we must be generous in providing experiences during their student years.

One of the most important issues to which we must address ourselves immediately is the question of appropriate proportions of professional vis-a-vis technical practitioners. How many of each type will we need to meet patient needs appropriately and adequately? Clearly, the cost of education for these two levels is quite different, but we must be certain that these initial fundings are spent wisely so that the return on the investment—the nurse's total career contribution—is worth the investment. In 1973 a total of 7,660 students graduated from registered nurse programs and 4,156 students graduated from practical nurse programs in New York State[8]. The ratio, then, was approximately 65 percent registered nurse to 35 percent practical nurse graduations. We must now begin to explore the future utilization of these two categories of personnel within our own settings and within the profession as a whole so that we can ensure the upgrading of the quality of care that the proposed revisions to the Nurse Practice Act promise. It should be remembered that many of our problems to date have arisen as a direct result of the incredibly small proportion of professional people among our ranks. We must not proceed to make that mistake again or we will find ourselves reiterating the old French proverb, "The more things change, the more they stay the same."

Closely related to the question of proportions is that of actual numbers of practitioners. Concerns are naturally being voiced regarding the ability of the baccalaureate programs to provide enough nurses to meet the needs of service settings across the state. Studies concerning this matter are underway; however, the council of deans of baccalaureate and higher degree programs expresses confidence that these demands can be met if we utilize our resources wisely and well.

One problem that will remain is the entire question of interstate mobility. Although nurses leaving New York will be expected to experience little difficulty, those who wish to enter the state will probably meet with some obstacles after 1984. There does appear to be evidence, however, that other states are considering changes in educational requirements very much like those outlined above; if this is the case, one can foresee that eventually the problem will solve itself, although admittedly the transitional period may be long and painful. It is important to bear in mind that this nation is one that was founded on a strong states rights philosophy, and therefore any major change can only be accomplished on a state-by-state basis.

In the final analysis, most directors of nursing are pragmatists and will therefore ask, "Will it work?" Those of us who have had the opportunity to employ large numbers of baccalaureate graduates in recent years can reply to this query with a resounding and emphatic "Yes." Experience has shown that these nurses make a significant difference in the quality of care that patients receive. On behalf of the consumer, then, we have an obligation to move forward in such a way as to ensure a better future for them.

REFERENCES

1 Montag, M. L. *The Education of Nursing Technician*. New York: G. P. Putnam's Sons, 1951, pp. 3–5.

2 Kubler-Ross, E. *On Death and Dying*. New York: The Macmillan Company, 1969.

3 Whitehead, A. N. *The Aims of Education and Other Essays*. New York: The Free Press, 1929, p. 48.

4 Hampe, S. O. Needs of the grieving spouse in a hospital setting. *Nurs. Res.*, Vol. 24, No. 2, 1975.

5 Beletz, E. E. Is nursing's public image up to date? *Nurs. Outlook*, Vol. 22, No. 7, 1974.

6 Ketefian, S. Application of selected research findings into nursing practice: A pilot study. *Nurs. Res.*, Vol. 24, No. 2, 1975.

7 Lewis, E. P. The two worlds of nursing. *Nurs. Outlook*, Vol. 23, No. 7, 1975.

8 *Educational Preparation for Practical and Professional Nursing in the State of New York 1973*. Albany: The University of the State of New York, the State Education Department, Office of Professional Education, Nursing Education, 1973, p. 12.

EDITOR'S QUESTIONS FOR DISCUSSION

What are the assumptions underlying the proposed legislation? What evidence exists that verifies or refutes these assumptions? What would be desirable in the curriculum for current registered nurses seeking a baccalaureate degree? How might it be possible to document differences in educational programs via patient outcome? Is it legitimate to evaluate an educational program in terms of patient outcome? Does the type of educational program from which one graduates make a difference in the quality of care provided? What societal forces and forces within the profession exist that may influence change for or against the proposed legislation? What obstacles exist in implementing the proposed legislation? What alternative legislative proposal for accreditation or licensure would you offer to ensure adequate professional education for the practitioner of nursing? Would these be different for varying educational programs? What alternative mechanisms would you propose for accreditation and licensure of nurses in the various nursing roles today, such as the independent nurse practitioner, clinical specialist, or staff nurse?

Chapter 9

Status Consistency and Nurses' Perception of Conflict Between Nursing Education and Practice

Norma L. Chaska, R.N., Ph.D.
Research Associate, Health Care Research Unit
Mayo Clinic and Mayor Foundation, Rochester, Minnesota

McClure's article also has implications for the conflict between nursing education and nursing practice. This conflict has been alluded to in the literature but has never been investigated. Because such a conflict presents a basic dichotomy within the profession, it seems valuable to include a portion of a study by Norma L. Chaska that deals with that issue and reveals how some nurses perceive the situation. By interviewing 303 nurses and recording responses to a series of statements, Chaska related type of status consistency (based on the variables of education, position, and income) to nurses' views of nursing education and nursing practice. Four of the statements showed significant relationships to the type of status consistency of the nurse. The findings reflect the tendency to consider the need for a degree or higher education in nursing of less value by the low-status-consistent and inconsistent-status nurses than by high-status-consistent nurses.

DEFINITION OF TERMS

The following definitions were used for this study.

Status An individual's place within a system of social ranking, measured on a three-dimensional scale consisting of education, position, and income.

Status consistent A high *or* low rank on all three dimensions of status (education, position, and income).

Status inconsistent A combination of a high *and* a low rank on any of the status dimensions of education, position, and income. Thus, for status inconsistent the following combinations are possible:

education high, position high, income low
education high, position low, income high

This investigation was supported in part by the Bureau of Health Services Research, Health Resources Administration from the Public Health Service, Department of Health, Education, and Welfare, Rockville, Maryland, based on work carried out elsewhere than at the Mayo Clinic, and was part of the unpublished doctoral dissertation, "Status Consistency and Status Inconsistency: Expectations and Perceptions of Role Performance Among Nurses," submitted in partial fulfillment of the requirements for the degree of Doctor of Philosophy, Boston University, 1975.

education high, position low, income low
education low, position high, income high
education low, position high, income low
education low, position low, income high
Expectations The anticipated performance of self and others in terms of some idealized norm.
Perceptions A view of performance of self or others, past or present, relative to an idealized norm.

CONSTRUCTION OF STATUS CONSISTENCY INDEX

Type of status consistency was determined by the following criteria. (1) In accordance with the standards set by the American Nurses Association and the National League for Nursing, as well as designated by the literature of the profession, subjects with a Bachelor's degree or less were categorized as "low" in *education*. (2) Subjects with monthly income of less than $1,200 were designated as "low" on the *income* scale, based on the income levels of nurses in an eastern metropolitan area. (3) Three professors of nursing with doctoral degrees and one nursing administrator with a master's degree and twenty-three years of nursing experience were asked to rate *positions* in nursing in terms of prestige. All four agreed to the following scale:

High prestige	Low prestige
Clinical specialists	Head nurses
Nurse practitioners	Staff nurses
Nurse educators	Public health nurses
Supervisors	Private duty nurses
Nurse administrators	Staff development nurses (in-service education)
	All other nursing roles

PURPOSE OF THE STUDY

The purpose of this study is threefold: (1) to analyze a problem of status in nursing in terms of the clarified theoretical construct of status consistency; (2) to report the findings regarding the conflict between nursing education and nursing prac-

tice; and (3) to add to the clarification of the theoretical concept of status consistency.

THEORETICAL FRAMEWORK

The theory of *status consistency* (also referred to in the literature as *status crystallization* or *status congruence*) holds that:

> Social status is multidimensional and hierarchical. Individuals are located in social space in terms of their positions on a variety of dimensions of status such as occupation, education, income, ethnicity, etc. Each person occupies a particular status configuration, determined by his location on each of the component dimensions. Thus, some status sets will be "crystallized" (consistent) in the sense that all of the component statuses give rise to similar values and expectations, while others will not.[1]

Inherent in this theory is the assumption that an aspect of a status position along a given status dimension consists of certain expectations for the behavior of the occupant of that position.[2] Thus, for example, a person ranking high in education may be expected to have certain behavior patterns, as would a person ranking high in position but low in education. The literature suggests the importance of empirical research directed toward identifying the expectations that correspond to the different positions of a status dimension.[3]

For the purpose of this study, not only is an individual's location on a status dimension important but more specifically the expectations and perceptions associated with that location.[3] For example, the nurse who has high consistent status may expect the status consistent nurse to function according to her level of education, whereas the status inconsistent nurse may evaluate the status consistent nurse as not performing up to the expectations of her educational level. This also suggests that performance expectations and perceptions of nurses within the group who rank low and high on consistent status will be different from those of nurses who are status inconsistent.

Furthermore, the difference may be related to the historical conflict between nursing practice and nursing theory. This conflict has made the coordination of the nursing profession an arduous task. The disparity between role expectations and role perceptions may be caused by the failure of the nursing profession to deal effectively with two different realities—the university setting where professional nursing education programs are based and the hospital organization where nursing is practiced.

RATIONALE FOR THE PROBLEM OF STATUS IN NURSING

Traditionally, nurse educators have been identified as the spokespersons for nursing theory and nurse practitioners as the proponents of nursing practice.[4] Rather than defining theory as a number of interrelated concepts from which hypotheses are deduced, nurses have more commonly used the term *theory* to mean a rationale for the basis of practice. At different times there have been varying degrees of prestige associated with the proponents of theory (nurse educators) and practice (nurse practitioners). The discrepancy, if any, between these two groups may be related to status consistency and status inconsistency. Levels of status consistency and status inconsistency may affect the expectations and perceptions of nurses in regard to the performance of nurses and may explain the conflict between nursing theory and nursing practice.

The status discrepancy between the nurse in practice and the nurse in education can be traced to the earliest years of the nursing profession. In 1874, Florence Nightingale said to her nurses:

> Shall we do everything in our power to become proficient, not only in knowing the symptoms, and what is to be done, but in knowing the "reason why" of such symptoms, and why such and such a thing is done? . . . many say, "we have no time: the ward work gives us no time!" But it is easy to degenerate into a mere drudgery about the wards, when we have good will to

do it, and are fonder of practical work than of giving ourselves the trouble of learning the reason why![5]

Since that time there has always been a specious distinction between nursing theory and nursing practice.[6] In the earliest history of nursing, learning was all practice—apprentice learning. Classroom study was intended primarily to make the nurse more effective in practice. However, these two aspects of nursing care have never been satisfactorily integrated.[7] Historically, nurses have tended to separate those who practice from those who teach, and the latter are generally accorded more status than the former.[6]

The quest for a theory base for nursing can be traced back to 1916 when several schools of nursing became associated with universities.[8] M. A. Nutting, one of the early nurse educators, visualized this achievement not only as a gain in status in nursing but also as an opportunity to develop the intellectual aspects of nursing.[9] Nutting, along with Isabel Stewart, another outstanding nurse educator of the 1940s, always believed that better instruction of nursing students would result in better nursing care.[10] Sheahan[5] believes that they were correct in asserting that professional education is fundamental to professional nursing practice but incorrect in assuming that given professional education, professional practice will follow. Thus, there is an historical basis for the dichotomy between those persons who have identified themselves with nursing theory and those who have identified themselves with nursing practice.

LITERATURE REVIEW

Low Education: Upward Mobility and Dissonance in Low-Status-Consistent and Status-Inconsistent Nurses

If one has low-status consistency or is status-inconsistent because of low education, presumably the lack of schooling could, in either case, affect one's perception of education. Individuals may try to compensate for their inconsistent status or their low investment on the educational dimension by lowering their perceptions of the status rank of the individuals with more education. Geschwender[2] postulates that if educational investment is the low dimension in the hierarchy of status, the group involved may attempt in an anti-intellectual way to criticize the educational level of others as being "ivory tower" and impractical. If this is true, then the status-inconsistent nurse, as well as the nurse who has low status consistency, would be more likely to undervalue the education achieved by nurses with higher degrees than would nurses who are high-status-consistent. Geschwender[2] further states that overrewarded inconsistent status individuals whose low investment dimension is educational will probably not be able to reduce dissonance through individual mobility. Because the status-inconsistent nurse or the nurse who has low status consistency may rank low on the educational dimension, she may find it more difficult to achieve status through upward mobility to positions that require higher education than would nurses with high-consistent status or those who rank high in education. Thus, a finding that the dissonance between the two groups cannot be equilibrated would contradict Benoit-Smullvan's suggestion that when dissonance exists on a status dimension there is a tendency for status equilibration.[11]

Low Education and Upward Mobility in Nursing

Exline and Ziller[12] purport that attempts at status equilibration may lead to conflict: one's overall status often depends on improving one's own standing at the expense of others on one dimension, while at the same time maintaining one's standing on other dimensions in the presence of equilibration attempts by others.

There may be an attempt at status equilibration in nursing today—a new position, the nurse practitioner, is being developed. The nurse practitioner may be defined as a nurse with a master's degree who has achieved in-depth clinical knowledge and expertise in patient care and who continues to function directly and somewhat autonomously with patients. The development of this position can be interpreted as an attempt by the nurse formerly interested in bedside nursing or direct patient care to attain equilibration in status. Heretofore, this equilibration could be achieved only by relinquishing the position of bedside nurse for an upward mobility position such as that of administrator or nurse educator.

Low Education and Dissonance in Nursing

When colleges and universities began to hire nursing faculty members who had had no lengthy bedside experience, or who had begun to withdraw from work with patients to teaching, differences of perspective between service and education were intensified.[6] The baccalaureate nurse became identified with the nurse educators. Many hospital colleagues began to view the baccalaureate nurse as needlessly overeducated or, as Davis et al.[7] comment, "long on theory and short on practice." Strauss[6] observes that the policing or raising of standards that educators have taken upon themselves augments the tension frequently found in professions in which the training programs are conducted partially or totally separate from the job.

Corwin,[9] Williamson,[8] and Keller[13] agree that much of the internal conflict in nursing is produced by the discrete differences in perspectives between practitioners and educators. Some writers[9, 13, 14] believe that professional education has given knowledge to the individual practitioner but has neither equipped her to apply it in the intended ways nor guaranteed the direction of her effort. As a result there is role discrepancy—a discrepancy between concepts and the actual work experience. Aydelotte[15] accuses faculty members of failing to extract from their knowledge base that which is relevant both to the purpose of nursing and to the care of the patient. She also emphasizes that teaching the *use* of knowledge in professional performance should be the focus of professional education.[16] The education of "supernurses" may tend to produce its own high-status-consistent hierarchy. At present there seem to be clear status divisions between those who have earned degrees and those who perform the practical tasks on the hospital ward. Will the nursing profession be able to withstand the pressures that may result from possible conflict among the different status groups?

Levine[4] warns that "there is enough anti-intellectualism in our society without allowing it to destroy the nursing profession." She is particularly alarmed about the fact that the best-educated nurses are the first to be declared surplus. Sheahan[5] expresses similar concern and states that doctors, hospital administrators, and many nurses maintain that a nurse does not need a college education. Furthermore, Sheahan believes that an investigation of the performance of the core workers in the hospital would verify their conviction. Aydelotte[15] observes that one group of nurses, who may be low-status-consistent or status-inconsistent, lives in a world of tradition, anti-intellectualism, and blind acceptance of constraints. The other group, composed of high-status-consistent nurses, believes in myths about what constitutes effective practice and denies the constraints that are real. As a result, the patient and the new graduate are caught between these two worlds.

Little research has been conducted to study the relationship between status consistency or status inconsistency and prejudice or discrimination,[2] although these judgments do exist and may affect the interaction between low- and high-status-consistent nurses. Presumably, low-status-consistent nurses would express their prejudice against high-status-consistent persons by downgrading their education or position. High-status-consistent nurses may discriminate against low-status-consistent nurses through bias in mobility practices. These relationships need to be examined.

Implications of Status Inconsistency for Coordination of the Nursing Profession

For nursing, the value system of a hospital is based more on performance and seniority than on amount of education. The hospital rewards conformity to administrative policies and procedures. Hospital status and positions are officially delegated through the authority mechanisms of the organizational system, whereas a value system based on higher education grants status and position through certification and professional peer group approval.[8] As a result, nursing students are confused in their role as professionals in the hospital and may be severely limited in practicing the tenets of professionalism. Removed to some degree from reality, the nursing educator may present an idealized version of hospital work. As a result, discrepancies may develop between the ideal and the actual practice of nursing.[9]

Technical nursing prevails in the hospital, and nurses are rewarded for performance of skills developed through practical experience rather than for the theory they may have learned at a university school of nursing.[5, 10] Keller[13] summarizes the present situation in nursing accordingly: educators are preoccupied with theory construction and practitioners are stymied by the multiple organizational impediments at all levels in the hospital. Despite equilibration attempts in nursing, a conflict still exists between the high-consistent-status nurse and nurses with inconsistent or low-consistent status. The conflict may be reflected by the manner in which they view nursing theory and nursing practice.

Status Inconsistency and the Development of Nursing as a Profession

Achieving professional status is a complicated process. The complexities involved in attaining this goal are evident in nursing. Etzioni[17] has observed that few professionals talk as much about being professionals as those whose professional status is in doubt. He states that nursing leaders, especially those teaching in university schools of nursing, talk a great deal about being professionals. That seems understandable because one of their objectives is to help nursing attain full-fledged professional status.

According to Hughes[18], the word *professional* in our society is more than a descriptive term; it is an indication of value and prestige. Perhaps people who are engaged in a certain occupation may attempt to revise the concept that the public has of the occupation and of the people in it. They also may attempt to revise their own conceptions of themselves and of their work. Nurses are attempting to create for themselves certain specialties and to proclaim that they have unique missions. Independent nurse practitioners, nurse practitioners, and clinical specialists now exist, and distinctions are being made between the technical and the professional nurse. Bucher and Strauss[19] point out that such distinctions are characteristic of the development of a profession. However, Hughes[18] reminds us that if any one group in a profession attempts to enhance its own status without some care for the status of others, the budding profession may have internal conflict.

Hughes[18] points out that one way for an occupation to gain prestige is for the training of its members for lower-status tasks to be discontinued. Such an attempt was made by the American Nurses Association by describing the differences between a professional and a technical nurse. (The *professional* nurse is a graduate of a baccalaureate degree program, whereas the *technical* nurse is a holder of an associate degree or is a graduate of a hospital-based diploma granting program.) There has been pressure by nursing leaders to terminate diploma programs, even though 32 percent of all nurses graduated in 1974 were educated in hospital-based programs.[20]

Most writers claim that the differences between professional and technical practice are differences in *kind*, not in level, amount, or degree.[21] However, Moore found, in her study of graduates of baccalaureate programs, that none of the respondents indicated that the baccalaureate graduate contributes a different *kind* of skill or knowledge to the care of the patient. Thus, Norris[22] says nurses from all three types of programs function in the same way, perform the same tasks, and take the same state board examinations. She concludes that nursing is still an occupation that depends on practical knowledge and good common sense.

Sheahan[5] emphasizes that labeling one nurse professional and another technical does not *make* one professional and the other technical. Without categorical distinctions in nursing practice, separate levels of nursing education are hardly justified. Every working group does some boundary watching in the performance of its roles, but the preoccupation with role distinctions found in nursing is greater than normal. Despite the nurse's attempt to professionalize her role, the physician's orders, as well as his expectations of the role of the nurse, are the principal source of social control and the chief determinant of the actions of nurses. To a large extent, nursing is dependent on the physician for the legitimation of whatever status it may try to achieve. The labeling of different types of nurses seems only to confuse the situation—not only for nurses and physicians but also for the patient.

Goode[23] suggests a possible correlation between the degree of community in a profession and the extent of differentiation between the values of the practitioners and those of the patients. One thing is obvious in nursing today: between members and nonmembers, and even among nurses themselves, role definitions are not agreed on. Goode states that it is critical for members of a profession to have a shared identity. This shared identity is the central element of a community. The profession cannot achieve status if it ceases to be a community. With so many divisions within the nursing profession, one wonders how effective a community can exist.

House[24] states that nurses often return to school for status associated with the degree rather than to improve their professional skills. Some nurses believe that the hospital is the only setting where one can become professionally competent, but because there is little status in the practice setting they decide to earn a degree. The implications of this situation are clearly dangerous for the nursing profession. Nurses must value education as a means of improving their professional competence, and nurse educators should devise new ways for applying knowledge to clinical practice. If such changes are not considered, improved status may still be denied to nursing as a profession.

HYPOTHESES

In the original study, there were no predictions made about a conflict in nursing, because the primary purpose of the study was to demonstrate empirically a relationship between expectations and perceptions of role behavior and status consistency or status inconsistency.* However, it was believed that status consistency might be related to the problem of status in nursing and perceptions of nursing education and nursing practice.

METHODS

Sampling Procedure

A purposive sampling design was used because it was not possible to obtain randomness. The sample was drawn from ten institutions in an eastern metropolitan city, which were chosen on the basis of representativeness in type as well as in regard to the nursing roles existing in the institutions. The institutions chosen were as follows: public health organization, Veterans Administration hospital, city hospital, nursing home, large private hospital, small private hospital, Jewish hospital, health maintenance organization, state mental hospital, and university school of nursing faculty.

The sample consisted of 303 registered nurses in various nursing roles (Table 9-1).

Instrument

An opinion-response questionnaire of seventy-two items was developed, pretested, and administered to each person in a face-to-face interview. It consisted of Likert-type scales and solicited responses along a continuum, designed to measure attitude

*These findings are reported in an article by N. L. Chaska, "Status Consistency and Nurses' Expectations and Perceptions of Role Performance," *Nursing Research*, in press.

Table 9-1 Nursing Roles and Number of Subjects Represented in Sample

Role	Number
Clinical specialists	9
Nurse practitioners	15
Nurse educators	20
Head nurses	36
Supervisors	29
In-service educators	19
Nursing administrators	11
Public health nurses	13
Private duty nurses	3
Staff nurses	141
Other roles	7
Total	303

on major variables of the study. Ten items about attitudes relative to nursing education and nursing practice were included.

Construction of Type of Status Consistency Index

Type of status consistency was determined by three items: education, position, and income. According to the responses about these three items, type of consistency was designated for each subject: high-status-consistent, low-status-consistent, or one of the six possible types of inconsistency (Table 9-2).

Because there were too few subjects in each type of inconsistent status for statistical analysis to be performed with the other variables included in this study, the inconsistent status categories were combined. Statistical analysis using the variable *type of consistency* thus included three groups: high-status-consistent (28), low-status-consistent (185), and status-inconsistent (90).

FINDINGS AND DISCUSSION

Table 9-3 shows the distribution of the type of consistency for each position held by respondents in the study. The seven errors in coding were believed to be insufficient to require recoding of the data. As expected, most low-status-consistent nurses were staff nurses. Most of the high-status-

Table 9-2   Type of Status Consistency of Subjects

Type	Number	%
High-status-consistent—education high, position high, income high	28	9.2
Low-status-consistent—education low, position low, income low	185	61.1
Inconsistent status—		
Education high, position high, income low	30	9.9
Education high, position low, income high	4	1.3
Education high, position low, income low	14	4.6
Education low, position high, income high	10	3.3
Education low, position high, income low	23	7.6
Education low, position low, income high	9	3.0
Total	303	100.0

Table 9-3   Type of Status Consistency of Subjects by Type of Position of Subjects

Position	Type of consistency		Inconsistent status*						Total
	High	Low	Ed H, posi H, inc L	Ed H, posi L, inc H	Ed H, posi L, inc L	Ed L, posi H, inc H	Ed L, posi H, inc L	Ed L, posi L, inc H	
Clinical specialists	3	0	4	0	2†	0	0	0	9
Nurse practitioners	4	0	9	0	1†	0	1	0	15
Educators	7	0	13	0	0	0	0	0	20
Head nurses	1	30	0	0	1	1†	1†	2	36
Supervisors	2	0	1	0	1	5	20	0	29
Staff nurses	1	131	1	1	3	1	0	3	141
In-service educators	0	11	0	3	2	1†	0	2	19
Nurse administrators	7	0	1	0	0	2	1	0	11
Public health nurses	2	9	0	0	2	0	0	0	13
Private duty nurses	0	2	0	0	0	0	0	1	3
Other roles	0	2	0	0	2	0	0	1	5
Error in coding	1	0	0	0	0	0	0	0	1
Error in coding	0	0	1	0	0	0	0	0	1
Total	28	185	30	4	14	10	23	9	303

*Abbreviations: Ed = education, posi = position, inc = income, H = high, and L = low.

†Error in coding.

consistent nurses were educators and administrators. The most common type of inconsistent status was education high, position high, and income low; most respondents in this group were clinical specialists, nurse practitioners, and nurse educators. Because all subjects in these three roles had master's degrees, they were expected by the investigator to be high-status-consistent; however, most were status-inconsistent. Apparently, nurses with higher education who are of inconsistent status are not being adequately compensated financially for their level of education. (However, it should be pointed out that status consistency in this study was not measured by performance.) This inadequate level of compensation may lead such a nurse to question the value of her education or to have low morale and lack of motivation.

Of the 303 subjects in the sample, 180 (59.4

percent) were graduated from a hospital diploma program, 24 (7.9 percent) from an associate degree program, and 99 (32.7 percent) from a baccalaureate degree program. Of the total sample, 153 (50.5 percent) had additional education beyond their basic program (Table 9-4).

Of the total sample, the total mean length of employment was 8.597 years. The subjects were asked in separate questions how many years they had been employed full-time and part-time, and the means were 7.578 years and 8.971 years, respectively. The most frequently reported monthly income was $800 to $1,199 (143 or 47.2 percent of the subjects). The mean age of the subjects was 31.25 years.

The data were analyzed to see whether the manner in which subjects viewed nursing education and nursing practice varied according to type of status consistency. There were no predictions made in the study, but it was believed that status consistency might be related to the problem of status and conflict in nursing. The responses to these statements that showed a significant relationship between these factors are shown in Tables 9-5, 9-6, 9-7, and 9-8.

There was high agreement (57.3 percent) among low-status-consistent nurses that nurses who have low education and a high position in nursing are more likely to function effectively in the practice of nursing than are those with higher education (Table 9-5). Most low-status-consistent nurses did not have a master's degree. According to Geschwender[2], if educational investment is the low dimension in the hierarchy of status, the group involved may perceive education as being impractical. Some inconsistent-status nurses (44.4 percent) also agreed with the statement. This is more difficult to understand, because many of the inconsistent-status nurses in this sample had master's degrees. Perhaps despite her high investment in education, this nurse has not been able to achieve desired status through upward mobility. The response of the inconsistent-status nurse, who has a master's degree, to this statement may also be related to the fact that she has a low income and may thus consider herself inadequately compensated for her education. The question remains as to how much the inconsistent-status nurse values her education.

Table 9-4   Type of Additional Education of Subjects Beyond Their Basic Program

Type of education	Numbers	%
Credits toward B. S. degree	49	32.02
B. S. degree but not in nursing	4	2.61
B. S. degree in nursing	11	7.19
Graduate of nurse practitioner program	7	4.58
Credits toward master's degree	13	8.50
Master's degree but not in nursing	5	3.27
Master's degree in nursing	48	31.37
Credits toward doctorate	9	5.88
Doctorate in education, sociology, anthropology, psychology	6	3.92
Doctor of Nursing Science	1	0.65
Total	153	100.00

Low-status-consistent and inconsistent-status subjects agreed more often than did high-status-consistent subjects with the statement that it was more important to have practical experience in nursing than a degree (Table 9-6). This response was expected from the low-inconsistent-status group. Those of the inconsistent-status group who have a master's degree may be experiencing a discrepancy between the ideal projected in the educational program and the realities of actual practice. Because some of those inconsistent-status subjects are nurse-educators, perhaps they suffer from a role conflict between their identity as nurse practitioners and their positions as educators. They may be identifying more with nursing practice than with nursing education. If nurses perceive that they can achieve the same status with or without a degree, they may not be motivated to obtain higher degrees and role confusion may ensue.

The findings presented thus far are further supported by the following responses. Low-status-consistent and inconsistent-status subjects agreed more often than did high-status-consistent subjects that if one is to have a high position in nursing it is not necessary to have higher educational prepara-

Table 9-5 Statement: Nurses Who Have Low Education (Bachelor's Degree or Less) and a High Position in Nursing Are More Likely to Function Effectively in the Practice of Nursing Than Are Those with a High Education Level (Answers Categorized by Type of Status Consistency)

	Type of consistency		
Response*	High-consistent (N = 28)	Low-consistent (N = 185)	Inconsistent (N = 90)
Agree	21.4%	57.3%	44.4%
Disagree	78.6%	42.7%	55.6%

*χ^2 = 14.1913; P < 0.0008.

Table 9-6 Statement: It is More Important to Have Practical Experience in Nursing Than a Degree (Answers Categorized by Type of Status Consistency)

	Type of consistency		
Response*	High-consistent (N = 28)	Low-consistent (N = 185)	Inconsistent (N = 90)
Agree	26.6%	64.9%	61.1%
Disagree	73.4%	35.1%	38.9%

*χ^2 = 15.1905; P < 0.0005.

Table 9-7 Statement: If One is to Have a High Position in Nursing It Is Not Necessary to have High Education Preparation (Answers Categorized by Type of Status Consistency)

	Type of consistency		
Response*	High-consistent (N = 28)	Low-consistent (N = 185)	Inconsistent (N = 90)
Agree	14.3%	41.6%	32.2%
Disagree	85.7%	58.4%	67.8%

*χ^2 = 8.7810; P < 0.0124.

tion (Table 9-7). However, in each category a higher percentage of subjects disagreed with the statement. Low-status-consistent nurses may detect that education has not made a significant difference in the quality of performance, the type of tasks performed, or the skills used by nurses who have master's degrees.

It is important to note that the majority of subjects in this sample are employed in hospitals. The practice setting of the hospital does not seem to require the theoretical knowledge possessed by the nurse with higher education. One cannot conclude from the responses to the above statements, however, that nurses do not apply their theoretical

Table 9-8 Statement: I Am Satisfied with my Job, Education, and Income (Answers Categorized by Type of Status Consistency)

	Type of consistency		
Response*	High-consistent (N = 28)	Low-consistent (N = 185)	Inconsistent (N = 90)
Agree	64.3%	49.2%	34.4%
Disagree	35.7%	50.8%	65.6%

*$\chi^2 = 9.3534; P < 0.0093.$

knowledge in their practice. Some persons, as clinical specialists, may be overqualified for positions available in the hospital. Even though the assessment of patient needs and the planning and evaluation of care may rightfully belong to the more highly educated nurse, the demands of technology in the hospital may reward technical skills rather than utilization of theoretical knowledge.

Among the types of status-consistency groups, high-status-consistent nurses are the most satisfied with their jobs, education, and income, and the inconsistent-status subjects are the least satisfied (Table 9-8)—an expected finding. As previously mentioned, low income may be one of the reasons the inconsistent-status subjects are dissatisfied (Table 9-3). As shown in Tables 9-2 and 9-3, the most common inconsistent status was the type in which education was high, position was high, and income was low. From Tables 9-5, 9-6, 9-7, and 9-8 one might conclude that, in general, the low-status-consistent and inconsistent-status nurses tended to consider the need for a degree or higher education in nursing of less value than did high-status-consistent nurses.

Subjects in all categories tended to agree with the following statements:

1 Nurse educators have great knowledge of theory but little knowledge of nursing practice.
2 Nurse educators are "ivory towerish."
3 There is a conflict in nursing between those in nursing education and those in nursing practice.

In addition, subjects in all categories tended to disagree with these three statements:

1 Staff nurses have great knowledge of nursing practice and little knowledge of theory.
2 The more education a nurse has the less likely she will be able to apply this to nursing practice.
3 I have been prevented from obtaining a job in nursing because of insufficient education.

There were no significant differences among the high-status-consistent, low-status-consistent, and inconsistent-status group responses to all of the above statements.

SUMMARY AND CONCLUSION

What ever conflict may exist in nursing today between those in nursing education and those in nursing practice is not necessarily related to the type of status consistency of the nurse. Only four of the questionnaire statements concerning nursing education and practice were significantly related to the type of status consistency of the nurse. The majority of nurses in this sample, regardless of type of status consistency, agree that there is a conflict between nursing education and nursing practice. Status-consistency theory does not explain this conflict in nursing.

REFERENCES

1 Treiman, D. J.: "Status Discrepancy and Prejudice," *American Journal of Sociology*, **81**:651–654, 1966.
2 Geschwender, J. A.: "Continuities in Theories of Status Consistency and Cognitive Dissonance," *Social Forces,* **46**:160–171, 1967.

3 Sampson, E. E.: "Status Congruence and Cognitive Consistency," *Sociometry*, **26**:146–162, 1963.

4 Levine, M.: "Nursing Educators—An Alienating Elite," *Chart*, **69**:56–61, 1972.

5 Sheahan, D.: "The Game of the Name: Nurse Professional and Nurse Technician," *Nursing Outlook*, **20**:440–444, 1973.

6 Strauss, A.: "The Structure and Ideology of American Nursing: An Interpretation," in Fred Davis (ed.), *The Nursing Profession: Five Sociological Essays,* John Wiley, New York, 1966.

7 Davis, F., V. L. Olesen, and E. W. Whittaker: "Problems and Issues in Collegiate Nursing Education," in Fred Davis (ed.), *The Nursing Profession: Five Sociological Essays,* John Wiley, New York, 1966.

8 Williamson, J. A.: "The Conflict-producing Role of the Professionally Socialized Nurse-Faculty Member," *Nursing Forum*, **11**:356–366, 1972.

9 Corwin, R.: "The Professional Employee: A Study of Conflict in Nursing Roles," *American Journal of Sociology*, **66**:604–615, 1961.

10 Corwin, R.: "Role Conception and Career Aspiration: A Study of Identity in Nursing," *The Sociological Quarterly*, **2**:69–86, 1961.

11 Hershey, N.: "Expanded Roles for Professional Nurses," *The Journal of Nursing Administration*, **3**:30–33, 1972.

12 Exline, R. V., and R. Ziller: "Status Congruency and Interpersonal Conflict in Decision-making Groups," *Human Relations*, **12**:147–162, 1959.

13 Keller, N. S.: "The Nurse's Role: Is It Expanding or Shrinking?" *Nursing Outlook*, **21**:236–240, 1972.

14 Gaynor, A., and R. K. Barry: "Observations of a Staff Nurse: An Organizational Analysis," *The Journal of Nursing Administration,* **3**:43–49, 1973.

15 Aydelotte, M. K.: "Nursing Education and Practice: Putting It All Together," *The Journal of Nursing Education,* **2**:21–27, 1972.

16 Sheahan, D.: "Degree, Yes—Education, No," *Nursing Outlook*, **22**:22–26, 1974.

17 Etzioni, A., (ed.): *Semi-Professions and Their Organization: Teachers, Nurses and Social Workers*, Free Press, New York, 1969.

18 Hughes, E. C.: *The Sociological Eye: Selected Papers on Work, Self, and the Study of Society,* Aldine-Atherton, Chicago and New York, 1971.

19 Bucher, R., and A. Strauss: "Professions in Process," *Nursing Times*, **69**:482, 1973.

20 National League for Nursing: *N.L.N. State Approved Schools of Nursing—R.N.*, 33d ed., Division of Research, National League for Nursing, New York, 1975.

21 Moore, M.: "The Professional Practice of Nursing: The Knowledge and How It Is Used," *Nursing Forum*, **8**:361–373, 1969.

22 Norris, C. M.: "Delusions That Trap Nurses," *Canadian Nurse*, **69**:37–40, 1973.

23 Goode, W.: "Community Within a Community: The Professions," *American Sociological Review,* **22**:194–200, 1957.

24 House, C.: "College-Education Tailor-made for Me," *American Journal of Nursing*, **73**:297–298, 1973.

EDITOR'S QUESTIONS FOR DISCUSSION

What alternative explanations might be offered for the finding that indicates a high level of agreement by inconsistent-status nurses that nurses who have low education and a high position in nursing are more likely to function effectively in the practice of nursing than are those with higher education? What further implications are there for nursing education in the findings that inconsistent-status subjects agreed more often than high-status-consistent subjects that it was more important to have practical experience in nursing than a degree? What evidence is there that nurses with newly acquired master's degrees experience "reality shock" as attributed to baccalaureate graduates? What other explanation(s) might be offered about why high-status-consistent nurses value higher education more than inconsistent-status nurses?

Chapter 10

The Development of Doctoral Education in Nursing: A Historical Perspective

Helen K. Grace, R.N., Ph.D., F.A.A.N.
Dean and Professor, College of Nursing
University of Illinois at the Medical Center, Chicago

Having read about the perceptions of some nurses concerning higher education, the reader may find an overview of the current trends regarding doctoral education for nurses helpful. The contribution of Helen K. Grace traces the problems in nursing and nursing education from their inception up to and including present-day trends. Grace localizes what may well be the critical problem inhibiting the development of nursing as a profession—that nursing is perceived solely as a practice discipline, devoid of a need for any scientific base for practice. Grace views doctoral education in nursing as a means of acquiring scientific authority for the foundation of nursing practice. The first form of doctoral education for nurses was to instruct them in functional specialties for teaching and administration. The second form was for nurses to be prepared in scientific disciplines related to nursing. The third form, currently emphasized, is the development of actual doctoral programs in nursing. Grace emphasizes the importance of such programs that are striving to prepare expert clinicians grounded in research skills.

The history of the development of doctoral education *for* nurses and *in* nursing is a reflection of the social forces that have surrounded the development of the field of nursing. Indeed, the struggles reflected in the development of nursing as a profession and doctoral education as a part of this developmental process mirror the struggles of women through the ages in defining a position of equality and worth. Doctoral education *for* nurses and *in* nursing is part of a political process to secure for nurses a position of authority within the larger health care system. This paper traces first the problems affecting the development of nursing, and second the evolution of nursing education within this context. Research in nursing provides further evidence of developmental trends. Finally, current models for doctoral education in nursing are described and future directions advocated.

PROBLEMS IN THE DEVELOPMENT OF NURSING

A consistent problem through the years has been that of the development of nursing within the constraints of the medical care domain. The origins of modern nursing serve to place these struggles into a proper perspective. In *A Century of Nursing*, Woolsey describes the origins of European and

American nursing. Prior to the late 1800s, nursing was entirely managed by religious orders assisted by "nurses" recruited from the lower strata of society. It is of interest to note that at that time considerable conflict existed between nursing, which was run by religious orders, and hospital administration and medicine. Referring to Davenne, a French writer, Woolsey describes the situation: "Being subject to their own religious superiors—an authority outside the hospital—and being bound by their own rules, the sisters never cooperate with the secular administration as heartily as secular subordinates (1950, pp. 10–11)." Contrary to seeing this lack of subordination as problematic, Florence Nightingale spoke of the positive aspects of this conflict:

Great have been the scrimmages from time to time between the administration and the religious orders, and great have been the benefits accruing to the sick from such scrimmages. The administration complains of the sisters, and the doctors wish the sisters were under them. The sisters complain of the administration, and wish that the sisterhood had it completely under itself. But the balance is kept up; all are the best possible friends, and the collision and competition do the greatest possible good (Woolsey, 1950, p. 27).

Nursing, instead of viewing these inherent conflicts as positive, has tended to allow these forces to impede its development.

The struggles described in the early history of nursing are not too dissimilar from those of the current situation, with the exception that the sisters were in a stronger position than nurses are today in that they could claim that their authority came from God. Present-day nursing, needing to lay claim to higher authority to secure its place, now looks to education and the *scientific* as its basis for practice instead of God. It would appear that the sisters, with their ties and claims to Divine authority, were remarkably successful. Hopefully, laying claim to scientific authority as the basis of further nursing practice will be equally successful. In effect, the development of doctoral education may be viewed as an attempt to solidify and expand the body of scientific knowledge and to use it as leverage in securing an equitable position within the health care system.

Nursing through the ages has had difficulty in developing a professional identity in its own right. Rather, it has tended to be associated with other purposes such as those derived from its religious origins and secondarily as a profession appropriate to women. The development of nursing under religious orders served a dual purpose; the sick and outcasts of society were cared for, but, perhaps more importantly, nursing was viewed as a means of spiritual development for nurses. Moving nursing out of this context was viewed as problematic. As Woolsey describes the situation:

It is claimed that the plan of putting the ward nurse directly under the ward doctor insures good nursing, i.e., nurses that please the doctor. But if patients are better nursed than they would be where nursing is under the oversight of a woman superintendent or a sister superior, which the writer will not admit, the nurses run the risk of destruction, body and soul. There is not a single element of moral supervision in this plan (1950, p. 38).

It is important to note that then, as now, nursing and the quality of nursing care was not the central aim of the profession. Nursing was directed toward benefits accruing to the nurse, namely, the moral development of her character.

The nature of nursing work is such that it has been considered menial labor. A consistent problem has been that of getting a higher class of women into the nursing profession. Even the sisters in the religious orders were from the lower strata of society. This problem was even more acute in countries such as England, where the religious orders were not as strong an influence. In many instances paupers were recruited as nurses and did nursing in exchange for room and board. Nurses of this time were described as:

. . . feeble old women, who know nothing about nursing, who cannot read the printed labels on medicine bottles and whose love of drink often leads them to beg or rob the stimulants which they should give the sick, and because their treatment of the sick is not characterized by either judgment or gentleness (Woolsey, 1950, p. 90).

To correct these ills, it was advocated that "A money allowance for pauper helpers should be made instead of beer or gin, and a badge of honor and whatever else can excite emulation and promote self-respect should be introduced. Ability to read is an essential requirement in a nurse (Woolsey, 1950, p. 90)." Nursing could be considered to have been a learned profession in its early stages.

Given the nature of nursing as "dirty work" one way of recruiting a refined class of women into the profession was to appeal to womanly virtues and the "fit" between women's roles and nursing. Woolsey, quoting Dr. Henry W. Ackland in his preface to Miss Lee's *Handbook for Hospital Sisters*, claims that:

Nursing is a department of the profession of medicine and surgery; it is the MEDICAL WORK OF WOMEN, and a fit object for the employment of the practical ability, and for the exercise of high moral qualities. It furnishes an outlet for the tender power and skill of good women of almost every class, as superintendents of hospitals or as ward sisters or nurses (Woolsey, 1950, p. 96).

Nursing through the years has been described as a woman's profession. Indeed, much of the early literature speaks of the lack of ability on the part of men to provide nursing care. Men were considered slovenly, unfeeling, and therefore unfit to be nurses. They were, however, considered fit to be doctors.

It is doubtful whether nursing would have advanced the way it has had it not been for the influence of wars upon the development of the profession. Through the years wars have provided opportunities for nursing to make progressive developmental steps that probably would not have occurred under peacetime conditions. Florence Nightingale, herself a member of the middle class, entered nursing on the basis of a "call" to some form of higher service. Responding to this call, she left home, contrary to the norm for middle class girls of her time, and began the pursuit of an independent career in nursing. Seymer summarizes the problems that Florence Nightingale had to overcome, and in so doing laid the foundation for the development of the profession. First, those in authority perceived her coming to the battlefield as an expression of lack of confidence in their ability. She was faced with the hostility and opposition of medical staff and other officers. Second, she had to deal with the unreliability of her nursing staff; and third, she was faced with the religious antagonisms of Protestant and Catholic nurses. Her methods of dealing with these problems included (1) winning over the officials by endless tact and patience, (2) improving the nursing staff by weeding out incompetents and keeping the others under her strict supervision, and (3) overcoming the religious antagonisms by distributing Catholics and Protestants throughout the wards (Seymer, 1949, pp. 85–86). Miss Nightingale demonstrated her abilities to deal with the political problems that to this day plague the profession—those of the relationship between nursing and medicine, of policing a profession that has minimal technical training and little professional identification, and of dealing with conflicting loyalties that interfere with commitment to the development of the nursing profession.

Cast within this historical framework, the evolution of the nursing profession has occurred within a political context that has placed many constraints upon the developmental process. Conflicts within administrative hierarchy, the effects of sexism, and circumscribed roles for women are but a few of the constraints. In this context, doctoral education *for* nurses and *in* nursing is but another step in the overall struggle for independence and recognition of worth.

NURSING EDUCATION AND ITS PLACE IN THE DEVELOPMENT OF THE PROFESSION

Throughout the history of nursing, education has been viewed as the vehicle for gaining strength in the political arena that surrounds the field. Doctoral education in nursing is the most recent step in this struggle and its development is faced with similar hurdles. Matarazzo summarizes the prevalent attitude of many:

> I simply do not understand why a nurse would want to give up taking temperatures, making beds, and otherwise comforting patients—the *real* nursing—which she does so well to fool with the business of research, which she clearly does so poorly. Can you honestly tell me why you would want to give up nursing for science? (1971, pp. 88–89).

Nursing is viewed solely as a practice field; the need for developing the scientific basis of this practice is not considered. This theme is repeated consistently throughout the history of nursing education.

Nursing education originated in hospitals as a source of cheap labor. A quote from a paper delivered at the World's Fair of 1893 by Lavinia L. Dock, the director of nursing at Johns Hopkins, clearly depicts the climate surrounding the development of training programs:

> The organization of a training school is and must be military. It is not and cannot be democratic. Absolute and unquestioning obedience must be the foundation of the nurse's work, and to this end complete subordination of the individual to the work as a whole is as necessary for her as for the soldier . . . if the military idea is the basis of the school, the members of the medical profession being undoubtedly the superior officers should properly control the school throughout its entire course, and even in its internal management, and the whole subject of the teaching, training, and discipline of nurses should be at the discretion of medicine. . . . There is much evidence to show that the material prosperity of the hospital is largely due

to the work of the training school. . . . The discipline and strict subordination of the school make it possible for the hospital to exact from it an amount of work which it would be quite impossible to demand from women over whom it had no special hold; while the chain of responsibility and the careful supervision of the school secure an average quality of work as good, if not better, than that which would be obtained from nurses working mainly as employees (1893, pp. 16–18).

This early picture of nursing education not only reflects its total subservience to the medical profession, but also provides a picture of the role of women in the late nineteenth century. In that era, schools of nursing were developed to reform hospitals by providing a dependable labor force. Those initial goals had little relationship to educational goals for the preparation of nurses. Improvement of nursing was viewed as being dependent primarily upon the rigid control of students and secondarily upon an improved system of education.

The first graduate education available to nurses was developed at Teachers College, Columbia University, in 1899 in the fields of hospital economics and educational administration. This particular development in education reflects the managerial goals of the early training schools. A major aim was to prepare nurses to train other nurses to meet the goals of hospitals.

Mary Adelaide Nutting was among the first to advocate reforms in nursing. In 1908 she stated:

> There is no place in its [the hospital's] strenuous scheme of life for the machinery of a school. All the space, the effort, the means which the hospital can provide are needed to carry out its immediate purpose, which is the care of the sick, and any scheme of education must, of necessity, take a secondary and insignificant place . . . the hospital has full power to restrict . . . teaching in various ways; it may reduce the ground covered in a certain subject to the barest outline. . . . The individual who thinks "this idea of teaching nurses so much is all nonsense, anyway" will not view with

favor anything which carries the pupil nurse
very far from her long hours of practical work
in the wards and he will be especially suspicious, and apt to shy violently at the mention
of bacteriology, for instance, or the still more
dangerous subject of pathology (1926, pp.
18–39).

The education of nurses was not encouraged in
such a milieu; indeed it was feared that nurses
might become too knowledgable and thus pose a
threat to the established medical hierarchy. The
development of nursing education *as education*
could occur only with great difficulty in so hostile
an environment.

In 1923 the Rockefellers supported a study,
*Nursing and Nursing Education in the United
States*, comparable to the Flexner report on
medicine. Known as the Goldmark Report, it
advocated removing the control of nursing education from hospitals, placing it within the educational system, and developing sounder educational
programs (1923). For the first time the move from
hospital-based training programs to the mainstream of American education had been suggested.

The report had little impact. A few schools of
nursing developed in universities with educational
programs organized in the same way as other disciplines, but until the middle of the twentieth
century, most schools of nursing were owned,
controlled, and operated by hospitals. They
remained the principal source of supply for hospital and other nursing services. The first noticeable
change in this pattern occurred in the mid-1940s
at the close of World War II. At this time large
numbers of nurses who had served in the armed
forces came home with aspirations to use the
G.I. Bill of Rights to attain a college education.
The post-World War II acceleration of the development of university schools of nursing was, at least
partially, a response to this demand.

Not surprisingly, the growth of university nurse
educational programs stimulated graduate study
in nursing to prepare nurses for teaching and
administrative positions in universities. Master's
degree programs in nursing were created and
expanded to meet this need. Then came the first
real wave of nurses with earned doctorates. They
received these degrees primarily in the field of
education: educational administration, educational psychology, curriculum and teaching, and
nursing education and administration. Following
this initial phase, increasing numbers of nurses
earned doctorates in the sciences to build for
themselves a solid base in clinical practice. By the
early 1960s, programs leading to doctoral degrees
in nursing began to be inaugurated. Figure 10-1
provides data depicting these trends.

The availability of federal funds has been a
factor in increasing the number of nurses earning
doctorates, particularly in scientific fields related
to nursing. The federal government developed two
mechanisms to accelerate the move of nurses into
doctoral education. In 1955, the United States
Public Health Service (National Institutes of
Health) started funding doctoral study through
Special Predoctoral Research Fellowships that
were applied for and awarded to the student
directly. As of September 1970, 156 nurses were
being supported through the Division of Nursing
fellowships (Matarazzo, 1971, p. 89).

A second source of federal funding has been
through the Nurse-Scientist Training Programs.
These grants were awarded directly to schools of
nursing to finance Ph.D.-level education in disciplines related to nursing. The intent underlying the
Nurse-Scientist Program was that of building a
critical mass of faculty for the development of
doctoral programs *in* nursing. A secondary function of the Nurse-Scientist program was that of
creating a receptive climate for the establishment
of doctoral programs in nursing. Nurses studying
in other areas of the university have demonstrated
their competence as scholars; interdepartmental
programming has served to develop collaboration
between nursing and other academic departments.
As doctoral programs in nursing develop, it is
anticipated that significant numbers of nurses will
continue seeking doctoral education in related scientific disciplines.

In speaking of the need for nurses prepared in
disciplines related to nursing, Schlotfeldt argues:

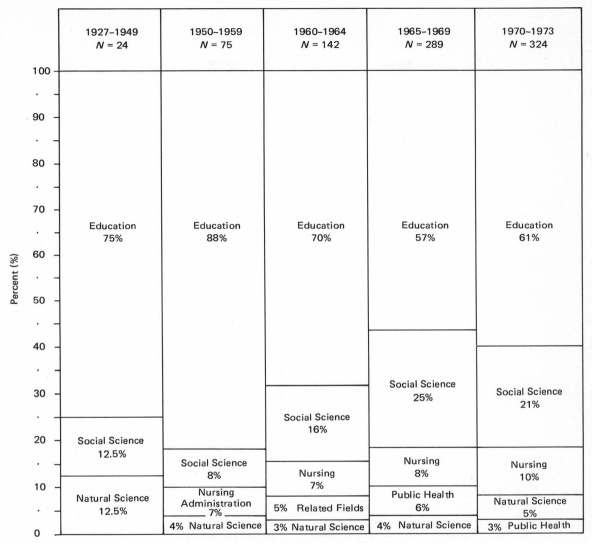

Figure 10-1   Distribution of field of preparation of doctorally prepared nurses.

There will, however, always be a need for some nurses to have training in disciplines relevant to nursing. Support for this position derives from the following considerations: (1) from the fact that nursing is an applied science needing investigators competent in the several sciences relevant to nursing practice, (2) from the need for nurse investigators competent to use, adapt and develop research procedures, tools and devices requiring knowledge of the basic sciences, (3) from a set of practical circumstances, and (4) from the generally accepted notion that advancement of knowledge is a desirable goal to which all able persons should have opportunity to contribute in accordance with their interests (1971, p. 123).

As doctoral education in nursing develops, the need for diversity of educational models becomes increasingly apparent.

Nursing education has obviously made the transition from its early origins in the hospital service structure to a secure position in the educational mainstream. Doctoral education for nurses has developed logically, first preparing them for education and administration, and then making them knowledgeable about the field and the research methodology used in basic scientific disciplines upon which the science and art of nursing rest. The development of doctoral programs *in nursing* is the third step in this logical progression. As a result of such diversity in the preparation of nurses, contemporary doctoral programs *in nursing* reflect the richness of this heritage. They encompass varying degrees of integration and synthesize related scientific fields into what is now a substantive field of nursing.

TYPES OF DOCTORAL PROGRAMS IN NURSING

The first form of doctoral education most readily available to nurses was that of the *functional specialty*. As has been noted in the history of the development of nursing education, doctoral education for nurses was first initiated by Columbia Teachers College in 1899 to prepare nurses to teach in nurse training programs. Throughout the years, nursing as a practice discipline has had a major need to prepare nurses for occupying functional roles as teachers and administrators in the profession. In programs of this type the emphasis is not upon substantive content of the discipline, but upon the methodologies and knowledge base necessary for teaching and administering of the discipline.

The second form of doctoral education for nurses was that of preparation in scientific disciplines related to the nursing field. A large number of nurses first sought preparation in the social sciences, and more recently increased emphasis has been placed upon biological sciences. As has been noted, the federal government, through the Nurse-Scientist program and through its programs of research fellowships, provided the impetus for

large numbers of nurses to gain doctoral preparation in basic scientific disciplines, with the anticipation that they would return to faculty positions in nursing and would provide the much needed input of basic science content and research into nursing.

Currently, considerable emphasis is being placed upon the development of doctoral programs *in* nursing. There are approximately ten such programs now operational throughout the country. Considerable controversy surrounds the nature of doctoral education in nursing. First and foremost, nurse educators hold differing views on the nature of research and theory development in nursing, with some viewing nursing as a pure science and others arguing that nursing is an applied field. Martha Rogers, for example, argues that "Nursing Science is a science of man. . . . Education for nursing's scholars and scientists requires that doctoral programs have as their core the critical and creative study of nursing (1971, p. 76)." Following this argument, doctoral level courses are structured around the science of man. In the research realm, the theoretic importance of research is stressed rather than the applicability of research findings to nursing settings.

A contrasting view, articulated by Erickson and Rubin, stresses integration of varying scientific perspectives into nursing. They argue that:

> The origin and destination of systematic investigation is in the nursing care of patients. Clinical practice, clinical teaching, and clinical research are inseparable components in academic learning at progressively higher levels (1971, p. 21).

In this framework, the primary purpose and organizing principle of doctoral education centers around the integration of knowledge from related disciplines, and research related to clinical practice. Perhaps the most problematic facet of doctoral education *in* nursing surrounds the clinical component and its place within a doctoral program. The difficulty of theory building in an applied field is described by Dickoff and James:

To consider what type of theory is needed for a professional discipline requires articulating professional purpose. A true professional, as opposed to a mere academic, is action oriented rather than being a professional spectator or commentator . . . . A true professional—as opposed to a mere visionary—shapes reality according to an articulate purpose . . . . a theory for a profession or practice discipline must provide for more than mere understanding or describing or even predicting reality and must provide conceptualization specifically intended to guide the shaping of reality to that profession's professional purpose. . . . Nursing must have an action that aims to shape reality, not hit or miss, but by a conception of ends as well as means (1973, p. 28).

The challenge in doctoral education in nursing is to move nursing theory from a descriptive level to one of intervention, and then to build this into the theoretical base of the profession.

MODEL FOR FURTHER DEVELOPMENT OF DOCTORAL PROGRAMS IN NURSING

How can these ambitious ends be attained within the nursing profession? The need for doctoral programs in nursing arises from an identification of gaps in currently existing bodies of knowledge and the need to integrate these bodies of knowledge to facilitate the investigation of and intervention in patient care situations. The history of nursing education reflects a pattern of drawing upon many bodies of scientific knowledge. The theoretical base on which nursing currently rests has been built from an amalgam of social and biological sciences. As these bodies of knowledge are brought together in nursing, gaps between scientific fields become increasingly apparent. Recognition of these gaps and the need for new knowledge provides the raison d'être for the development of doctoral programs in nursing. Perhaps an example will most clearly illustrate this point. Let us imagine a high-risk nursery in which care for premature infants is provided.

A common problem of premature infants is hyaline membrane disease. Research related to this problem may serve to illustrate significant gaps in the scientific knowledge base. Physician researchers are primarily interested in the disease process itself—its etiology, symptomatology, and treatment—and they are directed toward the immediate goal of keeping the infant alive. A physiologist may logically investigate such matters as the oxygen content of the blood under varying incubator conditions. The psychologist might be interested in the effect of hyaline membrane disease upon subsequent developmental processes, such as impairment of intelligence as a result of lack of adequate oxygen, while a sociologist's interest might be that of ascertaining the incidence of the disease in varying cultural groups under differing socioeconomic conditions. As all these scientists pursue their research interests, valuable knowledge is developed, but, at the same time, significant gaps occur. It is toward these gaps that research in nursing is directed.

What might a nurse-researcher focus upon that some of the others might not? A nurse-researcher is likely to focus upon the infant as a whole being within the context of his early living conditions and within the framework of his family. Taking the research findings from related scientific fields as to the nature of the disease, the conditions necessary to preserve life, and some of the long-range social and psychological effects of prematurity, nurses are raising questions about the long-range effects of spending the early days and weeks of one's life in an environment devoid of stimulation and human contact. Furthermore, nurses using research findings are beginning to experiment in altering the early living environment for such infants through the development of tools such as rocking devices, ticking instruments that simulate the mother's heartbeat, and other similar types of equipment. Testing out the long-range developmental progress of those who have been provided early stimulation compared with those who have not yields data useful in the development of new types of high-risk nursery settings.

Thus, nursing is building a body of knowledge that is uniquely nursing's. This is but one example of a multitude of problems that demand the investigation of highly skilled nurse-researchers and that encompass multiple variables in considering the total person within the context of his environment, whether it be a hospital, home, or community setting.

Given this perspective as to the need for development of a knowledge base for nursing, what types of doctoral programs are necessary to develop nurse researchers and practitioners? At least two distinctive models for doctoral education *in* nursing are needed to move the field to its next logical development phase. Current terminology in higher education would differentiate these degrees as professional in contrast to the academic degree. While in nursing there are differences in the name of the degree offered at various schools throughout the country, the objectives are not clearly differentiated and the end products are not clearly distinguished.

Of first priority is the development of research programs *in* nursing directed toward building the knowledge base upon which nursing practice must ultimately rest. The primary purpose of the research doctorate in nursing, from my point of view, is to develop a cadre of critical thinkers with the ability to analyze, synthesize, and test theories and to bring research findings from other areas of knowledge to bear upon nursing problems. Given these objectives, what is the program design for accomplishing these ends?

Of first importance is the assumption that the student entering a career of research in nursing has a firm footing in nursing and its practice. This is essential in providing the focal point around which the entire learning process is organized. The problems that nursing, as a practice discipline, must of necessity be concerned with, are not currently in the theoretic or abstract world, but should arise from the real world of nursing practice.

A critical look at the current state of health care delivery should serve to emphasize this point.

In examining our health care delivery system, one is immediately struck by the extent of scientific knowledge on the one hand, and the inadequate quality of health care available to the majority of Americans on the other. Bringing this closer to nursing, there are many areas of which we have extensive knowledge, such as the effects of over-stimulation upon sensory perception, but one look at the intensive care setting of any hospital will serve to illustrate how little of this knowledge is considered in the design of such settings. Nurses, in their research endeavors, can ill afford to constantly rediscover the wheel, but it is imperative that their research endeavors be directed to problems related to nursing.

With this focus in mind, doctoral education in nursing builds upon the assumption that nurses entering doctoral programs have a sound base in nursing. The focus of the research doctorate, then, is upon developing the research capabilities to investigate and generate knowledge directly pertinent to nursing. Second, the development of this base for nursing involves the integration of knowledge drawn from other scientific fields in a logical and consistent manner.

In constructing a doctoral program based upon this model, the first step consists of enabling the student to clearly conceptualize nursing in its current state of development. Through critically analyzing nursing theory, through critiquing the current state of nursing research, and through exploring the methodological problems of investigating clinical problems, the student gains the necessary focus and organizational perspective. A second step in the process consists of critically analyzing related scientific fields and applying these bodies of knowledge to nursing problems. Concepts such as systems, stress adaptation, and motivation are treated in many basic science disciplines. By seeing these concepts in the context of a variety of disciplines, the student can then systematically and logically fit these newly required perspectives into a better conceptualization of nursing. In the research realm a similar process of identifying varying approaches to the investigation of problems from related scientific disciplines and modifying these approaches to nursing situations provides the matrix for the development of the nurse researcher. With this as a base, students have the background for developing their own unique approaches to studying nursing problems by using what is applicable, modifying and adapting methodologies that might be useful, and in other instances developing new approaches to the study of specific problems.

In the theory realm, the final phase of the process is that of theory development. At this stage of our profession it is critical that theory be developed out of the practice setting rather than in the abstract. To accomplish these ends, field experiences designed to force the student to make actual observations of nursing, and from these observed practices to develop appropriate theory seem valuable and necessary. In this way, theoretical formulations are based not upon abstractions but upon the realities of the clinical practice setting.

These experiences in research and theory are designed specifically to develop a particular thinking style in the conceptualization of nursing and nursing research. Added to this must be the content of substantive knowledge necessary to allow students to build in the direction of their own research interests. This content includes the nurse's depth of knowledge of related scientific disciplines, as well as the necessary statistical base to be a competent researcher. With this type of programmatic structure researchers within nursing may be developed who in turn will build a knowledge base upon which nursing practice, education, and administration may build.

But it is not sufficient, given a field such as nursing, to have a corps of nurse researchers building such a knowledge base without also paying attention to the clinical field. As Dickoff and James pointed out earlier, not only must a profession be concerned with building a knowledge base, but its parallel concern must be that of applying this knowledge in intervening and changing situations. It is for this reason that there is an acute need for the development of clinical doctorates that clearly have different objectives in mind than those outlined for the research doctorate. While it may be argued that it is possible to prepare both researchers and clinicians within one program model, others argue that the skills of the researcher and those of the clinician are dichotomous. Indeed, this is a research question that sorely needs to be investigated. Until this question is addressed, it appears that there will be a critical need for doctorally prepared nurses in clinical practice settings who are engaged in modification of practice as their primary goal. For want of a better term, I would characterize nurses in such positions as the *social engineers* of the patient care system, whose function is that of taking knowledge generated by nurse-researchers and testing it out within a broader clinical context. At present, I do not see such a doctoral program model clearly delineated.

Clinical practice and nursing research are proceeding on two separate and parallel paths that do not intercept. As nurses move up a clinical career ladder, their mode of practice increasingly parallels that of the physician. While the quality of care may be improved by introducing nurses with such clinical preparation into the hospital system, the overall problems that are systemic in nature will not be addressed by nurses following a private practice model. What I am advocating is the development of a cadre of doctorally prepared nurses in clinical practice who are expert clinicians, but who also have a grounding in research enabling them to test out the effects of clinical interventions within the patient care setting, be it hospital, home, or community. With such a group of doctorally prepared nurses, it is at last possible to conceptualize the movement of the profession to a place of stature in its own right.

In summary, it is not enough to develop a core of nurse-researchers who are directed toward developing a body of nursing knowledge. This core must be coupled with a group of equally prepared expert clinicians who take this body of knowledge into the clinical practice arena, apply it in the care of patients, and test out the effects of new approaches in the patient care situation. In this systematic way, nursing can begin to demonstrate that application of nursing knowledge does make a profound difference upon the quality of the life experience.

The road ahead for nursing offers many challenges. It is not sufficient to be caught up in the wrongs of the past; rather, it is important to use past history as a stepping stone to the future. Nursing must garner a position of identity and independence in the heatlh care arena, the discipline must be built upon scientific knowledge that has applicability to the patient care situation, and the application of nursing knowledge must demonstrate that nursing indeed does make a measurable difference. Modern nursing no longer may appeal to God as its source of power to counter medical and administrative authority. Rather, the primary source of this type of authority in the current health care system is derived from scientific knowledge. This knowledge base can only be built by nurses actively engaged in research related to the patient care situation. The challenge is great. The task is arduous and can only be accomplished by those with a clear vision of the work to be done and the goals to be attained. Nursing can no longer exist in the shadows of medicine but must become an entity in its own right. It is time that nursing move away from its sexist self-identity problem and begin to assume full responsibility and authority as an equal participant in the health care arena. This can only be achieved through the authority of knowledge and through scholarly discipline, coupled with a clear sense of history and purpose.

BIBLIOGRAPHY

Dickoff, James, and Patricia James: "A Theory of Theories: A Position Paper," in Margaret E. Hardy (ed.), *Theoretical Foundations for Nurs-*

ing, MSS Information Corporation, New York, 1973.

Dock, Lavinia L.: "The Relation of Training Schools to Hospitals," in Isabel A. Hampton and others (eds.), *Nursing the Sick,* Chicago, 1893. A paper given before the International Congress of Charities, Correction, and Philanthropy at the Chicago World's Fair, 1893. Reprinted under the sponsorship of the National League for Nursing Education, Lucille Petry, consulting editor, McGraw-Hill, New York, 1949.

Erickson, Florence, and Reva Rubin: "Conference Overview," in *Future Directions of Doctoral Education for Nurses*, Conference held at National Institutes of Health, Bethesda, Md., January 20, 1971.

Goldmark, Josephine: *Nursing and Nursing Education in the United States*, Macmillan, New York, 1923.

Matarazzo, Joseph: "Perspective," in *Future Directions of Doctoral Education for Nurses*, Conference held at National Institutes of Health, Bethesda, Md., January 20, 1971.

Nutting, Mary Adelaide: Address given before the American Hospital Association in Toronto, Canada, in 1908 and later reprinted in *A Sound Economic Basis for Schools of Nursing*, Putnam, New York, 1926; and quoted in Bonnie and Vernon Bullough (eds.), *Issues in Nursing: Selected Readings*, Springer, New York, 1966.

Rogers, Martha E.: "The Ph.D. in Nursing," in *Future Directions of Doctoral Education for Nurses,* Conference held at National Institutes of Health, Bethesda, Md., January 20, 1971.

Schlotfeldt, Rozella: "Ph.D. in Science," in *Future Directions of Doctoral Education for Nurses*, Conference held at National Institutes of Health, Bethesda, Md., January 20, 1971.

Seymer, Lucy R.: *A General History of Nursing*, Macmillan, New York, 1949.

Woolsey, Abby Howland. "Hospitals and Training Schools: Report to the Standing Committee on Hospitals of the State Charities Aid Association," New York, May 24, 1876, in National League of Nursing Education, *A Century of Nursing*, Putnam, New York, 1950.

EDITOR'S QUESTIONS FOR DISCUSSION

What social forces have surrounded the development of doctoral education for nurses? What should be the focus of the content in doctoral programs in nursing? How can the skills of a researcher and clinician prepared in doctoral programs be dichotomous? What obligation, if any, do nurses who have received their doctoral education in another discipline have to that discipline versus an obligation to nursing? How might nurses with a doctoral degree in another discipline contribute to both nursing and the discipline of their doctorate? What requirements would you suggest for candidates admitted to doctoral programs in nursing?

Chapter 11

The Proper Environment for Educational Advancement: Academic Freedom

Eileen M. Jacobi, R.N., Ed.D.
Dean, School of Nursing
University of Texas at El Paso

Having reflected on the nursing programs available today, we wll now consider the environment, methods, and means conducive to facilitating learning in nursing educational programs.

Eileen M. Jacobi emphasizes the importance of a basic philosophy of academic freedom in education as a primary concern for the development of professional performance and a climate for the discovery of truth. She views education as an instrument for social change. To bring about social change, the educator and student alike must reserve the right to question tradition and to examine current beliefs in order to formulate a coherent, logical plan for action. Jacobi concludes by suggesting that academic freedom is associated with certain responsibilities for both the teacher and the student.

According to Alvin Toffler, we live in an era characterized by accelerated change. Higher education and professional education, in particular, occupy vulnerable positions in this revolutionary period. The educational institution is expected to keep pace with the explosion of knowledge, to make learning relevant, to respond to innovation, and to search for new ideas and arrangements as well as to keep costs down and to expand enrollments—in short, educational institutions must continually revitalize existing programs. The compelling responsibility of those who determine the character and substance of professional education is to design curricula that will prepare the individual student concurrently for a specialized calling and for the other varied activities of life.[1]

The increasing complexity and rapidly changing characteristics of our society demand that knowledge and skills be continually updated. Between 1900 and 1950, the total body of knowledge known to mankind doubled every fifteen years. Between 1950 and 1975, this body of knowledge doubled approximately every seven years. In the next ten years, it is estimated that the total body of knowledge known to mankind will double *every two years*. This means that knowledge that a student receives in school will be largely obsolete by the time he is 25 to 30 years of age. Toffler points out that, as the result of such an accelerated rate of change, knowledge will grow increasingly perishable. In essence, today's *fact* will become tomorrow's *misinformation*. Toffler observes that society places an enormous premium on learning efficiency. Therefore, tomorrow's schools must teach students to discard old ideas and how and when to replace them. A significant new dimension can be added to the educational process by instructing students how to learn, unlearn, and relearn.[2]

In his latest book, *Learning for Tomorrow*, Toffler speaks of the "future deprived," individuals who have been excluded from opportunities for professional advancement. He suggests that if individuals are to avoid being "future deprived," they must start today "learning for tomorrow."[3]

The goal of nursing education must be to prepare persons for professional practice who understand and are guided by its code of ethics, who know and understand the fundamental principles upon which nursing is based, and who can effectively apply these principles in the performance of their nursing activities. If nursing is to remain a viable profession in the health care field, educators must teach the fundamental principles of nursing not as ends in themselves, but as means of solving significant social and health problems.

Education is viewed as an instrument of social change. Consequently, the curriculum must be a reflection of what a profession can or should be rather than a reflection of current practice. The educational system must prepare students to conceptualize, document, and test the efficiency, effectiveness, and economics of their practice at a degree of sophistication consistent with their preparation. Educators must take a leadership role in reviewing practice and they must contribute heavily to the revisions necessary to meet emerging demands. This course of action demands that educators and the entire system become involved in a substantive way in practice. Conversely, practitioners must be prepared to evaluate the contents of curricula and propose significant revisions.

In the past, the majority of students of nursing were taught to rely on authority rather than to search for answers. They were taught to behave in certain prescribed ways rather than to develop the kind of self-awareness and self-understanding now believed to be crucial in establishing relationships with patients and colleagues. In essence, they were taught to value a high degree of skill in performance of nursing techniques rather than to search for knowledge and understanding that underlies effective performance.

Shall collegiate schools of nursing follow in the footsteps of the older generations and help maintain the status quo, or shall they develop independent, thoughtful citizens capable of contributing to the solution of the world's health problems?

Today, educator and student alike must reserve the right to question tradition and to critically examine current beliefs in order to formulate a coherent, logical philosophy of life and a plan for action. The goals of the professional nurse must include the development of social and intellectual competencies as well as professional performance. This must take place in an environment where education is the primary concern and where academic freedom is understood and practiced.[4]

If nursing is to take its rightful place in society, the boundaries of nursing knowledge must be expanded. Educational programs should anticipate the enlarging scope and increasingly sophisticated nature of practices that accompany advances in knowledge through technology and research. This can only be accomplished through freedom in teaching, experimentation, and research. Faculty in nursing programs must develop curricula and teach students in an atmosphere of freedom, within which the search for knowledge permeates all aspects of the curriculum.[5]

The exercise of academic freedom is the key to maintaining a relevant and worthwhile educational system in today's society. Academic freedom is the freedom to seek and impart knowledge without external or arbitrary interference.

Although academic freedom can be traced to Plato, who believed in the right of the teacher to follow an argument wherever it might lead, the roots of academic freedom were founded in the medieval universities in Europe. These institutions maintained their independence on the grounds that it was necessary to their corporate function and in order that education fulfill its obligations to society. The professors were persons dedicated to the conviction that the fear of God was the beginning of wisdom.[6]

During the colonial period the concept of academic freedom was not well understood in America and the control exerted on the university greatly inhibited freedom. Religious dogma and rigid theological discipline dominated education. Students were exposed only to what was considered consistent with Christian doctrine. Faculty members endangering the piety of students by presenting new ideas were dismissed by the trustees of the colleges. Students were not allowed to freely inquire into unorthodox writings. This restriction of thought characterized the American college until the nineteenth century, when the emphasis gradually changed from religious to political and economic issues.[7]

In the late nineteenth century, faculty educated in the German universities introduced to the American scene the concept of allowing the professors to teach and publish ideas that would not necessarily meet with public acceptance.[8]

Following the Civil War the universities became more secular. The leaders in the university movement were men of science with broad interests. This secularization was only part of a larger process as the revolutionary doctrines of Spencer and Darwin were sweeping the country.[9]

During the latter quarter of the nineteenth century the university became vitally concerned with science and social problems. The growth of academic freedom was affected by the personal character of the scholar, the research method through which men sought the truth, the services that the university contributed to the community, and the professionalization of the academic man. The contribution of science to the achievement of academic freedom can be condensed into three factors: a set of positive values, the formula for tolerating error, and limiting the power of administration.[10]   These were enhanced by the academic norms of tolerance and truth that were present in the institution.

The fundamental aim of academic freedom is to provide a climate for the discovery of truth and the energetic pursuit of excellence for individual development as well as for devotion to worth and progress. In this sense academic freedom applies to all scholars, whether they be members of the faculty or the student body.

The teacher and student should have the freedom to express and to defend views and beliefs, and the freedom to question and to differ, without authoritative repression or scholastic penalization. In the relationship between the student and teacher, each gives to the other and both are stimulated to search for the truth. This search is the essence of academic freedom.

Academic freedom demands of nursing instructors a research approach to the development of nursing theory, investigation of problems in nursing, and an expression of conclusions through publications as well as in the instruction of students without interference from administrative authority either inside or outside the educational institution.[11] I firmly believe that a responsible faculty should claim, as its professional privilege, the right to review all that bears upon the education of students and to take the initiative to evaluate and propose innovative measures.

Educators must seek to inculcate in students of nursing an awareness of their responsibilities and obligations to the public and to the profession. A social conscience and concern for the public good must be fostered. Members of the profession must also stand ready to protect nursing standards in order for the nursing profession to acquire, for the first time in full measure, the character, aspirations, and standards of a learned profession.[12]

Educators must provide opportunities for nursing students to learn to function interdependently and to learn the interdependence of those within the total field of nursing. As physicians and nurses become increasingly interdependent, it is imperative that nurses develop strong working relationships with physicians and other members of the health disciplines. The curricula should reflect increased emphasis on interdisciplinary practice. Moreover, teachers need to face the issue of adjusting curricula to demands of increasing specialization in our complex society and to pressure resulting from the explosion of knowledge.

The current organizational structure in American higher education provides a degree of insulation for the academic community that has proven congenial to the exercise of freedom of thought, inquiry, and expression. Since the college or university must be an institution without intellectual controls, this freedom is essential if higher education is to perform its unique function. New facts, new ideas, new methods of inquiry, and new information are the structural elements upon which progress depends. It is the function of higher education to ascertain and refine those elements essential to progress and to advise and assist other segments of society in their ultimate incorporation.[13]

Freedom within a society, however, cannot be maintained without certain obligations being assumed by the individuals of that society. To abuse a freedom is to betray it. Rights cannot exist without obligations if those rights are to continue to be distributed equally for all. The individual, in exercising his or her own freedom, has an obligation to the free society, of which he or she is a part, to respect the fact that the freedom within the teaching institution implies that certain obligations exist for both the teacher and the student.

An individual has freedom only if he or she is willing and able to judge the value and meaning of freedom and assume responsibility for it. Freedom rests on three principles: freedom from restraint, opportunity for belief and action, and moral and ethical responsibility. Without a sense of moral and ethical responsibility on the part of the individual, no true freedom is possible.[14]

Arthur Lovejoy, one of the founders of the American Association of University Professors, offered a definition that called attention to the responsibility inherent in ethical principles:

Academic Freedom is the freedom of the teacher or research worker in institutions of learning to investigate and discuss the problems of his science and to express his conclusions, whether through publication or in the instruction of students, without interference from political or ecclesiastical authority, or from the administrative officials of the institution in which he is employed, unless his methods are found by qualified bodies of his own profession to be clearly incompetent or contrary to professional ethics.[15]

The assemblage of scholars within the university sustains and reinforces in each member the standards necessary for the fulfillment of its primary function—the dissemination of knowledge. Dissemination of knowledge is possible only if scholars are free to pursue truth and thus render to humanity inestimable services. The indispensable requirement is *academic freedom*.

The nursing profession must have freedom to educate practitioners of nursing if the goals determined by contemporary patterns of health care are to be achieved. Professional autonomy customarily provides for setting standards of practice that includes educational standards for the profession. If the profession does not provide for meeting the needs for which it was established, then social forces will determine its destiny.

If we are to surmount the challenges that face the nursing profession, more creative, effective, and economical methods of teaching nursing must be sought in order to stimulate intellectual integrity and freedom of both faculty and students. The profession must be prepared to accept sustained and accelerated innovation and improvement in educational programs.

We need to persuade our legislators to appropriate sufficient funding to enable institutions to provide basic and advanced nursing education and continuing educational programs so that the practitioners can deliver the type of quality care demanded by citizens in this enlightened age.

Higher education recognizes that knowledge is gained in a variety of situations and is not limited to the classroom or laboratory. Transfer of knowledge and the application of knowledge is a continuing process. Testing individuals for advanced placement in nursing programs is a challenging, formidable task that cannot be avoided. Today, we live in the computer age. It is hypothesized that the computer can be utilized in the testing of individuals to determine their ability to apply knowledge. The problem of testing the application of knowledge has plagued the applied sciences, primarily the professions, from their inception. Every effort must be made to interest the government and foundations in investing money in this enterprise.

Not all students learn at the same rate. We must recognize that motivation is a primary force in learning. Have we in nursing identified the difference between reinforcement and boring repetition in our educational program? How can we exploit the nonclinical laboratory so that the technical component of practice can be developed in a more controlled environment? Can we identify the learnings that must take place in the clinical laboratory so that the technical component of practice can be developed in a more controlled environment? While clinical situations are rich in learning experiences, the psychological climate of the health care institutions is not always conducive to optimum learning. How much clinical practice is necessary for the preparation of a qualified practitioner? Does it not, in fact, differ for individuals? The old adage of practice makes perfect is only half true. Aristotle is reported to have said, "One learns to be a good flute player by practicing the flute; one also learns to be a poor flute player by practicing the flute."

New and innovative methods in nursing education will only be achieved through freedom in teaching, experimentation, and research. There can be no doubt that the proper environment for educational advancement is a setting that fosters academic freedom—academic freedom for both the teacher and the student.

NOTES

1 Eileen M. Jacobi, "Academic Freedom in Baccalaureate Programs in Nursing," unpublished Ed.D. dissertation, Teachers College, Columbia University, New York, 1964, p. 7.

2 Alvin Toffler, *Future Shock*, Bantam, New York, 1970, p. 414.

3 Alvin Toffler, *Learning for Tomorrow,* New York, Random House, 1974, p. 89.

4 Jacobi, op. cit., p. 5.

5 Ibid., p. 8.

6 Russel Kirk, *Academic Freedom: An Essay in Definition,* Regency, Chicago, 1955, p. 20.

7 John S. Brubacher and Willis Rudy, *Higher Education in Transition*, Harper and Brothers, New York, 1958, p. 269.

8 Ibid., p. 298.

9 Richard Hofstadter and Walter P. Metzer, *The Development of Academic Freedom in the United States*, Columbia, New York, 1955, p. 34.

10 Ibid., p. 364.

11 Jacobi, op. cit., p. 7.

12 Ibid., p. 6.

13 Ibid., p. 18.

14 Ibid., p. 1.

15 Arthur Lovejoy, "Academic Freedom," in Edwin A. Seligman (ed.), *Encyclopedia of Social Science,* Vol. 1, Macmillan, New York, 1930, p. 384.

EDITOR'S QUESTIONS FOR DISCUSSION

Are there implications for practitioners within a profession when educational curricula reflect what a profession *should be* rather than what it is? What social or health problems should be included in nursing educational curricula as an initial step toward their resolution? To what extent might or should the principle of academic freedom exist or be applied within the organization or setting of health care delivery? How is the search for *truth* conducted in a practice setting? Is there a conflict between the search for truth in education and the search for truth in practice?

Chapter 12

Nursing Practice and Nursing Education: Realism Versus Idealism

Dorothy J. Douglas, R.N., Ph.D.
Professor, School of Nursing
University of Wisconsin at Madison
Associate Director for Nursing Research,
University of Wisconsin Hospitals

Dorothy J. Douglas describes various types of modeling or methods of teaching, indicates typical objectives for education, and elaborates on characteristics of teachers. She emphasizes that there can be no single set of expectations and no one ideal method or model for teachers and students. Modeling is an educator's tool that can be used as a curricular technique, a dialectic to unite a didactic system of theoretical concepts with the practical (or real) situation.

Today there is a perceived lack of fit between what is taught nurses and what nurses do. Leave aside for the moment whether this statement represents a part or the totality of reality. It is almost as if nursing education had one model of what a professional nurse does and nursing practice another. Analytically, the terms *nursing* and *nurse* admit of no single referent. Perhaps the simplest definition of an American professional nurse is: an individual licensed as a registered nurse in a particular state. The difficulty with this is that it defines the minimum qualifications an individual must have to practice professional nursing within the boundaries of a state. Note that the federal services usually specify only that the nurse be licensed in a state, not necessarily the one in which she is practicing. This definition says nothing about what qualities, skills, and knowledge individual nurses must possess in order to fill a particular type of nursing position. Nor does it take into account the impact of nurses on the field of nursing who for one reason or another are not registered and are presumed not to be practicing. It also does not take into account the rich historical connotations of the terms, nursing and nurse, the technological development that has and will continue to change the practice and the education of nurses, and the changing mores and legal parameters surrounding and embedded in the profession that affect practice and education.

Education is another term that has rich connotations. We commonly think of education for something (nursing), but there are those who would argue that the infinitive *to educate* requires no modifier. An underlying tenet of either persuasion, often unstated, is that general principles can be taught and learned. This is not always the same process. The student is to apply the principles in a particular setting which results in unique and classifiable solutions to practical problems. In nursing education, as in most education for the health professions, there is still a large amount of apprenticeship training, which is one type of educational model for nursing education. There are historical reasons for the apprenticeship system but it persists because it works. In any field with an applied component, the easiest way to teach "how to" is to show the student "how to" or, at least, provide him or her with a model for selected classes of behavior. Even the most abstruse fields of study have some degree of apprenticeship incorporated into their educational framework, if only as a model for the student to see the correct utilization of setting variables.

Among the objectives of an education for an applied field, the following appear to be of importance and are often cited when attempting to typify the ideal graduate:

1 To train for specific tasks—imparting skills.

2 To provide and inculcate general principles of a field in the belief that the individual can make appropriate applications as needed.

3 To impart *facts* (this is close to imparting skills; these facts are mutable and can change).

4 To impart an underlying philosophy with or without a code of behavior.

5 To permit *controlled* access to a field of study (academic, professional, technical).

6 To impart a specialized language, culture, and mores that will distinguish the "finished" member from the student member, who gradually achieves an identity distinct from the nonmember.

7 To provide a framework, setting, and environment in which new knowledge (facts), theories, techniques, technologies, systems, and distinctions can develop.

8 To provide a functional *unit* superordinate to and distinct from the profession (occupation). The client and the practitioner can therefore act as an arbiter of *quality* in an applied field. Sometimes this results in the unit becoming the accreditor of minimum acceptable education.

The characteristics of those who work in institutions dedicated predominantly to the preparation of beginning entrants to an applied field can also be typified. The teachers are usually members of the occupation or profession who have *either* achieved a high level of skill/expertise in a defined portion of the field, or achieved higher education

in their field or a cognate field that qualifies them to impart a portion of their specialty to a learner, *or* (more rarely) individuals who possess some combination of these qualifications. In a few cases, especially where there is on-the-job training, the teacher may be simply an older person. This person may be one who has worked many years and earned the right to teach as an expected and natural privilege. This does not mean that these teachers are therefore less expert and experienced. It simply means that the reason they are selected as teachers is different. Often they may use a *straight lecture* approach. This, a second type of model for nursing education, can be distinguished from the first even though the teachers may also participate in on-the-job training.

There is a third type of model that also focuses on the teacher. *Ideally*, from the standpoint of the profession/occupation and the student, a teacher in an applied field is presumed to know a subject or specified part of it; be or have been a capable and therefore skillful practitioner (unless there is a compelling reason for the teacher to be from another field); be capable of contributing to the development of a field; be skilled at imparting his or her knowledge; exhibit the accepted or an acceptable philosophy and code of behavior the student is expected to internalize; and be familiar with the school and the community on a micro- and macrolevel. In actuality, there is no one set of unified expectations of a teacher or of the educational entity, or for that matter of a practitioner. Rather, the expectations are different depending on the goals, values, background, and *set* of the institution, group, or individuals with whom the teacher interacts. To compound the problem, an individual can have one set of expectations of a teacher, or an educational institution, *as an individual* and quite a different set of expectations *as a member* of a group. Also, the individual student can have quite different expectations depending on which facet of his or her education he or she is attending to.

Thus, a nursing student interested in the care of a particular patient with tetrology of fallot might want to learn very specific information and skills. At another time, while considering a career as a clinical nurse specialist in neonatology, he or she might be totally dissatisfied with a concrete, "this-is-what-you-do-when" approach and want a more theoretically based explanation of the cardiovascular system and its derangements. While a student is interested in the latter, any practical skill information, especially if it is too detailed or long, might be rejected as too concrete, too practical. At still another stage, the student might be preoccupied with the more existential question of whether such a child should be resuscitated if it ceases to breathe on its own. At another time, obtaining a "good" grade may be an all important consideration. In any given class, the students may, and indeed probably will, exhibit a range of these and other objectives in the learning situation. In fact, personal and social goals may well replace professional student goals at any given time.

No instructor can achieve the ideal goal of skillfully imparting his or her knowledge at every moment and all the time. The would be students' goals for learning sometimes will not mesh with the format of the instruction. The instructor, no matter how skilled, can only approach, but never meet, the ideal of being all knowledgeable about a field, skilled in it, skilled in imparting it, and able to anticipate and meet practice setting expectations. Therefore, especially in applied fields, we discuss and try to implement curricula that will facilitate the instructor's attempts to present a *model* for desired behavior and skills, to introduce multimedia techniques for imparting knowledge (facts), and to develop self-paced learning. The student is to be in control of his or her education so that he or she can learn what is needed when it is needed and at the time a need to learn is perceived. This is often presented as a new concept in education, but actually it is the apprenticeship system dressed up in institutional garb and usually removed from the real setting if not from the real pressures.

There is nothing intrinsically wrong with this manner of instruction, nor with straight lecture,

nor with full apprenticeship. The problem is that educators tend not to realize the discrepancy between educational techniques and the application of what is learned, including future applications, by the student. Educators tend to think, therefore, to believe, that they actually operate in the ideal way just described. In reality, they are externalizing an internalized model of nursing education, nurse and/or nursing practice that influences their selection of subject matter, teaching methods, objectives, and expectations. This internalized model can usually be traced to one of the three basic educational models mentioned above but by the time it is internalized it has been elaborated on by current knowledge, norms, and experience. Such models allow the teacher, the student, the patient, the accrediting body, and society in general to place nursing in a context that can be understood. However, there is no way of assuring that all of these parties to nursing education have an identical model of nursing in mind. It is not necessarily desirable that one model be a goal for which to strive. The very diversity of available models stimulates growth and development.

The description and classification of these internalized models is beyond the scope of the present paper. Rather, I would like to analyze the major ways in which models can be employed in delineating a profession or occupation. In the first place, models serve to elucidate a problematic area. Whenever a gap between education and practice presents itself within an occupation or profession, it is often helpful to try to find a model from another field that might explain it analogously. For example, in some of my own research, when the pressures, responsibilities, and viewpoint of ambulance drivers could not be fully understood by studying the medical and health-related side of their occupation, the truck driver was viewed as a model for some aspects of the ambulance driver's role. A major portion of a truck driver's job is packaging, either by doing it himself or insisting that it be done properly before accepting the consignment, loading, and transporting. Most truck drivers are expert at all three and have pride in these abilities. They have a specialized vocabulary to express nuances of each of these subroutines and carefully initiate apprentice drivers into the expertise and the language that connote this expertise. This information solved much of the conflict previously perceived by the researcher in the ambulance driver's role. The problem initially seen was that the *ideal type* conjured by the term *ambulance driver* did not fit the real driver whom I, as the investigator, was riding with, talking to, and observing. Once his primary task was perceived as packaging, loading, and transporting, other aspects of his role came into focus. This included an understanding of the educational and training objectives a program must have to produce a good ambulance driver.

Second, models can serve to control any given occupation or profession. For example, the behavioral expectations the military has of women it is currently enrolling in the service academies are based on a military model expressed, tested, and historically elaborated in an all-male context. Over time, the women will probably modify this model both as it applies to themselves and their male counterparts, but initially it will provide guidelines for the curriculum and will have a lasting effect on the way these young women come to view their profession.

A third use of modeling purportedly serves to illustrate modes of integrating the theoretical (ideal) with the applied (practical). This method of model building often approaches propaganda and stereotyping. Marcus Welby, the kindly family physician, is a good example. Television viewers see him behave in a certain manner. The plot leads them to believe that his behavior results in an attainment of the modeled professional goal, for example, a patient's cure. If they then *assume* that medical education effected the behavior and the desired cure, as most do, they have accepted the portrayal as a model on which to base their expectations of physician education, physician behavior, physician abilities, and physician competencies. Their real knowledge about and insight into the profession of medicine has not increased.

This third sort of modeling can and does take place through all the media including newspapers, radio, television, plays, movies, books, traditional folklore, and the like. It is probably the most persuasive but the least enlightening of the three kinds of modeling discussed, but it does serve as an interest catcher, a point of departure, and a way of expressing the collective idealized expectation of a group. Interestingly, the degree of exposure the media gives to an occupation or profession correlates well with the growth of stereotypes about that group. Stereotypes about teachers, nurses, housewives, physicians, policemen, detectives, scientists, and private secretaries are both represented in the media and fairly well entrenched in real life. Even if the modeled behavior that the stereotype symbolizes were to change, it would take time to alter them appreciably. For example, the stereotype of the black man or woman is gradually changing in accord with the current models presented in the media, but elements of the former stereotype remain and will be hard to eradicate.

An understanding of the types of modeling and the ways modeling may be used in defining a professional role can help us to understand the gap between nursing practice and nursing education, and indicate a clue as to what may be necessary to close that gap to a degree that is profitable for the profession. One method of using modeling—delineating a problem area—is the most useful to us. Through this means we can attempt to gain insight into the diversity of nursing education, the demands of various nursing practice settings, and the best correspondence to strive for between education and practice. For example, one method used in the past to decrease the gap between education and practice frequently was the apprenticeship model. There are historical antecedents to this model and today educational programs for nurses still include apprenticeship elements to a greater or lesser degree. If these elements are not present in programs, it is assumed they will be provided in the first year of practice. The apprenticeship model probably results in the most congruence between education and practice since the student learns predominantly on the job and can be expected to be socialized into his or her occupation by the end of the training period.

Another method used today in education is to use the model of a skilled mechanic. This model requires mastering the facts and skills in an organized and hierarchical order. The assumption is that the facts and skills together with the underlying technology have some degree of temporal permanence. Once learned, the facts and skills can be utilized with assurance in the practice setting. Still a third method introduced to align education with practice is that of the liberal education model. The assumption is that a nurse broadly educated in the arts and sciences and indoctrinated in the principles of practice will infallibly apply generalized knowledge to particular cases in a practice setting.

Most nurses could add to the list illustrating modeling. The point is that no model offers a foolproof blueprint for educating nurses for practice settings. All models, including those yet to be developed, simply provide paradigms for the development of portions of a curriculum. Continuous feedback loops from practice settings and research to education are essential in order to modify and keep current educational requirements to meet the needs of those in practice. Nurse educators, researchers, and leaders in practice settings need to be constantly on the lookout for useful models from other fields that could provide innovations in nursing curricula.

The nurse practitioner movement, for example, is modeled in part on medical education as we know it today. One basic assumption is that if nurses are grounded in some of the arts and skills of medical problem solving, they can apply this to the *nursing* care of their patients. Again, the correspondence is not perfect but the model has been useful in that it has opened new vistas in both nursing education and nursing practice.

It was pointed out that models can be a means of limiting a profession and occupation. This can be difficult to detect and counter, but can be found within all facets of nursing as well as applied to nursing from outside the profession itself. One example is the hierarchical model. A basic assumption is that the health care arena is a unique whole composed of workers, hierarchically organized and ranked. Each level gives orders to the rank below and takes orders from the rank above. The top rank answers to no authority but accepts responsibility of a sort for the final result of coordinated action.

Although this model rarely exists as a single model for nurse education, it is a familiar and easily applied model used by other professions. A more subtle form of this model is found in conjunction with the *hierarchy-of-subject-matter* model in which it is assumed that certified mastery of the applied basic sciences, as taught in the first three or four semesters of medical school, establishes precedence in the health care hierarchy. This model assumes that if a health care occupation or profession does not have the basic minimum of education in the applied basic science then the profession will be positioned lower in the hierarchy. That a health profession has in-depth knowledge in allied but different fields does not increase or change the profession's hierarchical position in the view of those who depend on this type of model.

Models applied to elucidate a problem area can masquerade as models to control a given profession. The difference is that the first type permits growth and development while the second type constricts and limits. Take the apprenticeship model for instance. If the model is introduced as the result of a recognized need for practice in any applied field, then it should lead to improved development of skills while protecting patients from unskilled practitioners. If, on the other hand, the model is advanced with the stated or implied condition that all or most of the education be apprenticeship in nature, then it becomes controlling and therefore limiting. In the first case, the assumption to be tested is, Is skill acquisition necessary? If skill acquisition is necessary, is some form of apprenticeship the best way to attain it?

In the second case, the assumption to test is, Is skill acquisition all there is to nursing? The third use of modeling to stereotype roles needs little discussion. Some thought needs to be given to providing the media with alternative models for nursing and nurses. It is a long slow process and it has not yet really begun.

Concerning this discussion of modeling, it should be emphasized it is not easy to apply this form of analysis. Attempting to perceive the model we are externalizing in our teaching and our practice in terms of its underlying assumptions may allow us to be aware of what we are doing or proposing to do in preparing nurses for today's—and tomorrow's—practice settings. Modeling can be a curricular technique on the one hand, an educator's tool. On the other hand, it can become the pattern that directs the teacher consciously or unconsciously. Mere labeling is not enough. Underlying assumptions must be made explicit and accepted as assumptions, not as immutable truths.

Modeling can be the dialectic that unites any given didactic system that imparts practical (applied and applicable) knowledge. It can also be a useful alternative at the curriculum level to the theoretical-practical techniques utilized such as the lecture and apprenticeship. How can nursing analyze a model to elicit and use it's component parts in an educational setting? First it is preferable that nursing utilize models that function as a curricular technique, a dialectic to unite a didactic system, and that provide alternatives to past techniques. One suggestion might be to regard modeling as a curricular technique that can cope successively with increasing abstract learning goals, in relating theoretical concepts to the practical. In summary, model analysis can be a useful tool in closing the gap between nursing education and nursing practice, in expanding and developing the profession of nursing, and in better understanding and correcting the stereotypes and erroneous concepts others have of the profession.

EDITOR'S QUESTIONS FOR DISCUSSION

How might the ability of students to apply principles of nursing care be tested? How can a student govern his or her education so that he or she can learn what is needed? (Should the student be the controlling force?) How can models limit the scope of a profession? What alternative models can be proposed as teaching tools? How might the effectiveness of a model be evaluated?

Chapter 13

Issues in Allied Health Education

Carol J. Willts Peterson, R.N., Ph.D., F.A.A.N.
Dean and Professor, College of Nursing
South Dakota State University, Brookings, South Dakota

The concluding chapter in this section is concerned with seven major issues in allied health education that also apply specifically to nursing education. Carol J. Willts Peterson presents explicit types of modeling and explains how they can be applied to nursing education. The importance of the development of a conceptual framework for education is emphasized and guidelines are presented for the development of such a framework as the basis of modeling. Peterson defines the meaning of individualized instruction and discusses its essential elements. The various forms of modularization of curricula, a number of critical issues and problems relevant to clinical education (the setting, economic forces, and the patient), the process of nursing education, and evaluation of the process are discussed.

Peterson also defines simulation and demonstrates its efficacy as a means of clinical education. It is apparently valuable in bridging the ideal world of the classroom and the practical milieu of the hospital. Four conditions are identified as necessary components for simulated experiences.

Peterson discusses at length the issues of educational mobility and suggests combining the two systems of challenge examinations and the ladder approach. Six issues are raised about continuing education for nurses. Peterson concludes that the challenge for educators is not to provide more nursing personnel for the profession but rather to incorporate new perspectives and new experiences in the curricula.

It is impossible in a paper of this length to treat in depth all of the major issues in the education of allied health practitioners. Seven major concerns— *health* as the coming perspective, curriculum development, individualized instruction, clinical education, continuing education, educational mobility, and maldistribution of personpower—are discussed at some length. A concluding section of the paper lists a number of other highly significant issues, making only a few comments about each.

HEALTH: THE COMING PERSPECTIVE

This may well be *the* issue of the late 1970s in the education of health personpower. Before discussing it, some generalizations seem both safe and appropriate to make.

1 The term *health care system* is a misnomer. What we really have is a medical care system, and an incomplete, maldistributed one at that.

2 Although we refer to *allied health profes-*

sions it is probably more accurate to describe most of these occupations, as they now exist, as *allied medical professions.*

3 With the exception of several of the health professions (for example, nursing, occupational therapy, health education), most of the so-called allied health occupations are patterned after the medical model and focus more on pathology, dysfunction, and cure than on health and prevention.

4 In general, we have never really grappled in this society with the concept of health—its definition, description, preservation, and promotion.

5 In spite of the significantly increased supply of personpower in health-related occupations, the overall health status of the nation has not improved proportionately. Increase in supply of personnel is not the answer to either the maldistribution problem or the maintenance of health issue.

6 Without a change in focus—from cure and "delivered" care to prevention and self-care—a national health care system will be economically impossible. [One author (1) has so appropriately stated, "Our current preoccupation with the health care system is motivated by our commitment to health care as a right, and by our fear that this commitment will bankrupt the country if we are not careful."]

These generalizations are only mildly critical compared with the charge by Ivan Illich in his recent book *Medical Nemesis.* Illich views modern medicine as a threat to health. Medicine has reached a point of counterproductivity. Instead of assisting society, it is detrimental to individuals' coping abilities, thereby expropriating their health. In spite of increasing budgets associated with medical care, society is not becoming healthier (2).

The consumer is the target of this nation's expensive and elaborate medical care system. However, little attention has been given to *keeping* the consumer healthy (prevention); *educating* him on health matters (health education); and *teaching* him to care for himself, to know when he needs professional help, and to know how to use the system for his maximal benefit (consumer education on self-care).

Jonas Salk (3), well known for his important role in fighting a devastating disease, shares some interesting perspectives on health. He states:

I regard health not as an abstraction but as something specific and concrete, not in terms of the absence of a negative condition (i.e., disease) but as a positive state (i.e., health). By this I mean a state in which the potential of the individual is developing in a balanced way, that he may cope with the vicissitudes of life and function fully in the service of life in evolution (p. 1).

Salk further suggests that we might think of health as being transmissible and the potential for health endogenous. Of particular relevance is the idea that we need to be concerned about both the reduction of disease and the enhancement of health as two different but related activities. Encouraging is his comment that increasing amounts of scientifically acquired knowledge will come to influence the practice of health in society much as scientific knowledge has improved the practice of medicine. One of Salk's concluding comments is that "What is needed is not only the art and science of healing of disease . . . but the art and science of health enhancement, in which the individual himself becomes his own practitioner" (p. 3).

This idea about health enhancement is integral to the concept of *patient activation* being developed at Georgetown University's Center for Continuing Health Education (4). There, laypersons/consumers are being taught basic knowledge about health and simple assessment skills so that they can be active participants in maintaining their health. Although not without its opposition from established medicine, the concept of patient activation is gaining interest as a potential countermeasure to the now exorbitant medical care costs and as a means of truly changing the focus from illness care to health promotion in this country.

All of this concern about medical care versus health care and treatment of diseases versus promotion and maintenance of health has profound implications for health professions. Although nurse educators probably have moved farther than most health occupation educators in incorporating primary care and health education/promotion concepts into their curricula, relatively few nursing programs are fully based on health-oriented conceptual frameworks. Health, as Salk, Illich, and Sehnert view it, is in reality an unfamiliar concept to most educators in the health professions. The various health occupations, with their heavy emphasis on care and intervention, will literally need to be revolutionized to share in concepts such as patient activation, self-care, and health as a transmissible entity. It must begin with the education of the new practitioners.

SOUND CURRICULUM DEVELOPMENT

Curriculum development in both nursing and in the allied health occupations has been and continues to be a significant challenge. This position reflects a number of historical elements.

1 Educational programs in all of the health professions have been profoundly influenced by medical education—particularly the pathology-body systems model, the modified apprenticeship approach, the student-extern-intern-resident cycle, and the allegiance to hours and hours of work-type clinical experience.

2 The heavy requirements in physical and biological sciences, in physio-pathology, and in clinical practice have fostered problems in curricular design, particularly as related to integration of general and professional/technical education, to sequencing, and to offering some choice or option to the student.

3 Teachers in the health professions are first practitioners and second educators. Depending upon the occupation, the person may or may not have formal preparation in the discipline of education. Curriculum and instruction may lack the mark of educational soundness because of this.

In spite of these concerns, progress during the past few decades is worthy of respect. Nursing has achieved national recognition among all of the professions (health and nonhealth) for its advancements in curriculum design, improvement of instruction, and general movement away from service settings into the mainstream of higher education. With the support of groups such as the American Society of Allied Health Professions and the Council on Medical Education of the American Medical Association, accreditation guidelines have been improved, preparation of teachers has been emphasized, improving clinical education has received attention—all with the outcome of improved allied health education.

Curriculum development in nursing education has recently been characterized by concern about conceptual frameworks (5). Basing nursing programs on carefully articulated conceptual models has had a number of benefits: better organized curricula, more careful selection of content for a given program, movement away from the medical model toward health-oriented models, and beginning description of parallel models for nursing practice. A review of allied health curricula quickly supports the generalization that allied health education would benefit greatly from this trend toward conceptual framework development in nursing education.

One can think in terms of five major elements interacting to determine the design of a curriculum. These are:

1 The conceptual framework
2 A philosophy of teaching and learning and related principles of learning
3 Practical academic realities
4 Application of the systems model (input, throughput, output) to the curriculum as a whole and to its various subdivisions (courses, units, modules)
5 The latticework composed of the various level objectives

The first of these, *conceptual framework*, can be defined as a loosely organized set or complex of ideas (some single concepts, some parts of developed theoretical formulations) that provides the overall structure of a curriculum (6). Faculty members often ask, "What is a conceptual framework; what does it look like?" To develop one's conceptual framework it is helpful to answer these key questions about the given health profession:

1 What is the nature of the service being pro-

vided to the client—that is, how is the service described?

2 What is the goal or outcome to which the service is directed—that is, how is health or well-being viewed?

3 Why does the client need the services that this profession provides?

4 How is the practitioner or giver of the service described?

5 Who is the client—that is, how is the client described?

6 What is the context in which the service is given?

What is accomplished by answering these six questions? When a faculty has arrived at a clear and common understanding of the answers to these questions, it has described six major *concepts* that are key elements in any conceptual framework. Using nursing as an example, these key concepts are: nursing/nursing process, health, nonhealth or illness, nursing practitioner, patient/client, care setting or environment. As a conceptual framework undergoes further development, subconcepts under these six areas will be described and thus facilitate increasingly greater implementation of the conceptual framework and clarification of the relevant content in that program. Explanations of how these concepts relate to each other form the *framework* aspect of the conceptual framework.

This type of thinking and questioning will help to stimulate allied health educators to think of curriculum development with new perspectives. Answering these questions for one's own discipline and practice facilitates thinking in terms other than in the traditional medical model.

INDIVIDUALIZED INSTRUCTION

We hear much these days about individualized instruction in education in general. This trend has also affected the education of health care practitioners. Nursing education has made considerable use of individualized approaches and would have to be regarded as the pioneer among the health professions in the use of multisensory, modular

approaches (7, 8, 9). Other health professions have pursued this trend, using modular and/or mediated approaches either as primary or supportive methods. Several aspects of individualized instruction warrant discussion in this paper.

Individualized instruction can be defined as *instruction that is designed, delivered, and/or evaluated in such a way as to account for variations in learner characteristics* (10). These variations among learners may relate to individual goals, personal learning styles, previous learning, past experience, and other such factors that contribute to what educators often refer to as a "heterogeneous student body."

Why individualization in the health fields? In our traditional approaches to instruction we have often assumed covertly, yet operationally, that all students approach a given course with the same competencies, the same interest, and with the same learning styles. Further, our habitual ways of delivering a program have implied that the end of an academic term represents closure to learning in a given area and that academic credit could be given only for a total course that fits a somewhat arbitrary time period. Individualization in education recognizes learner differences and focuses on finding flexible ways to accommodate these individual needs (11).

What is needed in a program setting to accommodate individual differences among students? That is, what are the key elements in individualized instruction? First, the content of a program needs to be organized into small, manageable subdivisions. As one moves away from large blocks of content such as semester or quarter-length courses and utilizes small blocks of content (minicourses, modules, learning packages) it becomes easier to select and sequence topics to meet individual students' unique needs. A second key element in individualized instruction is the concept of diagnosis, remediation, and/or exemption. There must be a perspective of assessing the student and planning with him or her, based on that educational assessment. Third, there is the opportunity for flexible use of time and individual pacing to accommodate variations in learning styles and life patterns. A fourth key element is the availability of content options, given that students enter a learning situation with differing competencies. Flexible evaluative approaches that include both formative (ongoing feedback for growth purposes) and summative (terminal evaluation to indicate level of performance/degree of achievement) evaluation make a fifth key element. Choice in the location where learning takes place and alternate teaching methods are the final two elements.

When conceptualizing individualized instruction, one can think in terms of these seven key elements as variables that can be manipulated by either the student or the teacher (13) (see Figure 13-1).

Perhaps of all the key elements, *small content blocks* have received the most attention in the form of modularization of curriculum. Concurrent with the recent emphasis on individualization is the interest in the modular approach. A module (minicourse, learning package) is a well-defined, self-contained instructional package that deals with a small segment of content or a single subtopic. As a minimum, it must contain behavioral objectives, a sequence of learning activities designed to achieve those objectives, and a method for pre- and post-testing to evaluate the achievement of the objectives.

Individualization is commonly pursued by reorganizing a total program into modules that are smaller curricular building blocks than the traditional large units or total courses. Combined with other features of individualization, such as alternate teaching strategies and self-pacing, the module permits a flexibility unknown to us in traditional education. Dr. S. N. Postlethwait, the pioneer in the development of the minicourse approach in biological sciences, has so appropriately captured the essence of the small unit of content in individualized instruction. Raising some concern about the use of the term *module* and discussing the merits of the alternate term *minicourse*, he states:

> My own bias is that education needs a term for a unit of subject matter relating specifically to content. Instructional strategy, time elements,

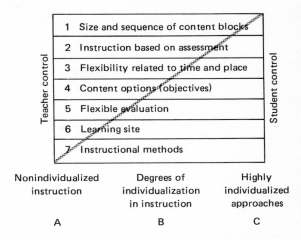

A Traditional approach such as a highly structured lecture approach with essentially no choices left to the student.

B The seven variables (key elements) may be manipulated in varying ways by the teacher and student. For example, in the typical multisensory, modular approach, the objectives (content) are controlled by the teacher, but the student is allowed some selection of teaching strategies and often controls his or her own pace of learning.

C Independent learning where the student essentially controls all variables and utilizes the teacher as a resource person or consultant—for example, independent study projects, interim projects.

Figure 13-1

study programs, and media components are secondary considerations and relate to the acquisition of knowledge rather than a unit of knowledge itself. . . . Because the course as a unit of knowledge is large and vague, the present and future generations need a new unit or subdivision of subject matter to provide greater flexibility and adaptation to individual requirements for content, instructional strategy, study habits, and credit assignments. The obvious need is to increase the "resolving power" of the present educational unit through the use of smaller units or smaller courses (14).

A concept often associated with a modular approach to individualization is *mastery*. Mastery, as described by Bloom, implies that most students can master what we have to teach them, provided the quality and type of instruction is appropriate, adequate time is allowed to meet individual needs, and the "perseverance" of the student is sufficient (15). Applied in a modularized curriculum, a mastery approach would be characterized by:

1 Clearly stated levels of expected performance/achievement (the level of mastery expected)
2 Achievement of the curriculum via progressive mastery of the individual units or modules at the specified levels
3 Flexible pacing and timing to accommodate student differences
4 Ongoing formative evaluation to provide the student and teacher with diagnostic feedback so that student remediation and/or enrichment needs can be met
5 Carefully developed summative evaluation so that the student and teacher clearly know when the student has in fact mastered certain objectives at the expected level

Individualized instruction, in spite of its benefits, is not without its adjustment concerns. For example, the teacher's role changes from information giver to diagnostician, facilitator, and interpreter of evaluation. If "giving information" via a lecture approach has been part of a faculty member's reward system, his or her new role in individualized instruction may be frustrating. One cannot assume that faculty members will automatically adapt to this new role. They may need assistance from the institution or their colleagues in this area of concern.

Student reward systems need to be respected, too, in individualized instruction—particularly if the mastery concept is applied. When utilized with a competency-based focus that deletes the traditional grading system, students may become frustrated. Simply being told that they have mastered the expectations satisfactorily and can move on to the next step often irritates students who have been socialized to compete for B's and A's that reflect "better than just satisfactory" performance. Faculty members using an individualized, mastery-of-competencies approach may have to retain

some remnants of the traditional letter grade system to facilitate student adaptation to the approach.

Educators exploring individualized instruction in the health professions need also to avoid some of the *erroneous* assumptions that get passed around in education circles. Some of these, which might be titled "Inappropriate Conclusions About Individualized Instruction," are listed here.

1 Individualized instruction is synonymous with independent learning.
2 Modular instruction reduces the number of faculty required.
3 Modular instruction is less expensive than traditional instruction.
4 Modular instruction fragments the delivery of a curriculum.
5 Modular instruction is appropriate for teaching skills but is not applicable to the teaching of concepts and processes.
6 Modular instruction is appropriate in technical education but is not appropriate for professional education.
7 Students do not need any special orientation to the modular approach since they will readily adapt.
8 Teaching is teaching—whether in the classroom or in the modular approach.
9 Modules can be any size the teacher chooses.
10 Modular instruction interferes with the notion of basing a curriculum on a conceptual framework.
11 Using modular instruction implies that one will use multimedia.

CLINICAL EDUCATION

It occasionally happens that at night over swampy ground a mysterious light appears. Sometimes it hovers, sometimes flits and dances. When one approaches it, the light seems to disappear. Although some persons have undoubtedly mistaken this mischievous light for an unidentified flying object, the usual scientific explanation for it is that it is the result of spontaneous combustion of swamp gas generated by rotting organic matter.

History suggests that the light occasionally misled travelers, thus it came to be known as *ignis fatuus*, a Latin term that translates to "foolish fire."

The educational rationale and practice of clinical education in the health occupations have often had this ephemeral, hard-to-define quality. From a distant vantage point, the merits of clinical education seem unassailable. How better to learn than by doing? Yet this portion of the curriculum of any health program is plagued with problems. Faculties struggle with trying to define essential clinical education, with clarifying the role of the clinical instructor, and with developing means to evaluate clinical performance. A number of issues and problems are relevant to cite here.

1 The Setting Educational institutions are extremely dependent upon clinical sites for providing significant and crucial portions of their educational programs, yet they have minimal control over this aspect of health occupation education. The clinical site's primary obligation is to the patient, and it must make decisions in that framework. The educational institution is usually the "guest" or "borrower" of resources in the clinical agency and realistically does not have much influence on decision making in such settings. If a hospital's census drops sharply (as is the case in various parts of the country), the decision to close one or more stations may have profound effects on an affiliating educational program, yet the educational institution has no voice in the decision. Consolidating and/or redesigning services that comes with a community's efforts to improve the planning of health care services has equally profound effects on the education of selected health care personnel.

2 Economic Forces Powerful economic forces, controlled neither by the clinical agency nor by the educational institution, alter the plans of both. The federal government, the general health of the nation's economy, the changing policies of third-party payers—all these and numerous other factors shape and alter the directions and plans of both institutions. An extremely important factor is the continuing search for means to control the high cost of health services. Discussions continue regarding the "true" cost to the clinical agency of having clinical students on the premises and the possibility of referring these costs back to the educational institution rather than on to the patient. Increasing pressures on educational institutions to pay for use of clinical sites have serious implications. The viability of health occupations programs and in some instances the very viability of a total institution are at stake.

Also, in many parts of the country an acute shortage of clinical sites exists. The expansion of clinical sites has not kept pace with the explosive growth of educational programs. The results of this nonalignment have been numerous: the facilities of many hospitals are tightly scheduled and allow no flexibility in planning or usage of various resources; the patient has become an "over-cared-for" individual whose welfare may at times be threatened by fragmented care and overstimulation; educational administrators have been forced to lengthen considerably the geographical radius in which they must seek sites; and smaller and more varied sites are being utilized, prompting a heavier investment of administrative time, an increased amount of travel time and expense by students and faculty, and a less homogeneous experience for the same level students.

3 The Patient The primary reason for using the actual clinical setting in health occupation programs is the access to the real patient and his or her problems. This positive factor, however, must be weighed against inherently negative ones. Although he or she is believed to be central to the process of clinical education, the patient is perhaps the most unpredictable and difficult to control variable in the learning situation for a variety of reasons. There may be:

a Cancellation of the specific treatment, diagnostic test, or therapeutic plan that was considered an important aspect of the learning experience and influenced the choice of a specific patient over others

b Changes in the patient's condition, making the care an inappropriate learning experience or creating an extremely high-risk situation for patient, student, and the clinical agency

c Unanticipated discharge or transfer of the patient, leaving the student without an assignment

d Interruptions in the patient's plan of care during the time the student is present, confusing the overall learning experience by extraneous factors and poor timing

e Significant variations in patient census, seasonal variations, and fluctuations in intrahospital patient distribution

4 The Process It is generally believed that the "goodness" of the instructional process has a high correlation with the amount of control exerted by the educational planners. Both the typical college classroom and the more innovative learning resource center have some built-in certainties that facilitate the teacher's control and the student's learning. Scheduling, environment, institutional policies, and location of resources are among the many variables that the teacher knows reasonably well due to being "part of" the educational institutional institution. There is not a direct parallel in clinical teaching. An instructor hired by the educational institution is usually the guest in the clinical facility and, depending upon the climate there, may or may not be a welcome one.

When a wide variety of clinical sites is used, it may become virtually impossible for the instructor to provide the direct guidance needed for effective clinical instruction. Since educational institutions simply cannot afford to hire multiple instructors, who function at various sites with only two or three students each, agency personnel are often called upon to provide much of the clinical supervision. Faculty then become itinerant instructors, seeing the students infrequently and perhaps meeting with them in clinical conferences weekly. A variation of this approach is to hire an additional, often less well prepared faculty member, who is used for clinical instruction only, having no responsibility for teaching the theoretical aspects of the course. The consequence of any

of these approaches is that the objectives of the clinical experience may not be achieved, since a well-qualified instructor who knows all aspects of the course is not constantly present at the clinical site.

5 Evaluation No problem in clinical teaching has received as much attention as the evaluation of clinical performance. Historically, evaluation in apprentice-style programs emphasized efficiency and organization. More sophisticated current efforts stress measurement of specific student behaviors that indicate student achievement in applying clinical knowledge and skill in performance of a patient-oriented service.

Use of behavioral criteria in evaluation of clinical performance, however, is not without its problems. Some instructors have tried to assess the student's achievement of various objectives by keeping anecdotal notes on student behavior. This is often time-consuming and incomplete as a valid, reliable means of evaluation. Further, the question of when clinical experience is practice or new learning and when it is performance for testing purposes enters into this approach. An increasingly common methodology is to develop rating tools based on the criteria and to use these to evaluate planned, specified clinical situations. Again, this approach is not without its problems. Some of these are:

a Difficulty in finding a patient situation that will provide an opportunity to observe the specified criteria

b Unanticipated patient problems or reactions that complicate the observation process

c Unreliability due to observer biases or inaccuracies

d The time-consuming nature of observing each student

e Limited sampling of the total range of behavior

f Difficulty in finding varied situations that will demand differing levels of behavior from students at varying levels of development

g Inconsistencies among evaluation experiences for students in the same lab group

h The challenge of accurately evaluating the higher cognitive levels, such as synthesis, evaluation, and related problem solving and decision making

i The difficulty of finding ideal clinical experiences for assessing interpersonal relationship skills and the relative difficulty in actually measuring them

In an effort to standardize the evaluation process, some health fields have moved to controlled situational tests or practical examinations. Often these evaluation situations are staged in a practice laboratory or learning resource center. Although these approaches are viewed as more valid and reliable than measurement in the clinical setting, the single situational test has often been criticized because it does not assess interpersonal relationship, decision making, and the student's ability to synthesize various knowledges and skills.

These various issues/problems are forcing educators in health occupation programs to scrutinize clinical education. Infante (16) has helped nursing educators consider the *essential* elements of the laboratory concept in her recent book *The Clinical Laboratory in Nursing Education*. Of particular importance are her comments about the use and misuse of clinical laboratory. Although nursing education has often been referred to as an apprenticeship-type system, a true apprenticeship was not modeled. Infante reminds us that the nursing student has traditionally not been aligned to a master practitioner to learn by doing, which is the case in a true apprenticeship situation. Nursing education has involved a "worker-type experience" where essentially the student works in order to learn. It is probably safe to say that this "work to learn" (or at best, "do to learn") practice is common to all of the health occupation programs. Nursing has, in fact, progressed to a greater degree of sophistication in clinical education than most of the so-called allied health occupations.

Infante's ideas about the clinical laboratory have vast implications. It is essential that all health occupations scrutinize their clinical education, clarifying what really needs to be accomplished in the clinical laboratory and what can be taught elsewhere. As Infante and others stress, we must get the perspective that the clinical laboratory is a place for some unique "learning to do," not a place to "do or work to learn."

Searching for this same clarity about clinical education, simulation has been explored extensively at St. Mary's Junior College, Minneapolis, Minnesota, as an adjunct to clinical education (17). Simulation is defined as the creation of lifelike staged activities or games that resemble as closely as possible the actual clinical situation with its variety of problem-solving experiences. In simulation the actual experience is analyzed, and from that analysis a model is derived. The simulation is then based on the theoretical model. Thus, simulation does not represent reality directly; rather, it represents the model of reality (18). In applying this conceptualization to the clinical situation, it would first be necessary to analyze the "real world" experience and produce a model based on that. For example, one might analyze a certain patient care situation and isolate the primary dimensions of that situation as a problem-solving episode. Having done this, a simulated problem-solving experience could be designed around the key dimensions extracted from the real clinical situation.

Simulated experiences can be described as having four crucial characteristics (19). The first is that of *analogous circumstances*, or a setting that is close enough to a real environment to permit lifelike problem solving to occur. A second and extremely important characteristic of simulation is that it involves minimal risk, both for the student and the teacher. Another characteristic of a simulation is that it provides almost immediate feedback and thus reinforcement related to the consequences of the learner's response. This benefit, like the low-risk feature, occurs without modification of the original physical or psychological learning climates. Finally, the simulated experience is replicable, a control factor that very few actual clinical experiences can incorporate.

The advantages of simulation parallel, to some extent, the problems related to clinical education. Obviously, the primary advantage is that the simulated portion of a course is under the control of the educational institution and not subject to the decision making of the clinical facility. Similarly, the individual simulation can be a controlled experience, one whose variables are carefully selected and are predictable and one where the environment is controlled.

Another benefit of simulated clinical experiences is their low-risk quality. Reactions occur, decisions can be made, and mastery can be achieved without threat to a real patient. Such experiences would provide an ideal context for students beginning to make decisions about patient care. Immediate feedback on the consequences of the student's actions and decisions is also a consistent feature of simulated experiences. Although there may be some question about the amount of factual content that can be learned via simulation, this methodology is particularly well-suited to teaching processes, primarily the problem-solving or decision-making process. The key elements of the process can be built into the model and then implemented in the actual simulation. Cost may also be an advantage. The initial planning, development, testing, and revision of the simulated package or experience would obviously be costly. A simulation used over a period of time, however, becomes a relatively low-cost model of the high-cost environment. Simulation also offers considerable opportunities for effective evaluation. The control feature, replicability, and the low-risk nature of simulated situations enhance validity and reliability in the evaluation of clinical performance.

Perhaps the chief challenge to this methodology as an alternative for much of the teaching in the actual clinical setting is that simulation is *not* reality, nor is it based directly on reality. As discussed earlier, a simulated situation is based on a model of reality, the model being a representation of reality (20). The simulated experience is consequently removed several steps from the real-life situation. Obviously, it is a constant challenge to achieve a valid parallel to the real situation so that variables learned can be transferred to the real world. Much hinges on how good the intermediate model is. Creation of simulations that closely parallel the real situation is time-consuming and requires a capable designer who can develop a valid model and then build the simulated experience patterned after this model.

In addition to concern about accurate portrayal of reality, faculty often argue that students in health fields must have frequent "exposure" to the real clinical setting. Although these individuals may not be able to provide descriptions of the specific learnings that are obtained in the clinical setting, they hold firmly to the belief that students need "adequate" time (whatever that means) in the clinical experience. This allegiance to the clinical aspects of the course, however, may be related more to positive feelings about clinical experience and the rewards received through patient care than to specific awareness of the learnings that take place in the clinical experience.

Another objection to simulation is that it cannot provide the variety of patient cues that students must respond to and therefore cannot elicit an appropriate repertoire of behavior from the student. A related concern is whether the unexpected variables that the student must learn to deal with in real life can be built into the simulation model. Further, the real clinical setting is believed to be essential to having the student "put it all together," or synthesize, in patient care.

These objections cannot be ignored. At the same time simulation should be considered as a viable alternative to present difficulties in clinical education. The challenge is to design simulations with varying degrees of complexity to serve as alternate ways of achieving objectives that are now assumed to be part of the clinical content of a course. A second challenge to the educator is to describe specifically the objectives or learnings that can be learned in no other setting but the real clinical area. The ultimate consequence, then, would be the extremely effective use of clinical sites.

EDUCATIONAL MOBILITY

The term *educational* was chosen rather than *career* because it seems more accurate in the discussion of this next issue. Presently we are emerging from an era in nursing and allied health education where it was very difficult for an individual to move from one level of educational preparation in a given field to another level. Generally, such a career decision meant considerable loss of time with little recognition of previous education and experience. The recent quest for "relevance" in higher education and the various trends in society pertaining to nontraditional study, growth, and equality of persons have fostered the establishment and acceptance of a new (perhaps revived) principle of higher education. That principle is that previous formal education at another level, informal education, work experience, life experience, and education outside the structured collegiate setting, *do* provide significant learning.

Career mobility, career ladder, challenge exams, open curriculum, career lattice—in reading the recent literature on educational mobility, one becomes acutely aware of the variety of terminology used. Of these, the term *open curriculum* has received considerable attention in recent years.

The idea of an open curriculum suggests that a practitioner can move from one level of education to another with a minimum of repetition and loss of time. More broadly, this term implies movement from one health occupation to another with recognition of commonalities and past learning. Several alternatives are available to achieve the concept of an open curriculum: challenge or equivalency examination systems, career ladder and career lattice systems, or a combination of these two approaches.

It is essential to thoroughly understand the dif-

ference between a challenge system and a career ladder approach to mobility. A challenge system recognizes that practitioners prepared in various programs do have some knowledge, skills, concepts and processes in common. However, proponents of the challenge system idea would view each level of education as a *unique* one, where the practitioner has learned a process that differs in depth, breadth, and perspective from that used by other types of practitioners. Thus, in a challenge system, the baccalaureate program would define its practitioner as the "professional." Essentially it would say to the associate degree or vocational graduate: You have some things in common with our product but you also differ from it. We have developed evaluation tools that measure selected aspects of our curriculum. You may use your past education and experience and independent study to challenge parts of our curriculum. Those areas in which you demonstrate knowledge, skill, processes, or perspectives equivalent to our specified levels need not be repeated.

What is different about a career ladder? The career ladder idea suggests that the *beginning stages* of *all the levels* of practice in a field are equivalents. Thus, nurse assistant training is comparable to the basic course in an LPN (licensed practical nurse) program, the LPN program is equivalent to the first year of the associate degree level, and the associate degree equals the first two years of a baccalaureate program. It implies that one layer of education is built on another. In contrast, the challenge idea supports the basic premise that a program is a group of interrelated, integrated, carefully selected experiences that produce a defined end product.

The distinction between a challenge system and a career ladder has been explained skillfully by Moore (21). She disagrees with the ladder approach because she does not believe the whole is simply the sum of its parts. She says:

As someone moves on to a higher level of nursing, I claim there should be not only addition of new knowledge, but also new organization of old knowledge. From such a combination can come new relationships, new insights into nursing, and more important, new responsibilities. The essential factor is a new synthesis or composition of knowledge, not merely adding more of the same.

Strict adherence to a challenge system is often criticized because (1) it discounts the quality of another institution's program and (2) does not yield enough gains or "payoff" for the mobilist. On the other hand, the ladder approach is sometimes viewed as educationally unsound because it *assumes* that persons have certain knowledge and skills, and fails to consider the differences in vocational, technical, and professional levels of practice and the differing backgrounds that underlie each of these. There is merit in combining the two systems. Initial assessment of the candidate will validate his or her skill and knowledge level; transitional experiences such as a special module or summer session can then be used to facilitate placement at the next step. Combining the two approaches—challenge/equivalency testing and laddering—avoids unnecessary duplication for the student, yet maintains quality control of the curriculum involved.

CONTINUING EDUCATION

A decade ago continuing and adult education (often under the umbrella of extension education) were still the low prestige departments in most institutions of higher education. The 1970s have brought a new perspective on continuing education. Increasing respect for nontraditional education, technological achievements, knowledge advances, more active consumers demanding quality service, and the maturation of health professions themselves are a few of the reasons that continuing education in the health occupations has become an issue.

As each of the professions considers continuing education, various questions must be addressed:

1 Should continuing education be mandatory or voluntary? Proponents of the first would say

that this is the only way for a profession to police itself and be certain that its practitioners keep updated. Those favoring voluntary continuing education would argue that being a professional implies automatic responsibility for maintaining quality practice. These persons believe that more effective learning will take place if the person is not forced by law to accrue a certain number of hours, points, or continuing education units (CEUs).

2 Who should provide continuing education: service agencies, established educational institutions, professional organizations, industrial corporations? Further, what is the relationship between in-service education in one's work setting and continuing education?

3 How will quality control be maintained in continuing education if a wide variety of agencies become sites for workshops, conferences, and the like? Related to this is the complex issue of accreditation. Should institutions be accredited by some national organization to offer continuing education or should individual offerings be reviewed and approved by local agencies?

4 How should continuing education be described within a given profession: in terms of hours, CEUs (the nationally accepted term that is a unit representing ten content hours of planned continuing education), as "growth credits," in terms of academic credits, or by some other means? Although the CEU is the common means for designating amount of continuing education, a variety of measures is used among the various professions leading to some confusion. Even where the CEU is used, it may not be well understood.

5 In what way can we assess the impact of continuing education on clinical practice? Does mandatory continuing education provide assurance that a practitioner will in fact maintain a safe level of practice?

6 Who should pay for continuing education: the employer, the employee, or both?

Of particular concern is the issue of acquiring the appropriate perspective about adult education. The adult learner seeking continuing education is different from the student in a basic health occupation program. Knowles (22) refers to teaching adults as *andragogy*. Andragogy is characterized by these assumptions. The adult learner:

1 Is essentially a self-directing person

2 Has, because of his maturity, a reservoir of experience that serves as a resource for learning

3 Illustrates a relationship between readiness to learn and the developmental tasks of his social roles

4 Is interested in immediate application of knowledge with emphasis on problem-centeredness

Careful needs assessment to determine what practitioners in a given health occupation really need in the area of continuing education is also essential to the success of a continuing education endeavor. Effective needs assessment usually involves skillful use of advisory groups, establishing linkages with the appropriate professional organizations, working closely with key persons in the given health profession, and finally establishing strong linkages with one's cooperating clinical agencies. Often these linkages yield more accurate information about needs in continuing education than do elaborate formal questionnaire surveys.

MALDISTRIBUTION OF PERSONPOWER

Hatch (23) reports that in 1960, about 6,000 persons graduated from collegiate programs for allied health occupations. Five years later, an 86 percent gain was evident when over 10,000 graduated. By 1970 there was another 144 percent increase with about 26,000 more persons graduating from such programs. Proliferation of new occupational categories paralleled this rapid growth in supply. Many established health professions have developed community college associate degree programs for preparation of technical level workers. Vocational-technical institutions have also become active in allied health education, usually preparing persons at a 1-year or assistant level.

In spite of significant gains in the supply of health personpower, distribution of personnel still remains an issue. Areas most needing improved health care services—for example, small outlying communities, sparsely populated states, deteriorating neighborhoods in metropolitan areas—have not benefited in proportion to the overall increase in

supply of personnel. Often, the health care professional does not want to practice in these areas. Even if he or she is enticed to do so through financial assistance, he or she leaves the community after completing the obligatory service period, returning to a larger community.

Another factor is economics. Small health care agencies in rural communities often cannot afford to hire persons representing all of the specialties, subspecialties, and units within the various health professions.

What are the implications for education? Often allied health and nursing programs are too oriented toward acute care, specialties in medical/health care, and the conveniences and practices in large metropolitan medical centers. For example, certain factions in nursing have argued during the past decade that basic nursing programs cannot teach team leading and prepare new graduates for beginning management responsibilities. Yet, the real world is that this country has numerous thirty- to fifty-bed hospitals in which RNs must assume extensive management responsibility, if such hospitals are even fortunate enough to have adequate RN staffing.

Some recent trends bring hope for alleviating the maldistribution. During the past few years, we saw a number of students at St. Mary's Junior College, Minneapolis, Minnesota, equip themselves with two technical majors (for example, nursing and physical therapy or respiration therapy and nursing) because they plan to move to small northern Minnesota communities and feel they need knowledge and skills in several areas. Within allied health education circles there has been some discussion of the need to prepare a general technical level health worker who might have the basic skills in a variety of areas (for example, occupational therapy, physical therapy, respiratory therapy, biomedical electronics, and so on) and be able to meet a variety of needs of a single service agency in a rural setting. Persons with a strong sense of professionalism about their disciplines often frown on such an idea, saying it erodes away the very essence of a profession. Yet this strong sense of professionalism in the health occupations has failed to meet the real health care needs of this country.

Another hopeful trend is the incorporation of a rural practicum or preceptorship into some programs. Cady and Anderson (24) report such a project involving nine health disciplines that were involved in a planned summer experience in rural primary care situations. Student attitudes toward and interest in working in such settings were strengthened by the experience. The associate degree nursing program at Dakota Wesleyan University in Mitchell, South Dakota, has developed an exciting interim experience in surrounding small hospitals. Evaluative results indicate that this is a very stimulating experience both for the students and the institutions involved (25). Another exciting trend in South Dakota includes the extension of the associate degree program of the University of South Dakota, Vermillion, to several of the Indian Reservations in South Dakota. This endeavor focuses on educating Native Americans in their own community so that they are likely to remain there in the work force.

In conclusion, preparing more people, developing more levels within an established field, and creating more types of health care workers are not the answers to improving health care in this country. Educators in the health professions will need to take bold steps to incorporate new perspectives and new experiences into curricula, hopefully increasing the probability that some practitioners will find the small, outlying, rural area an exciting place to practice.

OTHER RELEVANT ISSUES

National Health Policy What will it be? Will a policy evolve that will achieve coordination of the now disorganized system and bring a health care (instead of illness care) focus to services? Is it economically feasible to achieve the goal that health care is a right of all persons?

Licensure How can health professions education be flexibly regulated and continue to provide protection to the public? In what ways does licensure interfere with personpower utilization and career mobility? What should be the role of consumers on licensure boards? Does the concept of institutional licensure have merit or does it threaten the quality of care available to the consumer?

Certification Does certification lead to fragmentation rather than improvement of service? How can certification become better coordinated nationally within the health professions?

Accreditation In what way does accreditation perpetuate narrow professionalism that ignores the real needs of society? What is the role of lay members on accrediting bodies? What should be the continuing role of the American Medical Association (AMA) in the accreditation of allied health programs? The Study of Accreditation of Selected Health Educational Programs (SASHEP) recommended establishment of an independent group that would sponsor, coordinate, and supervise accreditation in allied health education. This group would be broadly representative of the health occupations and not be dominated by a single professional group. Will this recommendation yield new approaches to accreditation? (26)

Core Curriculum What are the benefits and disadvantages of this approach? Will it (does it) facilitate educational mobility? Are there economic advantages if a number of allied health programs share a common core or do programs end up reteaching certain concepts because of dissatisfaction with a core course in a core curriculum?

Professionalism What is the impact of the increased professionalism and independence of some health occupations on delivery of service? How can communication be improved between medicine, nursing, allied health groups, and hospital administration? Professionalism appears to interfere with the use of core curricula, with developing interoccupational/interdisciplinary approaches, with achieving health care teamwork, and with educational/career mobility. How can this barrier be effectively overcome?

Communication Between Service and Education Agencies The movement of nursing and allied health education programs into the mainstream of higher education has fostered strained relationships between service and education. What are some effective means for improving communications between these groups? What kinds of relationships need to exist to assure that competent practitioners are prepared for both the real world and for the future?

New Content Areas Health maintenance, health education, chemical dependency, consumer advocacy, and gerontology are a few of the content areas that may be more relevant than some currently included content areas in the preparation of health professionals. Are these topics being given adequate attention in present curricula?

Health Care Team How can the team function be effectively taught to health professions students? What is an ideal model for health team function?

The National Health Planning and Resources Development Act of 1974 What will be the outcomes of this act? Will the network of HSAs (Health Systems Agencies) that will be established and supported under this act really impact upon health services in some way so that the consumer is ultimately benefited?

Teaching Moral Decision Making What are the societal changes that affect this? How can ethical/moral decision making be taught in today's complex society? In what way do advances in technology and medicine affect this?

CONCLUSION

The issues are many and they all seem significant. Each of the concerns cited in this discussion could have been the singular focus of the paper. If one were asked to select the megaissue it would have to be health care delivery and the question of what will it be in the future. Will it be characterized by the health perspective described in the first issue discussed in this paper? Or will it follow old patterns and old perspectives? It seems there is no alternative but that it will change. Only with a new perspective will it be economically feasible to achieve the degree of health desired for the nation. Only with a new perspective will it be philosophically, educationally, and operationally feasible.

NOTES

1 Leon S. White, "How to Improve the Public's Health," *The New England Journal of Medicine,* **293** (15): 773, October 9, 1975.
2 Ivan Illich, *Medical Nemesis*, Pantheon, New York, 1976.
3 Jonas Salk, "What Do We Mean by Health," reprinted in *Readings in Health 76/77*, Dushkin Publishing Group, Guilford, Connecticut, 1976.
4 Keith W. Sehnert and Howard Eisenberg, *How to Be Your Own Doctor—Sometimes,* Grosset and Dunlap, New York, 1975.
5 Gertrude Torres and Helen Yura, *Today's Conceptual Framework: Its Relationship to the Curriculum Development Process*, Publication No. 15-1529, National League for Nursing, New York, 1974.
6 Carol J. Willts Peterson, "Questions Frequently Asked About the Development of a Conceptual Framework," unpublished paper.
7 Luis E. Folgueras, *The Use of the Auto-Tutorial Laboratory and the Mobile Tutorial Unit in Teaching Nursing Techniques*, Project Report: DIO-NU-00146-03, Delta College, University Center, Michigan, 1969.
8 Ada M. Lindsey, *Development of Multi-Media, Self-Instructional Study Units*, Third Annual Progress Report: DIO-NU-00353-03, University of Maryland School of Nursing, 1971.
9 Carol J. Willts Peterson, *Multi-Sensory Tutorial Instruction in Associate Degree Nursing Education*, St. Mary's Junior College, Minneapolis, 1973.

10 Personal communication with Larry Demarest, Coordinator of Individualized Instruction, St. Mary's Junior College, Minneapolis, Minnesota.

11 Robert M. Diamond et al., *Instructional Development in Higher Education*, Center for Instructional Development, Syracuse University, Syracuse, 1973, p. 14.

12 Ibid, pp. 3–11.

13 Pierre Woog and Dianne Berkell, "A Conceptual Model of Individualization," *Educational Technology*, **15**(9):33–35, September 1975.

14 S. N. Postlethwait, "Foreword" to James D. Russell, Modular Instruction, Burgess Publishing Company, Minneapolis, 1974, pp. v-vi.

15 Benjamin S. Bloom, "Learning for Mastery," RELCV Topical Papers and Reprints, No. 1 Reprinted from *Evaluation Comment*, vol. 1, no. 2, Center for the Study of Evaluation of Instructional Programs, University of California at Los Angeles, May 1968.

16 Mary Sue Infante, *The Clinical Laboratory in Nursing Education,* Wiley, New York, 1975.

17 Carol J. Willts Peterson, "Collaboration in Innovative Approaches in Health Care Education" in *Collaboration in Health Care Education,* Publication No. 23–1617, National League for Nursing, New York, 1976.

18 Paul A. Twelker, "Designing Simulation Systems," *Educational Technology,* **IX**(10): 64–70, October 1969.

19 Isabel H. Beck and Bruce Monroe, "Some Dimensions of Simulation," *Educational Technology,* **IX**(10):45–49, October 1969.

20 Twelker, op. cit.

21 Sister Anne Joachim Moore, "The Ladder and the Lattice," *Nursing Outlook,* **20**(5): 330–332, May 1972.

22 Malcolm S. Knowles, *The Modern Practice of Adult Education*, Association Press, New York, 1970, pp. 37–39.

23 Thomas D. Hatch, "The Changing Federal Role in Allied Health Professions Education, 1966-1972," *Journal of Allied Health*, introductory issue, pp. 20–24, November 1972.

24 John F. Cady and Carl T. Anderson, "The Preceptorship in Allied Health Education: Short-Term Results of a Program to Influence the Distribution of Allied Health Manpower," *Journal of Allied Health,* **3**(1): 34–39, Winter 1974.

25 Personal communication with Mrs. Faith Hubbard, Head, Department of Nursing, Dakota Wesleyan University, Mitchell, South Dakota.

26 Ruth Roemer, "Trends in Licensure, Certification and Accreditation: Implications for Health Manpower Education in the Future," *Journal of Allied Health,* **3**(1): 26–33, Winter 1974.

BIBLIOGRAPHY

"Allied Medical Education," *JAMA*, **234**(13): 1379–1388, December 29, 1975.

Barish, Nathaniel H.: "Professional Judgment and the Use of Auxiliaries," *American Journal of Public Health*, **65**(9):972–975, September 1975.

Barkin, Roger M.: "Directions for Statutory Change: The Physician Extender," *American Journal of Public Health*, **64**(12):1132–1137, December 1974.

Cathcart, H. Robert: "Solving the 1976 Health Issues Today," *Journal of Allied Health*, **5**(1): 7–13, Winter 1976.

Connelly, Tom: "Health Care Process Teaching Models for Allied Health Students," *Journal of Allied Health*, **4**(1):39–45, Winter 1975.

Creager, Joan G., and Darrel L. Murray (eds.): *The Use of Modules in College Biology Teaching*, Pub. No. 31 of The Commission on Undergraduate Education in the Biological Sciences, The American Institute of Biological Sciences, Washington, D.C., 1971.

Culliton, Barbara J.: "Health Manpower: The Feds Are Taking Over," *Science*, **191**(4226):446–450, February 6, 1976.

Flack, Harley E.: "The Self-Emancipation of Allied Health: Toward a Systematological Conceptualization," *Journal of Allied Health*, **2**(1):16–23, February 1973.

Holcomb, J. David, and Deborah K. Milligan: "Utilizing Self-Instructional Materials to Improve Clinical Education in the Allied Health Professions," *Journal of Allied Health*, **3**(3): 109–112, Summer 1974.

Holder, Lee: "Delivery of Health Care: Implications for Allied Health Educators," *Journal of Allied Health*, 2(2):68–75, Spring 1973.

Holland, Max G., Roland J. Knobel, and Idell Parrish: "The Health Field Concept: Its Implications for Educating Health Professionals," *Journal of Allied Health*, 5(1):47–53, Winter 1976.

Kinsinger, Robert E.: "What This Country Doesn't Need Is a Left Carotid Artery Technician or a Career-Based Response to the 'New Careers' Scramble," *Journal of Allied Health*, 2(1): 10–15, February 1973.

Life and Death and Medicine, A Scientific American Book, W. H. Freeman, San Francisco, 1973.

Light, Israel: "The Changing Baccalaureate in Allied Health Specialists: A Point of View," *Journal of Allied Health*, 3(3):94–99, Summer 1974.

Moore, Sister Anne Joachim: "Technical Level Education for the Health Fields: A Private College President's View," *Journal of Allied Health*, 3(3):100–103, Summer 1974.

Readings in Health 76/77, The Dushkin Publishing Group, Guilford, Connecticut, 1976. (Particularly sec. 8, "Health and Society")

Warner, Anne R.: "NHC's Manpower Distribution Project—Finding Ways to Interest Students to Practice in Shortage Areas," *Journal of Allied Health*, 4(1):27–34, Winter 1975.

EDITOR'S QUESTIONS FOR DISCUSSION

What social forces have influenced a change in perspective in health care delivery from cure to prevention and self-care? What health-oriented conceptual framework might be proposed for nursing curricula? What type of reward systems might be established or adjusted for a teacher and student in individualized instruction? What criteria might determine how much "practice" is sufficient for the student?

How (and under whose jurisdiction) are patients, students, and educators in a health care setting subject to social control? How can social control constrain or facilitate quality of care to the patient? What type of clinical experiences might be learned effectively through simulation models? What types of clinical experiences are best learned in the actual clinical setting?

What would be the advantages and disadvantages of combining a challenge examination approach with a career ladder for upward mobility in nursing education? How essential would it be to have a *demonstration of practice* examination included with the above approach? If a combined approach were to be encouraged, what would be the implications for nursing as a profession?

What implications are there for the profession of nursing if continuing education becomes mandatory? What should be the content of continuing education programs? Should continuing education focus primarily on the practice of nursing? Should different levels of practice have different requirements—for example, what should the requirements be for faculty members in university settings and those who are most likely to be involved in teaching? Should nurses be required to take a specific number of hours of course work only in the area of nursing in which they are employed?

Part Three

Nursing Research

The need for research to develop new knowledge and to expand existing knowledge has long been recognized by nursing leaders but perhaps this need has been less acknowledged by many in nursing practice. Until recently, a question frequently asked in regard to the master's thesis or doctoral dissertation of a nursing graduate student was, "Of what use is it?" Often the research was perceived as an intellectual exercise, the last ritual requirement to be completed before a student could obtain a specific degree. Knowledge for the sake of knowledge has not been considered useful by those in nursing practice. However, this negative attitude has begun to change.

An interesting phenomenon is now developing. Those in nursing practice are beginning to realize the richness of their roles. Many are looking for a way to document their actual performance and to establish the need for their role; many are also seeking to develop new strategies for intervention in patient care. Finally, the nurse in practice is beginning to realize the function of nursing research. At the same time, nurse educators are emphasizing the need to develop the first-level knowledge base of nursing as a profession. The views of practitioners and educators vis-à-vis the purpose and utility of research are becoming more compatible. The problems concerning research are not resolved, but nursing has progressed considerably; it now recognizes the need for relevant research and is planning for the development of research within the profession. The contributions in this section present a broad view of the topic of research in nursing.

Chapter 14

Why Research in Nursing?

Ida Martinson, R.N., Ph.D., F.A.A.N.
Associate Professor, School of Nursing
University of Minnesota, Minneapolis

A rationale for nursing research is presented here by Ida Martinson. First, she traces the early development of research in nursing. Martinson then identifies nursing research as a means of effecting change and of substantiating the theories and practices critical to health care. To illustrate this point, examples of research in nursing practice are offered.

For many the term *research* conjures up images of peering into microscopes, answering lengthy questionnaires, making observations—pencil and pad in hand—and computing and manipulating statistics. Although these are certainly part of the investigative process, research includes much more than these. Before making observations, for example, the investigator must decide what she is going to observe and where she will make these observations. She must have already articulated in her own mind why she is selecting certain factors for observation and rejecting others. Prior to making such decisions, she must formulate some ideas regarding her study. These ideas, whether in the form of vague hunches or clearly formulated propositions, will serve as a guide in determining what questions are to be addressed by the research and which procedures and tools are to be used in searching for the answers. As Webster defines it, research is a "studious inquiry or examination; especially investigation or experimentation aimed at the discovery and interpretation of facts, revision of accepted theories or law in the light of new facts, or practical application of such new or revised theories or laws." [1]

Because of the rapidity with which scientific knowledge is expanding today, continuing "studious inquiry" becomes critical to the professions based on such knowledge. This is true of all the health professions, nursing included, because the expansion of health care needs in our society and our increasingly complex health care systems demand the ongoing acquisition of scientific knowledge. If nursing is to effectively meet the needs challenging it, research by nurses is imperative.

The field of nursing research is of quite recent origin. Florence Nightingale, it is true, made outstanding contributions to the development of hospital records after her research studies conducted during the Crimean War in the 1850s. However, although there had been much talk of the need for research in nursing and for research training of nurses, only a very few studies were published prior to 1950. With the establishment in 1955 of the Special Nurse Research Fellowship Program in the National Institute of Health—Division of Nursing, nursing research received the impetus it needed to become firmly established. [2] Then, as the nursing field experienced growing independence, nursing research continued to develop and to meet with increasing recognition. Today, with nursing education programs moving from the hospitals into colleges and universities (the University of Minnesota being the first to set up its program of nursing in 1909), nursing research finds itself in a more natural setting for both research activity and research training. In this new setting, the need for research to develop new knowledge and to expand existing knowledge has become more obvious. Thus, the present curricula in most undergraduate nursing programs not only include a course in research but also provide the opportunity to participate in ongoing studies. At the graduate level, students spend a major portion of the program in research. Dr. C. Peter Magrath, president of the University of Minnesota, stated that "we must look at money spent on research more as investments than as expenditures."[3] This applies to the field of nursing as well as to the other disciplines.

Nursing research is the aspect of research related to the whole of nursing: nursing practice, nursing education, and nursing service. It attempts to develop new methods and techniques in patient care necessitated by the changes and expansion in nursing responsibilities; it deals with questions about the care and support of patients and their families during illness and the prevention of illness, and about coping when no cure is known; it attempts to identify community health needs so that nursing care will be appropriate to the community served.

Sometimes these needs can best be met by utilizing knowledge developed and provided by other disciplines. For the most part, however, this is not adequate, for many of the problems to be faced by researchers are unique to nursing and can be most efficiently investigated by nurses themselves. Nurses, with their patient contacts day and night and their insight into patient care needs, stand in an unusually advantageous position for identifying these needs and for determining effective ways to meet them. Moreover, in nursing research additional tools of measurement peculiar to nursing must be implemented. It is primarily

through the efforts of nurse-researchers that nursing practice can be improved and a higher quality of patient care obtained. The aim of much research, as Webster stated, is to update and revise already accepted knowledge according to newly discovered facts. Nursing research goes a step further, for its primary aim is to use this new knowledge as a means for effecting change. The National Commission for Study has stated that "we are confident that only through research can we begin to determine and fully exploit the capabilities of nurses to contribute to the health system."[4] It is also true that only through nurse-researchers can we begin to determine and fully exploit the potentials of research to contribute to the health system. It is the nurse-researcher whose position and experience enable him or her to best identify and develop the nursing theories and practices basic to health care.

The extent to which nursing research is steadily expanding can be seen in the increasing number of reports and analyses of its contributions to the health system. In a recent 5-year overview, the following categories of research in nursing practice (as distinct from nursing education and other subjects) in regard to content alone were developed:

1 Research relevant to nursing specialities, such as obstetrics and mental health
2 Research relevant to nursing procedures and techniques, including both physical and psychological or psychiatric treatment procedures
3 Research relevant to specific aspects of nursing care, such as assessing patient needs and administration of medications
4 Research relevant to the state or condition of the patient, such as pain, dying anxiety, or fear

In addition to studies in these content areas, investigations regarding methodology were categorized according to subjects, design of study, statistics, instruments, and variables manipulated.[5]

A few examples of recent studies in content areas (some already published) conducted by nurse-researchers underscore the importance of research for the improvement of nursing practice.

One study, "Human Wakefulness and Biological Rhythms," focuses on biorhythms, the cycles of an individual's sleeping patterns, his or her temperature fluctuations, his or her periods of of mental alertness and productivity, and so on. The purpose of this study is to determine the effects of biorhythms on the efficiency and effectiveness of hospital routines, and, conversely, the effects of the hospital routines on an individual's biorhythms. "Heart Rate, Perceived Exertion, and Energy Expenditure During Range of Motion Exercises of the Extremities" studies the range of motion exercises frequently used in hospitals, for example, to prevent stiffness after a stroke or other illness. In "Control of Shivering During Hypothermia" the patient's perception of shivering as most uncomfortable is acknowledged and methods of decreasing shivering when hypothermia is necessary are explored. The study "Body Heat Loss Under Various Environmental Conditions" researches the effects of body heat loss, the implications of which are important in Minnesota where outdoor sports such as cross-country skiing, snowshoeing, and ice skating are on the increase. Recognition that the ability to feed oneself leads to an increase in self-respect and independence is basic to the study, "Reestablishing Self-Feeding in a Nursing Home Resident." The study "Changes in Children's Attitudes Toward the Physically Handicapped" is especially relevant now in light of Minnesota's decision to include physically handicapped children in the public school system. Studies such as "Simulated Living Quarters in Which Rehabilitation Equipment and Structural Modification Needs Can Be Assessed for Handicapped Subjects" aim to help patients make the necessary adjustments at home following hospital discharge. "Topical Application of Insulin in the Treatment of Decubitus Ulcers" deals with a major problem in nursing practice: the appearance of bed sores resulting from prolonged bed rest. The significance of "Exploration of Comfort-Care Measures for a Terminally Ill Patient" is immediately evident.

In "Importance of Selected Nursing Activities," assessments of both nurses and patients were researched. Rating the importance of four types of nursing activities that included physical care and psychosocial care for three of their patients, the nurses showed greater concern for psychosocial needs. These patients, in rating the same activities evidenced greater concern for the physical care. In "Research in Nursing Practice," it was shown that nurse-researchers share the values indicated by these clinical nurses, and that there has been relatively little research of physical care by nurses.[6]

This is a small sample of studies conducted by nurses throughout the country. Even on the local scene widely varying research projects are under way, some of which are partially funded by a federal grant for the support and development of nursing research at the University of Minnesota. These studies are researching, for example, the effect on children of the body changes associated with cancer and cancer therapy, the needs of widows, nursing interventions following a myocardial infarction, identification of the problems of visually handicapped diabetics in insulin administration, and problems encountered in breast feeding. Two faculty members are studying the process of health through various stages of development, and others are concentrating on the areas of aging, the nursing needs of epileptics, and a critical examination of the nurse-midwifery service. The significance of these research efforts regarding nursing practice can be seen in the following examples. In a recent study, Dr. Barbara Walike,[7] nurse-researcher from the University of Washington at Seattle, together with several other researchers, determined that most of the diarrhea and cramps associated with tube feedings could be avoided by a lactose-free feeding. Until the report of her research findings, lactose had always been used as an ingredient. Now all major manufacturers make available a lactose-free solution, thus providing relief from these complaints formerly so common from patients receiving tube feedings.

Similarly, Dr. Jean Johnson's research[8] at Wayne State University in Detroit has also brought relief to patients through easing their fears associated with various laboratory tests and diagnostic procedures. Her study was based on the assumption that much of the responsibility for identifying and disseminating information necessary for patients to cope effectively with illness lies with the nursing profession. She states that "one way to influence a person's expectations about physical sensations caused by a threatening event is to give information which describes sensations typically experienced,"[8] things that are felt, seen, smelled, heard, and tasted. By selecting information relevant to the emotional response she substantiated her hypothesis that preparatory information describing the sensations typically experienced during a threatening event will reduce the discrepancy between expectations and experience and result in reduced emotional response. She was also able to conclude that giving patients this preparatory sensation information would not have the effect of suggesting that they experience the sensations. Moreover, she was able to demonstrate that sensory information reduced the length of hospitalization, a fact with potentially great impact on cost for hospitalization following surgery.

Finally, one research project I am currently conducting focuses on bringing changes into our health care delivery system. These changes hopefully will alleviate some serious problems not yet solved. It has been generally assumed that the hospital is the most appropriate setting for the chronically ill and dying. However, preliminary analysis of data from my study indicates that for the dying child, for whom any substantial medical help is no longer possible, the home may be the more appropriate setting. There is evidence that when there has been adequate preparation of the child's family and when there is a support system available to the parents, they are able to provide quality care for the child. The advantages are not limited to a substantial reduction of the financial burden on the family. The emotional and psychological benefits to the child and his family are great. The dying child's need for his parents' love and the security of their presence can be met more easily at home than in the hospital. The

parents whose child is hospitalized often suffer the strain of conflicting responsibilities—to be with their dying child at the hospital and to care for the rest of the family at home. Through home care, tension arising from this conflict may be lessened. Most parents who have experienced home care feel that the grief process is eased considerably by knowing that they were with their dying child when he needed them most, and that they had the opportunity to do all within their power to help him through his crisis. Documentation is being made in this study of some of these needs experienced by the dying child and his parents and family, needs that in the past have too frequently remained unrecognized and unmet.

Systematic documentation is being carried out in many such areas new to research. In another study, fourteen mothers who had a child in coma all reported both a change in their eating patterns and sleep disturbances. Eleven of these reported feelings of hopelessness, disbelief, anger, and guilt. Comments such as "If only I hadn't punished him" or "If only I had not allowed her to go out that night" were not uncommon.[9] Only through obtaining such base-line data can some fundamental health care problems be recognized as such and improvements in nursing care be conceived and accomplished.

The need for documentation of procedures in nursing practice is also evident. In the Twin Cities, for example, differing approaches are used for newborns in intensive care units. One practice dictates that before suctioning the newborns, an increase of nasal oxygen be adminstered for one minute; in the other practice there is no increase of oxygen prior to suctioning. Which practice is better? One nurse responded to the challenge presented by this question and is currently conducting a study of the two procedures. To ensure valid and reliable documentation of research results before implementation, replication of research studies is important. At the same time, care must be taken to avoid unnecessary and costly duplication of efforts.

To achieve this replication essential for substantiating a research finding without needless duplication, effective means of communication become crucial. In the field of nursing such communication is promoted through nursing journals, such as the *American Journal of Nursing, Nursing Outlook, R.N.,* and *Nursing Research.* In these publications nurse-researchers are able to share their concerns and report their research. Conventions are another effective means of communication. At the national conventions of both the National League for Nursing (NLN) and the American Nurses Association (ANA) sessions are held that are devoted solely to nursing research. In June of 1976 in Atlantic City, the annual ANA convention, titled "Knowledge for Practice," included research reports in the subject areas of patients' suffering, music therapy for schizophrenics, differing suctioning procedures, prediction of nurse staffing needs to meet patient needs, and studies in home care of the dying child. The Council of Nurse Researchers also meets annually, providing an opportunity for nurses to present and discuss their research efforts.

Locally, within the Midwest area, we are experiencing an increasing exchange of information and sharing of research resources. Several nurse-researchers have visited the University of Minnesota in the past few years. Faculty from the university have shared their research expertise at various nursing conferences, through continuing education programs, and in other schools of nursing. An annual Nursing Research Symposium has recently been established at the University of Minnesota under the sponsorship of the School of Nursing. At this symposium, students, faculty, and clinicians all have the opportunity to present their research, followed by group discussion.

There still remain, however, certain obstacles to the rapid development of nursing research. This was evidenced in one large university hospital when a nursing administrator suggested that the term *nursing research* not be used. When asked why, she replied, "Some staff nurses think and believe they are the last advocates of the patients and their families against use as research materials."[10] Such an attitude is tragic. It is also ironic, for it is the researcher's deep interest in safeguard-

ing human rights and values that promotes her desire to conduct research and thus improve health care. In fact, this is the major focus of all nursing research.

There is also the obstacle of action-orientation within the nursing profession. Primarily a service profession geared in general to doing and to facing problems with action, nursing tends to value immediacy rather than the time-consuming analysis and testing demanded by research before action is initiated.

Although these obstacles to research are very real, they are not insurmountable. With determination, patience, and a long-range view of the needs of patient care, nurses will increasingly adopt research as their approach to problem solving and nursing research will continue to expand and contribute to the improvement of health care. Nursing research is a worthy investment.

NOTES

1 *Webster's New Collegiate Dictionary,* Merriam, Springfield, Mass, 1974.

2 Margorie V. Batey, "Reflections—and the Way Ahead," *Communicating Nursing Research: Collaboration and Competition,* Western Interstate Commission for Higher Education, Boulder, Co., 1973, vol. 6, pp. 217.

3 Peter C. Magrath, in a speech to Phi Delta Kappa, University of Minnesota, May 15, 1975.

4 "Recommendation of the National Commission for the Study of Nursing and Nursing Education," *American Journal of Nursing,* 7:285-288, February 1970.

5 Kathleen Ann O'Connell, "Research in Nursing Practice: Its Nature and Direction," *Image,* 8(1):6–10, February 1976.

6 Ibid.

7 Barbara C. Walike, Geraldine Padilla, Nancy Bergstrom, Robert L. Hanson, Winifred Kubo, Marcia Grant, and Hilda Luna Wong, "Patient Problems Related to Tube Feeding," *Communicating Nursing Research: Critical Issues in Access to Data,* vol. 7, Western Interstate Commission for High Education, Boulder, Co., 1975, pp. 89-112.

8 Jean E. Johnson, "Altering Patients' Responses to Threatening Events: A Classic Research Plan with Pragmatic Significance," Paper presented at Council for Nursing Researchers, ANA Convention, Atlantic City, June 1976.

9 Joyce Anderson, "The Identification of Psychosocial Stresses Experienced by the Mother Whose Child Is in a Prolonged Unconscious State Due to Acute Injury to the Brain," unpublished paper, University of Minnesota School of Nursing, March 1976.

10 Ida M. Martinson, "Nursing Research: Obstacles and Challenges," *Image*, 8(1):3-5, February 1976.

EDITOR'S QUESTIONS FOR DISCUSSION

How might research in nursing and the results of research be made more acceptable and meaningful for nurses at all levels? What research in nursing practice is needed? In what type of settings should research in nursing be done?

Chapter 15

Research in Nursing Practice: Its Present Scope

Kathleen A. O'Connell, R.N., Ph.D.
Midwest Research Institute, Kansas City, Missouri

Margery Duffey, R.N., Ph.D.
Professor and Associate Dean, School of Nursing
College of Health Sciences and Hospital
Kansas University Medical Center, Kansas City, Kansas

To establish goals and direct future efforts in the development of research programs, periodic reassessment of past achievements is beneficial. Kathleen A. O'Connell and Margery Duffey present an analysis of research in nursing practice published in *Nursing Research* during a 6-year period. To be included in this review, a study had to deal with the interaction of nurses, acting as nurses, and patients. The 88 studies reviewed were done by 161 investigators, the majority of whom had Master's degrees in nursing. Surgical patients were the most frequently studied. Studies seldom dealt with patients who had chronic illnesses, acute medical diagnoses, orthopedic problems, or communicable diseases. Fewer than one-third of the studies dealt with physical needs. O'Connell and Duffey indicate that there is a need for more concern about the reliability and validity of data-collecting techniques and the accurate replication of research, and they recommend the establishment of a system for the interchange of research instruments so that investigators could test the reliability of newly-developed instruments.

This chapter presents an analysis of the research in nursing practice that has been published by the journal *Nursing Research* during a 6-year period. The research is described according to (1) the characteristics of the investigators, (2) the content of the studies, and (3) the research methods employed. The results of this analysis enable us to identify the nature and direction of the research in nursing practice. The content areas that researchers emphasized as well as those that they neglected are described. In addition, the analysis gives some indication of the relative sophistication of the research methods.

In an article in a 1975 issue of *Nursing Research*, Dickoff, James, and Semradek contended that nursing research has left nursing practice virtually untouched. As if to prove the point, *Nursing Research* editors followed the article

This article is a revised and updated version of the original article "Research in Nursing Practice: Its Nature and Direction," published in *Image*, 8(1), February 1976. Because the sample has been increased and some of the categories redefined, the results are not equivalent to those published in the original article.

with a study by Ketefian, in which only one of eighty-seven nurses knew the correct placement time for taking oral temperatures. Experiments by Nichols and others (1966, 1967, 1972) that determined the correct placement time had been reported in *Nursing Research* and in the *American Journal of Nursing.*

The lack of impact of nursing research was attributed to different causes in the two articles. Ketefian held that there was a lack of communication between researchers and practitioners. Dickoff, James, and Semradek, on the other hand, maintained that nursing-researchers were so preoccupied with "pseudotechnical research methodology" that they lost sight of the real problems in nursing. The research findings, they said, are either obvious generalities, inapplicable, or unapplied minute points. This indictment of nursing research is sweeping and serious.

This chapter enumerates and describes a sample of studies that concern the practice of nursing. The information presented here provides a factual basis from which to react to the charges made by Dickoff and his associates. The sample includes all studies of nursing practice published in the journal *Nursing Research* from 1970 through 1975. *Nursing Research* is not the only publisher of studies of nursing research, but it was felt that the studies published there would be representative of the best studies in nursing.

A study of "nursing practice" was defined as a study that in any way dealt with the interaction of nurses, acting as nurses, and clients, be they well or ill. This definition was designed to include studies of nurses in extended roles, and studies that dealt with the use of nursing assessment tools. The definition excludes studies of nurses in isolation from patients, and studies of patients in isolation from nurses.

The variables of the studies were examined to determine if any of them related to the interaction of nurses and patients. If no such variables were found, the study was excluded from the sample. For instance, a study by Muhlenkamp, Gress, and Flood (1975) dealt with the perception of life

change events by the elderly. Since the study is focused on clients (rather than nursing personnel, students, or educators) it met one criterion of the definition. However, because the variables considered did not include interaction between the clients and nurses, the study was excluded from the sample. Similarly, studies that correlated patients' preoperative anxiety with variables such as number of days in the hospital, number of complications, and number of analgesics were not included in the sample unless a specific nursing action, such as preoperative teaching by a nurse, was among the variables considered. Studies that concerned patients' attitudes toward specific nurses, or patients' satisfaction with care, were included in the sample, since these variables presuppose interaction with nurses. If a study encompassed many variables and at least one of them concerned the interaction between nurses and patients, the study was included in the sample.

It should be noted that a study of nursing practice is not necessarily a "clinical study." Some of the studies in the present sample were carried out in laboratories. The laboratory studies included research on the reliability of monitoring techniques, and methods of applying elastic bandages, of administering oxygen, and of increasing tolerance for pain. Such studies have direct relevance for nursing practice because they concern behaviors that are generally recognized as nursing care. However, they may be considered laboratory rather than clinical studies. On the other hand, some of the studies that might be of a clinical nature, for example, the study of the perception of life change events by the elderly, cannot be considered studies of nursing practice.

The sample of studies was classified along a number of dimensions. The investigators were categorized according to whether or not they were nurses and according to their educational attainment. Each study's content was classified according to four different perspectives: general diagnostic category of the subjects; the procedure or technique investigated; the specific needs of patients that the research focused on; and the state or condition of the subjects. The studies were also categorized according to the research methods that were employed. These methods included the types of subject samples; the design of the studies; the types of variables manipulated; and the statistics used and the instruments employed.

During the 6-year period from 1970 through 1975, *Nursing Research* published about 325 studies. For purposes of this analysis, eighty-eight or 27 percent were deemed studies of nursing practice. Table 15-1 shows the number of studies of nursing practice each year.

As the table shows, the number of studies of nursing practice has been quite stable over the period with a slight increase in 1975. The editor of *Nursing Research*, Elizabeth Carnegie, stated (1976) that the number of articles of a clinical nature increased 100 percent between 1972 and 1974. It is not entirely clear what her definition of an "article of a clinical nature" is. However, the increase in articles of a clinical nature was not accompanied by an increase in studies of nursing practice.

Table 15-1 Number of Studies of Nursing Practice—by Year

Year	Number of studies
1970	14
1971	16
1972	15
1973	12
1974	14
1975	17
Total	88

Table 15-2 Educational Attainment of Investigators at the Time Studies Were Published

	Bachelor's or less	Master's	Doctorates	Total
Nurses	19	91	28	138
Non-nurses	0	4	19*	23

*Includes four investigators with M.D.s

The 88 studies were carried out by 161 investigators, 86 percent of whom were nurses. Of the nurse-investigators, twenty-eight (20 percent) had doctoral degrees. Only two of the nurses with doctoral degrees had doctorates in nursing science, and thirteen had earned a Ph.D. Of the non-nurse investigators, 83 percent had doctoral degrees. The majority of nurse-investigators had master's degrees at the time the studies were published. This fact is both encouraging and discouraging. It shows that nurses with master's degrees are capable of carrying out the bulk of research in nursing practice and that the doctoral degree is not a prerequisite as it is in some fields. However, there is little indication that these nurse-investigators hold positions that emphasize doing research on nursing practice.

CONTENT

Diagnostic Category of the Subjects

The eighty-eight studies in the sample were all classified according to the diagnostic category of the subjects. Studies in which *all* of the subjects were children were categorized in the "pediatrics" category, regardless of the diagnosis of the subject. Studies in which the subjects were healthy or in which subjects did not fit in any of the other categories, were placed in the "other" category. The "diverse" category included studies in which the subjects were in more than one diagnostic category. Some of these studies had both children and adults as subjects. The categories are mutually exclusive.

As Table 15-3 shows, the investigators frequently chose clients with diverse diagnoses as subjects for their studies. The "diverse" category accounted for 30 percent of the studies, a greater proportion than any of the discrete diagnostic categories. "Surgery" was the most frequently studied discrete diagnostic category. It accounted for 16 percent of the studies. "Pediatrics" accounted for 15 percent of the studies.

The fact that many of the studies concern

...ostic Category of Subjects

	1975	1970–75 (Total)	Percent
...	2	5	6
Pediatrics	5	13	15
Acute medicine	0	1	1
Surgery	1	14	16
Orthopedics	0	2	2
Communicable disease	0	0	0
Chronic illness and disability	1	6	7
Mental illness	3	11	12
Other	1	10	11
Diverse	4	26	30
Total	17	88	100

subjects with varied diagnoses may indicate that nurse-researchers are striving to investigate problems that are common to all patients. When specific types of patients are studied, however, surgical patients are studied far more frequently than any other type. This is not surprising since surgery is a dramatic intervention into a person's life, and its potential complications are similar for all patients who undergo surgery. Perhaps the most telling finding in this classification is the lack of studies dealing with chronic illness, acute medical diagnoses, orthopedics, or communicable disease. The lack of studies in the "communicable disease" category is probably indicative of the few communicable diseases (among adults) nurses deal with in current nursing practice. The same cannot be said for the "chronic illness" category, which included studies of patients with heart disease, diabetes, and spinal cord injuries. Patients with these conditions, along with patients with orthopedic conditions, present some of nursing's most difficult problems, because of the length of time such patients require nursing care. The few studies in the "acute medicine" category probably reflect the heavy weighting of the sample with clients who were hospitalized rather than outpatients. Outpatient clinics are more likely to deal with acute medical problems such as noncommunicable infections.

Procedures and Techniques

The eighty-eight studies were categorized according to the procedures and techniques that the studies investigated. "Monitoring techniques" refer to procedures for measuring physical indexes such as vital signs. "Physical care techniques" include studies that are concerned with specific nursing care procedures such as bathing, moist soaks, catheterization, and so on. "Psychiatric treatments" refer to specific treatments of psychiatric patients such as group therapy. "Assessment techniques" refer to the process of assessing an individual patient's nursing care needs. The assessment category does *not* refer to the assessment of the quality of nursing care, nor does it refer to assessment of patients' satisfaction with nursing care. The category "organization of staff" refers to studies of the effect on patients of special nursing care programs or staffing procedures, for example, primary care. "Other" refers to various techniques or procedures that are not described by the previously mentioned categories. Most studies in the "other" category have to do with techniques for giving emotional support and with techniques for increasing pain tolerance.

The categories are not mutually exclusive. Three of the studies concerned more than one type of procedure or technique. As Table 15-4 shows, 20 percent of the studies do not deal with any type of nursing procedure or technique. Most of these studies have to do with patients' attitudes toward nursing care. The studies that are concerned with procedures and techniques are evenly divided among most of the categories with relatively fewer studies in the "organization of staff" and "psychiatric treatments" categories.

Specific Needs of Patients

The eighty-eight studies were classified according to the specific needs of patients with which the studies were concerned. The category "protection" refers to the need for prevention of infection and of complications such as infusion phlebitis. The category "emotional support" includes studies that the investigators stipulated were

Table 15-4 Number of Studies of Procedure and Techniques

Procedure or technique	1975	1970–75 (Total)	Percent
Monitoring techniques	0	11	12
Physical care techniques	2	13	15
Psychiatric treatments	2	6	7
Teaching techniques	1	13	15
Assessment techniques	3	12	14
Organization of staff	2	5	6
Other	4	13	15
None of the above	3	18	20

Table 15-5 Number of Studies Focusing on Specific Needs of Patients That Were Studied

	1975	1970–75 (Total)	Percent
Physical needs	3	28	32
Food and nutrition	1	4	4
Rest and sleep	1	4	4
Cleanliness	1	3	3
Exercise	0	1	1
Elimination	0	3	3
Respiration	0	5	6
Relief of pain	0	5	6
Protection	1	9	10
Medication	0	0	0
Nonphysical needs	8	26	30
Emotional support	4	15	17
Communication	3	10	11
Recreation	1	1	1
Religious	0	0	0
Family	2	2	2
No specific needs studied	7	37	42

concerned with the relief of anxiety or tension. The "communication" category includes studies of verbal and nonverbal communication that do not expressly relate to the relief of anxiety and are not considered teaching. Included in the "communication" category are studies concerning the effect of touch on the seriously ill patient and the effect of preoperative visits by operating room nurses. The categories are not mutually exclusive. Nine of the studies concerned more than one type of need.

As Table 15-5 shows, 42 percent of the studies could not be classified in any of the categories relating to patients' needs. Most of these studies concerned studies of monitoring techniques, assessment techniques, measurement of attitudes, and teaching techniques that are not directed at any specific needs. In addition, studies concerning organization of staff wherein the variables reflect overall needs—such as quality of nursing care— were counted in the "no specific needs studied" category. Approximately 32 percent of the studies concerned physical needs, while 30 percent of the studies concerned nonphysical needs. Four of the studies concerned both physical and nonphysical needs. Most · of the studies concerning nonphysical needs had to do with emotional support and communication. Before 1975, there were no studies in the sample that concerned needs of the family of the client. In 1975 two studies appeared that dealt with this area. Protection from infections and complications was the

most frequently studied physical need. There were no studies that had to do with the patients' needs for medication or with religious needs.

The most frequently studied need was the need for emotional support. There is no doubt that this is an important need. Nevertheless, one wonders why relatively little attention is given to physical nursing care. Clinical nurses spend much of their time administering medications, helping to bathe, feed, and move patients, and trying to promote rest and comfort. Yet, few of the studies investigated these areas of concern. In fact, the twenty-eight studies of physical needs represent less than 9 percent of *all* the studies published in *Nursing Research* over the 6 years.

States or Conditions of the Subjects

The studies in the sample were also classified with reference to the actual states of the subjects in

Table 15-6 Number of Studies That Focused on Specific Patient States

State	1975	1970–75 (Total)	Percent
Anoxia	0	0	0
Anxiety and fear	1	12	14
Bedfastness	1	3	3
Dying	0	0	0
Fever	0	6	7
Healthy	2	9	10
Hyperactivity or hypoactivity	0	1	1
Incontinence or constipation	0	1	1
Infection, inflammation	0	6	7
Insomnia	1	5	6
Malnutrition	1	1	1
Nausea	0	0	0
Pain or distress	1	11	12
Prematurity	1	2	2
Preop, postop states	1	15	17
Reactions to nursing	4	14	16
Psychological maladaptation	3	12	14
Shock	0	0	0
Unconsciousness	0	4	4
None of the above	4	14	16

Table 15-7 Number of Studies by Status and Age Group of Subjects

	1975	1970–75 (Total)	Percent
Status			
Inpatients	12	67	76
Outpatients	4	12	14
Healthy clients	2	11	12
Age			
Neonates	1	4	4
Children	4	9	10
18 to 64 years old	3	29	33
65 and over	1	1	1
Age not specified or spans above categories	8	45	51
Total	17	88	99

the studies. The categories are not mutually exclusive since twenty-two of the studies were concerned with more than one patient state. For instance, some of the studies concerned patients who were about to undergo surgery and who were anxious.

The category "bedfastness" has to do with studies of patients who are confined to bed. The "pain or distress" category is concerned with studies of patients who are experiencing pain. The category "reactions to nursing" identifies studies that have to do with attitudes of patients toward nurses or nursing care. The category "none of the above" contains studies that did not deal with a particular patient state as a variable of interest. Most of these studies had to do with teaching, assessment, and organization of nursing care.

The emphasis on the surgical patient is evident. Preoperative and postoperative states are the most frequently studied category. Other frequently studied categories are "anxiety and fear," "reactions to nursing," and "psychological maladaptation." Studies concerning patients experiencing pain or distress also appear with relative frequency. There were no studies in which the clients were anoxic, dying, nauseated, or in shock, and few studies concerned with problems of hyperactivity and hypoactivity, incontinence and constipation, malnutrition, and bedfastness.

RESEARCH METHODS

Characteristics of Subjects

The studies of nursing practice were classified according to whether the subjects were inpatients, outpatients, or healthy, and according to the ages of the subjects. Two of the studies used healthy clients and patients as subjects; therefore, the categories are not mutually exclusive.

Only 14 percent of the studies used outpatients as subjects. With the increasing emphasis on outpatient care, and with the participation of nurse clinicians and nurse practitioners in outpatient services, there should, perhaps, be more concentration on outpatient care. However, outpatients are more difficult to study since, unlike inpatients, they are not a captive population.

The great majority of studies had to do with adults. However, as the table shows, the studies appear to span the age groups rather well. This situation is important, especially when compared to the large number of studies in other fields that are done with college-age subjects. Only one study in the sample concentrated on persons over the age of 64. But, a number of studies did focus on patients that were both under and over 65. However, the lack of studies relating to the special health and nursing problems of the elderly is quite real. It is ironic that only one of the eighty-eight studies took place in a nursing home. Indeed, nursing care, rather than medical care, is the primary activity of nursing homes and extended care facilities. Yet, research in nursing practice as represented by the sample reviewed here has barely touched on topics of special interest to such nursing domains.

The eighty-eight studies comprise a wide range of sample sizes. Only one of the studies in the sample was a single case study. Case studies have been quite common in medical research and are often useful in illustrating rare cases, or in generating ideas and hypotheses. The rarity of the case study in this literature may have something to do with the trend toward investigations that produce findings that can be generalized. As Table 15-8 shows, approximately one-fourth of the studies had between eleven and thirty subjects. Another fourth of the studies had over 100 subjects.

Although the appropriateness of the sample size depends on the nature of the research, the fact that more than half of the studies in the sample use fewer than fifty subjects indicates that the researchers have tended to deal with small samples. In clinical research, it is sometimes impractical or impossible to deal with samples greater than fifty subjects. However, it is more difficult to

Table 15-8 Number of Studies of Various Sample Sizes

Number of subjects	1975	1970–1975 (Total)	Percent
10 or less	1	10	11
11 to 30	5	22	25
31 to 50	1	17	19
51 to 70	2	8	9
71 to 100	3	9	10
Over 100	5	20	23
Not reported	0	2	2
Total	17	88	99

detect statistically significant differences with small samples. In addition, because we rarely are able to select subjects at random, findings based on small samples are not convincingly generalized to other groups. Thus, replication is a necessity.

RESEARCH DESIGN

The studies in the sample were also categorized according to the research designs used. "Experimental" studies were those that manipulated one or more of the variables. "Correlational" studies were those that showed relationships between variables but did not manipulate them. "Descriptive" studies present frequency counts and percentages as findings without relating the variables studied. "Reliability" testing had to do with studies that were *solely* for the testing of the reliability of measurement instruments.

If a study was both experimental and correlational, it was considered an experimental study. If a study was both correlational and descriptive, it was categorized as a correlational study. And, if a study tested the reliability of an instrument in addition to manipulating variables, or demonstrating relationships, it was categorized in the "experimental" or "correlational" category, rather than in the "reliability" category. Therefore, the categories are mutually exclusive.

A little over half of the studies were experimental. Before 1975, *Nursing Research* published an average of seven studies of nursing practice a year that were experimental. In 1975, thirteen of the studies in nursing practice were experimental. While it is true that experimental studies are not necessarily superior to descriptive or correlational studies, the increase probably reflects increased sophistication in research techniques. But, increased sophistication in research techniques does not imply that the investigators have lost sight of the real problems in nursing, as Dickoff and his associates have charged. The experimental method is well suited to determining if there is a difference between two types of treatments. It would seem that if the practice of nursing is going to be affected by nursing research, it will be those studies that use experimental designs that will contribute most to constructive changes in nursing practice.

Approximately one-fifth of the studies were correlational. Most of the studies in the "reliability" category were concerned with the reliability of monitoring techniques. Only two of the studies in this category concerned the reliability of paper-and-pencil instruments.

Variables Manipulated

As reported above, forty-six of the studies were experimental. These studies were classified according to the nature of their independent variables. Some of the studies manipulated more than one type of variable.

As the table shows, most of the manipulated variables were classified in the "other" category. Most of these studies dealt with nonphysical aspects of care, such as techniques for reducing anxiety, or for increasing pain tolerance. "Teaching techniques" and "physical care techniques" were manipulated with greater frequency than "psychiatric treatments" or "assessment techniques."

Statistics

The studies were classified according to the types of statistics used. The "nonparametric" category

Table 15-9 Number of Studies According to Research Design

Design	1975	1970–75 (Total)	Percent
Expermiental	13	46	52
Correlational	1	17	19
Descriptive	1	13	15
Reliability	2	12	14

Table 15-10 Number of Studies by Types of Variables Manipulated

Independent variables	1975	1970–75 (Total)	Percent
Physical care techniques	4	12	14
Psychiatric treatments	1	4	4
Assessment techniques	2	5	6
Teaching	1	12	14
Other	6	16	18
None	4	42	48

Table 15-11 Number of Studies Using Various Types of Statistics

Type of statistic	1975	1970–75	Percent
Parametric	11	51	58
Nonparametric	10	31	35
Descriptive	2	17	19
Not reported	0	6	7

includes chi-square tests and Fisher's exact probability test. Some of the studies used both parametric and nonparametric statistics.

Most of the studies used inferential statistics, either parametric, nonparametric, or both. There was some indication that the investigators were becoming more careful about how they reported the statistics used. Prior to 1975, there were six studies in the sample that did not report what type of statistics were used. In 1975, however, there were no studies that did not include this information.

Instruments

The instruments that investigators use to measure the phenomena they study are critically important to the validity of their findings. The studies were classified according to the types of instruments employed. Thirty-one of the studies used more than one type of instrument; therefore, the categories are not mutually exclusive. "Physical measures" are those used to determine physical characteristics like height, pulse, galvanic skin response, and serum levels of cortico-steroids.

As Table 15-12 shows, over one-third of the studies in the sample used some type of physical measure. The measures were approximately equally divided between those that nurses usually perform, for example, central venous pressure readings, and those not usually performed by nurses, for example, galvanic skin responses.

The interview is a technique that is familiar to most nurses. Over one-fifth of the studies in the sample used the interview as a data-collection technique.

The remaining instruments are referred to as paper-and-pencil measures. Included in the paper-and-pencil measures are two types of self-report instruments, and two types of observer report measures. Sixty percent of the studies in the sample used some type of paper-and-pencil instrument. Approximately one-third of the studies in the sample used a self-report measure of attitudes or feelings. Only 4 percent of the studies used a self-report of knowledge measure. This finding is interesting in light of the emphasis on teaching techniques in this sample. The dependent measure in many of the teaching studies was not an objective test of the patients' knowledge, but a subjective measure of some sort, for example, anxiety, or a physical measure. Perhaps some of the negative findings in this area relate to the fact that the patient did not, in fact, learn what he or she was taught. With great emphasis on self-care for most patients, it may be crucial for nurse-researchers to develop nonthreatening tests of knowledge in order to determine if patients really have the knowledge basic to their self-care.

Table 15-12   Number of Studies Using Various Research Instruments

Type of instrument	1975	1970–75 (Total)	Percent
Physical measures	4	31	35
Interviews	5	19	22
Self-report of attitudes, opinions, feelings	10	29	33
Self-report of knowledge	1	4	4
Observer rating scales	12	36	41
Report of family member	2	3	3
None reported	0	6	7

Over 40 percent of the studies in the sample used some type of observer rating scale in which an observer—usually the investigator, but sometimes the nurse taking care of a patient—rates the subject on the variables in question. The second type of observer rating scale—one in which the objectivity is left more open to question—is a scale that family members complete about their relatives who are patients. These scales are most often used in a pediatric setting and represented only a small proportion of the instruments used.

Reliability of instruments is a critical question in all research. A factor that may indicate the reliability of an instrument is whether the instrument has been used in previous studies. While it is possible to test the reliability of newly-developed instruments, a small fraction of the studies actually did so. It is probably (although not necessarily) true that previously published instruments have greater reliability and validity than instruments developed for a particular study. While fifty-three of the eighty-eight studies used paper-and-pencil instruments, only twenty-one studies used at least one previously-developed instrument and thirty-two studies used original instruments exclusively. The use of previously-developed instruments increased dramatically in 1975. In the years 1970 to 1974 only 17 percent of the studies used at least one previously-developed instrument. In 1975, however, 53 percent of the studies used at least one instrument that was previously developed. Most of the previously-developed instruments were developed outside the nursing context. Only six of the eighty-eight studies in the sample used instruments previously developed by nurses. Four of these studies appeared in 1975.

SUMMARY AND CONCLUSIONS

Over a 6-year period, eighty-eight studies of nursing practice appeared in *Nursing Research*. Most of the studies were carried out by nurses who had master's degrees. The group of studies represents research on patients of different ages who had a variety of diagnoses, needs, and conditions. More than half of the studies used experimental designs, and nearly three-fourths of the studies used some type of inferential statistic.

The group of studies showed a heavy concentration on inpatients, especially those who were undergoing surgery. There were few studies on patients with chronic illness. One of the most telling findings was the lack of concentration on physical needs and physical care. Less than one-third of the studies dealt with physical needs. Only 15 percent of the studies concerned physical care procedures, and only 12 percent of the studies used a physical care technique as an independent variable.

One of the most disconcerting aspects of the research presented here is the lack of concern about the reliability and validity of the instruments used to collect data. While some researchers did try to establish reliability on their own instruments, few seemed to have consulted the literature to find instruments that were already constructed. Each investigator seemed to find it necessary to invent a new instrument. This practice may be appropriate for studies in new areas, but researchers should be more concerned with the reliability and validity of their data-collecting techniques. Without such concern the ability to generalize findings is greatly compromised. This problem could be remedied if some system were established for the interchange of research

instruments so that investigators in different parts of the country could test the reliability of the newly-developed instruments.

Dickoff, James, and Semradek contended that nursing research has been irrelevant and inapplicable to the practice of nursing. This review challenges that contention, by pointing out that eighty-eight studies, or 27 percent of all the studies published by *Nursing Research* in the last 6 years have direct relevance to the practice of nursing. Dickoff and his associates also charged that nurses were so preoccupied with research methodology that they lost sight of the real problems in nursing. There are indications in the studies reviewed here that research designs are becoming more sophisticated. However, an inspection of the types of instruments used in the studies reveals that there is, perhaps, too little rather than too much concern with methodological issues such as reliability of instruments.

Therefore, it must be said that the indictments made by Dickoff, James, and Semradek are not completely grounded in fact. Nevertheless, those who have given the matter consideration must admit that research in nursing has not appreciably changed the behavior of nurses. Part of the reason for this is that not enough research has been undertaken. How can the physical care that is rendered by nurses be affected by nursing research when only 11 of 325 studies published during a 6-year period actually compared different techniques for physical care?

Another reason for the lack of impact of research on practice is the lack of replicated research. Nursing practitioners should be reluctant to adopt procedures that are based on findings of a single research study. Such findings may be peculiar to the particular characteristics of the sample, the location of the study, or experimenter effect. Only replication of the research in different localities by different researchers on larger samples will insure the reliability of the findings.

This chapter has presented an analysis of research in nursing practice that has been published in the last 6 years. It is hoped that this analysis will influence the future direction of research in nursing practice. The approach of analyzing the past as a base for projecting the needs of the future is a pragmatic one. Alone, it is insufficient as a guide for planning future directions for research in nursing. However, when nurse-theorists integrate findings such as these with the conceptual systems they develop, it is hoped the ensuing nursing research will have a profound effect on the practice of nursing.

BIBLIOGRAPHY

Carnegie, M. Elizabeth: "The Editor's Report—1976," *Nursing Research,* vol. 25, p. 3, 1976.

Dickoff, J., P. James, and J. Semradek: "8–4 Research Part 1: A Stance for Nursing Research—Tenacity or Inquiry," *Nursing Research,* vol. 24, pp. 84–88, 1975.

Ketefian, S.: "Application of Selected Nursing Research Findings into Nursing Practice: A Pilot Study," *Nursing Research,* vol. 24, pp. 89-92, 1975.

Muhlenkamp, A. F., L. D. Gress, and M. A. Flood: "Perception of Life Change Events by the Elderly," *Nursing Research,* vol. 24, pp. 109-113, 1975.

Nichols, G. A., and D. H. Kucha: "Taking Adult Temperatures: Oral Measurements," *American Journal of Nursing,* vol. 72, pp. 1090-1093, 1972.

——, and P. J. Verhonick: "Time and Temperature," *American Journal of Nursing,* vol. 67, pp. 2304-2306, 1967.

——, et al: "Oral, Axillary, and Rectal Temperature Determinations and Relationships," *Nursing Research,* vol. 15, pp. 307-310, 1966.

APPENDIX

Research Studies of Nursing Practice in *Nursing Research* by Year

Nursing Research, vol. 19, 1970:

Bluemle, Madeline L.: "Tracheal Bacterial Counts of Patients Following Suctioning," no. 2, pp. 116-121.

Cohen, Roberta: "The Effect of Specific Emotional Support on Anxiety Levels Prior to Electroconvulsive Therapy," no. 2, pp. 163-165.

Forster, Brenda, Diance C. Adler, and Mardell Davis: "Duration of Effects of Drinking Iced Water on Oral Temperature," no. 2, pp. 169-170.

Glor, B. A. K., and Zane Estes: "Moist Soaks: A Survey of Clinical Practices," no. 5, pp. 463-465.

——, E. F. Sullivan, and Zane E. Estes: "Reproducibility of Blood Pressure Measurements: A Replication," no. 2, pp. 170-172.

Graffam, Shirley R.: "Nurse Response to the Patient in Distress-Development of an Instrument," no. 4, pp. 331-336.

Guberski, Thomasine, and Mary Ellen Campbell: "The Effects on Leg Volume of Two Methods of Wrapping Elastic Bandages," no. 3, pp. 260-265.

Hamdi, Mary Evans, and Carol M. Hutelmeyer: "A Study of the Effectiveness of an Assessment Tool in the Identification of Nursing Care Problems," no. 4, pp. 354-359.

Larson, Elaine: "Bacterial Colonization of Tracheal Tubes of Patients in a Surgical Intensive Care Unit," no. 2, pp. 122-128.

Lowe, Marie L.: "Effectiveness of Teaching as Measured by Compliance with Medical Recommendations," no. 1, pp. 59-63.

Putt, Arlene M.: "One Experiment in Nursing Adults with Peptic Ulcers," no. 6, pp. 484-494.

Triplett, June L.: "Characteristics and Perceptions of Low-Income Women and Use of Preventive Health Services," no. 2, pp. 140-146.

Waligora, Sr. Barbara Marie: "The Effect of Nasal and Oral Breathing upon Nasopharyngeal Oxygen Concentration," no. 1, pp. 75-78.

Whitner, Willamay, and Margaret Thompson: "The Influence of Bathing on the Newborn Infant's Body," no. 1, pp. 30-36.

Nursing Research, vol. 20, 1971:

Aiken, Linda H., and Theodore F. Henrichs: "Systematic Relaxation as a Nursing Intervention Technique with Open Heart Surgery Patients," no. 3, pp. 212-217.

Ankenbrandt, Margurerite D., and Linda K. Tanner: "Role-delineated and Informal Nurse-Teaching and Food Selection Behavior of Geriatric Patients," no. 1, pp. 61–64.

Balthazar, Earl E., George E. English, and Ronald M. Sindberg: "Behavior Changes in Mentally Retarded Children Following the Initiation of an Experimental Nursing Program," no. 1, pp. 69–74.

Bliss, Ann, Lila Decker, and Wayne O. Southwick: "The Emergency Room Nurse Orders X-Rays of Distal Limbs in Orthopedic Trauma," no. 5, pp. 440–443.

Chastko, Helen E., Ira D. Glick, Edward Gould, and William A. Hargreaves: "Patients' Posthospital Evaluations of Psychiatric Nursing Treatment," no. 4, pp. 333–338.

Cleland, Virginia, Frank Cox, Helen Berggren, and M. R. MacInnis: "Prevention of Bacteriuria in Female Patients with Indwelling Catheters," no. 4, pp. 309–318.

Cross, Joanne E., and Carol R. Parsons: "Nurse-Teaching and Goal-directed Nurse-Teaching to Motivate Change in Food Selection Behavior of Hospitalized Patients," no. 5, pp. 454–458.

Foley, Mary F.: "Variations in Blood Pressure in the Lateral Recumbent Position," no. 1, pp. 64–69.

Lagina, Suzanne M.: "A Computer Program to Diagnose Anxiety Levels," no. 6, pp. 484–492.

Lindeman, Carol, and Betty VanAernam: "Nursing Intervention with the Presurgical Patient—the Effects of Structured and Unstructured Preoperative Teaching," no. 4, pp. 319–332.

McCaffery, Margo: "Children's Responses to Rectal Temperatures: An Exploratory Study," no. 1, pp. 32–45.

McFadden, Eileen H., and Elizabeth C. Giblin: "Sleep Deprivation in Patients Having Open-Heart Surgery," no. 3, pp. 249–254.

Mikulic, Mary Ann: "Reinforcement of Independent and Dependent Patient Behaviors by Nursing Personnel: An Exploratory Study," no. 2, pp. 162–165.

Nield, Margaret Ann: "The Effect of Health Teaching on the Anxiety Level of Patients with Chronic Obstructive Lung Disease," no. 6, pp. 537–542.

Palmer, Edwina M., and Elizabeth W. Griffith: "Effect of Activity During Bedmaking on

Heart Rate and Blood Pressure," no. 1, pp. 17–24.

Van Meter, Margie, and Patricia W. Mitchell: "Reproducibility of Blood Pressures Recorded on Patients' Records by Nursing Personnel," no. 4, pp. 348–352.

Nursing Research, vol. 21, 1972:

Brink, Pamela J.: "Behavioral Characteristics of Heroin Addicts on a Short-Term Detoxification Program," no. 1, pp. 38–45.

Diers, Donna, Ruth Schmidt, M. A. B. McBride, and Bette Davis: "The Effect of Nursing Interaction on Patients in Pain," no. 5, pp. 419–428.

Elms, Roslyn: "Recovery Room Behavior and Postoperative Convalescence," no. 5, pp. 390–397.

Harper, Mary, Betty Marcom, and Victor Wall: "Abortion—Do Attitudes of Nursing Personnel Affect the Patient's Perceptions of Care?" no. 4, pp. 327–331.

LaFargue, Jane P.: "Role of Prejudice in Rejection of Health Care," no. 1, pp. 53–58.

Lindeman, Carol: "Nursing Intervention with the Presurgical Patient," no. 3, pp. 196–209.

Marshall, Jon C., and Sally S. Feeney: "Structured Versus Intuitive Intake Interview," no. 3, pp. 269–272.

Nichols, Glennadee A.: "Time Analyses of Afebrile and Febrile Temperature Reading," no. 5, pp. 463–464.

——, Rosemarie Mahoney, and Delores Kucha: "Rectal Thermometer Placement Times for Febrile Adults," no. 1, pp. 76–77.

——, Ruth Kulvi, Nancy Christ, and Hazel Life: "Measuring Oral and Rectal Temperatures of Febrile Children," no. 3, pp. 261–264.

Ross, S. A.: "Infusion Phlebitis," no. 4, pp. 313–318.

Walker, Betty Boyd: "The Postsurgery Heart Patient: Amount of Uninterrupted Time for Sleep and Rest During the First, Second, and Third Postoperative Days in a Teaching Hospital," no. 2, pp. 164–169.

White, Marguerite: "Importance of Selected Nursing Activities," no. 1, pp. 4–14.

Williams, Anne: "A Study of Factors Contributing to Skin Breakdown," no. 3, pp. 238–243.

Woods, Nancy F.: "Patterns of Sleep in Postcardiotomy Patients," no. 4, pp. 347–352.

Nursing Research, vol. 22, 1973:

Anderson, Catherine J.: "Use of Videotape Feedback as a Psychotherapeutic Nursing Approach with Long-Term Psychiatric Patients: A Pilot Study," no. 6, pp. 507-515.

Chamorro, Ilta L., Mary L. Davis, Dora Green, and Marlene Kramer: "Development of an Instrument to Measure Premature Infant Behavior and Caretaker Activities: Time Sampling Methodology," no. 4, pp. 300-309.

Cornell, Sudie A., Laura Campion, Susan Bacero, Judith Frazier, Mary Kjellstrom, and Susan Purdy: "Comparison of Three Bowel Management Programs," no. 4, pp. 321-328.

Gosnell, Davina J.: "An Assessment Tool to Identify Pressure Sores," no. 1, pp. 55-59.

Hedberg, Allan G., and Audrey Schlong: "Eliminating Fainting by School Children During Mass Inoculation," no. 4, pp. 352-353.

Lindeman, Carol, and Steven L. Stetzer: "Effect of Preoperative Visits by Operating Room Nurses," no. 1, pp. 4-16.

Mansfield, Elaine: "Empathy: Concept and Identified Psychiatric Nursing Behavior," no. 6, pp. 525-530.

McPhetridge, L. Mae: "Relationship of Patients' Responses to Nursing History Questions and Selected Factors: A Preliminary Study," no. 4, pp. 310-320.

Midgley, Jan W., and Sr. Ruth Ann Osterhage: "Effect of Nursing Instruction and Length of Hospitalization on Postoperative Complications in Cholecystectomy Patients," no. 1, pp. 69-72.

Mulcahy, Rae Anne, and Nancy K. Janz: "Effectiveness of Raising Pain Perception Threshold in Males and Females Using Psychoprophylatic Childbirth Technique During Induced Pain," no. 5, pp. 423-427.

Pienschke, Sr. Darlene: "Guardedness or Openness on the Cancer Unit," no. 6, pp. 484-490.

Schmitt, Florence E., and Powhatan Wooldridge: "Psychological Preparation of Surgical Patients," no. 2, pp. 108-116.

Nursing Research, vol. 23, 1974:

Budd, Suzanne P., and Willa Brown: "Effect of a Reorientation Technique on Postcardiotomy Delirium," no. 4, pp. 341-348.

Burgess, Ann W., and Lynda L. Holmstrom: "Crisis and Counseling Requests of Rape Victims," no. 3, pp. 196-202.

Castle, Mary, and Suydam Osterhout: "Urinary Tract Catheterization and Associated Infection," no. 2, pp. 170-174.

Cornell, Sudie A.: "Development of an Instrument for Measuring the Quality of Nursing Care," no. 2, pp. 108-117.

Drake, Joyce Johnson: "Locating the External Reference Point for Central Venous Pressure Determination," no. 6, pp. 475-482.

Eoff, Mary Jo Fike, Robert S. Meier, and Carol L. Miller: "Temperature Measurement in Infants," no. 6, pp. 457-460.

Foster, Sue B.: "An Adrenal Measure for Evaluating Nursing Effectiveness," no. 2, pp. 118-124.

Jensen, Judith L., and W. Leona McGrew: "Leadership Techniques in Group Therapy with Chronic Schizophrenic Patients," no. 5, pp. 416-420.

Johnson, Jean E., and Virginia Hill Rice: "Sensory and Distress Components of Pain," no. 3, pp. 203-209.

McCorkle, Ruth: "Effects of Touch on Seriously Ill Patients," no. 2, pp. 125-132.

Murray, Jacquelyn E.: "Patient Participation in Determining Psychiatric Treatment," no. 4, pp. 325-333.

Nunnally, Diane M., and Martha B. Aguiar: "Patients' Evaluation of their Prenatal and Delivery Care," no. 6, pp. 469-474.

Pender, Nola J.: "Patient Identification of Health Information Received During Hospitalization," no. 3, pp. 262-267.

Rodgers, Beckett, Julian Ferhold, and Carol Cooper: "A Screening Tool to Detect Psychosocial Adjustment of Children with Cystic Fibrosis," no. 5, pp. 420-426.

Nursing Research, vol. 24, 1975:

Aspinall, Mary Jo: "Development of a Patient-completed Admission Questionnaire and Its Comparison with the Nursing Interview," no. 5, pp. 377-381.

Beard, Margaret T., and Patsy Y. Scott: "The Efficacy of Group Therapy by Nurses for Hospitalized Patients," no. 2, pp. 120-124.

Brown, Marie Scott, and Joan T. Hurlock: "Preparation of the Breast for Breast Feeding," no. 6, pp. 448-451.

DeWalt, Evelyn M.: "Effect of Timed Hygienic

Measures on Oral Mucosa in a Group of Elderly Subjects," no. 2, pp. 104–108.

Durand, Barbara: "Failure to Thrive in a Child with Down's Syndrome," no. 4, pp. 272–286.

Dyer, Elaine D., Mary A. Monson, and Maxine J. Cope: "Increasing the Quality of Patient Care Through Performance Counseling and Written Goal Setting," no. 2, pp. 138–144.

Felton, Geraldene: "Increasing the Quality of Nursing Care by Introducing the Concept of Primary Nursing: A Model Project," no. 1, pp. 27–32.

Hampe, Sandra O.: "Needs of the Grieving Spouse in a Hospital Setting," no. 2, pp. 113–120.

Hefferin, Elizabeth A., and Ruth E. Hunter: "Nursing Assessment and Nursing Care Plan Statements," no. 5, pp. 360–366.

Johnson, Jean E., Karin T. Kirchhoff, and M. Patricia Endress: "Altering Children's Distress Behavior During Orthopedic Cast Removal," no. 6, pp. 404–410.

Keener, Mary Lou: "The Public Health Nurse in Mental Health Follow-Up Care," no. 3, pp. 198–201.

Kramer, Marlene, Ilta Chamorro, Dora Green, and Frances Knudtson: "Extra Tactile Stimulation of the Premature Infant," no. 5, pp. 324–334.

Leonard, Calista V.: "Patient Attitudes Toward Nursing Interventions," no. 5, pp. 335–339.

Moore, Diane S., and Karen Cook-Hubbard: "Comparison of Methods for Evaluating Patient Response to Nursing Care," no. 3, pp. 202–204.

Risser, Nancy L.: "Development of an Instrument to Measure Patient Satisfaction with Nurses and Nursing Care in Primary Care Settings," no. 1, pp. 45–52.

Volicer, Beverly J., and Mary Wynne Bohannon: "A Hospital Stress Rating Scale," no. 5, pp. 352–359.

Wolfer, John A., and Madelon Visintainer: "Pediatric Surgical Patients' and Parents' Stress Responses and Adjustments," no. 4, pp. 244–255.

EDITOR'S QUESTIONS FOR DISCUSSION

How might you explain the lack of attention given to studying physical nursing care? What differences in research should be expected from investigators with master's degrees compared to those with doctoral degrees? What problems specific to nursing domains should be studied? How might research pertaining to the documentation of nursing care be proposed? What qualifications for research should an investigator possess? What percentage of nursing research done is published and thus made available for others to examine and build on?

Chapter 16

Critical Issues in Access to Data

Patricia Marchman MacElveen, R.N., Ph.D.
Assistant Professor, Department of Psychosocial Nursing
University of Washington, Seattle

Research is most often conducted in an open-system environment. Investigators seldom indicate the limitations under which their studies were conducted. Consequently, replication of studies is difficult and misinterpretation or misrepresentation of findings is possible. Patricia M. MacElveen considers the research process as undertaken by nurses. She outlines an interactional systems model and identifies and dicusses four phases of it: development and planning, initiation and entrance into the research setting, implementation, and conclusion and exit from the research setting. MacElveen points out that the relationships that a principal investigator establishes with those who participate in his or her research may be implications for that investigator's access to data.

Research does not occur in a vacuum; it is an open subsystem in society. Factors of the social climate determine the possibility of doing major research and often the phenomena to be studied. How highly research is valued in society at a given time relates to official and public concern with the topic of inquiry, economic priorities, and the prevailing attitude toward intellectual activities. Research requires interaction with other subsystems and persons external to the research itself, which influence the research process. Particular influences may be supportive or obstructive. Of special concern to us here are influences that impede the access to data.

Unexpected obstacles to data accessibility are experienced by many investigators during the process of implementing well-designed research projects. My own experiences in two investigations of psychosocial aspects of home dialysis, dialogues with other nurse-researchers at the University of Washington, and the literature have yielded many problems highlighting the importance of the investigators' dependence on interactions with numerous people, groups, agencies, and institutions in the process of research. Thus, I will propose a model in which the research process is viewed as a dynamic interactional system. The model incorporates sources of strengths and stresses that influence access to good data and the outcomes of any research endeavor. Before

This paper was developed during a study associated with the conduct of DHEW, Division of Nursing Research Grant NU00472-02, and a previous study conducted under the Nurse Scientist Fellowship Grant 5T01-NU-05008. I also acknowledge the numerous dialogues with Dr. Jeanne Q. Benoliel that stimulated articulation of the model described in this paper.

Reprinted from M.V. Batey (ed.), *Communicating Nursing Research*, Western Interstate Commission for Higher Education, Boulder, Co., 1975, vol. 7, pp. 1–16.

presenting the model and its phases, I will discuss briefly two societal issues presently exerting considerable pressure on the research process as undertaken by nurses: first, the nurse as principal investigator and, second, the protection of human rights and welfare.

THE NURSE AS PRINCIPAL INVESTIGATOR

Because 98 percent of the nursing profession is female, most nurse-researchers are women operating in a male-dominated research world. According to Benoliel (3), male researchers place high value on the attributes of strength, cognition, objectivity, intelligence, and analytical skills. Intellectually, they have dominated research methods, conceptual models, and substantive knowledge. The ideal model of male-dominated research is the experimental, highly controlled manipulation of one or a few variables. Traditionally, women have been thought to value the attributes of nurturance and caretaking and have been viewed as weak, inferior, and subordinate to men (3:2-4).

All the attributes mentioned are not sex determined, of course, but are distributed unequally in the population as a result of the socialization process from early childhood. Benoliel and Stevenson have agreed that women have greater flexibility of operation and the capacity for intuitive awareness of personal and social phenomena (3:11-13; 11:1-2). Intuition has a magical connotation to it; however, I believe intuition is not magical, but rather is a function of women's ability to absorb and process large amounts of stimuli or date in social situations without analysis of the sources of their conclusions or "intuitions."

Stevenson expressed that women are socially conditioned to "deal better with ambiguity and complexity" (11:2). She proposed that nurses as scientists maintain these "feminine" attributes and take on the challenge of exploring new ways to research the complex processes of reality in their natural environments. This proposal, of course, assumes that nurses will resist the powerful pressures during their advanced education to

fashion their research activities after the "male" model. Alternatives to that model need not be inferior. Indeed, knowledge is more likely to advance under pluralistic approaches and methodologies. The burden of proof that their activities are valuable is on the shoulders of the nurse-researchers: "By their works shall you know them."

In the effort to secure funding (a male-dominated arena) the nurse-researcher confronts the problem of being both a woman (i.e., unscientific) and a nurse (i.e., a caretaker, not a researcher). Even when she is successful in obtaining funding, she and her staff are frequently called upon to defend data defined by males as "soft, irrelevant information." The areas of interest favored by many nurse-researchers, as the efforts to build a research-based discipline evolve, frequently may be individuals, agencies, and institutions subject to public accountability. This issue of public accountability may help to legitimize nurse-researchers, their topics of inquiry, and their research approaches.

HUMAN RIGHTS AND WELFARE

Closely related to accountability are concerns about human rights and welfare. Professional and societal concern about research ethics was generated in response to experiments carried out in Nazi Germany. A basic tenet that emerged from the debate was that contributions to the advancement of knowledge could never be used to justify research methods that denied subjects' rights to safety and human dignity. Other research has been publicly recognized to have negative consequences for subjects. The Tuskegee syphilis study is an example. Another example is provided by research findings used for social engineering or control contrary to the self-interest of the participants. Deceptive research strategies have been severely criticized by Erikson (7) and Rainwater and Pittman (8); an example is the use of prisoners in pharmaceutical and biomedical studies without their truly informed consent.

The right not to be researched is a principle

defined by Sagarin (9), who stated that "any group other than a publicly accountable one has the right to withhold information from investigators." When an investigation is conducted without informed consent, the researcher takes on the role of an invader of privacy. That cannot be ethically justified.

Issues raised about research ethics, subject risk/benefit ratio, and informed consent have sensitized federal funding agencies to their own responsibility and to their vulnerability to public criticism as financial supporters of many research projects.

Stevenson (10) described the Department of Health, Education, and Welfare's response to these problems as a system overcorrection. In the effort to reduce abuses and errors, the human rights guidelines developed at DHEW are counterproductive. They consume tremendous amounts of time and energy, which substantially increase the workload while decreasing the output. In reducing research efforts, the public, whose rights are being protected, may be denied its right to research findings and resulting progress. The guidelines also control access to certain kinds of data by eliminating specific populations from study; restricting the use of cadavers, tissues, and records; and requiring complex consent forms. Stevenson optimistically regarded this system overcorrection as temporary, advising investigators to go along with the guidelines for now, expecting a new, more mature position on human rights to emerge.

A human rights issue of personal concern to me is the dilemma of subject-object relationships. When a person is used for the purpose of data collection to achieve project goals, does that person become a means to an end? If so, then does he or she become an object in the interaction with the interviewer? How much more profound this issue becomes when we approach patients and families who are under great stress. My own efforts to solve this dilemma have centered around ways of maintaining the humanistic quality of the interaction. Home dialysis patients and families, for example, are the only source of in-depth data for how it is to live with home dialysis. My field interviewers and I emphasize this and acknowledge the information respondents share with us as the only means by which professionals can gain a more comprehensive understanding of that life, which is necessary if we are to be able to help others with home dialysis. In this way, we recognize the contribution respondents make and its value to both them and us. We also believe that people are basically more important than data. Occasionally when, as nurses, we see that the patient is fatiguing or not tolerating the interview well, we terminate it. Thus, we make every attempt to do our interviews in good faith.

AN INTERACTIONAL SYSTEMS MODEL OF THE RESEARCH PROCESS

Discussion of the research process has traditionally emphasized the steps of conceptualizing the problem, creating an appropriate research design, implementing the study, and writing the final report. The interactional systems model proposed here attempts to incorporate aspects of major research efforts that are affected by the relationships between the principal investigator and her or his staff and the many people with whom they all interact in the process of the research project. The following list is not exhaustive and all the groups defined might not be included in every research effort:

1 *Colleagues* are resources in the researcher's own environment or in the community of scholars who provide opportunity for dialogue and intellectual feedback.

2 *A research facilitation office* provides support, resources, and advice for the development of the proposal; this is invaluable when present.

3 *Institutional legitimators* are members of the investigator's institutional system whose approval is necessary for institutional support and whose approval also gives legitimacy to the investigator carrying out the project. Examples are institutional directors, deans, and department chairmen.

4 *Institutional reviewers* are individuals and members of groups in the investigator's system who must be convinced that the proposal satis-

fies institutional policies and specifications, e.g., human rights review boards, grants, and contract offices.

5 *Sponsors* are persons and groups whose influence and collaboration facilitate access to others whose acceptance is important to the project's success, e.g., administrators, physicians, agency directors, professional groups, and public officials.

6 *Gatekeepers of the sample* are those who control access to the population from which the sample is to be selected, e.g., physicians, department heads, institutional and agency directors, and persons responsible for records.

7 *Funding agents* are those who provide the financial assistance necessary to implement the research project, e.g., federal departments, public and private foundations, and philanthropic persons or organizations.

8 *Sample members* are those who are the sources of the data.

9 *Research staff* are those whose major responsibility is to the principal investigator and the project, e.g., research assistants and associates and secretarial staff.

10 *Members of the research setting* are those in the environment in which the research is conducted, who may or may not be actively involved in the research activities, e.g., clinic, hospital or agency staff, institutional personnel, and families of subjects.

11 *Professional peers* are those to whom the findings of the research efforts are addressed for purposes of sharing theory development and empirical findings and for peer review.

12 *The general public* comprises those who may benefit from the findings of the research, e.g., patients, families, high-risk groups, or generally well people.

Counterproductive interactions with any of these people during the research process can affect the access to data through withdrawal of support, withdrawal from the sample, lack of cooperation, or conscious or unconscious sabotage of the research efforts. These people all interact with the researchers and are vital to the successful conduct of the study. If we follow the principal investiga-

tor through the research process over time, we can identify the points at which these interrelationships are critical. Four phases are identified in the model of the research process: (1) development and planning, (2) initiation and entrance into the research setting, (3) implementation, and (4) conclusion and exit from the research setting. These phases may be summarized as follows:

Phase I. Development and Planning

A Articulation of the research proposal
B Generation of sponsorship
C Establishment of relationships with gatekeepers
D Acquisition of funding

Phase II. Initiation and Entrance into the Research Setting

A Recruitment and training of research staff
B Introduction of staff into institutional structures
C Education of gatekeepers of the sample
D Education of members in the research setting
E Identification and utilization of consultants

Phase III. Implementation

A Sample selection and acquisition of consent
B Collection of data
C Analysis of data

Phase IV. Conclusion and Exit from the Research Setting

A Completion of report to funding agency
B Presentation of feedback to participants
C Publication of findings for professional peers
D Communication to the general public

PHASE I. DEVELOPMENT AND PLANNING

At the start, the research problem must be conceptualized and the research design articulated. Interaction with colleagues often helps the researcher to clarify and crystallize ideas, assess feasibility, and generate alternative strategies. The form of the research proposal is often dictated by the potential funding agents to be approached and the specific format they may require. If the investigator intends to conduct the research in a setting where she or he is a known member, relationships with those who can act as sponsors may already exist, and these require minimal energy to formalize, depending on their previous history. Special characteristics of the study might require links with additional persons of influence outside the setting in which the investigator is known. If she or he is new to the environment, the establishment of many of the needed relationships requires investment of time and energy to involve people who may be crucial in the research interactional system. Those persons in key positions of potential sponsorship or gatekeepers of the sample are especially important. Where possible, early contact with these people, before completion of the proposal, is beneficial. It creates opportunities for the exchange of ideas and information valuable to the articulation of the proposal. The early contact also helps to generate interest, involvement, and identification with the study. Securing these relationships with contracts and written communications contributes to the feasibility of the research from the funder's point of view; such contracts may be valuable at a later time as reminders of the agreements.

Research requiring the support and participation of a large group to which the investigator is unknown or marginal is a special problem. In that case it is advisable to create opportunities to make oneself and the proposed study visible. For example, if it requires the participation of doctors in the community, discussion of the study—both during its development and after funding is obtained—at local medical societies and hospitals the doctors use is very advantageous. Such visibility and opportunity for dialogue with them about the research helps to legitimize it and lay the foundation for cooperation.

Given the importance of establishing these relationships, what kinds of strategies are available to us? Benoliel (2:4) used the term "collabo-

ration" to define the above relationships as joint efforts, often in intellectual enterprises; voluntary cooperation with the enemy in one's own country; and cooperation with an agency or entity with which one is not directly connected. She reported (4:7), for example, that developing a proposal as a joint project of the schools of nursing and medicine greatly facilitated her mastectomy study. Sponsorship by key persons is a form of collaboration (2:4–7).

Besides insuring access to situations, expertise, and the sample, collaboration also helps to gain identity and legitimacy to do the research. This issue was identified by Barber (1) as a special concern when the researchers were seen as lacking comparative prestige and power in a sociological study of biomedical researchers. Strategies used in that study applicable to nursing research were the use of countervailing power (a concept similar to Benoliel's collaboration) and the appeal to shared roles, goals, and values. We used this approach in our dialysis study by identifying our common health care concerns with those of the Northwest Kidney Center and its community physicians: the need for more knowledge about home dialysis families and the identification of factors that might improve patient outcomes. We are able to share with those people in our sample who were already living with home dialysis the goals and values of wanting to make it easier and better for new dialysis patients and families.

Negotiations with the gatekeepers of the sample for access to the population they control require that they have a good understanding of the project and see it as valuable and not conflicting with their own or organizational goals. Procedures for obtaining the sample should be explicit and definitions of their role or the active role of any of their subordinates in sample selection should be clarified. General evidence of cooperation alone is not enough. Access to hospital records, as a case in point, may be highly regulated and may involve the medical records librarian as another gatekeeper. Patient records, particularly for previous years, may be inadequate for data needs or unavailable, according to the kind of record-keeping system operating presently and in the past. Assumptions that the records are easily accessible and adequate are dangerous.

Acquisition of funding determines whether the proposed research project becomes a reality. Nurse-researchers are an unknown entity to many organizations that support research. Philanthropic groups and individuals, industry, and manufacturers are often interested in supporting research especially when it addresses populations of their concern. Generation of this kind of support requires a different approach from that of appealing to the federal or state funding agencies with which we are more familiar. Initial contact by letter to determine the research interest areas of nongovernmental funding sources is a small, first step. Knowledge of who makes the funding decision and what kinds of individuals are involved in that process is important information to guide presentation of the project. Establishment of personal contact with a person in the review group is very valuable. Eliciting the opportunity to make a face-to-face presentation and answer questions may have great influence on the funding decision. The use of well-prepared audiovisual materials appears to enhance communication about the study. (One very expensive medical education project funded by a foundation is known to have used a color movie with background music for the presentation of the proposed project.) Once the research proposal is articulated, sponsorship obtained, access to the sample negotiated, and funding secured, the research moves into the second phase.

PHASE II. INITIATION AND ENTRANCE INTO THE RESEARCH SETTING

The research assistants must be recruited and trained for their respective roles. Nurses interested and prepared to do research are in scarce supply. Without previous experience in research, the probability of efficient performance is difficult to predict. The roles they play in the study should be clearly defined so as to reduce role ambiguity and amorphousness, which are potential sources of stress and tension. Role responsibilities of the principal investigator should also be clearly defined to the staff.

Regular staff meetings are invaluable for providing opportunities not only for the exchange of information, but also for the staff to become accustomed to the way each person thinks, solves problems, and feels about her or his work and staff interactions.

Allocation of adequate time for this stage of the study is critical and requires much of the principal investigator. Before cooperative relationships among those working together can develop, several factors are essential: identification with the study's goals and resolution of any conflicting goals; consensus on means to achieve the goals; evolution of trust; and knowing how individuals on the staff can work together efficiently and comfortably. This all takes time. Cooperation of varying intensities relates not only to the staff, but also to all those involved in the research as insurance against future difficulties and problems that might jeopardize the study.

Staff training in my own project focused on review of the literature, interviewing schedules, and observation skills. In addition, discussion was devoted to potential sources of conflict between the role of interviewer and the role of nurse. During the first six months of field work, the two research associates experienced three major incidents of role conflict. During one family interview, the patient went into severe shock while on dialysis. The research associate temporarily abdicated the role of interviewer and assumed the role of nurse, assisting the spouse in responding to the emergency. The two other incidents involved communication of suicidal intentions, once from a patient and once from a spouse. In the first case, the interviewer was present when the spouse notified the doctor, who did not respond with any assistance. Her concern for the patient's cry for help prompted her to call the doctor upon return to the office to reinforce with him the spouse's evaluation of the situation. The patient was promptly hospitalized for a day or so for a better assessment of physical and emotional status. In the second case, the spouse was inundated with a crisis external to the dialysis situation. The nurse-interviewer carefully assessed the situation and provided the respondent with support while he talked out his problem, reinforcing his intent to possibly seek local counseling. This extended the interview considerably, and later the nurse-interviewer sought consultation to confirm her own assessment of the situation and exploration of her own responses to it.

The above examples illustrate role conflicts encountered by nurse-interviewers in our dialysis study and also the emotional toll experienced by them in researching families and patients involved in crisis, dealing with life-threatening illness, disfigurement, poverty, or demeaned statuses. Especially where in-depth interviews are repeated and heavy or emotionally laden content is part of the data, the interviewers themselves need support from within the research project. If the principal investigator cannot provide this support, a consultant should be engaged for this purpose on a regular basis. Interviews should be paced well within the interviewer's tolerance if good data are to be obtained, i.e., too many interviews per week may seriously impede field work efficiency. Recognition of these issues raises questions about the necessary qualifications of field interviewers for this kind of research.

Introduction and integration of the staff into the institutional structures associated with the study are also important. Research associates, for example, may become part of a hospital unit, agency staff, or university faculty. Participation in these structures through orientation to the setting, attendance at meetings, and the spending of time in the setting helps to establish relationships between the research staff and the others they will be encountering in their work.

In addition, staff must be oriented to other structures to which the study relates. In our study,

the sample was derived from the Northwest Kidney Center. Orientation to the center and attendance at meetings there helped to establish our relationships with people in that setting at several levels and facilitated our interactions around selecting the sample, requests for consultation, and access to data from patient charts. During the field work phase, our contacts with the center were reduced. Intermittent verbal and written reports to the center of our research progress maintained the communications and the relationships. These progress reports will continue until completion of the project.

Similar interaction occurs between the principal investigator and the funding agency, which usually requires annual progress reports and financial accountability. These annual reports necessitate interaction again with the institutional legitimators and institutional reviewers. The research staff may also be visited by persons from the funding agency to insure that the project is in order.

Gatekeepers of the sample are likely to need reeducation about the project during the second phase. An extended period may elapse between original negotiation with them, the time during which funding is acquired, and the point at which the sample is to be selected. Subordinates of the gatekeepers of the sample who will be involved in the acquisition of the sample should be approached and their cooperation elicited.

Continued investment of resources in the relationships between the investigators and sponsors, gatekeepers of the sample, and members of the institutional structures associated with the study is mainly a function of the degree to which those persons remain actively involved in the ongoing research activities. Sponsors who help to legitimize the investigator and the project to others or who facilitate access to other people necessary to the research may require minimal contact with the investigator at this time until conclusion of the project. Sponsors may also act as gatekeepers to the sample, as when sponsors are physicians and the sample is composed of their patients. In this instance, continued interactions are likely to be maintained. Gatekeepers of the sample who only provide access to patient rosters or specimens would require little ongoing interaction until conclusion of the project. Where the research is conducted in a setting shared by the gatekeepers, contact and interaction will be sustained, as when the data are collected in a clinic or hospital unit. Education and involvement of members of the research setting is often a challenge. Blau's experience in studying a bureaucratic organization led him to believe that introduction of a study to members of the research setting should focus on concrete examples of similar studies to demonstrate the potential value of the proposed investigation. Such an approach is more meaningful to the people and "not only affirms his [the investigator's] professional identity but also helps to command respect for his research and to motivate respondents to cooperate with it" (5:27).

If staff on a hospital unit or in a clinic is to participate in data collection, the principal investigator must be aware of how well these additional tasks fit into the regularly scheduled work load. Clinical personnel participating in data collection need to feel comfortable with the research staff, who must be accessible when questions arise. If, for example, a unit nurse does not obtain an hourly urine specimen on time due to other pressures on the unit, does she mark it with the actual time of the collection, omit that collection, or call a research staff member? Has she been instructed how to deal with that problem, or if not, does she feel comfortable in asking for help? If she tries to call for assistance, is she likely to be able to contact a member of the research staff? Or is she likely to make her own decision, feeling little involvement or commitment to the study, which she perceives as additional work. There are many conscious and unconscious ways that unwilling participants can sabotage the study, e.g., collecting incomplete, inaccurate, or no data, or departing from sample selection procedures. If data collection imposes a considerable burden on the unit staff, alternatives to involving them should be considered if additional unit staff cannot be provided by the research project during the time of data collection.

Researchers must accept that in some settings service or care has the highest priority. Personnel may not have an orientation to value research activity, especially if their education does not exceed the bachelor's degree level. This can sometimes be predicted by talking directly to those people who would be assigned to assist with data collection. Cooperation obtained from upper levels of an agency or hospital does not guarantee the same degree of cooperation from subordinates who will be required to carry out the tasks. In this situation data or the sample itself may be at great risk. Recognition of these factors requires consideration of alternatives, e.g., hiring someone to collect the data or possibly offering financial incentives to members in the setting by paying for each interview or each unit of data obtained.

Assessment of the impact of the project on the research setting and its system is extremely important. Carnevali and Little's description of the effects of a clinical research study on a hospital is a classic (6). In their study, using two wards in a 400-bed hospital, the range of personnel who eventually were affected by their project included the medical director, physicians, hospital administrative staff, nursing service administrators, pharmacists, medical records librarian, director of central service, business manager, ward nursing staff, ward coordinator, ward clerk, patients, and nursing students. Project demands on time, energy, space, personnel, and other resources of the hospital increased costs and often created conflicts of interest for hospital staff at all levels. The authors advised that the environment *must* be prepared prior to the actual implementation of the study for the impacts on the system.

The identification and use of consultants may occur at any point in the research process, on a formal or informal basis. Colleagues, sponsors, gatekeepers of the sample, and personnel in the research setting may make contributions in a consulting way during Phase I. Consultants who assist with computer analysis prefer to be involved early in the process if their expertise is to facilitate expeditious handling of the data. Special expertise may be needed at any point in the research process and may require consulting services.

PHASE III. IMPLEMENTATION

Sample selection and the acquisition of informal consent for participation in the study have become a major source of investigator stress in certain types of populations. Some sample losses are predictable; others are not. Failure to achieve the desired "N" may result from overestimation of the population or its availability by the gatekeeper of the sample; sample selection overly controlled by a member of the setting; poor response to the invitation to participate; or attrition from the sample.

The last problem may occur due to death, change of residence, change of physical or mental status, or withdrawal from the project. An example of the latter is the special case where community physicians themselves are participants either as sources of patients' data or as members of the sample and are strangers to the nurse-researcher. In our dialysis study, a few physicians who did not value the psychosocial factors relating to patients and their families defined our project as irrelevant to their concerns and not worth their valuable time. Where a physician had several patients in the study it was necessary to negotiate the number of patients on whom he would provide data, especially since there was a series of three interviews to collect data at intervals. Some physicians were uncomfortable in the role of member of the sample and became anxious when they thought their performance was being evaluated or compared to that of other physicians. They found it difficult to accept that we were looking for change over time in patients, spouses, and physicians rather than comparing physicians to physicians. We had not anticipated this resistance, believing that endorsement by the Northwest Kidney Center would legitimate us. In

contrast, many physicians were most cooperative. Thus, inclusion of physicians at large in the community in the sample is apt to add risk to sample loss if data collection requires much time and effort from them. Sponsorship of the research by more than one medical group is probably necessary.

Once the field work is completed and all data are in, efforts of the research staff focus primarily on data analysis. The rhythm of the work changes considerably from the comings and goings involved in interviewing out in the field. This is a significant shift, and staff meetings should be used to define the current division of labor and responsibilities of the research associates and other project staff. Untroubled data analysis is obviously expedited by good relationships among the project staff, among the staff and consultants, and among people at the computer center when that facility is used.

As analysis moves toward completion, the preparation of reports ensues. The third phase of the research process is finished, and the final phase begins.

PHASE IV. CONCLUSION AND EXIT FROM THE RESEARCH SETTING

Access to data is obviously not a critical concern during this final phase, but the conclusion of the study and the exit from the research setting influence data accessibility for future research.

Reports to the funding agents are the immediate returns on their financial investment in the study. The principal investigator is evaluated by these reports and relationships with the funding agents for future support are greatly influenced by the project outcomes.

Satisfying feedback to all participants in the study is important if we are to expect them to value research, recognize their contribution, and be willing to participate in future research efforts. Providing participants with access to the formal report does not necessarily meet their needs or achieve the desired results stated above. Brief reports tailored to their particular interests and written without professional jargon are more apt to be meaningful. Where members of the setting have assisted with data collection or otherwise made substantial contribution to the research process, a meeting with the principal investigator is in order. Research findings should be shared and discussed; recognition should be given for participation and cooperation.

While the researcher may be excited about the theoretical and more abstract aspects of the study, it is sometimes necessary to translate them into pragmatic implications for use by participants whose priorities are service or care. This can be the thrust of the reports and/or the meetings in which the researcher discusses the findings with groups who have particular interests in the implications of the findings for their practice or their delivery of services.

Special care must be taken when findings of the research are likely to be disappointing to the participants or interpreted as negative evaluation of their efforts. Honest sharing of the findings in this case requires much tact and reinforcement of positive aspects of the findings or the researcher's observations. Emphasis may be turned to problem solving and contributions the study may make toward that end.

Negative findings raise the issue of what rights involved institutions or agencies have in the publication of findings. Should the participants be identifiable in the literature? Certainly publicly supported enterprises are fully accountable. Research in the private sector raises similar issues that cannot be pursued in depth here. In addition, do researchers have any obligation to allow review of articles before submission for publication? Does the researcher "own the data" and have all rights to use it as she or he chooses? These issues are important, I believe, and need to be addressed in terms of our relationships with those who participate in our research.

Publication of the research in professional journals is the opportunity to share empirical findings and contribute to the development of theory and knowledge. Such activity also provides for peer evaluation and for interaction in the community of scholars.

Communication with the general public is an area in which I think nursing has been remiss. Doctors, psychologists, anthropologists, psychiatrists, dieticians, and other professionals are well represented in the mass media. Do nurses really have nothing to say? By not communicating with the general public about our research we deny ourselves visibility and deny the public the opportunity to observe the concerns we have and the work we do.

In summary, I have proposed an interactional systems model of the research process and its phases. The many relationships that a nurse, as principal investigator of a research project, is likely to encounter and the implications that these relationships have for the access to data have been identified. This effort has been made primarily to assist future nurse-researchers in avoiding what others have learned to avoid only through experience and informal sharing with colleagues. Awareness of these issues in data accessibility will help us to assure and protect our access to data in future research.

REFERENCES

1 Barber, B. "Research on Research on Human Subjects: Problems of Access to a Powerful Profession." *Social Problems* 21 (1973): 103–112.

2 Benoliel, J. Q. "Collaboration and Competition in Nursing Research." In *Communicating Nursing Research*, edited by M. V. Batey. Boulder, Colo.: WICHE, 1972.

3 ——. "Scholarship, A Woman's Perspective." Paper presented at a Graduate Faculty Retreat, School of Nursing, University of Washington, Seattle, June 1, 1973.

4 ——. "Research Related to Death and the Dying Patient." In *Research in Nursing Based on Psychosocial Data,* edited by P. J. Verhonick. Boston: Little, Brown and Company, in press.

5 Blau, P. M. "The Research Process in the Study of the Dynamics of the Bureaucracy." In *Sociologists at Work*, edited by P. H. Hammond. New York: Basic Books, 1964.

6 Carnevali, D. L., and Little, D. E. "Effects of a Clinical Nursing Research Study on a Hospital." *Hospitals* 39 (Sept. 1, 1965): 70–80.

7 Erikson, K. T. "A Comment on Disguised Observation in Sociology." *Social Problems* 14 (1967):366–373.

8 Rainwater, L., and Pittman, D. J. "Ethical Problems in Studying a Politically Sensitive and Deviant Community." *Social Problems* 14 (1967):357–366.

9 Sagarin, E. "The Research Setting and the Right Not to Be Researched." *Social Problems* 21 (1974):52–64.

10 Stevenson, J. S. "Protection of Human Subjects and the Phenomena of Overcorrection." *CNR Voice*, Ohio State University School of Nursing Newsletter No. 3 (1974): 1–3.

11 ——. "Women Scientists." *CNR Voice*, Ohio State University School of Nursing Newsletter No. 4 (1974):1–3.

EDITOR'S QUESTIONS FOR DISCUSSION

How does a nurse legitimize her position as a principal investigator? How does one elicit the cooperation of a team of multidiscipline coinvestigators in a research project? What strategies can an investigator use to gain entrance into a research setting? What strategies might be used in proposing research in a health care setting? What obstacles concerning the "territorial" rights of the patient might present themselves in research? What obligations does an investigator have to the subjects being studied, his or her coinvestigators, the setting or organization where the research is being conducted, the funding agency, and the professional community?

Chapter 17

The Phenomenological Approach in Nursing Research

Anne J. Davis, R.N., Ph.D., F.A.A.N.
Associate Professor, Department of Mental Health and Community Nursing
School of Nursing, University of California, San Francisco

This chapter and the one that follows by Carol A. Soares present new approaches to research, other than the experimental model, that are applicable to nursing. Davis discusses the use of the phenomenological approach. This approach primarily considers the meaning social acts have for persons who perform them and who live in a reality created by their subjective interpretation of such acts. Because nursing is predominantly a social act between nurse and patient, the phenomenological approach may enable nurses to better understand patients by entering into fields of perception and thus see life, as well as their illnesses and the implications of their illnesses from the patients' points of view.

A number of new currents have evolved recently in the social sciences. One of these currents is the phenomenological movement, which has the potential not only for providing an approach to research different from the experimental model, but for aiding nurse-researchers and clinicians to better understand experimental studies.

The following discussion is based on a philosophical stance that supports this phenomenological approach and which, therefore, by its very nature, cannot at the same time support the so-called naturalistic approach to research. This is not to say, however, that there is any one royal road to truth. All research approaches, including the phenomenological one, combine assets and limita-

tions and, because human beings are so immensely complex, no one research approach at this time is sufficient to provide all the knowledge needed.

THE FOCUS OF DISCUSSION

Most discussions of the social sciences in graduate nursing education focus on social sciences as disciplines that provide additional wealth of formulative notions with which to encounter experience. However, they can, but not necessarily do they always, encourage the act of holding up to the light for examination one's basic assumptions regarding the nature of man and the philosophy of science. Taking this latter function of the

This article is a reprint from Esther A. Garrison (ed.), *Doctoral Preparation for Nurses with Emphasis on the Psychiatric Field*, University of California, San Francisco, 1973, and supported by Training Grant–M H 11890 from the National Institute of Mental Health, United States Public Health Service, Department of Health, Education, and Welfare.

social sciences (examination of basic assumptions), this paper focuses on a relatively recent development in both psychology and sociology. It is a reaction to what a growing number of social scientists view as unsatisfactory states of today's mainstream in these two behavioral disciplines.

The majority of students who enter doctoral programs in nursing have arrived there by way of clinical preparation. The doctoral level in nursing combines some mixture of clinical nursing, research, and biological and/or social sciences, culminating in a dissertation. Taking this into account, the focus of this paper is twofold:

1 A critical examination of the so-called positivistic approach to the content and research in the social sciences, particularly in the fields of psychology and sociology
2 An attempt to present an alternative view, the phenomenological approach

In my opinion, phenomenology provides a more perfect fit conceptually with the functions of clinical nursing and with many of the research questions that evolve from clinical practice.

The phenomenological approach originated in Europe and is a relatively new approach to human studies. It breaks with traditional empiricism. One needs to understand that the field of phenomenology contains many subperspectives that have not been reconciled, yet, within the larger phenomenological movement.

The phenomenological movement is an attempt to understand empirical matters from the perspective of those who are being studied. Central to this development is the realization, at least by some, of the social nature of the research act. According to them, the view of the human subject-as-object is no longer meaningful when considered in light of current thinking in physics and philosophy of science, which recognizes the subjectivity of all knowledge and fusion of the observer and observed in the very act of observing. This development has immense implications for clinical researchers in nursing: (a) for those who develop clinical expertness by integrating knowledge from clinical nursing with knowledge from the sciences,

and (b) for those who generate new clinical knowledge through research.

Fundamentally, the phenomenological approach is different from empirical methods in that it argues that the phenomena of the social sciences are not qualitatively continuous with those of the natural sciences, and, therefore, different methods need to be employed to study social reality (Natanson, 1968). This approach maintains that looking at social phenomena requires a way that takes into primary account the meaning social acts have for actors who perform them and who live in a reality built out of their subjective interpretation (Natanson, 1968). The unique characteristic of this approach lies in the questions about its own methods and procedures, which become an integral part of its structural content. It does not eliminate bias but, rather, attempts to recognize and incorporate it.

BACKGROUND

Although many sociologists and psychologists do not regard the problem of how to study man as significant, a growing number regard this as today's most important problem confronting these disciplines. The major reason underlying the disregard of this fundamental problem can be easily understood if one believes that the problem has already been solved, in that the essential character and principles of scientific procedure have been firmly established. In this opinion, the steady development of physical and biological sciences during the last four hundred years has forged rudiments of the method of science. Those who hold this opinion regard the difficult task of applying already established knowledge of scientific procedure to their area of social science research as their major problem, but, obviously, this is of a different genre than that of challenging the known nature of scientific method per se.

The view that the only real task in social and psychological science is to apply the established principles and criteria of scientific procedure needs critical examination. The method of science is seen fundamentally as the scientific method that has been worked out in the physical and biological sciences. But one needs to ask what is the social scientists' conception of that scientific method that has been developed and established in the natural sciences. The answer does not reflect a unitary and firmly established view. Rather, we find ourselves faced with differences, ambiguity, confusion, and controversy.

> Some see scientific method in terms of a set of logical procedures, such as are outlined in conventional treatises on logic or scientific method. Others identify scientific method with given forms of general procedures, such as quantification or the use of laboratory experimentation. Others feel that its essence is to lie in certain special procedures, such as "operationalism" or the use of "input-output" models. Others view it in terms of the presumed composition of the "world" addressed by science, as in the case of a probabilistic model, a mechanical model, a "system" model, or an aggregate of variables (Bruyn, 1966, p. iv).

The conclusion to be drawn is that no consensus exists regarding scientific method.

These extensive differences are obscured by the historical tendency for a particular conception to gain prestige and dominance. One such idea is current identification of scientific method with research design bearing a relationship between independent and dependent variables under conditions of a control group. We need to be cautious not to be deceived by what appears as a consensus at the present or any other time. Nor can one accurately assume this disarray is due to social scientists' lack of knowledge and understanding of the scientific method as developed in the physical and biological sciences. When one views the history of the natural sciences over the past two hundred years, a comparable picture of differences, change, shifts, and new versions appear.

These remarks lead to the point I want to make, namely, that the nature of the scientific method has not been and is not now a fixed, established datum. Therefore, ". . . *the problem of how to study human beings and their group life cannot be handled by the simple dictum to apply the true and tested principles of scientific study as they have developed by physical and biological science. Such 'principles' have not been clearly and firmly established* (Bruyn, 1966, p. v)."

Nevertheless, naturalistic methodology is held applicable to the problems of the social sciences. According to Ernest Nagel (1952), such methodology in the social sciences would have to be continuous with theories from the natural sciences.

In contrast to naturalistic methodology, the phenomenological approach of Edmund Husserl[1] concerns itself with the foundation problems of knowledge in the broadest and most inclusive sense. Further, Husserl's approach heeds the prescientific and pretheoretical experience that we have of the surrounding perceptual world and by which we are guided in our everyday life (Natanson, 1969).

The term "phenomenological" is used to include all positions that stress the primacy of consciousness and subjective meaning in the interpretation of social action. To conclude that the problems of the social sciences are basically phenomenological means, then, that social action is understood as founded on the intentional[2] experience of the actors on the social scene. The distinctive feature of the phenomenological

---

[1] Husserl was a trained mathematician who acquired his doctorate in mathematics on the basis of a thesis dealing with the philosophy of arithmetic. It was his contention that none of the so-called rigorous sciences can lead toward an understanding of our experiences of the world—a world, the existence of which they uncritically presuppose, and which they attempt to measure by yardstick and pointers on scales of their instruments (Natanson, 1969, p. 24).

[2] Any of our experiences as they appear within our stream of thought are necessarily referred to the object experienced. There is no such thing as thought, fear, fantasy, remembrance as such; every thought is thought *of*, every fear is fear *of*, every remembrance is remembrance *of* the object that is thought, feared, remembered. Husserl coined the term "intentionality" to designate this relationship (Natanson, 1969, p. 26).

approach rests with its claim to see knowledge directly through immediate human experience. This method of seeking original knowledge involves what is called by these philosophers as "bracketing" preconceptions,[3] which literally means suspending assumptions or the "reduction" of concepts to a point where the observer can obtain a pure apprehension of experience. This approach *"represents a species of knowledge and a method of knowing that are not within the naturalistic traditions of science. . . . Phenomenology serves as the rationale behind efforts to understand individuals by entering into their fields of perception in order to see life as these individuals see it* (Bruyn, 1966, p. 90)."

The psychiatrist, van der Berg (1955), describes the attitude of the phenomenologist who sees this kind of perceptual knowledge when he refers to the writer of a treatise on swimming who first must learn the sea, the river, and the lake by swimming before undertaking his writing task.

After this brief overview of the scientific method and the phenomenological approach, we proceed to this paper's focus: the relatively recent development in both psychology and sociology which attempts to confront empirical experience from the perspective of those who are being studied.

Psychology: A View of Man

Of great importance in the development of science was the realization that all science is relatively subjective. Physicists like Planck, Bohr, von Weizssaecker, and Heisenberg have made us aware

of this. Their work in quantum physics makes clear that the ideal of absolute objectivity and of an absolutely objective view of the universe remains a dream and one never to be realized. Every so-called scientific view of the world is extremely limited. Every scientist selects, of necessity, one out of many available viewpoints, and this selection is based on relatively subjective choices and assumptions.

Some physicists and other thinkers point to the relative subjectivity of science. The phenomenologist, mentioned earlier, studies man's primary experiences. These are more comprehensive than the conceptual knowledge that man later selects analytically from his original experience.[4] This original experience antecedes clear conceptualizations.

In his primary experience, man is still open to the universe, he is in contact with all the nuances of experiences. This experience essentially differs from the scientific way of knowing since the latter involves man's subjectively limiting his original view. Scientific thinking foregoes primary experience rather than penetrating it—that is, science modifies experience fundamentally by means of what may be a subjective choice by the scientist.

Psychology does not assimilate these new realizations easily. The fact remains, no matter how one argues against it—there is no escape from assumptions in psychology. Psychologists, regardless of their school of thought, always make an ultimate and absolute judgment as to the nature of man and the way in which man can be understood. These assumptions are not derived from psychological research but are the point of departure for the research one will undertake. Since there is no escape from assumptions, the question arises, "What assumptions are operant with the

---

[3] Husserl himself was well aware of the impossibility of a truly presuppositionless understanding of knowledge. He realized that we presuppose implicitly in all questioning and answering. As Langer (1951) says, the exploration of any situation begins with its first expression as a question, and the manner in which "a question is asked limits and disposes the way in which any answer to it, right or wrong, may be given (p. 15)." What Husserl insists be suspended are assumptions which extend beyond these questions so that the researcher does not enter the situation that he has defined according to his own perceptions prior to any understanding of the situation as it is defined by those experiencing it.

[4] To reiterate the point made previously, the phenomenologist seeks to understand experience from the point of view of those being studied which makes for broad parameters rather than imposing a structure on these experiences a priori by such means as hypotheses which structure not only the research design but force the researcher into overlooking the fact that multiple realities exist.

mainstream of research psychologists?" According to Van Kaam:

> It briefly comes down to this, that the more positivistic psychologist still adheres implicitly to the two assumptions of mechanism and determinism which were characteristic of early physics. Mechanism implies a wholly quantitative theory of atoms-without-qualities. This implicit assumption is more and more in contradiction with the facts discovered by physicists. The same is true of the development in psychology. The implicit assumption that man can be understood by analyzing him into elements which are statistically the same is basically in contradiction with reality. . . . Another assumption of the early physicists, namely that of determinism, was that every situation of primordial particles at any given moment was determined by an inner law and by the situation at another moment. This assumption in its psychological form is still of great influence on the thinking of the positivist psychologist. The physicists are far more cautious since the principle of uncertainty was formulated by Heisenberg (Schultz, 1970, pp. 28–29).

The assumptions of phenomenological psychologists are the contrary to an absolute mechanism and an absolute determinism. They are the psychological counterpart of recent assumptions in quantum physics. Terms such as becoming, creativity, growth, self-actualization, and emergence indicate the direction in which these assumptions are developing.

Continuing with the matter of presuppositions, Douglas raises the question whether or not there are certain presuppositions to which the commitment to do scientific investigation binds us. He responds to this question by saying:

> The answer given by the positivistic scientist is that there are and that, in fact, we are committed to an experimental and quantitative (that is, absolutist) method and theory. The problem with this absolutist approach is that it confounds the tools of science, that is, the methods of investigation and the specific theories constructed, with the (essential) nature of science, so that any investigation or explanation that does not make use of these tools is seen as unscientific. But this confounding can be avoided if we recognize that there are certain more fundamental aspects of science about which we can all agree. These aspects seem to be (1) a commitment to discovering truths about the world as experienced by human beings, (2) a commitment to grounding or testing any idea proposed as truths in empirical observations of some kind at some stage, and (3) a commitment to accepting such tests as valid only when at some stage they can be made (publicly) shareable, that is objective (Douglas, 1970, p. 23).

Douglas makes the further point that much argument has occurred among social scientists over whether or not phenomenology is truly a science, because so many of these social scientists continue to think of science as necessarily positivistic, although this view has long been discredited in the natural sciences.

Rendezvous with Validity

This phrase is taken from Friedman's *The Social Nature of Psychological Research*, in which he raises the larger question: How precise and how valid is our knowledge being accumulated by our rigorous methods? The answer to this, of course, depends on how rigorous the methods really are. He then raises the more specific question: What does happen in a psychological experiment?

Friedman begins his examination of the psychological experiment by noting that little work has been done on the mediation of experimenter effect and experimenter bias. Within the traditional philosophy of psychology the experimenter is "understood," experimental conditions are controlled, experimenters behave standardly. He goes on to conceptualize the psychological experiment as a "particular type of interaction in a particular social situation." By filming and then examining what went on during the encounter of nineteen experimenters engaged with 107 subjects in a person-perception task, Friedman drew the conclusion that experiments are not controlled since they do not take into account the way the experimenter behaves kinesically and paralinguistically, which is not standardized.

Psychologists traditionally consider that the variance in the responses of subjects in the same treatment conditions results from individual differences among subjects and these differences are conceptualized as intervening variables, the sole source of error variance in experiments. Friedman, however, demonstrates that there is much variability in the interaction between experimenter and subject. On this point he writes: *"Recognizing that the unstandardized aspects of the interactions of experimenters and subjects represent interpersonal "intervening variables" allow us to reduce the explanatory burden placed on the statistical intervening variables by putting some of the variance in experimental results back into the social environment* (1967, p. 108)."

This leads to his conclusion that the philosophy of the psychological experiment must come to terms with the social nature of the psychological experiment: *"I am trying to say that although an experimenter-subject dyad may be viewed as a tight little island of social interaction cut off from the mainland of everyday social gatherings, it is an island to which the population of two carries its entire interpersonal repertoire* (p. 109)." And, finally:

> . . . here is one of the fundamental implications of founding our conception of psychology upon the real rather than the ideal psychological experiment. Psychology's hitherto most "applied" discipline (social psychology) becomes, in many ways, its most basic. For in the constant talk about extrapolating from the experiment to the "real" or the "social" world, we must never forget that the experiment is itself a part of that real and that social world (p. 169).

In summary, the subjectivity of the more phenomenological psychologists seems to be more accessible, flexible, and open. Less inclined to believe that his assumptions are absolutely objective, he is more aware of what determines his scientific work and this awareness prevents subjective influences from becoming too fixed and rigid. He is more inclined to reflect on his relatively subjective assumptions and to ask himself after a time whether they are still tenable, whether they can be expanded or reconciled with the relatively subjective viewpoints of others who study the human in a variety of ways. Early in its development, psychology separated from philosophy with Wundt leading the way toward experimental science emphasizing measurable stimuli and responses. As a result, consciousness ceased to be of importance since it was not amenable to objective experimental methods of study. While psychology has continued to reject philosophy, postnewtonian physics came to strongly interact with it. According to its critics, psychology holds to *"an outmoded view that causes it to be too bewitched by methodology, analysis, and operational definition* (Schultz, 1970, p. 30)." Critics, many of whom are psychologists themselves[5] of this state of affairs, urge that psychology *"develop a theory of man based not on an obsolete physical model but rather on an existential richness of full, and distinctly human, living* (Schultz, 1970, p. 20)."

Sociology: A View of Man

Sociology emerged with Auguste Comte and his contemporaries as a science of society cast in the mold of scientific method of the natural sciences.

> Sociological theory began in the creative synthesis of two sets of theoretical poles. The model of society, a synthesis of the organic and physical dimensions of knowledge whose terms were applied to society, was combined with a method for studying society, a synthesis of the empirical and rational modes of knowing, called by Comte the positive, or scientific method (Bruyn, 1966, p. 58).

[5] Adrian Van Kaam, Carl Rogers, Duane Schultz, Sigmund Koch, Robert Rosenthal, Abraham Maslow, Nevitt Sanford, Henry Murray, to name a few.

These components, which Comte called the positive method, go back to the Greeks but became especially important through the writings of Francis Bacon. He wrote that there are two ways of searching into and discovering truth. One way begins with general axioms and proceeds to judgments and to the discovery of middle axioms. The other way derives axioms from the senses and particulars, rising by a gradual broken ascent, so that it arrives at the most general axioms last of all (Bacon, 1936, p. 27). Bacon recommended the latter be developed, which he called empiricism, while the former was referred to as rationalism and its development was not pushed. Not until Immanuel Kant were these two polar forms of knowing reconciled as two independent, but interdependent, ways of knowing truth, and together they came to form the scientific method.

Two major research approaches are apparent in sociology as demonstrated in the work of Durkheim and Znaniecki. In his book, *The Rules of Sociological Method,* Durkheim laid out the positivistic approach to follow in order to discover empirical knowledge: "*The first and most fundamental rule: Consider facts as things* (p. 14)." Later he clarified what he meant by "things" in the following fashion: "*A thing differs from an idea in the same way as that which we know from without differs from that which we know from within* (Rules, 2d Ed., p. xliii)." For Durkheim, "*every object of science is a thing* (Rules, p. xliv)," and he introduced a corollary establishing preconceptions, "*The subject matter of every sociological study should comprise a group of phenomena defined in advance by certain common external characteristics, and all phenomena so defined should be included in this group* (p. 35)."

In this statement we have the essence of nineteenth-century naturalism in its social form, and the beginning of one major approach to research.

In distinct contrast, the other major approach came some forty years later with the work of Florian Znaniecki (1934), in which he saw value in quantitative studies but went on to say that the data in social research are always "somebody's" data and their essential character he referred to as the "humanistic coefficient." It was his opinion that if the social scientist attempted to study the cultural system in the same way he studied a material or natural system—that is, as though it existed separately from human experience—"*the system would disappear and in its stead he would find a disjointed mass of natural things and processes, without any similarity to the reality he started to investigage* (p. 37)." Znaniecki (1934) identified two fundamental ways of viewing scientific data:

> One is the way of the naturalist who, even while recognizing that cultural objects are human values and that cultural systems are constructed by human activity, believes that human activity can nevertheless be studied as a natural process given to him (like other natural processes) without any reference to how it appears to anybody else; and also that a human value viewed in the light of a naturalist theory of activity can be simply analyzed into a natural thing. . . . The other way of obtaining an inductive knowledge of human activity would be to use consistently the humanistic coefficient in dealing with it and take it as it appears to the agent himself and to those who cooperate with him or counteract him (pp. 44–45).

A more recent critic of Durkheim has summarized it:

> Durkheim and the other positivists found their solution in treating all social phenomena *as if* they were objects. That is, they looked for a way by which they could study and analyze social phenomena using the traditional methods of classical science (experimental controls, quantification, hypothesis testing, and so on). A way was found. They imposed their "scientific" presuppositions upon the realm of social phenomena, but in doing so they so distorted the fundamental nature of human existence— they bootlegged commonsense meanings into

their object-like data and theories and created an *as if* science of man (Douglas, 1970, p. 1x).

In the works of Durkheim and Znaniecki, hallmarks in the history of sociological research, we find the two major pillars of research methodology in the discipline. The one pillar, which represents quantitative research, includes the positivist and the behaviorist, and the other includes the more phenomenological types of inquiry such as participant observation. However, the physical model came to be accepted as primary in the exploration and explanation of society and the emphasis of this model as the guide for studying social phenomena is very much in evidence today (Bruyn, 1966, p. 59). While this model has continued to dominate sociological theory, there have been a number of significant deviations from it. One such departure from the Comtean tradition can be found in social phenomenology. The theoretical bent here in the United States, which to some extent parallels the phenomenological trend in Europe, is work of the group of symbolic interactionists[6] who study what can be termed the inner perspective (Bruyn, 1966, p. 62). This school stresses the processual character of human behavior and the need for "sympathetic introspection" in the study of human behavior.

Although not entirely new, interest in phenomenological sociology has grown rapidly in the past few years among many research workers and theorists,[7] all of whom share ideas about the scientific inadequacies of conventional sociology. According to their stance, all sociology necessarily begins with the understanding of everyday life. Yet, until recently, few sociologists either realized or acted in accord with the realization "*that the understanding of everyday life must be the foundation of all sociological research and theory* (Douglas, 1970, p. 3)."

[6] Charles H. Cooley, W. I. Thomas, Florian Znaniecki, George Herbert Mead, Herbert Blumer, Manford Kuhn, Anselm Strauss, Irving Goffman.
[7] Jack Douglas, Thomas Wilson, John Heeren, Don Zimmerman, Melvin Pollner, Severyn Bruyn, and Norman Denzin, to name a few.

However much some sociologists today may be constrained in their thinking by the tatters and remnants of nineteenth-century positivism, there is no doubt that almost all of them agree that social actions are *meaningful* actions, that is, that they must be studied and explained in terms of their situations and their meanings to the actors themselves. The disputes over the kinds of meanings involved and the ways in which they are to be determined are fundamental, but there is now little dispute among sociologists over the proposition that social meanings are in some way the fundamental determinants of social action (Douglas, 1970, p. 4).

Taking this stance, the first and most fundamental methodological commitment of phenomenological sociologists is: ". . .*to study the phenomena of everyday life on their own terms, or to make use only of methods of observation and analysis that retain the integrity of the phenomena* (Douglas, 1970, p. 16)."

At the most basic level this means that the phenomena to be studied must be those experienced in everyday life, not those created by, or strained through, experimental situations. This stance made central to its approach the idea that human actions are highly situational and human actors act in accord with their constructions of meanings for the concrete situations they face.

The Phenomenological Approach

Utilizing the phenomenological approach to obtain a grasp of the phenomena under study, the researcher must become extremely aware of his subject and its surroundings. The heightened awareness of the researcher's consciousness is critical to the approach, so he must approach his subject with a minimal number of structured expectations as to how an object should be described—that is to say, he must reduce his preconceptions to a minimum so that he will be able to receive an object as it is given to his consciousness. No hypotheses direct him as to what he should find in his investigation; rather, he goes into the situation to be studied with as open a mind as possible.

While the phenomenologist contends that although the general scheme of study can by systematically outlined by gathering the background information available in literature, he intends to open himself to the human realities he studies. He would argue that if, however, he kept an empirical hypothesis constantly in mind in the social situation where he functions, he probably would create that very reality that he defines in his research design. This results from his belief researchers unintentionally define reality as that which they seek without recognizing their own involvement in the creation of the product.

The phenomenologist assumes that there is something in the nature of human experience, beyond sheer reason or sensory observation, which will produce knowledge. The empiricist on occasion has had sudden revelations or has gained valuable insight from outside the scientific framework of knowing. No one has attempted to explain this process systematically. The phenomenological approach describes the process resting behind the revelation of new, testable knowledge; the revelation which Merton (1949) calls the "serendipity pattern" of social research: *"The serendipity pattern refers to the fairly common experience of observing an unanticipated, anomalous, and strategic datum which becomes the occasion for developing a new theory or extending an existing theory* (p. 98)."

What here is referred to as unanticipated data are sometimes produced when empirical researchers have unintentionally used the phenomenological method.

In summary, then, human meanings cannot be logically inferred from sense impressions, although this traditional method provides knowledge of a certain kind. Phenomenologists *"insist upon the importance of intuition in the development of knowledge which fulfills the scientific requirement of certainty as well as or better than traditional forms of knowledge* (Bruyn, 1966, pp. 278-279)."

IMPLICATIONS FOR NURSING RESEARCH

As mentioned earlier in this paper, the majority of students who enter doctoral programs in nursing have arrived there by way of clinical preparation in their previous professional programs. It is this clinical approach which emphasizes observation, interviews, interaction, and interpersonal relations in an attempt to understand the patient's definition of the situation. In my opinion, this clinical research approach more perfectly fits conceptually the phenomenological approach.

In discussing the historical roots of nursing education and nursing research, Olesen (in press) indicates that one consequence stemming from the historical roots of nursing education and research is that nursing researchers inherited perspectives from educational psychology and have given allegiance to the experimental model. Thereby, they often deflected attention from other possible research styles, such as particular observation. This allegiance to the experimental model has overlooked the fact that the research observer's skills are the same skills central to clinical nursing. Differences may exist; however, the similarities are there.

Recognizing this similarity, a nurse-researcher could, for example, use her skills in observation and interviewing to study a given phenomena within the symbolic lives of the people involved. To accomplish this end, she has to enter into the process itself and interpret it as it appears to the people engaged.

Let it be understood that such a personal, concrete explanation, even though it is widely applicable, is not wholly sufficient in itself for the purposes of social science any more than is the impersonal abstract type of analysis, traditional to the physical sciences. Each is sufficient for certain levels of understanding, but cannot serve as a model for all of psychological, social, or nursing theory. Separately, these approaches illustrate different principles and levels of inquiry, selecting what is important to study, while together these approaches help explain the human perspective. Much remains to be done to define and clarify the conceptual approach of the phenomenologist, but this approach, as it now presents itself, may provide the basis for building one systematic perspective capable of embracing the factual realities revealed in the work of the clinical nurse-researcher.

SUMMARY

This paper has examined the so-called naturalistic approach to the content in psychology and sociology and has presented one alternative approach—namely, the phenomenological. It takes as a point of departure the realization that these two approaches to research rest on philosophical presuppositions that widely differ from one another. In developing this alternative approach the author is fully aware of both the usefulness of all research approaches to the study of man as a psychological and social being and, also, of the necessity for nurse-researchers, interested in extending nursing knowledge, to realize that the nature of the scientific method is not a fixed, established datum. In addition, however, they need to understand the social nature of the research act (Pearsall, 1965, and Poulos and McCabe, 1960). Clinical interest and involvement implies concern for the individual and, especially, for experiential life. This genuine, fundamental attention to man's experience may lead to a realization that his relatively subjective experience is the source of all his endeavors, even in science. It is with this attitude that the clinician approaches modern thinking and the perceptivity of contemporary existence. One result is researchers' increased awareness of their assumptions and an attempt to make them explicit.

The humanities tell us what man is outside the framework of traditional science and how to know man in a human sense. Phenomenology developed historically for the same purpose. From this philosophical stance, the scientist's interest in manipulation, prediction, and control tend to obscure man's individuality and freedom. Therefore, they cancel the value of science to the individual and to society. In the final analysis, we must assume truth is a constantly growing reality in man's consciousness and science is a major contributor.

REFERENCES

Bacon, F. *Novum organum*. In B. Rand (Ed.), *Modern classical philosophers*. Boston: Houghton-Mifflin, 1936.

Bruyn, S. R. *The human perspective in sociology*. Englewood Cliffs, N. J.: Prentice-Hall, 1966.

Douglas, J. D. (Ed.), *Understanding everyday life*. Chicago: Aldine Publishing, 1970.

Durkheim, E. *The rules of sociological method*. New York: Free Press, 1950 (1st ed., 1895).

Friedman, N. *The social nature of psychological research*. New York: Basic Books, 1967.

Langer, S. *Philosophy in a new key*. New York: Mentor Book, New American Library, 1951.

Merton, R. K. *Social theory and social structure*. New York: Free Press, 1949.

Nagel, E. Problems of concept and theory. In *Science, language, and human rights*. Philadelphia: American Philosophical Association, 1952.

Natanson, M. *Literature, philosophy and the social sciences*. The Hague: Martinus Nijhoff, 1968.

Natanson, M. (Ed.), *Essays in phenomenology*. The Hague: Martinus Nijhoff, 1969.

Natanson, M. (Ed.), *Phenomenology and social reality*. The Hague: Martinus Nijhoff, 1970.

Olesen, V. L. Naturalism in nursing research: Participant observation and studies of students. In P. Verhonik (Ed.), *Research in nursing based on psychosocial data*. Boston: Little, Brown, in press.

Pearsall, M. Participant observation as role and method in behavioral research. *Nursing Research*, 1965, **14**, 37–42.

Schultz, D. (Ed.), *The science of psychology: Critical reflections*. New York: Appleton-Century-Crofts, 1970.

van der Berg, J. H. *The phenomenological approach to psychiatry*. Springfield, Ill.: Charles Thomas, 1955.

Znaniecki, F. *The method of sociology*. New York: Holt, Rinehart and Winston, 1934.

BACKGROUND READING

Berger, P. L., and Luckman, T. *The social construction of reality*. Garden City: Anchor Book, Doubleday, 1966.

Berkhofer, R. F. *A behavioral approach to historical analysis*. New York: Free Press, paperback, Macmillan, 1969.

Boss, M. *Psychoanalysis and daseinanalysis*. New York: Basic Books, 1963.

Cassirer, E. *An essay on man*. New Haven: Yale University Press, 1944.

Goffman, E. *Encounters*. Indianapolis: Bobbs-Merrill, 1961.

Husserl, E. *Phenomenology and the crisis of philosophy*. New York: Harper Torchbooks, 1960.

Husserl, E. *Ideas: General introduction to pure phenomenology*. New York: Collier Paperback, Macmillan, 1962.

Husserl, E. *The phenomenology of internal time-consciousness*. Bloomington: Indiana University Press, 1964.

Jarvie, I. C. *The revolution in anthropology*. Chicago: Gateway Edition, Henry Regnery, 1964.

Kockelmans, J. J. (Ed.), *Phenomenology*. Garden City: Doubleday, 1967.

Lawrence, N., and O'Connor, D. (Eds.), *Readings in existential phenomenology*. Englewood Cliffs, N.J.: Prentice-Hall, 1967.

Lyons, J. *Psychology and the measure of man: Phenomenological approach*. New York: Free Press, 1963.

McHugh, P. *Defining the situation*. Indianapolis, Bobbs-Merrill, 1968.

Merleau-Ponty, M. *The phenomenology of perception*. New York: Humanities, 1962.

Meyerhoff, H. (Ed.), *The philosophy of history in our time*. Garden City: Anchor Book, Doubleday, 1959.

Natanson, M. *The journeying self: A study in philosophy and social role*. Reading, Mass.: Addison-Wesley Co., 1970.

Ogden, C. K., and Richards, I. A. *The meaning of meaning*. New York: Harvest Book, Harcourt, Brace, 1923.

Perry, S. E. *The human nature of science: Researchers at work in psychiatry*. New York: Free Press, 1966.

Poulos, E. S., and McCabe, G. S. The nurse in the role of research observer. *Nursing Research*, 1960, **9**, 137–140.

Read, K. E. *The high valley*, New York: Charles Scribner's, 1965.

Reymert, M. L. (Ed.), *Feelings and emotions*. New York: McGraw-Hill, 1950.

Sarte, J. P. *Transcendence of the ego*. New York: Noonday, 1957.

Scheler, M. *On the nature of sympathy*. London: Routledge and Kegan Paul, 1954.

Schutz, A. J. *Collected papers I: The problem of social reality*. The Hague: Martinus Nijhoff, 1962.

Spiegelberg, H. The essentials of the phenomenological method. In *The phenomenological movement: A historical introduction,* vol. II. The Hague, Martinus Nijhoff, 1965.

Strasser, S. *Phenomenology and human sciences*. Pittsburgh: Duquesne University Press, 1963.

Straus, E. *Phenomenology: Pure and applied*. Pittsburgh: Duquesne University Press, 1964.

Thevenaz, P. *What is phenomenology?* Chicago: Quadrangle Books, 1962.

Van Melsen, A. G. *Science and responsibility*. Pittsburgh: Duquesne University Press, 1970.

Editor's Note:

In accord with publishers' specifications, we acknowledge permission to excerpt from:

Severyn T. Bruyn, *The Human Perspective in Sociology: The Methodology of Participant Observation* © 1966. Reprinted by permission of Prentice-Hall Inc., Englewood Cliffs, New Jersey.

The Social Nature of Psychological Research: The Psychological Experiment as a Social Interaction by Neil Friedman. Basic Books, Inc., publishers, New York.

The Science of Psychology: Critical Reflections, edited by Duane P. Schultz. Copyright © 1970. By permission of Appleton-Century-Crofts, Educational Division, Meredith Corporation.

EDITOR'S QUESTIONS FOR DISCUSSION

What specific phenomena of the role of the patient might be studied through the phenomenological approach? What is the value of the participant observation method in research? What are the advantages and disadvantages of qualitative and quantitative research methods? What type of problems may be more effectively studied through qualitative methods? What are the limitations in regard to objectivity when using qualitative and quantitative methods in research?

Chapter 18

Low Verbal Usage
and Status Maintenance
Among Intensive Care Nurses

Carol A. Soares, R.N., Ph.D.
Associate Professor, School of Nursing
Boston University

Carol A. Soares draws on Goffman's dramaturgical model to analyze verbal usage in an intensive care unit. By means of the method of participant observation, Soares utilizes the language of the theater—actor, scene, and production—to describe the drama and behavior of nurses in a specialized unit. First, Soares defines the norms of behavior in the unit. The importance of language, tone of voice, and gestures is then illustrated by the interaction of nurses in a patient care situation. Throughout, the reader witnesses the nurse as an agent of social control.

This article reports on a study of how a particular nursing staff, in a particular clinical unit, maintains the status, or more specifically gives off the impression of being actors whose behavior is defined as "snobbish, cold, and unfriendly" by other staff nurses who are not located in this particular unit on a regularly assigned basis. This problem was made manifest to me when I was assigned on a regular basis to participate in the everyday activities of this particular unit as a clinical staff nurse for a period of 6 weeks. The staff nurses in the unit made it known that they felt that the other nurses regarded them as "snobbish, cold, and unfriendly." They supported their perception of the situation by referring to several nurses who had refused to "float" into the unit to work. Other nurses

had been known to say that they did not like working in the unit because of the attitude of the staff nurses who were assigned there on regular basis.

Factors in this problem are: nurses in the unit (inside staff nurses), nurses floated into the unit (outside staff nurses), the clinical unit (intensive care unit—ICU), patients, visitors (noncontrolling participants), and the head nurse (controlling participant). The primary methodology employed in this study was that of participant observation. Observations were noted at various times of the day—morning, afternoon, and evening—over a period of 7 days. Tape recordings of the information that was given to the evening nurses by the day nurses—the unit report—were made. Also,

Permission to study this problem was secured from Nursing Service Administration and the individual nurses involved in this particular intensive care unit. No effort to disguise the researcher's intent was made.

each member of the day staff was interviewed individually to ascertain his or her perception of the situation.

Attention was focused on the usage of language particularly on the verbal structuring of messages and their meanings as conveyed between staff members and between staff members and other participants who may have entered the scene during the period of observation. The interpretations resulting from this research reveal generalizations that may apply to other isolated, remote, specialized units in voluntary 24-hour service institutions.

The following sociological analysis will be based in part on the heuristic device of Irving Goffman's dramaturgical model, which utilizes the language of the theater—actor, scene, and production—to describe behavior which expresses and gives off the impression of role performance (Goffman, 1959, pp. 239-242).

DESCRIPTION OF THE SITUATION

This particular intensive care unit is an isolated, remote unit that renders specialized public service. The physical location of this unit in a remote, isolated area of the hospital maintains the impression of its being a place in which activities are of a secretive nature, i.e., not readily made known to those outside the unit. Other remote and isolated areas of the hospital are delivery rooms, operating rooms, recovery rooms, coronary care units, and the morgue.

To participate as an actor or audience in these settings, one must either give the impression of being in control of a particular skill, or maintain the status of a patient by being in need of a particular skilled service. The only other participants who may enter the scene are carefully cued into their parts. They are the controlled ones, namely, the visitors. In order to become a visitor, one must be a blood relative or spouse of the patient and one must follow the rules of behavior prescribed for the role of visitor. For example, one may not enter the unit unless one first rings a buzzer, and then

announces the "password" through a two-way speaker system. The password, i.e., the formal name of the patient, signifies that the visitor wishes to enter this secret room, and will comply with the rule of staying no longer than 5 minutes. The legitimacy of the password may be challenged by the staff nurse who may ask the visitor, "Are you a relative?" If the visitor succeeds in giving off the impression that he has a legitimate right to be there, the nurse may still continue to express her control of the situation by stating, "O.K., but no more than 5 minutes!"

One maintains the status of visitor by (1) not asking any questions regarding the patient, and (2) displaying facial gestures and body posture that convey the message of grave seriousness and concern. One does not ask, "How are you, today?" nor does one bring into the definition of the situation any outside information, such as the weather, Johnny's grades, or Aunt Helen's rheumatism. The rules of the game seem to be: see no evil, hear no evil, and speak no evil, i.e., say nothing and look helpless and completely out of control of the situation.

The interpretation here is that the patient's visitor, by his acquiescence to the nurses, confirms the status of the skilled workers in the unit as the only ones who can control the situation. Therefore, the patient must place his trust in the staff as being the only ones who can get him out of the unit alive.

By participating in the kind of communication implicitly forbidden to the visitor, e.g., conversation such as "How are you, today?" and "How is your Aunt Helen's rheumatism?" the staff nurses maintain their status as controllers. The implication is that by discussing such lighthearted topics, the staff nurse as controller cannot be too concerned about the serious business at hand. If this is so, from the patient's point of view it follows that things are not as serious as they could be, i.e., "I (the patient) am going to live!"

Therefore, patients' tensions are decreased by staff nurses acting in a way as to convey that there is nothing to be tense about. One deals with "serious business," i.e., life and death situations, by behaving as if they were "nonserious business." To the extent that the actor can carry through a performance of nonserious business, i.e., staging activities of lighthearted carefreeness, the audience (the patient) will perceive the actor (the nurse) as performing a highly competent role. In giving definition to the situation as "being under control," the actor performs as if the situation were a manageable one.

Staff nurses who are floated into the unit under emergency conditions do not seem to be aware of how to stage a highly competent role performance. From another perspective, the character that is fashioned by outside staff nurses is not the one that is typically expressed in the unit. Outside nurses tend to conceal their fears through a highly technical performance. They maintain their character portrayal through the manipulation of props, e.g., by adjusting intravenous equipment and other such tubing and machinery, and through kinesics, facial gestures, and body movements that give off meanings of alertness and serious business.

Patients test the status of the nurse as competent or incompetent by calling into question her ability to carry off a "cool " performance. It was noted on several occasions that at the change of shift, especially when new personnel arrived in the unit, the patients tended to "act out." Goffman suggests that the acting-out behavior of patients may be related to their ability to carry through their performance as defined by the staff nurses who are leaving the unit.

> . . . the new frame of reference. . .often provide[s] a context in which it is especially difficult to maintain the previous suppressions. And so the participants flood out in regard to a definition of the situation which has just been displaced, it being safe to offend something no longer credited as reality (Goffman, 1961*a*, p. 60).

However, this "flooding out" behavior may also be viewed as the manner in which patients challenge the new staff's ability to redefine the situation as nonserious business. One example of this is a patient with a cervical fracture (broken neck) who asked a nurse to hold his head while he moved about in bed. The patient had been allowed to perform this type of activity. The manner in which the nurse acted in response to this request conveyed different meanings to the patient. If the nurse gave no outward gesture that would imply hesitancy, and if her activities conveyed the message that this was as serious as flipping a pillow, then the patient would perceive her performance as being cool, and accept the former definition of nonserious business. If, on the other hand, the actor did give signs of hesitancy, e.g., by saying such things as "Wait a moment, I'll check that," "I'll get some help," or "You shouldn't move, it can be dangerous!" then the audience would perceive her performance as not being legitimate, and therefore he would not accept the definition of the situation as nonserious business. The audience would continue to flood out until someone changed his definition of the situation.

Patients who flood out are frequently labeled by staff nurses as "uncooperative," meaning that they are persistent in their flooding-out performance. The role of the uncooperative patient calls into question the legitimacy of the nurse's role and her ability to maintain her status as controller of the situation. An actor who is unable to carry off a cool performance avoids the uncooperative patient. In so doing the actor reinforces the audience's impression of the actor as being out of control of the situation.

> Coolness, then, refers to the capacity to execute physical acts, including conversation, in a concerted, smooth, self-controlled fashion in risky situations, or to maintain affective detachment during the course of encounters involving considerable emotion (Lyman and Scott, 1968, p. 93).

Stanford M. Lyman and Marvin B. Scott, in discussing coolness in everyday life, note that one is more likely to give off the impression of coolness in hazardous situations if the actor displays stylized affective neutrality, *savoir-faire*, aplomb, and *sang-froid* (Lyman and Scott, 1968, p. 95). Coolness is therefore an expression of being in control during a performance. "To successfully pass coolness tests one must mobilize and control a sizeable and complex retinue of material and moral forces" (Lyman and Scott, 1968, p. 97). Goffman further notes that one may pass audience tests by successful impression management. He describes an actor's performance as a communicative act that can be translated into a moral act. Moral acts are labeled as such by virtue of the fact that the audience can and does attribute credibility to the claims and promises of the actor's performance. As the audience can never know all of the relevant social data pertaining to the actor, it becomes necessary for them to rely upon appearances (Goffman, 1959, pp. 249-251). "It is always possible to manipulate the impression the observer uses as a substitute for reality because a sign for the presence of a thing, not being that thing, can be employed in the absence of it" (Goffman, 1959, pp. 250-251). Goffman (1959, p. 251) elaborates on this point when he writes:

> In their capacity as performers, individuals will be concerned with maintaining the impression that they are living up to the many standards by which they and their products are judged. Because these standards are so numerous and so pervasive, the individuals who are performers dwell more than we think in a moral world. But, *qua* performers, individuals are concerned not with the moral issues of realizing these standards, but with the amoral issue of engineering a convincing impression that these standards are being realized.

During the participant observation period, an emergency situation did occur when several outside staff nurses were reassigned to the intensive care unit. If one can accept that the "floats" into the unit disrupt the organization of everyday activities for the members of the regular staff nurses, then one may be able to discern some of the taken-for-granted expectations around these routine activities that inside staff nurses normally hold.

The area of disorganization that was imme-

diately noted was that of communicative acts. Communication between inside staff and outside staff, particularly in the asking for and the giving of information, became problematic. When the head nurse, sitting at her desk and without lifting her head asked, "How many cc's in that thing?" meaning "Miss A, how much liquid is there left in that container that you are now measuring?," there was no response from Miss A. On another occasion, an inside staff nurse explained to an outside staff nurse, "The bile filters itself through that thing and if it gets blocked, just push it back to number one." The meaning of that statement would require several pages of detailed description of technology and physiology. The inside staff nurse returned the following day to find that the outside staff nurse did not carry through the procedure as she had explained it.

In order to come off as cool to a testing audience, the inside staff nurse must be in possession of certain information regarding equipment, drugs, and machines. Without this information, the outside staff nurse maintains the status of visitor, i.e., as one out of control of the situation. In order to maintain the status of being an inside staff nurse, therefore, one must perform as if the activities at hand are not serious business and give off the impression of being in control in a rather carefree impersonal manner. On the other hand, to maintain the status of being an outside staff nurse, one must act as if the activities at hand are serious business and approach the situation in a manner of helplessness and fear, e.g., by giving off appropriate changes in voice tone, hurried speech, clumsiness, and a look of panic.

The problem of how outside nurses perceive and define the situation of inside staff nurses is further complicated when an outside staff nurse is floated into the unit and becomes an inside staff nurse. Outside staff nurses are floated into the unit under conditions of extreme emergency and, therefore, are under a great deal of stress. When an outside staff nurse becomes an inside nurse she simultaneously enters the situation as a visitor. She thus brings to the definition of the situation the conflicting performance expectations of an actor who as visitor is out of control of the situation.

The inside staff nurses in this particular unit were maintaining their status of being in control of the situation by decreasing the amount of information given to the outside nurses.

> The image that one status grouping is able to maintain in the eyes of an audience of other status groupings will depend upon the performers' capacity to restrict communicative contact with the audience (Goffman, 1959, p.241).

Thus, through giving information in "low verbal usage," the inside staff gave off the impression of being "cold, snobbish, and impersonal." In Goffman's terminology, one could say that the inside staff nurses through their role performance were creating the impression of social distance.

LOW VERBAL USAGE

Having concluded that the inside staff nurses were indeed giving off the impression of being "cold, snobbish, and impersonal," and were creating social distance from the outside staff nurses, I then focused my attention on the low verbal usage that was creating these impressions. My chief concern at this time was to investigate whether or not these inside staff nurses employed low verbal usage among themselves, and if so, to see whether these messages or meanings were peculiar to this unit.

Although previously I was both a participant and an observer, I found that at this point I was creating the *impression* of participant. By this I mean that although I wore the symbolic paraphernalia—uniform, cap, and pin— that legitimatized my entry into this situation, I did not actively participate in the activities of the unit. However, I created the impression that I was by pretending to be securing information from the patients' charts. This provided me with a strategic position from which to observe the verbal interac-

tion among the staff members. Verbal interactions were noted between staff and patient, staff and staff, and staff and head nurse, which were audible from this position (see Fig. 18-1).

In recording the flow of interaction, I, as investigator, became quite perplexed. How did the various actors know who was being addressed when no names were being utilized? Interaction flowed back and forth between the staff and the head nurse, who was visibly present at the main desk. All the staff nurses were behind curtains and were neither visible to each other nor to the head nurse (except at bed 2), yet they continued to talk with each other. For example, X asked, "Are you touching a lead?" to which *a* replied, "One just came off."

After taking notes for a while, I was able to discern differences in the nurses' tones of voice when they addressed, i.e., nurse, head nurse, and patient. When a staff nurse addressed a patient it was in a loud voice and structured in the form of a simple command, such as, "Turn over." When this staff nurse addressed another staff nurse in the same physical proximity as she had been to the patient, she did so in a very light, conversational tone of voice (*a* and *b* at bed 2). Thus, *a*'s and *b*'s tone of voice conveyed the message to the patient A, "This conversation is not for you." No patient participated in staff nurse conversation even though the interaction took place within the patients' auditory and visible range. The head nurse did, however, participate in nearly all verbal interactions between staff nurse and staff nurse, even when the staff nurses were not visible to the head nurse. Whenever a staff nurse addressed the head nurse, the voice tone was louder than that of conversational speech and softer than that of a loud command.

The conclusion is that in order to be able to carry off a performance with the actors in this unit, one must know the rules of verbal communicative acts and how they are characterized by tonal differences. Through the use of tonal differences, messages could be conveyed while em-

CODE: A - E, patients   - - - - interaction
         a - d, staff nurses   _____ drawn bed curtain
         X , head nurse
         x , observer

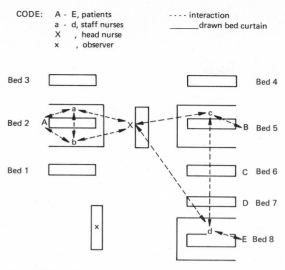

Figure 18-1 Flow of interaction

ploying a lesser quantity of words, i.e., with low verbal usage.

One particular tonal message seemed to have a consistent response from the actors. When a nurse addressed another person by name in an exclamatory tone of voice, whoever was in the area immediately responded by moving toward that particular location. In one instance, the head nurse said "Mr. Jones!"—which was followed by the observer running to Mr. Jones as the head nurse jumped over the desk, and then, working together, we both caught Mr. Jones before he hit the floor. In all situations noted where a name and exclamatory tone of voice were used, the meaning was always *emergency*. It is also worth mentioning that the code for the two major emergencies that are anticipated throughout the hospital are coded in names. Mr. Red means fire and Mr. Blue means a cardiac arrest. When announced over the loudspeaker, both names result in specified behavior from actors throughout the entire hospital. Rules of emergency behavior are explicitly stated and posted on all clinical units. They define exact step-by-step procedures, which all personnel are expected to be able to carry out should either

name be called. Emphasis is placed on each person in the institution knowing what he or she must do under these conditions, and all hospital orientation programs include these rules of emergency behavior for actors of every status.

However, in the intensive care unit, where staff are continuously anticipating emergency situations other than fire and cardiac arrest, little attention has been given to *how* one announces an emergency or to what rules of behavior one should adhere to in order to carry out a cool performance, such as saving a life.

In summary, inside staff nurses give off the impression of being "cold, snobbish, and impersonal" to outside staff nurses, who may be floated into the unit. This impression is conveyed through the use of low verbal communication between inside and outside staff nurses. During emergency situations, inside staff nurses' communicative acts are characterized by low verbal usage among themselves, as well as between them and outside staff nurses. Inside staff nurses have been exposed to the informal rules of interaction within this particular unit, and they have learned the taken-for-granted meanings that are known to the members of the inside group. Since outside staff nurses do not appear to understand the meanings conveyed in the unit, as seen by the lack of response to action messages, it seems feasible that these messages and meanings are peculiar to this particular unit.

It should be noted that because of the physical layout of this intensive care unit, one of the factors that may be influencing the solidarity of the inside staff group is that the nurses' station is within the patient care area. Therefore, backstage and frontstage areas share the same physical location.

For further study, I recommend the following: First, there should be participant observation studies in other similar units where there are clearly defined frontstage and backstage areas to ascertain if members of these units employ low verbal usage. One possibility is the coronary unit, which is situated in a remote part of this hospital where emergency situations are routinely anticipated, and which has a distinct front- and backstage area. Second, the isolation of extensive taken-for-granted codes of messages and corresponding responses that are peculiar to each individual clinical unit is possible and warranted. The outcomes of this type of future research will enhance the development of nursing practice theory.

BIBLIOGRAPHY

Church, J.: *Language and the Discovery of Reality,* Harper & Row, New York, 1961.

Cicourel, A.: *Method and Measurement in Sociology,* Free Press, New York, 1969.

Garfinkel, H.: *Studies in Ethnomethodology,* Prentice-Hall, Englewood Cliffs, N. J., 1967.

Goffman, I.: "Symbols of Class Status," *The British Journal of Sociology,* 2:294–304, 1951.

——: *The Presentation of Self in Everyday Life,* Doubleday, New York, 1959.

——: *Asylums,* Doubleday, New York, 1961(*a*).

——: *Encounters,* Bobbs-Merrill, Indianapolis, Ind., 1961(*b*).

——: *Behavior in Public Places,* Free Press, New York, 1963(*a*).

——: *Stigma,* Prentice-Hall, Englewood Cliffs, N.J., 1963(*b*).

Hall, E.: *The Silent Language,* Fawcett Publications, Greenwich, Conn., 1967.

Lyman, S., and M. Scott: "Coolness in Everyday Life," in Marcello Truzzi (ed.), *Sociology and Everyday Life,* Prentice-Hall, Englewood Cliffs, N.J., 1968, pp. 92–101.

Messinger, S. et al.: "Life as Theater: Some Notes on the Dramaturgic Approach to Social Reality," *Sociometry,* 25:98–110, 1962.

Psathas, G.: "Ethnomethods and Phenomenology," *Social Research,* 35:500–520, 1968.

Truzzi, M.: *Sociology and Everyday Life,* Prentice-Hall, Englewood Cliffs, N.J., 1968.

EDITOR'S QUESTIONS FOR DISCUSSION

What are the implications for patient care in intensive care units in light of this study? How might the patient define the situation in this intensive care unit? To what extent may the findings of this study be typical of other intensive care units and general hospital nursing units? What factors are likely to encourage low verbal usage on any nursing unit? What are other examples of symbolism in patient care that may have meaning for a patient?

Part Four

Nursing Theory

The development of a scientific knowledge base on which to establish nursing practice has been a desired goal of the profession for many years. The attempts of nursing to formulate nursing theory have met with controversy over both the types of theory that might be developed and the purposes of developing such theory. Nurses in nursing practice often question the need for nursing theory since for decades patients have been given excellent care without it. The contributions in this section attempt to answer that question.

Chapter 19

Development of Theory: A Requisite for Nursing as a Primary Health Profession

Dorothy E. Johnson, R.N., Ph.D.
Professor, School of Nursing
The Center for the Health Sciences, University of California at Los Angeles

Dorothy E. Johnson is aware of many of the questions and concerns of nursing practitioners as she presents alternative routes to theory development in nursing. She points out that the development of a theoretical body of nursing knowledge is a means of acquiring a distinctive professional identity for nursing. The basic assumption is that the formulation of theory will make a valuable difference in patient care. Johnson discusses the different conceptual models that may be used for theory development and presents three social criteria for evaluating models: congruence, significance, and utility.

Since its first recorded use in the midfifteenth century, the word "profession" has been defined as a learned vocation (Cogan, 1953). While scholars may differ to some extent on the distinguishing characteristics of a profession, there is universal agreement that a theoretical body of knowledge is an essential attribute (Cogan, 1953; Goode, 1960; New, 1965). A profession's service to society is an intellectual one, and a sound, scientific basis for that service is indispensable. Moreover, a profession is responsible for creating the constantly increasing body of knowledge upon which its service depends (Goode, 1960; New, 1965). If nursing is indeed an emerging profession, nurses must be able to identify clearly and develop continually the theoretical body of knowledge upon which practice must rest.

THE STATUS OF NURSING SCIENCE

Progress toward this end is not an easy task, however, as many a sincere and industrious nurse-scientist has discovered. Investigators in other disciplines forge ahead, building on the work of their founding fathers. But there are no scientific giants in nursing's heritage on whose shoulders present-day investigators can stand. There is no circumscribed body of knowledge. There is not even a particular group of facts or empirical generalizations widely recognized and accepted as offering the rudiments of nursing science that can provide a foundation for further work. Even the focus of scientific concern considered appropriate for this profession varies markedly among investigators and within the profession at large.

Reprinted from *Nursing Research,* **23**(5): 372–377, September–October 1974.

Given such a situation, the prospective scientist in nursing is left without support and without direction. Small wonder then that our scientists tend to be relatively unproductive and our research reports, though increasing in numbers and producing a variety of findings, have yet to reflect a cumulative effect to any degree.

The prospective nurse-investigator might well search for direction, consciously and rationally, by attempting to answer two relevant and related questions, at least to her own satisfaction, before she sets about her work. The seeker of answers will recognize that in each instance more than one alternative exists and must be examined and that the answers selected will reflect underlying social decisions. The most obvious question is: For what purpose is a theoretical body of knowledge intended? Or, what is the nature of the service nursing offers, for which knowledge is needed? Secondly, given this responsibility, what phenomena must be studied and what kinds of questions must be asked to develop the needed knowledge?

EVOLUTION OF SCIENTIFIC DISCIPLINES

Nurses and nursing probably are rarities in the scientific world in facing such questions so deliberately and self-consciously. Indeed, the necessity for doing so is questioned not only by individuals in other disciplines but also by many nurses. But nursing has not followed the path of evolutionary progress characteristic of other scientific disciplines. Scientific endeavor began thousands of years ago, with observations of the natural world generated by innate curiosity or pragmatic concern. Later, but still centuries ago, the search for truth was strengthened and stimulated by the rise of philosophy. Over the years, as facts were uncovered and relationships established concerning man and his universe, the several natural and social sciences emerged gradually as independent and distinct fields of inquiry. Each of the sciences developed by seeking partial understanding of the world through a focus on selected phenomena from a particular perspective. Each emerged as some investigators addressed the phenomena of concern to a parent discipline from a new perspective or turned their attention to a different kind of phenomenon with still other questions. Because a different kind of phenomenon was studied or a different perspective (or frame of reference) was used as a basis for the observations and interpretations made, a new body of theoretical knowledge was developed and a new science was born. From a pragmatic interest in metals and in the heavenly bodies gradually emerged the sciences of chemistry and astronomy, while interest in all material phenomena under the rubric of natural philosophy led to the disciplines of physics and biology. And, eventually, the concern for understanding man manifested so early by the Greeks was rounded out by the births of the several social sciences in the seventeenth, eighteenth, and nineteenth centuries.

Sciences, then, become differentiated from one another on the basis of what is studied and the perspective used to raise questions, make observations, and interpret evidence. Since several sciences may, and often do, study the same phenomenon, it is the distinctive perspective of each science which most clearly discriminates it from others. Emergence of the now recognized and accepted basic disciplines is an historical product, brought about by the more or less arbitrary decisions of investigators, as phenomena for study were selected and the particular questions to be asked were identified. The emergence of the professional disciplines is also an historical product, and these disciplines generally have followed the same evolutionary path in that there was a gradual growth of knowledge through the study of selected phenomena from a distinctive perspective. The direction of growth for these disciplines, however, has been governed to an extent by logic—or at least by social responsibility. Professional decisions of what to study and what questions to ask necessarily have gone hand in hand with social decisions about the profession's realm of responsibility.

THE PROFESSIONS AS SCIENCES

The focus of any profession's scientific concern is interdependent with the profession's service, its social function. Given the task of safeguarding some significant social value for the members of society, the members of a profession are obligated to develop the theoretical and technological means by which this responsibility can be met. Ascribed long ago, medicine's social responsibility has been stated aptly and colorfully by the historian, Lynn White (1963, p. 52): "to free mankind from the ills of the flesh." Given this task, physicians have created over the years a large and continuously growing body of knowledge as a means of understanding and controlling man's bodily ills. They have done so by identifying, describing, and explaining all manner of disorders or disturbances in man's biological being and by developing the rationale necessary to their prevention and management. In essence, this statement of an explicit, ideal goal in patient care for the physician established for the medical investigator the proper object for study—the living human body—and pointed to the socially relevant perspective—the identification and control of biological system disorders.

If nursing's social responsibility has been clearly and precisely formulated as an ideal goal in patient care many years ago, perhaps we, too, would have been building upon previously established theory. But nursing's history is quite different from that of medicine, despite a certain similarity in the ages of the two fields. The significant differences are many; I will mention only two. First, nursing is an occupation whose form of service, until recently, was not considered particularly socially valuable and certainly not very critical in social life. What matter the quality of life if biological survival could not be insured? Furthermore, the service given was practical, not intellectual in nature, requiring in the main strong legs, strong arms, and a certain amount of human compassion. This service with its underlying pragmatic concern—the care of the sick, the injured, and the helpless (Bullough and Bullough, 1964)—did not lead easily to the development of knowledge. Unlike the case with metals or heavenly bodies, or even disease, nursing's service encompasses a wide range of objects and events of a less tangible nature and its purpose has been difficult to identify or describe in symbolic terms. As a concern focused on essentially social objects and events, nursing antedated the social sciences. But the possibility of theoretical knowledge in nursing could scarcely be envisioned when there has been little or no development in a significant component of its basic science foundations. Nursing stands today, as a field of practice without a scientific heritage—an occupation created by society long ago to offer a distinctive service, but one still ill-defined in practical terms, a profession without the theoretical base it seems to require.

There is a controversial point which should be mentioned here although it is somewhat unrelated to the preceding discussion. The issue concerns the nature of an applied science and the relationship of knowledge in an applied science to that of a basic science. At the most fundamental level, all professions (and that includes the professional outgrowths of the basic sciences) are applied sciences in that theoretical knowledge is developed and used to achieve practical ends. Moreover, theory construction in the professions usually draws upon and builds from the foundation provided by one or more of the basic sciences. In general, however, a theoretical body of professional knowledge cannot be developed simply by the testing of basic science theories; or, to put it another way, professional knowledge does not consist of basic science theory which has been validated in practice.

The professional fields also are in the business of describing and explaining selected aspects of reality, a reality that with few exceptions differs from that considered by any one of the basic sciences.[1] Furthermore, as Dickoff and James (1968) pointed out, professional discipines are obligated to go a step further than explanation and prediction in theory construction, to the development of prescriptive theory. Specifically, the phenomenon of interest and the perspective utilized in the several professions differs from those of the several basic sciences, and so different and unique bodies of theoretical knowledge are developed. Each of the biological sciences, for example, focuses on the biological organism, and each has added partial understanding of the structure and function of that organism. Only medicine, however, has focused on disturbances in the system as a whole and on their management.

This issue would be no trouble at all, were it not for the fact that many prospective nurse-scientists have had advanced education and research training in one or another of the basic sciences rather than in nursing. In this process, they have necessarily acquired the scientific orientation of that discipline; that is, they have learned to direct their attention toward those aspects of the world of interest to that discipline and to use the discipline's frame of reference in raising questions about the world. Moreover, it is a reasonable observation that more than a few basic scientists tend to be somewhat prejudicial in their judgments and somewhat limited in their understanding of the professions and their research tasks. Consequently, a not uncommon view among them is that the professions, as applied sciences, convert basic science laws into principles of practice through the testing of these laws (Greenwood, 1961). This point of view has been transmitted to many nurses who then limit their research efforts to those seen as appropriate in the discipline of orientation. While this may be productive for the basic discipline, it will not necessarily further the cause of nursing. And to the extent that it clouds

[1] Those professional fields that are applied branches of only one basic science, e.g., applied physics, or the counseling-psychotherapy branch of psychology, are exceptions to this generalization.

the thinking, it creates a potentially serious problem for nursing.

ALTERNATIVE ROUTES TO THEORY DEVELOPMENT

The would-be nurse-scientist as well as a faculty contemplating curriculum development at the highest level face problems for which several choices are possible. There is the laissez-faire alternative; that is, either intentionally or unwittingly letting the future course of events evolve as it will. Each nurse-scientist would continue to follow her own scientific orientation, whatever its origin; and educational programs would continue to emerge and expand within a more or less rational, explicit, and cohesive framework. It is conceivable, of course, that our unconscious ties and strong commitment in common to our heritage will lead most of us along at least parallel educational paths and to scientific findings that eventually reveal a cohesive and cumulative effect and provide a substantial basis for a professional form of practice.

Progress, via this route will be very slow, if it comes at all. Certainly a deliberate, relatively widespread emphasis on the necessity for theory development for more than two decades has yielded little in the way of a circumscribed body of nursing knowledge. In fact, in only two schools in the country do faculty and students seem to share a common research orientation and whose reports reveal orderly, even sequential progress in theory development. There probably are not more than a dozen nurse-scientists whose work reveals a central focus and an effort to build. Nonetheless, many nurses appear to think this is the most desirable route and perhaps the only route. When reasons are given, they often include the difficulties in obtaining a faculty consensus on nursing's reasons for being (and this is very real); a strongly held belief that a scientist should be "free" to follow his own destiny (as if any scientist is really free of some kind of mental image to guide empirical research, or as if he did not have the "right" to change his images); and an insistence that we already know what we are about and where we are going (and no rational counterargument serves any purpose here).

A second alternative is to follow medicine's path, a route nursing has used in the past often without overt recognition of the significance and the consequences of doing so. Moreover, it is a route that today is increasingly sanctioned and well rewarded. A number of nurses have chosen this path willingly and deliberately—some because they do not think nursing has a destiny of its own and that the occupation's identity rests on a specialized competence within medicine; some, because they are simply seeking greater intellectual challenge and personal responsibility than is currently available in most practice settings today; and some, motivated largely by altruistic aims, because they want to bring better medical care to the poor and to the geographically isolated.

The proportion of nurses who would willingly "give up nursing" entirely to follow the medical path is very small, it seems, for most nurses who have taken this route in practice or in research are attempting to maintain identification as nurses while adopting actual practice or scientific orientations that vary on a scale of mixed orientation from partly nursing to largely medical. These nurses can be found in hospitals, often in intensive care units, and in outpatient clinics and other community settings. In the latter setting, they sometimes operate under the guise of providing "health care" as a synonym for nursing care. Nurse-scientists who use medicine's research orientation in empirical investigations tend to study problems rather directly related to nursing activities in the diagnosis and treatment of disease. Others, many of who claim the laissez-faire attitude, appear to use the medical model indirectly to determine the appropriateness or significance of a particular problem area, but actually identify and study the problem from the orientation of one of the basic sciences, both the natural and social sciences being involved.

Progress toward a theoretical body of *nursing*

knowledge via this route is inconceivable to anyone who envisions a distinctive professional identity for nursing. And without such an identity, there is little reason to be concerned about theory development at all. If nursing represents simply an area of specialized competence in medical practice, then whatever theoretical contributions nurse-scientists, who do not have a medical education, might make to *medical science* are likely to be restricted along much the same lines as would hold for the basic scientist, or to be limited to technological advances. This is, however, a safe and rewarding option for nurses in practice, and it appears to have certain benefits for patients. For investigators, it provides clear direction and does not require a great deal of risk-taking in research. And, certainly, there is no guarantee that other options available will lead to a circumscribed body of knowledge that can be called the science of nursing and support an increasingly well-defined and distinctive professional service.

The third alternative does involve risk-taking, a good deal of it; it also requires another choice among still other options. It is, of course, to accept as a premise that nursing has a distinctive professional service to offer and to attempt to answer the question posed in that light. Available to assist in making such a decision are nursing's history, observatons drawn from current practice, and the ability to analyze the kind of service patients require that nursing might provide. History suggests that the nurse's primary concern has been for the person who is ill, rather than the illness itself, and that in particular her concern has been for the part played by the ambient environment in fostering illness or in preventing recovery (Nightingale, 1860). That same concern appears prevalent today, although it is perhaps less evident in practice at times than in clinical and research reports in the literature. It is a concern that is expressed in the attention give to patient adjustments and adaptations under the changed circumstances of illness, to coping abilities and strategies, to personalized care and patient comfort during illness, to the development of lifestyles and behavior patterns conducive to a sense of physical, psychological, and social well-being, and the like. And, most significantly, reason suggests that within the organization of relationships and the way of life found especially in today's society, patients require precisely that which nursing, by heritage and current interest, seems uniquely qualified to give: concern for the person and assistance in living and coping with his circumstances and his environment in such a way that illness may be prevented or recovery may be facilitated.

Building the Conceptual System

The majority of nurses today probably hold to this view of nursing's general purpose. Moreover, this purpose represents a significant social responsibility and, when formulated as an explicit ideal goal, the service will make a valuable and valued difference in the lives of people. Implicit in this last sentence is the rub, however, for nursing's difficulty is not eased appreciably by acceptance of this general statement. There remains the necessity of building a focused and cohesive conceptual system of the person to be served and of deriving from that system an abstract model for practice that will allow such a purpose to be fulfilled. We must proceed in much the same fashion as was the case in medicine, when physicians, focused on bodily ills, both sought in the basic sciences and helped to create a conceptual system which explains the person to be served as a biological system subject to inefficiencies and disorders in operation as a consequence of internal difficulties or environmental forces. From this they were able to project medical practice as consisting of the recognition and treatment of biological system problems.

Any number of individuals in nursing now are attempting to do just this. Some are focused primarily on practice and are working on more goal-directed approaches to nursing diagnosis and treatment by developing diagnostic protocols and typologies of nursing problems (Gebbie and Lavin, 1974; McCain, 1965). Others, concerned with curriculum development and revision, have attempted to formulate theoretical frameworks that would give clear direction to the selection and organization of courses and learning experiences and provide a diagnostic and treatment orientation for practice (Lum and Kim, 1967; McDonald and Harms, 1966; Vaillot, 1970). A growing number of expositions of practice models, both published and unpublished, are becoming available as well. Since these have been more completely developed and are accompanied by the underlying rationale, and since they also are more general and more abstract, they may well be nursing's greatest source of assistance.

Most, if not all, of these individual efforts to conceptualize the consumer of nursing service appear to have started from about the same point of view of nursing's general purpose. Nonetheless, if the various routes were followed to their logical conclusions not only would practice and the nature of curriculum offerings differ now, but, at some future point the research undertaken to support different forms of practice would provide differing bodies of knowledge also. For example, the two most common types of models now available are developmental models and system models. If the person is conceptualized as a developmental process of some kind, and nursing's goal is seen as the maximization of development along specific lines, then the research task is to identify and explain potential problems in that course of development and to develop the theoretical and technological means of preventing or controlling these problems or of otherwise fostering developmental progress. On the other hand, if the person is conceptualized as some kind of system, and nursing's goal is seen to be the maximization of effective system operation, then the research task is to identify and explain potential problems in the functioning of the system and to develop relevant rationale and means of management. Clearly these two different classes of approaches to understanding the person who is a patient, not only call for differing forms of practice toward different objectives, but also point to different kinds of phenomena, suggest different kinds of questions, and lead eventually to dissimilar bodies of knowledge.

CONCEPTUAL MODELS

The conceptual models now utilized or discussed include, among the developmental models, models based on the developmental theories of Erikson (1963), Freud (1949), Maslow (1954), Peplau (1952), C. Rogers (1959), Sullivan (1953), and of the behaviorist school (Bijou and Baer, 1961). Among the system models are found the adaptation system model of Roy (1970), the triad system of Howland and McDowell (1964), the life process system of M.E. Rogers (1970), and Johnson's behavioral system model (1968). There are no doubt others in each of these general categories; and still others might well be developed since man's development proceeds along many dimensions, and it is possible to conceptualize man as a number of different kinds of systems. Then, in addition, there is another type of model for nursing practice, called an interaction model, since its conceptual system is dependent upon symbolic interaction theory. The most well-known model in this group is that of Orlando (1961) and Wiedenbach (1964).

A number of these specific models have been used as a guide to practice and as a basis for curriculum development. Several—specifically the M. E. Rogers and Johnson system models, Peplau's developmental model, and the Orlando-Wiedenbach model—have been used as a framework for theory construction. Most are commensurate with the general purpose of nursing but are far more specific, clearly goal-related, and reducible to concrete terms. None of these models can be judged at this point in time as the best model, or the right one for nursing. In this regard, it is particularly important to emphasize that as long as the conceptual system for understanding the person is reasonably sound, scientifically, the question of "truth" plays no part in judging a model for nursing practice, education, and research based on that conceptual system. The question of whether any model is right or wrong *for nursing*

is a social decision, and criteria extrinsic to the substance of the model must be utilized.

CRITERIA FOR EVALUATION

Three criteria may be helpful in evaluating models. The first is *social congruence*; that is, do nursing decisions and actions which are based on the model fulfill social expectations or might society be helped to develop such expectations? The last phrase here is included in full recognition that current nursing practice is not entirely what it might become and that society might come to expect a different form of practice, given the opportunity to experience it. The second is *social significance*; that is, do nursing decisions and actions based on the model lead to outcomes for patients which make an important difference in their lives or well-being? This criterion recognizes that a professional service is a highly valued one because it is critical to people in some way. The third criterion is concerned with the value of the model for the profession, its *social utility*; it asks whether the conceptual system on which the model is based is sufficiently well-developed to provide clear direction for nursing practice, education, and research.

The task for the nurse-scientist, practitioner, or educator who chooses the third alternative is to select one of the options now available or to develop another that will provide answers to such questions as: practice toward what goals? knowledge and skills for what purpose? theory about what? It is for the theory developer and postbaccalaureate educator that answers are most urgently needed, however, since both practitioners and basic service educators can continue to get along for a while, just doing what has always been done. The scientist in nursing has no past and she faces many difficulties in this old occupation, newly awakened to the need for a sound scientific basis for professional practice. Without the self-confidence and scientific respectability granted by parentage or ancient heritage, newcomers in the world of science—most often with research training not in their proposed field of study but in various other fields—our scientists, our founding parents, if you will, cannot share a common identity with one another, nor can they identify with nursing as a science. This in a time and in a world which does not look kindly, either professionally or scientifically, upon new founding parents, particularly if they are mothers, and illegitimate themselves, have questionable educational backgrounds, appear to share scientific interests loosely if at all, and seem to be encroaching on the boundaries of other disciplines. The best anchor for this group, as well as others in nursing, acting either individually or collectively, is self-conscious reflection, and decision about the purpose for which theoretical knowledge is intended. Only this will provide a rationale and open the door to a rational course in the development of theory.

The scientist in nursing also faces the exciting challenge of influencing nursing's direction and progress as a profession and a scientific discipline. Purposeful and goal-directed development of the theoretical knowledge of an emerging profession is a rare opportunity and one to be cherished all the more because of its unusual demands.

BIBLIOGRAPHY

Bijou, J. W., and Baer, D. M. *Child Development I: A Systematic and Empirical Theory.* New York, Appleton-Century-Crofts, 1961.

Bullough, Bonnie, and Bullough, Vern. *The Emergence of Modern Nursing.* New York, Macmillan Co., 1964.

Cogan, M. L. Towards the definition of a profession. *Harvard Educ Rev* 23 (1):33–50, 1953.

Dickoff, James, and James, Patricia. A theory of theories: A position paper. *Nurs Res* 17:197–203, May–June 1968.

Erikson, E. H. *Childhood and Society,* 2d ed. New York, W. W. Norton & Co., Inc., 1963.

Freud, S. *An Outline of Psychoanalysis.* New York, W. W. Norton & Co., Inc., 1949.

Gebbie, Kristine, and Lavin, M. A. Classifying nursing diagnoses. *Am J Nurs* 74:250–253, Feb. 1974.

Goode, W. J. Encroachment, charlatanism, and the emerging professions. *Am Sociol Rev* 25: 902–914, Dec. 1960.

Greenwood, Ernest. The practice of science and the science of practice. In *The Planning of Change,* ed. by W. G. Bennis and others. New York, Holt, Rinehart and Winston, 1961, pp. 73–82.

Howland, Daniel, and McDowell, W. E. Measurement of patient care: A conceptual framework. *Nurs Res* 13:4–7, Winter 1964.

Johnson, Dorothy, *One Conceptual Model of Nursing.* Lecture given at Vanderbilt University, 1968. (Unpublished)

Lum, J. L., and Kim, H. T. A faculty undertakes a major curriculum revision. *J Nurs Educ* 6:19–21, 24–25, Aug. 1967.

Maslow, A. H. *Motivation and Personality.* New York, Harper & Row, 1954.

McCain, Faye R. Nursing by assessment—not institution. *Am J Nurs* 65:82–84, Apr. 1965.

McDonald, F. J., and Harms, M. T. A theoretical model for an experimental curriculum. *Nurs Outlook* 14:48–51, Aug. 1966.

New, P. K. M. Another approach to professionalism. *Am J Nurs* 65:124–126, Feb. 1965.

Nightingale, Florence. *Notes on Nursing.* New York, Appleton and Co., 1860.

Orlando, I. J. *The Dynamic Nurse-Patient Relationship.* New York, G. P. Putnam's Sons, 1961.

Peplau, Hildegarde. *Interpersonal Relations in Nursing.* New York, G. P. Putnam's Sons, 1952.

Rogers, Carl. A theory of therapy, personality, and interpersonal relations as developed in a client-centered framework. In *Psychology: A Study of a Science,* ed. by J. Koch. New York, McGraw-Hill Book Co., 1959, vol. III.

Rogers, M. E. *An Introduction to the Theoretical Basis of Nursing.* Philadelphia, F. A. Davis Co., 1970.

Roy, Sr. Callista. Adaptation: A conceptual framework for nursing. *Nurs Outlook* 18:42–45, Mar. 1970.

Sullivan, Harry. *The Interpersonal Theory of Psychiatry.* New York, W. W. Norton & Co., Inc., 1953.

Vaillot, Sister M. C. Nursing theory, levels of nursing, and curriculum development. *Nurs Forum* 9(3):234–249, 1970.

White, Lynn. Humanism and the education of engineers. In *Studies of Courses and Sequences in Humanities, Fine Arts, and Social Sciences for Engineering Students.* (EDP Report No. 7-63) Los Angeles, Humanities Sub-Committee,

Education Development Program, College of Education, 1963.

Wiedenbach, Ernestine. *Clinical Nursing: A Helping Art.* New York, Springer Publishing Co., 1964.

EDITOR'S QUESTIONS FOR DISCUSSION

What is meant by a conceptual model? Are there specific types that might be used for investigating different nursing problems? What is the difference between inductive and deductive reasoning in theory development? Is there one method of theory development that might be more applicable to nursing than another? How might nursing theory be helpful in nursing practice? How might a meaningful dialogue be established between the nurse scientist and the nurse practitioner for the purpose of formulating a rationale for the development of theory?

Chapter 20

Theory Development:
A Challenge for Nursing

Edna M. Menke, R.N., Ph.D.
Assistant Professor, School of Nursing
Ohio State University, Columbus

Edna M. Menke answers many of the questions raised previously about the development of nursing theory. The issues she considers are the importance of theory development, the present status of theory development, and strategies to facilitate theory development. Theory may be considered as a conceptual framework for deriving, accounting for, and explaining relationships in nursing practice that can be used to predict outcomes in patient care. Menke discusses four levels of theories: factor-isolating, factor-relating, situation-relating, and situation-producing. She emphasizes the importance of lower-level theory development as a sound basis for theory development for nursing and proposes consideration of theories *about* nursing rather than *of* nursing. She points out that the lack of theory development may have been caused by the lack of systematic direction and collaboration among theory developers. Menke emphasizes the need for an eclectic approach to methods of theory development.

Nursing as a discipline is in the evolutionary process of becoming a science. Nursing can only become a science if nurses develop a highly organized and specialized field of knowledge and concomitantly continue to be seekers of knowledge. The body of knowledge required is theories about nursing. In the past decade many nursing scholars have discussed theory development in nursing. (1-6) The discussions have focused on why nursing does not have many theories, strategies for the development of theories, and the factors hindering theory development. However, theory development in nursing has progressed slowly. Theory development must become the responsibility of nurses in all areas of nursing—practitioners, educators, administrators, and researchers. The purpose of this paper is to deal with several issues related to theory development in nursing. The issues that will be considered are the importance of theory development, the present status of theory development, and strategies to facilitate theory development in nursing.

THE IMPORTANCE OF THEORY DEVELOPMENT

Theory development is important for any discipline because it prescribes the conceptual framework for describing, explaining, and predicting phenomena.(7) Theory serves as a means to isolate and classify facts and points to gaps in the available knowledge. Theories embody propositions, principles, syntactical structure, and theoretical constructs that are not completely interpretable through observation. Theories vary in their preciseness in describing, explaining, and/or predicting phenomena. However, all theories attempt to be systems of inference for deriving confirmable hypotheses.(8) Theory can never be known to be entirely true.(9) Hempel contends that it is of paramount importance for science to develop a system of concepts that is suited to the formulation of general exploratory and predictive principles. Likewise, he stresses the importance of operationalism in theory development.(10) Bronowski compared the development of theory to the unraveling of a coded puzzle.(11) Thus, theory may be considered as a conceptual framework for deriving, accounting for, and explaining relationships of constructs that can be used to predict outcomes in a specialized system.

Jacox has delineated three stages in the development of a theory. The first stage is a period of specifying, defining, and classifying the concepts used to describe the phenomena of the field. A *concept* is an abstraction of the empirical world that can only be indirectly observed. In the first stage of theory development the parameters of each concept must be established. The second stage consists of developing statements that propose how two or more concepts are related. The last stage is that of specifying how all of the propositions are related to each other in a systematic way.(12) Each stage in theory development should be tested through research. Research lends support to the theory or assists in the identification of how the theory needs to be modified to accord with the phenomena in the empirical world.

Dickoff and James describe theory as a conceptual system or framework invented for some specific purpose. Dickoff and James say:

A theory is a set of elements in interrelation. All elements of a theory are at the conceptual level, but theories vary according to the number of elements, the characteristic kind and complexity of the elements, and the kind of relation holding between or among the theory's

elements of ingredients. The factor (or concept) is the simplest element; a proposition or law is a certain relation among concepts. Theory at one level might be a coordinate set of factors or a coordinate set of propositions. But theory at its highest level has elements that differ from one another in level of complexity and even some elements that contain whole theories as elements. (13)

Also, Dickoff and James identify four levels of theories. The levels are factor-isolating, factor-relating, situation-relating, and situation-producing. *Factor-isolating* is the lowest level of theory and focuses on identifying pertinent factors or concepts in a situation. *Factor-relating* consists of determining relationships between the factors. *Situation-relating* theory involves predicting what will occur in the situation and assumes a causal relationship exists between the factors. *Situation-producing* theory, which is the highest level, is prescriptive in that it tells how to alter aspects of a situation in order to have a specified outcome. (14) Dickoff and James contend that nursing should develop situation-producing theory.

Dickoff and James are idealistic when they propose that nursing develop situation-producing theory. It is more realistic for nursing to concentrate on developing lower-level theories initially and then use these as a base to develop situation-producing theories. The purpose of lower-level theories should be to obtain knowledge about the phenomena rather than to try to determine how the knowledge can be used in nursing practice. At present the majority of theory development in nursing has been either factor-isolating or factor-relating. Empirical relationships need to be shown that can withstand the rigors of scientific inquiry before it is possible to attempt conceptualization of desired situations and how they may be achieved. Trying initially to develop situation-producing theory may lead to hastily developing lower-level theories without subjecting the theories to rigorous testing. This would be disastrous as the lower-level theories serve as the basis for more sophisticated theories. Situation-producing theory should be the long-range objective for any theory developed for nursing. It would serve as a means to assure only the development of theory that has utility for the practice of nursing.

Nursing may have more difficulty in developing theory because it is an applied discipline operating in a complex situation of organism-environment interactions that may be unpredictable; however, the behavioral sciences have similar situations and it has not stopped them from developing theories. Other models of theory development need to be used rather than only the models of the basic or natural sciences. The basic science models have a tendency to reduce the phenomena to a point that is not always useful to the discipline of nursing.

The theories that are developed must be considered theories *about* nursing. This may be questionable to some nurses who think nursing theory or theory *of* nursing is more appropriate. In the literature different theories of nursing have been proposed, such as those of Rogers, King, and Johnson, but none of them have achieved enough consensus to be considered *the* theory of nursing. (15-17) From a meta-theorist perspective each of these theories has shortcomings. No discipline has a grand theory but has many theories pertaining to the particular discipline. Nursing should not be searching for *the* theory of nursing but should be developing many theories that can be tested and used in the empirical world.

STATUS OF THEORY DEVELOPMENT

Thus far there has been a dearth of theory developed for nursing. Efforts have not been organized in any specific manner. The theory that has been developed has followed a laissez-faire route or has not necessarily been focused in any specific direction. This lack of theory might be attributed to the fact that nursing is a discipline without a scientific heritage.(18) However, nursing is evolving as a scientific discipline and is developing a community of scholars. Schlotfeldt states that "increasingly, nurses are being recognized as members of the scientific community; more significantly for the

development and enhancement of nursing's commitment to scholarship, some nurses are identifying themselves and their nurse colleagues as members of that community."(19) When one considers the total number of registered nurses, however, relatively few are involved in theory development.

Evidence of the insufficiency of theory development for nursing can be inferred from the literature. *Nursing Research* has been published only since 1952; a review of the journal reveals the lack of theory development, especially in the early years. It has only been within the last decade that many of the reported research studies have theoretical frameworks and provide evidence of testing concepts or theories. Simmons and Henderson's study, which provided a review and assessment of research in the areas of occupational orientation and nursing care up to 1955, showed that research concerning nursing administration and nursing education exceeded the study of nursing practice. Simmons and Henderson contended that research applied to practice is an essential link between discoveries of pure science and their successful utilization.(20) In 1956, Henderson reported that research studies about the nurse outnumbered studies on nursing practice ten to one. Less than 15 percent of doctoral dissertations dealt with nursing care.(21) In 1958, Fry reported that nurses were more interested in studying nurses rather than nursing care.(22) In 1959, Sheldon, Johnson, and Slusher described nursing research as being undeveloped and lacking theoretical orientation. They stated: "At present nursing research may be characterized generally by some broad erudition, little theoretical sensitivity, and the beginnings or even an adolescence—of meticulous attention to empirical detail."(23) In 1960, Schlotfeldt expressed the opinion that the primary task of nursing research was to develop theories that would serve as guides to nursing practice. Schlotfeldt stated that:

To date, a comprehensive body of nursing knowledge has not been amassed through scientific inquiry; instead, nursing continues to rely primarily upon the cumulative experiences of its practitioners and to make assumptions concerning the efficacy of its practices without subjecting them to scientific test.(24)

Schlotfeldt speculated that the lack of group attitudes toward nursing research might be attributed to the recent nature of scientific inquiry in nursing.

In 1962, Heidgerken presented a critical review of nursing literature published from 1860 to 1962. Her purpose was to assess the status of nursing knowledge and its relation to research. Her conclusions were that research in nursing was not yet scientific and that nursing knowledge was not yet cumulative and structured. Heidgerken found that most of the studies in nursing were problem-oriented rather than knowledge-oriented; were fact-finding and descriptive rather than experimental and/or predictive; were limited in their application of the scientific method; seemed to be isolated studies unrelated to other studies; and seldom dealt with nursing practice.(25) Heidgerken's findings reflect the lack of organization and orientation toward theory development in nursing. Nearly 15 years later the same laissez-faire trend in theory development continues.

In 1964, Brown assessed the progress of theory development in nursing. Again it was shown that nursing was lacking in theory. Brown pointed out that nurse-researchers had been urged to focus their studies on concept validation and theory testing, but there had been few instances in which the relationship of a study to theory had been made explicit. Concept formulation and validation can be considered an early phase of theory development. Brown contended that certain criteria must be utilized in the analysis and criticism of research studies if they are going to contribute to theory development. The criteria Brown offered were that the study should make explicit its relationship to theory, have as an aim the pursuit of knowledge for its own sake, use terms that have established meanings, show the association of its findings to the work of others, show logical but creative exposition of implications, and present hypotheses for further testing.(26)

Nursing has thus far relied heavily on other disciplines for its theory development. Most of nursing's early studies have been done primarily by other disciplines. In fact, some may think there is a great deal of theory for nursing since we are using theories that have been developed in related disciplines, such as the behavioral and natural sciences. However, the theories have often been taken out of their original context without testing them in the new context of nursing. There are not any definite criteria to use in deciding whether or not to adopt a theory from another discipline. At present this decision rests primarily with the nurse's personal judgments and preferences. It means that the nurse must be knowledgable about the other disciplines and consult with scholars in these disciplines before deciding if a theory might be applicable to nursing. Conant has expressed the need for caution in borrowing theory. She states:

> We, as nurses, are the people who should determine the value and specify the use of this borrowed knowledge for nursing practice. Too often in nursing we have sought somewhat blindly to obtain knowledge from other disciplines, without realizing the potentially valuable contribution that nursing can make to the general knowledge of human behavior.(27)

Within the past decade nursing has shown the most progress in theory development. Universities have had conferences and workshops on theory development, for example, University of Kansas Medical Center Department of Nursing, New York University Division of Nursing, Frances Payne Bolton School of Nursing at Case Western Reserve University, and The University of Colorado School of Nursing. The book *Concept Formalization in Nursing Process and Product* was written by a group of nurses at Catholic University.(28) Articles pertaining to theory development have appeared in the majority of nursing journals. An article that should be mentioned is Walker's "Toward a Clearer Understanding of the Concept of Nursing Theory."(29) Walker's article stimulated other scholars to react to her beliefs regarding theory development. Her article and the reactions to it represent a growth within the disciplines of nursing. Similar articles need to become more a part of nursing.

Nursing has evolved to a new stage in its theory development. Folta describes the present stage in the following way:

> Nursing is at a new stage of development. While recognizing clinical practice as its stated reason for being, nursing has generally accepted research as an integral aspect of its professional development. This acceptance while not without its own problems, has led the profession to a new degree of sophistication and prestige. Most research has been of the theory-testing nature with little concern from whence came the theories. Now nursing appears ready to move to the stage of developing its own theories and consequently the issue of nursing theory is of increasing importance in today's scene. Perhaps a degree of security within the profession in its ability to conduct its own research is a factor moving nursing in the direction of positing the development of nursing theory as a value which is seen as both necessary and desirable. The pinnacle of scientific disciplines is the development of theory and nursing is moving toward this pinnacle.(30)

STRATEGIES TO FACILITATE THEORY DEVELOPMENT

Theory development in nursing must become more organized. No longer can nursing afford to follow a laissez-faire direction in theory development. If nursing is going to evolve into a scientific discipline, theory development must have a systematic direction. The direction must evolve around concepts that have utility for nursing. Some concepts that might be used include health, coping, stress, adaptation, man, family, groups, systems, and community. Theories can be developed from the concepts. It is critical that the theories be developed and/or tested via research.

The theories that are initially developed should be factor-isolating and factor-relating. These theories would describe and explain the phenomena. Later, situation-relating theories could be developed in laboratories and/or simulated environments. The situation-producing theories would be the last kind of theories developed since they are the highest level.

The academic community should assume a leadership position in theory development as the majority of theory developers are housed in university settings. The theory developers are a hybrid group in terms of their educational backgrounds since doctorally-prepared nurses have attained their degrees primarily in higher education, the behavioral sciences, or nurse-scientist programs. As a result, each individual's approach to theory development reflects the discipline(s) in which she studied. Unfortunately, some of the doctorally-prepared nurses do not have the knowledge or desire to develop theory. Theory developers within a university must learn to collaborate with each other rather than everyone having a separate territory. Likewise, there needs to be collaboration between theory developers in different universities. Graduate programs in nursing should emphasize philosophy of science, theory development, and inquiry in their curricula. Early in their graduate study students should learn to value the search for knowledge and should master the tools necessary for theory development. Students must be encouraged to focus their graduate studies on specific concepts that can serve as the basis for clinical papers, master's theses, and doctoral dissertations, and these in turn would be sources for theory development. The papers should be shared with other students and theory developers via publications and/or presentations.

The individuals who graduate from master's and doctoral programs must continue to develop and test theories. These individuals are the potential cadre for the systematic direction of theory development. If they continue to work with the concepts and theories studied in graduate programs, a great deal could be done to advance the development of nursing theory. Likewise, these nurses would have the knowledge necessary to develop new concepts and theories. Until this state becomes an outcome of graduate education in nursing, nursing will continue to have a low productivity of theory.

An organized community of scholars in nursing should be developed. This group would consist of nurses from all areas of practice who are working on theory development. The community would serve as a "think tank" for theory development and meta-theory discussions. The groups would be responsible for developing strategies to get tested theory into the practice of nursing. This community would be another means for systematic direction in theory development.

An eclectic approach should be taken to theory development. No one approach is *the* way for theory development. As long as the theory developer can justify the approach, it has a place in theory development. Probably nurses will take two main approaches—developing theory within nursing and borrowing theory from other disciplines. Nursing needs to be open-minded in trying various approaches; but concomitantly, nursing needs to use scientific inquiry before accepting a theory. Theory can only evolve when nurses are willing to describe, explain, and make predictions about the phenomena in their practice. At present theory development is a challenge for nursing. Nursing has the potential to meet the challenge.

NOTES

1 Rosemary Ellis, "Characteristics of Significant Theories," *Nursing Research,* **17**:217–222, May–June 1968.
2 Margaret E. Hardy, "Theories: Components, Development, Evaluation," *Nursing Research*, **18**:100–107, March–April 1974.
3 Dorothy E. Johnson, "Development of Theory: A Requisite for Nursing as a Primary Health Profession," *Nursing Research,* **18**:372–377, September–October 1974.

4 Ada Jacox, "Theory Construction in Nursing: An Overview," *Nursing Research*, **23**:4–13, January–February 1974.
5 Rozella M. Schlotfeldt, "Research in Nursing and Research Training for Nurses: Retrospect and Prospect," *Nursing Research,* **24**:177–183, May–June 1975.
6 Lorraine Olszewski Walker, "Toward a Clearer Understanding of the Concept of Nursing Theory," *Nursing Research,* **20**:428–435, September–October 1971.
7 Carl G. Hempel, "Fundamentals of Concept Formation in Empirical Science," in Otto Neurath (ed.), *International Encyclopedia of Unified Science,* Foundation of the Unity of Science, vol. 2, no. 7, pp. 32–50, University of Chicago Press, Chicago, 1952.
8 Merle B. Turner, *Philosophy and the Science of Behavior*, Appleton-Century-Crofts, New York, 1967.
9 John G. Kemeny, *A Philosopher Looks at Science*, Van Nostrand, Princeton, N.J., 1959.
10 Hempel, op. cit.
11 Jacob Bronowski, "Science as Foresight," in James R. Newman (ed.), *What Is Science?* Simon and Shuster, New York, 1955.
12 Jacox, op. cit.
13 James Dickoff and Patricia James, "A Theory of Theories: A Position Paper," *Nursing Research*, **17**:198, May–June 1968.
14 Ibid., pp. 197–203.
15 Martha E. Rogers, *An Introduction to the Theoretical Basis of Nursing*, Davis, Philadelphia, 1970.
16 Imogene M. King, *Toward a Theory of Nursing*, Wiley, New York, 1971.
17 Dorothy Johnson, "A Philosophy of Nursing," *Nursing Outlook,* **7**:198–200, 1959.
18 Dorothy Johnson, "Development of Theory: A Requisite for Nursing as a Primary Health Profession," *Nursing Outlook,* **7**:373, 1959.
19 Schlotfeldt, op. cit., p. 178.
20 Leo W. Simmons and Virginia Henderson, *Nursing Research: A Survey and Assessment*, Appleton-Century-Crofts, New York, 1964.
21 Virginia A. Henderson, "Research in Nursing Practice—When?" *Nursing Research,* **4**:99, February 1956.

22 Vera Fry, "A Conference on Research in Nursing," *Nursing Research*, 7:52–56, June 1968.
23 Eleanor B. Sheldon, Dorothy E. Johnson, and
Margaret Slusher, "An Experimental Program in
Nursing Research," *Nursing Research,* 8:169,
Summer 1959.
24 Rozella A. Schlotfeldt, "Reflections on Nursing Research," *American Journal of Nursing*,
60:493, April 1960.
25 Loretta E. Heidgerken, "Nursing Research—Its
Role in Research Activities in Nursing," *Nursing Research*, 11:140–143, Summer 1962.
26 Myrtle Irene Brown, "Research in the Development of Nursing Theory," *Nursing Research*,
13:109–112, Spring 1964.
27 Lucy H. Conant, "A Search for Resolution of
Existing Problems in Nursing," *Nursing Research,* 16:115, Spring 1967.
28 The Nursing Development Conference Group,
*Concept Formalization in Nursing Process and
Product*, Little, Brown, Boston, 1973.
29 Walker, op. cit.
30 Jeannette R. Folta, "Obfuscation of Clarification: A Reaction to Walker's Concept of Nursing Theory," *Nursing Research,* 20:496,
November–December 1971.

EDITOR'S QUESTIONS FOR DISCUSSION

Why can nursing become a science only through theory development? What potential
does nursing have for becoming a science? Why should or should not nursing be defined as a science? What examples exist (or might be proposed) of factor-isolating and
factor-relating theories in nursing? What might be the next step in developing those
examples into situation-relating and situation-producing theories?

Chapter 21

Theory Development in Nursing

John F. Klein, S.M., R.N., Ph.D.
Associate Professor and Chairperson, Department of Sociology
John Carroll University, Cleveland, Ohio

John F. Klein clarifies some of the confusion surrounding theory development and its relationship to nursing. In an attempt to define the domains of nursing, he differentiates theory *of* nursing and theory *in* nursing, and suggests three possible sources for theory *in* nursing: drawing directly from many disciplines ("alphabet soup" theory), coming totally from within the activity scope of nursing as a closed system, and adapting theory from other disciplines to the nursing situation. Klein is more inclined to view the present development of theory *in* nursing as being *about* nursing, which results in "nursing practice theory." Thus, Klein appears to agree with Menke on the necessity for theory *about* nursing but he stresses the borrowing of theory from other disciplines and elevates the phrase "theory in nursing" to that of "nursing practice theory."

Klein explores some of the issues and problems of theory development and its implementation in nursing practice. He points to the failure of our basic educational programs to introduce the theoretical concepts of the traditional sciences as a limiting factor in the development of nursing practice theory. Another problem in nursing is the infrequent blending of adequate educational preparation and contact with clinical practice. A third problem is the lack of consensus concerning what constitutes the domain of nursing. Klein raises the question, "What benefit is theory to the patient?" He states that nursing can and should reciprocate and make a contribution in return to the basic sciences. Klein acknowledges that there has been greater sophistication in defining nursing and more discussion about nursing theory development but he concludes that nursing, as a profession, is just beginning.

The purpose of this chapter is to review the discussion that has taken place in regard to theory development and the practice of nursing, highlighting possible problems and issues that exist in nursing and their relationship to theory development. The past ten years have witnessed an increased activity directed to the nature of nursing theory, its use and misuse and many ensuing questions. The linkage between theory and research activity in nursing has been indicated (Meyer and Heidgerken, 1962, p. 248; Gortner, 1975, pp. 194) as well as in the established scien-

I am indebted to Margaret McDermott, R.N., M.S.N. and to Janice Noack, R.N., Ph.D. for prior discussion concerning many ideas disucssed in this article.

tific disciplines (Black, 1946, pp. 362-363; Merton, 1957, pp. 85-117). While this linkage between theory and research will be reinforced later in this chapter, a kind of analytical separation will be made between the two for the purposes of this section. This separation will hopefully permit a sharper focus on the theory development component in nursing for the purpose of strengthening its claim to a scientific and professional basis. Research activity in nursing is discussed elsewhere in the book (see Part 3).

DEFINITIONS OF THEORY

For many of us raised on the "classical" definition of theory, a heading indicating that there is more than one definition of theory may be strange at best and repugnant at worst. The rote definition of theory that for many has been associated with the established scientific enterprises is something like the following: *a logically interrelated set of statements with the power to explain and predict a facet of the real world.* Such an abbreviated definition of theory seems to capture the essence of the typical philosophy of science approach espoused by Northrop (1947), Nagel (1961), Kaplan (1964), and Rudner (1966). The use of such an approach in the nursing literature is briefly reviewed by Hardy (1974); she implies that the use of the classical approach should be sanctioned for nursing as it struggles with theory development in its research activity.

A variation of this classical approach to theory and its development is offered by Dickoff and James (1968) and Dickoff, James, and Wiedenbach (1968 a, b) as they forge beyond the strict interpretation of the classical approach to theory development. Their elaboration of theory development or, as they call it, "a theory of theories," provides special promise, at the generic level, for applied areas of human service and the professions.

The work of Dickoff and James (1968, pp. 420-422) divides theories into four levels: factor-isolating theories, factor-relating theories, situa-

tion-relating theories, and situation-producing theories. *Factor-isolating* is the process by which "conceptual unities" (ideas) invented or created by the mind are named (Dickoff and James, 1968, p. 421). "The kind of naming most often recognized as theoretical activity is called classifying" (1968, p. 420). To classify is to sort or to categorize in terms of belonging to one thing as opposed to another, and identify the subsets of each thing. For example, protozoa is a significant thing or factor biologically and ciliata are a subfactor (1968, p. 420).

Factor-relating is the process of "seeing things not in isolation but rather in relation" (Dickoff and James, 1968, p. 421). Factor-relating theories depict conceptions of interrelations or correlations among factors. An example of a theory at this level is anatomy (1968, p. 421).

Situation-relating theories state relationships between such situations as are depictable. This theory deals with either a prediction such as, "situation A causes situation B" or with what promotes or inhibits the relationship between A and B (Dickoff and James, 1968, p. 421). *Situation-producting* theories allow for the production of situations of a desired kind (1968, p. 421). This theory says "B is among the things conceived as appropriate to bring into being and so here is how to bring about A" (1968, p. 421). Each higher level of theory presupposes the existence of theories developed from the previous level (1968, p. 420).

Despite the painstaking clarity of Dickoff and James and their later collaboration with Wiedenbach, and the relative popularity of the classical philosophy of science approach to theory development, some confusion surrounds theory and its meaning for nursing.

Before discussing this confusion and its relationship to nursing, it would seem appropriate to explicate some basic assumptions upon which the discussions are based. First, it is assumed that nursing is a profession, with "profession" used in a classical sense. Second, it is assumed that some criteria are necessary by which to judge what occupational areas of nursing are professional. Specific criteria of what constitutes a profession will not be discussed to any extent, nor the degree to which nursing fits, approximates, or approaches such criteria. Third, it is assumed that the standard criteria of a profession include as one of their basic features the existence of a "body of theoretical knowledge that is dynamic" (Bixler and Bixler, 1945, p. 733; Pavalko, 1971, p. 18). It would appear that nursing's concern about theory and its development stems from this criterion.

THE PROBLEM OF THE PREPOSITION

Ellis (1968) has characterized the confusion surrounding theory and nursing as arising from the "stated or implied preposition used to connect the word theory, or the term theory development, to the word nursing." At the risk of oversimplification, it might be said that two common ways of connecting the word theory with that of nursing are: theory *of* nursing and theory *in* nursing. It appears that the phrase "theory *of* nursing" is an attempt to define and delineate the territorial boundaries of nursing, separating it from allied health/illness-related areas, so that the unique scope of nursing can be seen.

Such efforts to define the scope of nursing are seen in the works of King (1971), who proposes four universal ideas—social systems, health, perception, and interpersonal relations—and explores their relevance to nursing. Rogers states that nursing theory should "represent that unit of theoretical knowledge which differentiates nursing from other professional disciplines" (1961, p. 26). The work of Orem (1971) was directed toward identifying significant concepts in nursing for the purpose of providing general guides for use in "finding solutions to complex health care problems which individual nurses and patients are expected to solve within a system of daily living" (p. vii). The Nursing Development Conference Group (1973, pp. 67-68) was motivated by "its search of the order in nursing and from effort to work with a specific general concept of nursing and, therefore, to consider nursing in its broadest dimensions." These three works are examples of the efforts to identify relevant and specific concepts, which are usually indicative of action-orientation, in order to circumscribe the territorial boundaries of the professional area of nursing. This is an extremely important contribution to nursing itself and to theory building as well, but it neither represents the whole of theory building nor its final stages.

Those who connect the word "theory" with the word "nursing," by using the word "in," frequently take one of three positions. The first position would be that since nursing represents something of an applied science, it is dependent upon the traditional sciences, wholly and with little or no qualification, for both its direction and theoretical statements for specific action. Nursing theory derived from this position consists of various pieces pulled in from the social/behavioral sciences and the biological/physical sciences. The problems ensuing from this approach have been faced by the profession of social work (Boehm, 1959, pp. 96-101). If any profession were to be given directional activity from such a theoretical orientation, it would consist of one part biology, one part sociology, one part chemistry, one part psychology, and so on. This approach would seem to establish an "alphabet soup" theory basis for nursing at best, and a schizophrenic foundation for it at worst.

A second version of the theory-*in*-nursing conceptualization is that the development of theory would come wholly and entirely from within the activity scope of nursing. This position would basically deny any kind of contribution from external sources, such as the traditional scientific areas, and would probably be directed especially to the behavioral activity of nursing as it performs specified duties. This version has a great deal of pragmatism associated with its theory formulation—if it has worked often enough, it predicts. The explanation of the situation may be deemed irrelevant or unimportant, for the functional nature of the statements speak for themselves. Basically, this version denies that nursing is part of a larger reality that has been studied by established scientific disciplines which have something worthwhile to offer, and that nursing has traditionally assumed a technological basis for at least some of its activity from the biological/natural sciences. This approach is analogous to a rediscovery of the wheel, or at least part of it.

The third version of the theory-*in*-nursing conceptualization, which seems to have popularity, is that nursing theory consists of theories from various established scientific disciplines, that are selectively brought in to the nursing area. These theories then undergo some kind of transformation process as when they are adapted to the nursing situation. The work of Johnson (1974) suggests this, and the work of Dickoff, James, and Wiedenbach (1968a, b) has sketched it at the generic level. Wooldridge and his associates (1968) forcefully demonstrate such a relationship between nursing and sociology.

These works presume that nursing theory is dependent upon the development of theory in the traditional sciences. These developments are then transformed and incorporated into the nursing situation. The transformation process in significant part is based upon "the accurate prediction of the effects" of utilizing the theory for nursing practice (Wooldridge et al., 1968, p. 24). Thus, this method of utilizing theory in nursing results in capitalizing upon the theory developed from the traditional sciences. The theory is then further developed in nursing practice as it is directed to a body of clients seeking/needing nursing activity.

It should be pointed out, however, that this third position, which seems to be a favored one by many within the ranks of nursing, is dependent upon the definitional scope of nursing.

Thus, the so-called works and efforts directed at theory *about* nursing or the attempt to answer the question, "What is nursing?" is presupposed to be a basis for selectively choosing and adapting the concepts and theoretical statements that may help predict the outcome of nursing actions on the patient. It would seem, then, that the current status of the word "theory" as it is associated with nursing, has received sufficient support to elevate the phrase "theory in nursing"

to that of "nursing practice theory." The selection of concepts from the various sciences is guided by some kind of definitional scope of what nursing is and what its objectives are or should be. The "borrowed" theory and the "developed" practice theory can then adequately predict the accomplishment of stated nursing goals by stated means. However, lest the reader believe that the interpretation of nursing practice theory has been finalized see Walker's (1971) conceptualization of nursing theory, and the Commentary (1971) on it and also Walker's (1972) rejoinder.

The need for research, or the empirical verification of the utility of such formulated practice theory, has been referred to previously and should be self-evident. Empirical verification is necessary not only to validate the theoretical formulations, but also to specify the variations of the theoretical formulations and to expand the formulations in light of further developments in the basic sciences, the changes that take place within the health/illness setting, and the changes associated with the clientele toward which nursing directs its attention.

ISSUES AND PROBLEMS

The continuing discussion among nurses about the nature of theory development and its implementation into nursing practice is an activity that is potentially issue-laden and problem-producing within the profession of nursing. Attention will now be directed to a number of such problems, real and potential, since they are associated with the implications stemming from theory development and the nursing profession.

The Problem of Nursing Education

Two dimensions associated with the preparation of nursing practitioners have been perennial problems within the profession itself and are of significant importance to the development of nursing practice theory. The first dimension concerns the varied nature of the structure of nursing education. The current state of first-level nursing education features three competing structural arrangements for the preparation of the beginning practitioner—diploma programs, associate degree programs, and baccalaureate programs. While the American Nurses Association's position paper of 1965 recommended that "minimum preparation for beginning professional nursing practice at the present time should be baccalaureate degree education in nursing" (1965, p. 6), a distinction was made between professional nursing practice and technical nursing practice. Such a distinction may have precipitated more confusion than clarity within the nursing ranks. Additionally, of the 1,373 state-approved schools of nursing in 1973, 35.9 percent were diploma schools, 41.8 percent were associate degree schools, and only 22.2 percent were baccalaureate schools (*Source Book*, 1975). While the attempt is made to differentiate "technical" from "professional" nursing practice, a qualified practitioner emerges from some program that is *below* the graduate level of preparation. Although nursing is not unique in this regard among the professions, it neither helps improve its professional standing vis-à-vis other professions, nor helps to prepare broad-based practitioners equipped with sensitive analytical skills. Analytical skills are necessary at the basic level of nursing practice since it is at the practice level that theory needs to be developed and implemented.

The second dimension of the preparation of nursing practitioners that presents some problems is the traditional emphasis that nursing has placed upon the acquisition of technical skills, not only in the biological/natural sciences, but also in the social/behavioral sciences. This pragmatic tradition has not fostered among any significant cadre of practitioners a needed depth in the various traditional sciences. Superficial and pragmatic knowledge has not provided the in-depth background, even in one or a few selected traditional scientific areas, that is necessary to selectively relate theoretical developments in the traditional sciences to nursing practice for the development of nursing practice theory. In a sense, we might say that the

rank-and-file nurse is limited in her knowledge of those areas outside of nursing technology that foster exploration outside of nursing for relevant concepts and propositions that might be used in nursing in order to develop nursing practice theory. The scarcity of cosmopolitan, well-prepared nurses with a sufficient background to travel between the traditional scientific areas and nursing practice has contributed to the following issue/problem.

Elitism in Nursing

From the preceding there might appear to be a kind of elite group of nurses, located especially within the walls of academe, who have a broad enough education and background to travel between nursing practice and various scientific areas, allow for this intellectual exploration of pertinent material in order to develop nursing practice theory. Yet, this number is small and their relationship to rank-and-file nursing personnel is ambiguous at best and tension-laden at worst. In 1973 the American Nurses' Foundation could list only 1,019 nurses with earned doctoral degrees—a number that included 55 persons listed as living outside of the United States, in addition to an unknown number of deceased and retired nurses. Even if this number were to double by 1977, which is unlikely, it would represent such an infinitesimal number of the close to one million nurses throughout the United States as to be insignificant. Furthermore, in 1974 only 28,000, or 3.3 percent, of the 857,000 actively practicing RNs possessed graduate degrees of any kind.

This point is emphasized, since it is reasonable to expect that some of the more significant developments in nursing would come from such a well-trained and graduate-educated group. Yet, the number of these nurses is not only minuscule, but a closer examination of the situation would show that a certain number of such people are not involved in clinical practice or have only marginally been so involved for some time. It should be pointed out that full recognition is given to the fact that nurses prepared below the doctoral level and even the graduate level are, in many cases, more than adequately able to make significant contributions to nursing and especially to the development of nursing practice theory. However, the academically prepared elite and the academically placed elite are those in most contact with the supporting scientific disciplines; yet they may be removed from clinical practice, or place lower priority on it. Conversely, the nonacademically prepared nursing group and those located in nonacademic settings may reverse the priority for the sake of meeting the exigencies of everyday nursing practice. Not to be overlooked is the directive given by Dickoff and James (1968, p. 199) in which they indicate that the clinical area is especially fruitful for the preliminary stages of the development of nursing practice theory. Yet, this necessary blend of adequate educational preparation and contact with clinical practice is most probably limited to very few nurses.

The Problem of Consensus

Closely associated with the above-mentioned problems is the lack of consensus among both rank-and-file nursing and the academic elite about what constitutes the domain of nursing. We have already mentioned the problem of definition that nursing continues to face—the problem of how nursing shall be defined. Such differential answers cut across any lines of categorization of nursing personnel. Regardless of educational preparation, or even chosen specialty within nursing, a demonstrated lack of agreement concerning the definitional scope of nursing persists. Furthermore, even those nurses with preparation in one or more of the traditional sciences, and even those within the same science, cannot agree on the nature or content of a particular scientific area's theory to be articulated within the practice of nursing. This general lack of consensus in relationship to so many vital questions may not be all that startling when we consider the dramatic developments within nursing over the last 2 or 3 decades. Given these changes and the corresponding changes that

have taken place within the health field since World War II, we might even be so bold as to say that nursing as an academic discipline is only about 30 years old, or perhaps has only just come into its adult stage of development. In this sense, then, nursing as a young and rather immature profession can expect only the most rudimentary form of consensus about such important questions as those we have mentioned. No advancement toward further consensus may be obtained until nursing has both adjusted to its adult stage and become familiar enough with its present location within the health care disciplines to communicate both within its own ranks and with those disciplines and professions with which it is so closely associated. Nonetheless, in the here and now, this lack of consensus on so many fundamental issues is a barrier to the efforts directed to theory development for the practice of nursing.

The Problem of Client Payoff

Lest we neglect a most significant dimension of nursing, attention should be directed to the recipient of a good deal of nursing activity. While it should be emphasized that not all nursing activity is directly associated with human beings/clients, as Dickoff, James, and Wiedenbach (1968a, p. 425) have pointed out, some definitional body of clients is of prime importance to a good deal of nursing activity, either directly or indirectly. While the development of nursing practice theory is directly applicable when evaluating the *means* or activity used to achieve nursing practice goals, the question can be raised as to how, when, and where the patient benefits from such an expenditure of energy. If both nursing practice theory and the empirical verification of such theory are either overtly or even covertly left to the nursing elite previously discussed, or to some other group, it is questionabale whether theory development and research verification can take place at the rank-and-file level. What is being stressed here is not only the time factor delay—it takes time to formulate theory and verify it empirically—but also the additional dimension of implementation and the potential loss that can occur from the filtering-down process. Thus, a kind of cultural lag is possible; that is, the ideational and practice content among a nursing elite in some way can be distorted or diminished as it trickles down, over time, to the common nursing situation on a day-to-day basis. Attempts to avoid such lags and distortions should be carefully considered by means of the publishing mechanisms available to nursing personnel and, perhaps most importantly, through the nursing education process itself, both at the beginning level and at the ongoing staff development and continuing education level.

Returning the Gift

A final issue to be discussed is the debt that nursing owes to the basic sciences and how it might repay that debt in kind. Emphasis has been given to the real and potential contribution of theoretical material from the various basic sciences to the development of nursing practice theory. Indeed, a good deal of the traditional and commonly accepted kinds of nursing activity have come from the domain of the established sciences. As nursing continues to elaborate on such knowledge and expend energy in the search for relevant theoretical building materials (some of which will certainly continue to come from the basic sciences) consideration should be given to the contribution that nursing might and possibly should make in return.

The case for such reciprocity becomes all the more obvious if attention is given to the nurse-scientist program. While the number of nurse-scientists educated in the basic disciplines may be small compared to all nurses who receive graduate education, and even smaller compared to the total number of nurses, the case may still stand that nursing owes some kind of intellectual debt to the basic sciences. There has been some, although minor, criticism expressed in certain quarters of the basic sciences to the effect that the time and energy expended on educating nurse-scientists in a basic discipline is wasted. From the discipline's viewpoint, it is profitless if, upon completion of a program, the nurse-scientist returns to nursing

with a minimal commitment to contribute to the basic scientific discipline which provided the intellectual basis for the attainment of the doctoral degree.

An additional argument for reciprocity is the long-standing tradition of many scientific inputs, to say nothing of the professional contributions, that have been made to nursing education over the decades by individuals outside of nursing. While there is little doubt that some of this contribution was done from patronizing motives, it would seem appropriate that some kind of return should, if possible, be made. If the current trend toward increased graduate education and an increased activity in theory development and research continues, nursing may well be in a very viable position in the not-too-distant future to return some of the intellectual favors that have been, and are being, extended to it.

THE BEGINNING

It is traditional to end a work of this nature by reviewing what has been said and drawing some significant conclusions for the future. Considering the ferment of activity within the realm of nursing—activity especially directed at defining nursing's scope of operation and at developing in initial form nursing's practice theory as well as a variety of research endeavors—it seems appropriate to title this conclusion not "The End" but "The Beginning." Having been a marginal participant in the nursing scene for a number of years, this author was startled to see the expansion of activity in relation to the question of theory and its role in nursing.

A detailed study of this subject would have carefully scrutinized the published research in terms of its use of theory and its contribution to the verification and modification of such theory. The limited time for preparing this chapter did not permit such an analysis. However, a glance at the research activity as presented in *Nursing Research* did reveal a relatively sophisticated awareness of the role of theory in nursing research. A work such as McCarthy's (1972) is an example of the struggle to develop nursing practice theory, with the result that "theory loses its 'mystical' quality and the theorist (practitioner) views theory as a viable aspect of practice that, when tested, can be modified or discarded as new data emerge" (McCarthy, 1972, p. 409).

The increased attention given to theory development within the nursing profession, especially in the various conferences and nursing journals, indicates two very clear and distinct developments that are related to the purposes of this chapter. First, there has not only been an increase in activity but also a greater degree of sophistication in defining the scope of nursing in such a way as to both distinguish it from other health-related occupations and to permit a continual trend toward greater professionalization, especially in terms of the professional criteria of specifying the nursing body of theoretical knowledge. Second, there continues a vibrant and exhilarating dialogue concerning the formulation of practice theory for nursing and a willingness and ability to test such theory under the scrutiny of the research process.

One might be tempted to close this section by concluding that the current endeavors within the realm of nursing practice theory development are "modest" at best. A closer examination of nursing's history might serve to qualify this conclusion with the expectation that this, the contemporary scene, is only the beginning, with the best part of the show yet to come.

BIBLIOGRAPHY

American Nurses Association: "Educational Preparation for Nurse Practitioners and Assistants to Nurses," a position paper, New York, 1965.

American Nurses' Foundation: *International Directory of Nurses with Doctoral Degrees*, New York, 1973.

Bixler, Roy, and Genevieve Bixler: "The Professional Status of Nursing," *American Journal of Nursing*, **45**:731–735, 1945.

Black, Max: *Critical Thinking, An Introduction to Logic and Scientific Method*, Prentice-Hall, Englewood Cliffs, N.J., 1946.

Boehm, Werner: *Objectives of the Social Work Curriculum of the Future*, Council on Social Work Education, New York, 1959.

Commentary on Walker's "Toward a Clearer Understanding of the Concept of Nursing Theory," *Nursing Research*, **20**:493–502, 1971.

Dickoff, James, and Patricia James: "A Theory of Theories: A Position Paper," *Nursing Research*, **17**:197–203, 1968.

——, ——, and Ernestine Wiedenbach: "Theory in a Practice Discipline: Part I. Practice Oriented Theory," *Nursing Research*, **17**:415–435, 1968a.

——, ——, and ——: "Theory in a Practice Discipline: Part II. Practice Oriented Research," *Nursing Research*, **17**:545–554, 1968b.

Ellis, Rosemary: "Characteristics of Significant Theories," *Nursing Research*, **17**:217–222, 1968.

Gortner, Susan: "Research for a Practice Profession," *Nursing Research*, **24**:193–197, 1975.

Hardy, Margaret: "Theories: Components, Development, Evaluation," *Nursing Research*, **23**:100–107, 1974.

Haug, Marie, and Marvin Sussman: "Professional Autonomy and the Revolt of the Client," *Social Problems*, **17**:153–161, 1969.

Johnson, Dorothy: "Development of Theory: A Requisite for Nursing as a Primary Health Profession," *Nursing Research*, **23**:372–377, 1974.

Kaplan, Abraham: *The Conduct of Inquiry*, Chandler, San Francisco, 1964.

King, Imogene: *Toward a Theory for Nursing: General Concepts of Human Behavior*, Wiley, New York, 1971.

McCarthy, Rosemary: "A Practice Theory of Nursing Care," *Nursing Research*, **21**:406–410, 1972.

Merton, Robert: *Social Theory and Social Structure*, Free Press, Glencoe, Ill., 1957.

Meyer, Burton, and Loretta Heidgerken: *Introduction to Research in Nursing*, Lippincott, Philadelphia, 1962.

Nagel, Ernest: *The Structure of Science*, Harcourt, Brace & World, New York, 1961.

Northrop, F. S. C.: *The Logic of the Sciences and the Humanities*, Macmillan, New York, 1947.

Nursing Development Conference Group: *Concept Formalization in Nursing: Process and Product*, Little, Brown, Boston, 1973.

Orem, Dorothea: *Nursing: Concepts of Practice*, McGraw-Hill, New York, 1971.

Pavalko, Ronald: *Sociology of Occupations and Professions*, Peacock, Itasca, Ill., 1971.

Rogers, Martha: *Educational Revolution in Nursing*, Macmillan, New York, 1961.

Rudner, Richard: *Philosophy of Social Science*, Prentice-Hall, Englewood Cliffs, N.J., 1966.

Source Book—Nursing Personnel, Health Man-power References, Government Printing Office, Washington, D.C., 1975.

Walker, Lorraine: "Toward A Clearer Understanding of the Concept of Nursing Theory," *Nursing Research*, **20**(5):428–435, September–October 1971.

Walker, Lorraine: "Rejoinder to Commentary: Toward a Clearer Understanding of the Concept of Nursing Theory," *Nursing Research*, **21**(1): 59–62, January–February 1972.

Wooldridge, Powhatan, James Skipper, and Robert Leonard: *Behavioral Science, Social Practice, and the Nursing Profession*, Case Western Reserve University Press, Cleveland, 1968.

EDITOR'S QUESTIONS FOR DISCUSSION

How might concepts about theory development for nursing be introduced in baccalaureate nursing programs? What evidence is there of theory that has been developed within the activity scope of nursing? How might nursing resolve the problem of the insufficient blending of advanced educational preparation and contact with clinical practice in order to facilitate theory development? In what domain of nursing might theory be developed? What contribution can nursing make to the basic sciences? How can these contributions be made?

Part Five

Nursing Practice

Nursing practice has experienced more changes in the last decade than has any other area of the nursing profession; consequently, nurses in practice may have had the most difficulty in keeping up to date. The changes that have occurred were caused by many factors: the increased emphasis on prevention of disease in health care; changes in settings where health care is provided; nursing's progress in defining the unique role of the nurse; the development of new roles in nursing; increasing costs of health care delivery; government planning in providing for health care; the attempt by nurses to attain more autonomy in their roles; and the increased awareness and expectations of the patient for quality in health care delivery. The following section attempts to portray what nursing practice is today and to identify more clearly the role of the nurse and of nursing.

Chapter 22

The Social Context of Nursing

Sharon J. Reeder, R.N., Ph.D.
Associate Professor, School of Nursing
The Center for the Health Sciences
University of California at Los Angeles

Sharon J. Reeder examines the impact of social change on the health care delivery system and nursing in terms of contributing social issues. The influences on nursing of such social issues as proposed national health insurance, changing attitudes toward health care, and changes in work-leisure patterns and in the housing environment of the patient are discussed. The need for change in educational programs for the providers of medical care is stressed. Reeder attributes the position of nursing today to three historical factors: religion, the military tradition of nursing, and the female role image. She shows how these historical antecedents interact with the current forces in nursing of consciousness raising, role innovation, and the drive for professionalization. Nurses are encouraged to be agents of change for the health care system by collaborating with physicians and patients in order to plan innovations.

INTRODUCTION

Over a century ago, Charles Dickens expressed his philosophy regarding change in his novel, *Martin Chuzzlewit*: "Change begets change: Nothing propagates so fast . . . the wedge of change was driven to the head rendering what was a solid mass to fragments, things cemented and held together by the usages of years burst asunder . . . and what was rock became but sand and dust" (Dickens, 1953, p. 20). Our own age, perhaps more than any other, is experiencing Dickens's meaning as a social reality. Social change is occuring to such an extent and with such rapidity that many are finding themselves confused, and are hampered in meeting the demands of everyday living (Donahue, 1975, p. 26).

In recent years, writers from a variety of disciplines have echoed the above concerns and questioned whether change and increased technological sophistication necessarily result in an improved quality of life. Many would agree that rapid change can interfere with positive social development unless a strong consciousness of tradition directs the process of change (Donahue, 1975). It is with the relationship among change, tradition, and development that the health care professions in the 1970s continue to wrestle.

In this chapter we will examine the impact of social change on the health care delivery system in general and nursing in particular in terms of the social issues that are contributing to crisis and change within the system. The antecedents of nursing that have helped shape today's cross-pressures on the profession will be explored. In addition, the present forces from both within and without nursing that have to do with changing role relationships, consumerism, consciousness raising, and the drive to professionalization will be examined briefly for their impact on the field. Finally, some thoughts on the direction that nursing might take will be offered.

SOCIAL CHANGE AND THE CRISES IN THE HEALTH CARE DELIVERY SYSTEM

All health care delivery is practiced in a social context and is reflective of the state of flux of that context. Rapid urbanization together with the development of a high degree of technology linked to urbanization has been cited as a basic factor that is contributing to the flux (Orleans and Orleans, 1976). Throughout their histories and in all parts of the world, cities have been marked as unhealthy for man. Throughout the recorded history of the Western world we find accounts of illness contracted in the city—and cured in the country. In the United States, for example, mortality rates are highest in metropolitan counties with a central city, lower in outlying metropolitan counties, and lowest in nonmetropolitan counties. Moreover, this trend holds for both sexes and all races with only minor variations in some regions of the country (Kitagawa and Hauser, 1973, pp. 120-123).

Identification of the specific factors and circumstances responsible for higher morbidity and mortality in the city is difficult because of the complexity of urban assets and liabilities. Cities provide enrichment for some, stresses for others: proximity to elaborate health facilities and the wherewithall to use them for some, and for others, no access to any of the expertise (Orleans and Orleans, 1976).

The existence of a crisis in the American health care system was officially declared by President Richard M. Nixon in 1969. However, as Orleans and Orleans (1976) point out, we have been in a health care crisis in this country for far longer. The economist, Sumner Rosen, reviewed the findings of the Committee on the Costs of Medical Care, first published in 1932, and republished in 1970. He noted that the catalog of problems first delineated 40 years ago resembles almost exactly

the latest list: inadequate services, insufficient funds, and understaffing in various settings. Nothing had changed, on the urban scene (Alford, 1972, pp. 127-164). Thus, we still define "crisis" in terms of inadequate and poor quality services, blocked access to services, and maldistribution of health care personnel.

Terris (1973) states that one of the basic issues underlying the now full-blown crisis arises from the fundamental organization of the American health care system itself.

Many observers have characterized this system as a two-class system: private and charity. However, it seems more accurate to delineate three systems, since the private system has two rather major subdivisions. The first of these can be designated as the pediatrician—internist system. This arena is used by the wealthier and/or more knowledgable segments of the upper and upper-middle classes. Primary care is divided between two highly trained physicians whose services may be supplemented by additional specialists. The second form of the private system is that of the general practitioner/family medicine system used by the less sophisticated sections of the middle class and the more skilled and better paid segments of the working class. Primary care is obtained through a single physician who does not have the same degree of specialization as the internist or pediatrician. Specialist services may be delivered either through the general practitioner or through a qualified specialist if one is available. In rural and small communities all sections of the population may utilize this system since other alternatives do not exist.

Finally, there is the charity system that serves the unskilled and poorly paid sections of the working class, the unemployed, those on welfare, and the elderly poor. Here, primary care is provided in hospital and outpatient departments by interns, residents, and sometimes specialists—pediatricians, internists, and so on. Specialist services may be obtained from residents and interns with varying degrees of supervision from the various specialists (Terris, 1973).

Thus, these health care systems are essentially parts of a single system based on market relations where health care is bought and sold like any other commodity. The wealthy can afford the expensive specialist system; the poor must rely on the charity system. Hence the "crisis" in health care may not be so apparent for the affluent, unless catastrophic illness occurs, and/or critical long-term care is necessary. For instance, a year's hospitalization at approximately $150 per day, not counting physician's fees, would total about $54,750, which would render us all medically indigent even with major medical insurance coverage. For the poor, however, there is always blocked access, as well as poor quality and too few facilities and personnel.

In addition, there is another aspect of health care to be considered, that of quality; and here even the affluent may fare poorly. Like others with lesser means, they must shop in an open market with all of the problems of caveat emptor that that implies. The care they receive may be hard to evaluate, particularly if they choose the solo physician who is relatively free from supervison or peer review. Hence fees and procedures may multiply as well as mistakes that go undetected (Terris, 1973; Donabedian, 1969).

There have been a variety of responses to the crisis from both the consumers and providers within the health care system. Indeed, the notion of an individual as a "consumer" of health care services rather than as a "patient" or even "client" puts a very different connotation on the professional relationship.

Within this newer connotation we are finding that the patient may dominate negotiations with the provider as a paying customer in a buyer's market (Freidson, 1970b). However, as previously stated, he is subject to all of the caveat emptor restrictions and thus is taking formal, militant steps to see that his services are as complete and of as an acceptable quality as he can make them. Hence we have the response of militancy from the consumer that Reeder (1972) has noted is reaching the proportions of a social movement aimed at "solving collectively a problem which they (consumers) feel they have in common" (Toch, 1965). This militancy is manifested most prominently in the expression of satisfaction and disatisfaction with the amount and quality of health care given. In the usual practice of health care, patient satisfaction is particularly difficult to express in any way that will promote lasting change in the system (Notkin and Notkin, 1970; Reeder, 1972). As the larger society undergoes structural change, however, there may be greater opportunities for producing change in the health system as greater cognizance is taken of the increasing number of research articles dealing with the issue of client satisfaction and dissatisfaction that portend a much more far reaching issues—that of citizen participation in health care (Alpert, 1970; Campbell, 1971; Kane, 1969). The accumulation of knowledge concerning these areas of satisfaction/ dissatisfaction will contribute to the understanding of the social movement aspects of consumerism as a force for changing the professional-client relationship, particularly in bureaucratic settings.

Providers in their way are also responding to the crisis. There have been admonitions to "adapt or perish" (Hoerr, 1971) and recognition that changing societal attitudes are instrumental in contributing to changes and conflicts in medical identity and role relationships (Boname, 1975; Menke, 1971; Demond, 1971). While we do not wish to lose the salient aspects of this provider adaptation through oversimplification, it must be said that the provider response is perhaps less organized than that of the consumer in that there is still little consensus as to where the thrust for change and/or reform should be. Few physicians appear to embrace the notion of a national health insurance plan, fearing that their "professional" entrepreneurial status will be reduced to that of salaried employee. There is also no consensus regarding the development of qualified colleagues, particularly nurse practitioners, to supplement medical services. Indeed, even in the nursing profession itself, there is no solid front as to the legitimacy of this type of practitioner. However, the general expansion of the nurses' role has been perhaps the single most concrete response to the health care crisis that all providers have made—with strong encouragement from both the state and national legislatures.

In sum, then, there appears to be general recognition that a health care crisis does exist; and various adaptive responses have been undertaken by both consumer and provider to meet the current needs. What appears most necessary for a truly effective adaptation with definite positive change is a thorough overhaul of the existing three-class health care system into one that delivers quality health care to all irrespective of ability to pay. This will be accomplished, many feel, only by creative preparation and utilization of health manpower and concrete delineation of domains of practice and accountability for performance among the various providers.

Social Issues Having Impact on the Health Scene

A number of social issues and forces have been delineated by the Task Force on Social Issues (1972) that have implication directly and indirectly for the health care delivery system in general. Some of these issues will help alleviate the crisis; some will exacerbate it. It is important to note that these issues are only illustrative, not exhaustive, of the many that will affect the health care delivery system. Of necessity we can only provide a summary of the issues and their anticipated effects.

First among these forces is that of national health insurance and its concomitant legislation. It is anticipated that within the coming decade, Congress will pass legislation to provide for national health insurance coverage. Such legislation is aimed at the financing, delivery, and control of health services, as well as the establishment and promotion of standards of evaluating delivery of services by all health professionals. In addition there will be the regulation of the credentialing, licensing, and accreditation processes of the health professions. Attention will also be given to the supervision of health care providers and the

environments in which services are rendered, as well as to the definition of relationships and domains of practice among the various health providers. Hopefully, this legislation will contribute to an easing of the crises if proposals can be developed that reflect a need for a continuum of health services that include definitions of health and illness and an emphasis on health maintenance (Somers, 1972).

The next several social issues relate to the consumer of health services. These include changes in attitudes toward health care that mandate health care as a right rather than a privilege and concomitantly, emphasize prevention rather than cure. Within a preventive framework providers will be required to assure accessible and adequate services within one system that provides quality care to all, regardless of socioeconomic status. More public pressure will be brought to bear on the federal government to impose controls and provide financing for services; hence it is likely that there will be conflict in the area of states versus federal rights that must be resolved before equality in the provision of health services will be attained (Task Force on Social Issues, 1972).

Changing patterns in consumers' work-leisure patterns also will affect the health delivery system. As leisure time increases there will be the need to devise an "extended" health delivery where patients' records and conditions may be monitored long distance, which means sophisticated data retrieval must be instituted among the providers. Moreover, the salubrious use of leisure time will necessitate more emphasis on the health education aspects of health maintenance rather than on the curative aspects of care.

Closely associated with work-leisure patterns is that of the housing and environment of the consumer. With the shift to urbanization and the consequent increase in pollution more attention must be paid to determinations and evaluations of criteria for health living environments. These criteria must be directed not only at the pollution aspects of urbanization but also at building a healthy community organization that diminishes the feelings of social isolation, anonymity, and alienation so often experienced in highly urbanized settings (Orleans and Orleans, 1976).

The next set of social issues relate to the providers themselves. These include changing educational patterns for providers, the impact of a high degree of technology, and the need for sophisticated methods of transmitting knowledge. Traditional educational patterns are changing not only for health providers but also for society as a whole. With our highly technocratic society, there is a need for technical training at the subbaccalaureate level to ensure better fit between education and job skills. Professional education is striving to develop better utilization of challenge, equivalency, and proficiency examinations as substitutes for formal course work and accelerated movement through the educational system. Moreover, there is a growing recognition that continuing education is necessary for work competency as well as personal growth. Thus, there is the suggestion that educational programs, including professional programs, will move in the direction of developing a competency base where there is a strong relationship of curriculum to the defined output of the program (Task Force on Social Issues, 1972). The impact of these newer educational methods and emphasis needs to be critically researched to see if these innovations will indeed contribute to an improvement in the quality and competence of providers and services.

NURSING'S POSITION IN THE CHANGING HEALTH SCENE

As one of the most salient health care professions, nursing stands somewhat at a crossroads in today's health care dilemma. Moreover, the state of our profession is no less paradoxical than that of the health care scene in general. There are concerns about "shortages," yet as a whole nursing has increased in overall numbers. In fact, unlike the other health manpower spheres, nursing has actually exceeded the growth in the population as a whole (Reeder and Mauksch, in press). Yet, the career-withdrawal (Kramer, 1974; 1970) rate is alarming. In 1972, approximately 30 percent of nurses holding licenses to practice reported professional inactivity (American Nurses' Association, 1974, p. 2). Moreover, the problem of career withdrawals is compounded by the high turnover rate, in institutions of practice, of those who remain active in nursing. This turnover rate at times reaches more than 70 percent. In urban settings where job change is facilitated by a greater number of choices, the turnover rate may reach 150 to 200 percent (Jenab, 1973).

In addition, as with the general health care scene, there is the problem of quality in nursing care. Studies have indicated (Kramer, 1969; Kramer et al., 1972; Kramer, 1970) that nurses may spend 50 to 75 percent of their time in non-nursing functions and this proves to be a source of dissatisfaction for nurses and their patients alike. Graduates of baccalaureate and master's degree programs are both under- and overutilized. They are prepared to deliver high caliber nursing care to patients with complex nursing needs, yet for want of a career perspective and opportunities for advancement, they are often lured into positions of educational and administrative leadership for which they may not be fully prepared. When they do work as staff nurses and clinical specialists, they are forced into task-centered role functions dictated by bureaucratic organizational policies that allow little opportunity or support for patient-centered care.

Antecedents Shaping Nursing's Dilemma

In order to understand nursing's position in today's health care dilemma, it is necessary to look to the past as well as the present to trace the ties that bind nursing into the current social context. The historical antecedents that include the religious and military traditions of nursing together with the symbolic linking to female role images have all contributed to the structure and function of nursing as it is practical today. While these are not the only historical happenings that are important to nursing they represent perhaps the most important.

The forerunners of the modern nursing practitioner included both the servant hired to care for the sick as well as those who felt an obligation stemming from wealth and status who believed that charitable attention to the poor and sick was an appropriate activity for nobility.

The Christian belief system elaborated and cemented this orientation and lent an aura of sanctity to caring for those in need. Indeed, the religious tradition so prevalent in the inception of nursing has been possibly the one that, from earliest times to the present, has remained the most significant force both for the development and detriment of the profession. The combination of the ethic of service together with the traditional view of women as inferior and subservient to men, so prominent in the Christian ethos and dogma, have provided a double-edged sword under which the female providers of nursing services have labored for centuries (Reeder and Mauksch, in press).

The second early historical tradition that has had a profound influence in shaping the practice of nursing is that of the military. This root became most apparent at the time of the Crimean War, although its contribution can be observed throughout history, from the era of the crusades to its most recent impact during World War II (Griffin and Griffin, 1973; Bullough and Bullough, 1971).

It was in the Crimean campaign that Florence Nightingale made concerted attempts to establish formal standards for nursing practice and to organize the rendering of nursing care into an institutionally responsible delivery system. Hence, the establishment of nursing as a collectively organized, institutionally responsible system is primarily associated with Ms. Nightingale and is inextricably bound to the military. Moreover, the institutionalization of educational prerequisites for nursing that grew out of the efforts of Ms. Nightingale and others continued to reflect the influence of the military in its emphasis on what was essentially obedience training for nursing aspirants. It was not until the advent of the academic-based collegiate programs that this obedience, respect-for-authority orientation, was attenuated.

The war and the formalization of a specific educational curriculum also brought the physician into close contact with nursing. His supervisory status and his participation in the educational activities paved the way for his gradual assumption of control and jurisdiction over nursing activities—not only those relating to the patient's cure aspects but also those involving the patient's comfort, nutrition, and finally all other aspects relating to the "patient" status.

The final recent impact of the military on nursing occurred in World War II when the scarcity of manpower caused by the conflict and the need in the postwar economy gave rise to the development of ancillary nursing personnel. Thus, the nurse's aide, practical nurse, and nursing assistant remained and proliferated as permanent fixtures in the health care scene. Thus, the one-to-one primary nursing role gave way to a stratified nursing team that over the years gradually pushed many registered nurses away from the bedside and into supervisory and managerial roles. These new roles allowed for increased status and prestige but removed the nurse further from direct patient care (Reeder and Mauksch, in press; Bullough and Bullough, 1971).

The third historical strand that has had profound implication for today's nursing profession is that of the immutable link to female role images. This linkage has persisted through the centuries, although it is important to note that males have been involved in the performance of nursing activities since the time of the crusades (Dock and Steward, 1938).

In the English language, the word "nursing" implies the essence of a mother's relationship to her child. A clue to this connotation lies in the etymology of the word "nurse." "Nurse" was derived through the French language from the Latin *nutrix* that came from *nutrire*: to nourish or suckle. The word appeared in Middle English around the twelfth century as *nourse, norse,* etc. In this period a nurse was one who was retained to suckle or otherwise attend an infant and/or one who had general charge of young children (Donahue, 1975). As time went on the meaning of the word expanded to include all persons, male or female, who took care of all manner of persons and things, until by the 1700s the term had crystallized to mean "a person, generally a woman who attended or waited upon the sick" (Donahue, 1975, p. 28). Hence the quasi-innate qualities that have been perceived to be the attributes of the mother and female evoke images that influence the fate of nursing practice and education to this day. Thus, the tendency of a mother to care for her family without having formal parameters to her areas of competence, together with society's insistence that she perform the many managerial and supervisory tasks associated with homemaking, continue to underlie many of the overall expectations held today by both those within and without nursing regarding the appropriate role of the nurse. Hence, the spirit of serving, the strong sense of obedience, and the binding to the female role image are the immutable heritage of nursing.

Current Conditions: Change from Within and Without

Thus have historical factors set the stage for today's images and dilemmas for nursing. Tying into these traditions are current events that are influencing the changes experienced by the profession. The exigencies of space do not permit a discussion of all of the current factors having relevance for today's nursing scene. However, there are several related, simultaneously occurring events that have special importance in nursing's current life. The first of these, as we have stated, is that of consumerism.

There has been a long-standing concern with professional-client relations, particularly the doctor-patient relationship (Freidson, 1961; Bloom, 1963; Scott and Volkart, 1966; Mechanic, 1968). Most of the literature speaks of the client role in terms of "patient behavior" and this role is seen only as a contingency in the structure of medical

care. Review of the patient-practitioner role set indicates that as a distinctive type of occupation, professions and their incumbents have been successful in obtaining institutional powers that set limits on client freedoms and autonomy. Professional expertise becomes institutionalized in a form similar to that of the bureaucratic office (Freidson, 1970a; Wilson and Bloom, 1972). Hence the patient may be treated as an object, and may receive little information about his condition, treatment, and outcomes. Medical orders determine the entire gamut of patient activities and any breakdown in communication is blamed on the patient. There is insistence on faith and trust in the professional that neutralizes any threatening or demeaning of the status of the provider when the layman requests explanation or justification (Freidson, 1970a).

Earlier we noted that the mere use of the term consumer to replace that of patient initiates a very different perspective for viewing the relationship between provider and client. It might be said parenthetically that most discussions regarding this construct have focused on the *physician* and patient (Hochbaum, 1969; Campbell, 1971; Thursz, 1970). However, it is appropriate and germane that the discussion can be extended to all health providers including nursing.

When one utilizes the perspective of labeling theory of deviance, it can be expected that differential behavior will occur on the parts of the actors of the role relationship in question. Thus a patient delivers himself into the hands of the professional—who, by definition, is the sole decision maker regarding the services to be delivered. If, on the other hand, the patient is viewed as consumer, he purchases services for their amount and quality. Thus, he has more bargaining powers but is also limited by the amount of time and money he can spend (Titmus, 1963).

As the locus of professional-client interaction takes place increasingly in bureaucratic and organizational settings, the nature of the relationship will be altered further. More attention will have to be paid to the client's needs, wishes, and satisfaction. There are already demands for consumer representation on the governing councils of organizations within which the professional and client interact. Increasingly, these demands are being met and it is anticipated that pressures will continue for more and varied consumer participation as well as for the employment of the ombudsman format to mediate differences between professionals and consumers (Reeder, 1972). We see this latter concept already developing in nursing when we define one of the nurse's role functions as that of a patient advocate.

Proceeding from the above it is reasonable to anticipate that "the legitimate role definers," that is, physicians and by extension other health professionals, may no longer be the sole incumbents of those particular roles traditionally associated with this function. The consumer as an alter to the professional is well on his way to becoming another important source of that legitimation by having much more input into what constitutes legitimate patterns of interaction (Reeder, 1972).

Nursing in the expanding and shifting sands of the health care arena will do well to focus its attention, especially its research attention, on the forms, content, and symbols of the professional-client interaction, particularly with respect to the scope, depth, and timing of consumer roles in health maintenance and health care decisions. Out of these empirical observations we can gain a better understanding of the underlying processes involved in the changing professional-client relationship and therefore be able to make creative innovations and adaptations in our own roles.

There are several other changes within and without nursing that form a related constellation, each feeding into the other and impinging on nursing's future.

One noticeable happening in nursing is the amount of literature, directed at all levels of nursing, aimed at apprising the nurse of the efficacy of consciousness raising, not only for herself as a nurse but also for herself as a woman (Schorr, 1972; Levinson, 1976; McBride, 1976; Kaiser and Kaiser, 1974; Kravetz and Sargent, 1975). This

appears to be a process that is linked to emerging changes in the self-image of the modern nurse and even to the changing image of women in society. Few will dispute that women have not been socialized into the role of decision maker in our society; and nursing, as we have seen, being predominantly and historically female, has also suffered a debilitating suppression of intellectual activity. Current medical professional literature (Chesler, 1971; Marlow, 1973; Jeffcoate, 1967; Willson et al., 1975), sexist ideology couched in medical rhetoric (Ehrenreich, 1974; Scully and Bart, 1973; Barker-Benfield, 1972; Spock, 1971), and traditional sex-role socialization (Levinson, 1976; Feather and Simon, 1975; 1973) all have played their pernicious parts in keeping nurses and other women from achieving high levels of occupational and educational success. This has certainly been evidenced in nursing by the continual battle with medical colleagues to determine the scope and content of practice and hence the attainment of true professionalization. Hopefully, the new awareness and militancy engendered by consciousness raising will provide a sufficient counterforce to ensure continual impetus toward professionalization.

Tied to consciousness raising and the changing self-image of the nurse has been the concept of role expansion for nurses and changing physician-nurse role relationships. The temporal placement of these variables is hard to determine, that is, does changing self-image precede role expansion or does the idea of more autonomous, expanded functions encourage a more positive self-image? At this point we have no empirical evidence; however, this is an area that needs concentrated attention to determine the process of professionalization for our field.

We are all familiar by now with the concept of role expansion and the controversy that it has engendered since its inception in the late 1960s. This concept has been operationalized into the development of the nurse practitioner, nurse clinician, or nurse associate, as she has variously been called. Definitions of this practitioner have varied, but she has come to be known as a nurse who has physical assessment and clinical management skills in addition to a solid nursing orientation. She works in collaboration with the physician in devising treatment and health maintenance plans that have both a medical and nursing component. This newer role frequently involves placing the nurse into positions where she has primary contact with patients; hence she may function as the direct and primary resource of those who seek entry into the health care system (Januska, et al., 1975; Lurie, 1975). The heart of the controversy that centered around the development of these practitioners lay essentially in a concern that the nursing role would be abandoned and/or the medical role would be challenged or encroached upon (Osborne, 1975). A corollary concern has been that of the fear of proliferation of ancillary medical roles with ensuing confusion as to whether this role truly represented a more autonomous nursing role or merely a role that has been coopted into a physician's "assistant role" (Weiler, 1975).

Data to date indicate that the above concerns have not materialized when the educational programs have had a solid academic base with collaborative program planning by both physicians and nurses (Linn, 1975; Lewis et al., 1969); when the innovation has been hurriedly incorporated into an existing program then there has been genuine concern as to whether expansion did, in fact, mean "abandonment" (Silver and Ford, 1967).

Perhaps the salient point here is that the concept of role expansion has spurred the legislative drive to define the domains of practice and perogatives between medicine and nursing and to place parameters on the problem of accountability for nurses (Bullough, 1976). This in turn has helped sharpen the drive to professionalism and has been looked on by some as a creative response to a need for innovation in health provider roles that in turn has helped alleviate some of the crisis in health care.

Thus, in the later 1970s we see the historical antecedents that have shaped today's image of nursing interacting with the current forces of con-

sciousness raising, role innovation, and the thrust for professionalization. Given this interplay of variables within the larger societal context, what might be the direction nursing could take to continue positive growth and prevent obsolescence?

Directions

As we can infer from our discussion, one of the inevitable concomitants of social change is disequilibrium among the various groups contributing to the organization and functioning of the system undergoing change. As knowledge increases and new attitudes and values shift, forces emerge that require drastic accommodation in the system. This certainly appears to be the case in our current health care dilemma. Given the concern that nursing scholars, as well as many of the rank and file in nursing, feel about their field in terms of its possible disintegration and obsolesence (Zich, 1976; Fagin, 1976), it appears that planned change is one of the key issues. This type of change involves a deliberate collaborative effort involving a change agent and a client system (Reinkmeyer, 1970) that further involves specified effort to define ends and means for the system. Nursing has long identified itself with being a change agent for the health care system. Continuing to support both client and provider dissatisfaction with the existing delivery system, thereby helping both parties perceive the discrepancy between what is and what could be, can lead to increased levels of expectations that eventually lead to action. Research projects involving experiments and demonstrations in care-giving together with true collaboration with other members of the health care team, including the consumer, would be subsequent steps in long-term planned change. This collaboration would facilitate the appropriate diagnosis of the needs and problems of the client, and make possible an examination of alternative routes and methods of care delivery in order to arrive at some point of agreement between the needs of the client and the needs of the system at any given time (Reeder and Mauksch, in press).

It remains to be seen if educators and practitioners of nursing will be able to rise to the challenge of inviting and encouraging change while accepting the inevitable disequilibrium. As Reinkmeyer (1970) has stated, given a clear grasp of the ramifications of change, an intelligent control of the processes of change, and the conviction that resurrection requires dying, nursing can turn the present crisis into a tremendous opportunity that will allow the field not only to survive but also to gain a firm mastery over its destiny.

BIBLIOGRAPHY

Alford, R.: "The Political Economy of Health Care: Dynamics Without Change," *Politics and Society,* 1:127–164, Winter 1972.

Alpert, J. J. et. al.: "Attitudes and Satisfactions of Low-Income Families Receiving Comprehensive Pediatric Care," *American Journal of Public Health,* 60:499–506, March 1970.

American Nurses Association: "The Nation's Nurses," in *1972 Inventory of Registered Nurses,* 1974.

Barker-Benfield, B.: "The Spermatic Economy: A Nineteenth Century View of Sexuality," *Feminist Studies,* 1:5–10, 1972.

Bloom, S.: *The Doctor and his Patient,* Sage, New York, 1963.

Boname, J. R.: "Changing Attitudes Create Health Care Dilemma," *Association of Operating Room Nurses Journal,* 22(4):543–548, 1975.

Bullough, B.: "The Law and the Expanding Nursing Role," *American Journal of Public Health,* 66:249–254, March 1976.

———, and V. Bullough: "Career Ladder in Nursing: Problems and Prospects," *American Journal of Nursing,* 71:1938–1943, October 1971.

Campbell, J.: "Working Relationships Between Providers and Consumers in a Neighborhood Health Center," *American Journal of Public Health,* 60:97–103, January 1971.

Chesler, P.: "Women as Psychiatric and Psychotherapeutic Patients," *Journal of Marriage and the Family,* 33:753–762, November 1971.

Demond, E. G.: "A Crisis in our Time," *Missouri Medicine,* 68:868–869, November 1971.

Dickens, Charles: *Martin Chuzzlewit,* Collins, London, 1953, p. 20.

Dock, L., and I. Stewart: *A Short History of Nursing,* Putnam, New York, 1938.

Donabedian, A.: "An Evaluation of Prepaid Group Practice," *Inquiry,* 6:3–27, 1969.

Donahue, S.: "Humanist Traditions in Nursing Developments," *Australian Nurses Journal,* 4: 26–30, June 1975.

Ehrenreich, B., and E. Deirdre: "Complaints and Disorders: The Sexual Politics of Sickness," Glass Mountain Pamphlet Series, Feminist Press, New York, 1974.

Fagin, C.: "Can We Bring Order Out of the Chaos of Nursing Education?" *American Journal of Nursing,* 76:98–105, January 1976.

Feather, N., and J. Simon: "Fear of Success and Causal Attribution for Outcome," *Journal of Personality,* 41:525–541, 1973.

———: "Reactions of Male and Female Success and Failure in Sex-linked Occupations: Impressions of Personality, Causal Attributions and Perceived Likelihood of Different Consequences," *Journal of Personality and Social Psychology,* 31:20–31, January 1975.

Freidson, E.: *Patients' Views of Medical Practice,* Sage, New York, 1961.

———: "Dominant Professions, Bureaucracy, and Client Services," in William Rosengren and Mark Lefton (eds.), *Organizations and Clients,* Charles E. Merrill, Columbus, Ohio, 1970a, pp. 71–92.

———: *The Profession of Medicine,* Dodd, Mead Publishing, New York, 1970b.

Griffin, G. J., and J. K. Griffin: *History and Trends of Professional Nursing,* Mosby, St. Louis, 1973.

Hochbaum, G. M.: "Consumer Participation in Health Planning: Toward Conceptual Clarification," *American Journal of Public Health,* 59: 1698–1705, September 1969.

Hoerr, S.: "Adapt or Perish," *Archives of Surgery,* 103:103–107, August 1971.

Januska, C. et. al.: "Development of a Family Nurse Practitioner Curriculum," *Nursing Outlook,* 22:103–108, February 1974.

Jeffcoate, T. N. A.: *Principles of Gynecology,* 3d ed., Appleton-Century-Crofts, New York, 1967, p. 726.

Jenab, L. D.: "The Health Care Scene: Nursing's Dilemma," *West Virginia Medical Journal*, **69**: 328–332, November 1973.

Kaiser, B., and I. Kaiser: "The Challenge of the Women's Movement and American Gynecology," *American Journal of Obstetrics and Gynecology*, **120**:652–665, November 1974.

Kane, R. L.: "Determination of Health Care Priorities and Expectations Among Rural Consumers," *Health Services Research,* **4**:142–151, Summer 1969.

Kitagawa, E., and P. Hauser: *Differential Mortality in the United States: A Study of Socioeconomic Epidemiology*, Cambridge, Mass., 1973.

Kramer, M.: "Collegiate Graduate Nurses in a Medical Center Hospital: Mutual Challenge of Duels," *Nursing Research*, **194**:196–210, March–April 1969.

———: *Reality Shock: Why Nurses Leave Nursing*, Mosby, St. Louis, 1974.

———: "Role Conceptions of Baccalaureate Nurses and Success in Hospital Nursing," *Nursing Research*, **195**:428–439, September–October 1970.

——— et. al.: "Self Actualization and Role Adaptation of Baccalaureate Degree Nurses," *Nursing Research,* **21**:111–112, March–April 1972.

Kravetz, D., and A. Sargent: "Consciousness-raising Groups: A Resocialization Process for Personal and Social Change," *Supervisory Nurse*, **6**:26–27; 29–31, October 1975.

Levinson, R.: "Sexism in Medicine," *American Journal of Nursing*, **3**:426–431, March 1976.

Lewis, C. et. al.: "Activities, Events and Outcomes in Ambulatory Patient Care," *New England Journal of Medicine*, **280**:645–649, March 20, 1969.

Linn, L.: "Expectation vs. Realization in the Nurse Practitioner Role," *Nursing Outlook*, **23**:166–171, March 1975.

Lurie, E.: "A New Role in Health Care: Nurse Practitioner After the First 12 Months," unpublished paper, 1975.

Marlow, D.: *Textbook of Pediatric Nursing*, 4th ed., Saunders, Philadelphia, 1973, p. 61.

McBride, A. B.: "A Married Feminist," *American Journal of Nursing*, **76**:754–757, May 1976.

Mechanic, D.: *Medical Sociology, A Selective View*, Free Press, New York, 1968.

Menke, W. G.: "Medical Identity: Change and Conflict in Professional Roles," *Journal of Medical Education*, **46**:58–63, January 1971.

Notkin, J., and M. S. Notkin: "Community Participation in Health Services," *Medical Care Review*, **27**:537–543, December 1970.

Orleans, P., and M. Orleans: *Urban Life: Diversity and Inequality*, Brown, Dubuque, Iowa, 1976.

Osborne, O.: "Issues in Achieving Effective Professional Alliances," *Hospital Community Psychiatry*, **26**:207–213, April 1975.

Reeder, L.: "The Patient-Client as a Consumer: Some Observations on the Changing Professional-Client Relationship," *Journal of Health and Social Behavior*, **18**, December 1972.

Reeder, S., and H. Mauksch: "Nursing: Continuing Change," in H. Freeman, et. al. (eds.), *Handbook of Medical Sociology*, Prentice-Hall, Englewood Cliffs, N.J., in press.

Reinkmeyer, A.: "Nursing's Need: Commitment to an Ideology of Change," *Nursing Forum*, **9**(4):340–355, 1970.

"Report of the Task Force on Social Issues," *American Journal of Occupational Therapy*, **26**:332–359, October 1972.

Schorr, T.: "The Passing of the 'Its-Smart-to-Be-Dumb' Era," *American Journal of Nursing*, **72**: 249, February 1972.

Scott, R., and E. Volkart: *Medical Care,* Wiley, New York, 1966.

Scully, D., and P. Bart: "A Funny Thing Happened on the Way to the Oriface: Women Gynecology Textbooks," *American Journal of Sociology*, **78**:1045–1050, January 1973.

Silver, H., and L. Ford: "The Pediatric Nurse Practitioner at Colorado," *American Journal of Nursing,* **67**:1443–1444, July 1967.

Somers, H. M.: "National Health Insurance: Strategy and Standards," *Medical Care,* **285** (23):1288–1292, 1972.

Spock, H.: *Decent and Indecent*, Fawcett World, New York, 1971.

Terris, M.: "Crises and Change in America's Health System," *American Journal of Public Health,* **63**:313–318, April 1973.

Thursz, D.: *Consumer Involvement in Rehabilitation Service*, SRS-114 System of Documents, U.S. Government Printing Office, Washington, D.C., 1970.

Titmus, R. H.: "Ethics and Economics of Medical Care," *Medical Care,* 1:16–22, January-March 1963.

Toch, H.: *The Social Psychology of Social Movements,* Bobbs-Merrill, Indianapolis, 1965.

Weiler, P.: "Health Manpower Dialectic—Physician, Nurse, Physician's Assistant," *American Journal of Public Health,* 65:858–863, August 1975.

Willson, J. R. et. al.: *Obstetrics and Gynecology,* 5th ed., Mosby, St. Louis, 1975.

Wilson, R., and S. Bloom: "Patient-Practitioner Relationships," in H. Freeman et. al., (eds.), *Handbook of Medical Sociology,* Prentice-Hall, Englewood Cliffs, N.J., 1972, pp. 315–337.

Zich, C.: "News of American Nurses Foundation Grantees," *American Nurses Foundation Nursing Research Report,* 11:3, October 1976.

EDITOR'S QUESTIONS FOR DISCUSSION

What evidence is there of patients negotiating for quality care with the providers of that care? What bargaining power does a patient have? How have the providers of medical care and the patients adapted to the crises in health care delivery? Would one expect a tendency to reject the historical traditions of nursing in planning for the future? What role should nursing have in collaboration with physicians and patients in health care planning?

Chapter 23

Primary Care:
The Challenge for Nursing

Linda H. Aiken, R.N., Ph.D.
Program Officer, Robert Wood Johnson Foundation
Princeton, New Jersey

Linda H. Aiken discusses the factors that have led to new types of health care and describes the role of the nurse in ambulatory care settings. She believes that passage of a broad-coverage national health insurance program will increase the demand for outpatient care. For primary care (first-contact general health care), nurses can assume a major role, with physician back-up. The type of health problems encountered in primary care usually are not complex. In such settings, there is the possibility of fee-for-service and third-party reimbursement for nursing care, although the question remains as to what extent the care provided by nurses should substitute for care by other providers. To answer that question, however, nurses must develop methods to document their contributions in primary care. Aiken indicates how the unique skills of the nurse might be used in primary care in joint practice with the physician. She advocates provision of faculty role models and learning experiences in primary care as part of the nursing education program to prepare such nurses sufficiently.

There is increasing concern on the part of health care providers, policy makers, and consumers that the American health care system is not providing reasonably accessible health care for the more common problems of the population. The difficulty some groups experience in obtaining ambulatory care of acceptable quality on a continuing basis is thought by some to be one of the most serious problems we face in health.[1,2] Despite the fact that national health expenditures now exceed $100 billion a year,[3] or 8 percent of the gross national product, the public appears to perceive that there is a health care crisis. Consumer surveys[4,5] indicate concern that out-of-pocket costs

for medical care will soon exceed the capacity of the average person to pay. In addition, there is widespread concern that general front-line medical care is unavailable when needed, and that health care is becoming increasingly impersonal.

Problems of access to health care are not new. They have been brought to the attention of providers and consumers by developments both in the health sector and in the larger community. Two important changes have taken place in the health sector. There has been an increasing specialization of health manpower that has reduced considerably the number of primary care providers. For example, the number of physicians in general practice in the United States fell from 64 percent in 1949 to 27 percent in 1970.[6] Second, there is a serious geographical maldistribution of health manpower. Rural areas, particularly those in the South, and inner city ghetto areas have significantly fewer health professionals than the more affluent urban and suburban areas. The very areas with the lowest health professional-to-population ratios are also the areas of greatest need in terms of health problems.

In addition to the problems brought about by increasing specialization and geographical maldistribution, consumers' expectations have increased. Everyone wants a share of the wonders modern medicine has to offer. Medicaid and Medicare, for instance, have erased the traditional relationship between income and physician visits, but have also increased expectations in general. There is growing concern that there be equity in health services throughout all segments of the population.[7,8]

"The term primary care . . . is the current popular phrase for a form of medical practice said to be in small supply and large demand."[9] *Primary care* usually refers to first-contact general health care as opposed to *secondary care* that is usually provided in a hospital or by specialists, or *tertiary care* that is complex technological care provided for patients with complicated problems. The primary care practitioner is a generalist who is well prepared to deal with commonly occurring problems, referring on those patients requiring the knowledge and skills of the specialist. Continuity of care is an important component. Primary care practitioners assume ongoing responsibility for patients, particularly groups of patients. Many primary care practitioners care for both sexes and all ages. Their scope of practice tends to be broad since they serve as entry points and the locus of contact with the health care system. Their scope of practice includes psychosocial as well as physiological dimensions of care.[10,11]

Both nursing and medical education have undergone significant changes over the past several decades that have affected the practice and deployment of practitioners.[12] The Flexner Report

of 1910 that was highly critical of many aspects of medical education, particularly the use of part-time general physicians as primary faculty, brought about a number of changes in teaching institutions. As a result of this report, a strong biomedical research base was introduced in academic medical centers, and the faculty of schools of medicine began to bring special science skills to bear upon the care of patients rather than the skills of the generalist. The knowledge explosion that brought insulin, the antimicrobial drugs, and the other technological advancements rapidly turned teaching hospitals into referral centers that treated patients with complex medical problems. Thus, students trained in teaching hospitals were taught by specialists and cared primarily for patients with problems not often seen in general practice. As a result of their training, more and more practitioners elected specialties that required urban locations, and proportionately fewer chose general practice.

As the training of physicians changed, so did the training of nurses, since even before the advent of widespread baccalaureate nursing education, the training of nurses tended to take place in hospitals that served as major teaching centers. Prior to the Great Depression, nurses worked outside of hospitals in large numbers, many caring for the sick in their homes. Since that time, however, the vast majority of nurses have practiced within the walls of hospitals. Today, 70 percent of employed nurses are in hospital settings.[13] The character of nursing practice has therefore been highly influenced by the changing nature of hospitals and medical care. Nursing faculty have become more specialized in their knowledge and skills in an effort to teach more effectively in tertiary care centers. Further, the patients with whom students have greatest contact are not representative of patients in general. Even many ambulatory patient experiences involved medical or surgical subspecialty outpatient clinics instead of general care clinics. White and his colleagues[14] point out quite clearly the potential impact of using referral hospitals as primary training sites. They note that in an adult population of 1,000 people, 750 persons have some illness monthly, 250 of these see a physician, and only 1 is referred for care to a medical teaching center. To the extent that nursing students are primarily exposed to patients in tertiary referral centers, they will be less than adequately prepared or motivated to work in primary care settings.

There is no doubt that changes in medical and nursing education and accompanying technological advances in the diagnosis and treatment of illness have vastly improved the care of the seriously ill in American hospitals. However, there has not been the same level of improvement in the care of the ambulatory patient. In fact, it has been argued that the growing specialization and geographical maldistribution of health manpower has had a detrimental effects on the health care available for common illnesses and preventive health supervision.

From 1955 to 1970, the number of visits to hospital emergency rooms increased by over 300 percent. During the same period, hospital outpatient visits increased by over 130 percent, while hospital admissions increased by only 50 percent.[15] Further, bed occupancy rates in hospitals have been steadily falling off.[16] The significant increase in the use of emergency rooms and outpatient clinics has occurred at a time when third-party reimbursement still favors hospitalization. Some researchers predict that the passage of any broad-coverage national health insurance program will dramatically increase the demand for out-of-hospital care. A study at Rand, for instance, predicts that comprehensive coverage would increase demand by 75 percent, and that a 25 percent maximum coinsurance plan would increase demand by 30 percent.[17] Although the fate of national health insurance is unknown, it is probable that some form will be passed in the next decade that will provide additional coverage for out-of-hospital care. Experience with Medicare and Medicaid has demonstrated that removing the cost barriers to medical care significantly increases utilization of services, especially among groups whose access problems relate to income. Therefore, there is every indication that future manpower needs will be in the out-of-hospital sector, and that nursing should increasingly focus its attention on developing the country's potential for providing primary care.

NURSING INVOLVEMENT IN PRIMARY CARE

It has previously been pointed out that the demand for out-of-hospital care is growing faster than any other health care component, and that the country's manpower resources are inadequate to meet the demand. The only responsible position for nursing to assume given these trends is to increase the number of primary care nurses, and to facilitate the development of an environment in which primary care nursing can make a contribution. This is clearly in the interest of nursing in the future.

Since the 1950s, schools of nursing have been expanding rapidly with the help of federal capitation funds and other training monies. The associate degree programs in particular have mushroomed during this period. Much of this expansion was due to a perceived shortage of nurses. Today, however, there is evidence that there is no longer a shortage, and some predict an oversupply of nurses in the next decade.[18] For instance, from 1962 to 1972, the number of nurses per 100,000 people increased from 298 to 380, a gain of almost 300 percent over the previous decades.[19] There is already evidence that new graduates are having difficulty finding jobs in some areas of the country. The interaction of three trends, if continued, could severely jeopardize the economic gains made in nursing in the last decade: (1) the continued employment of the majority of nurses within hospitals; (2) the decreasing occupancy rates of hospitals, and the increasing pressure of planning agencies to reduce hospital expansion; (3) the continued expansion of schools of nursing. The evidence points very strongly to the fact that the primary care sector must be developed to provide employment opportunities for a significant number of nurses.

In addition to the evidence indicating that the demand exists for primary care and that the supply of nurses warrants more involvement in primary care, there are two additional factors of importance. The first is that the background, unique skills, and interests of nurses are particularly relevant to the needs of patients in ambulatory settings. The second is that out-of-hospital care offers nurses increased opportunity for autonomy and control over their practice because it lacks the bureaucratic structure of the hospital and the associated dominance of physicians. Although there has been increasing interest among physicians in recent years in the primary care sector due to the infusion of public and private funds, the reward system in medicine is such that under most circumstances physicians are likely to consider nurses welcome partners rather than a threat.

American medical care has traditionally focused on the cure of disease. However, it has been pointed out that many of the most prevalent health problems in this country tend to be problems that are either not curable by the medical interventions available, are the result of environmental or behavioral factors not influenced by traditional medical care, or are self-limiting in that they usually run their course with or without medical care.[20] Thus, health care providers are called upon to serve in many roles in addition to the cure of disease. The kinds of health problems encountered by primary care practitioners are, in general, not complex in terms of medical management but often represent significant discomfort to patients. Table 23-1 summarizes the types of problems seen by a general practitioner.[21] The medical management of the more commonly occurring problems is relatively straightforward as long as the "system" has the capacity to identify, from innocent-appearing situations, those few that are potentially serious, and to provide properly for them.[22]

There have been a series of demonstrations that nurse practitioners can provide health care of high

Table 23-1 Consultations per 2,500 Patients for a Hypothetical Average General Practice

Conditions	Consultations per 2,500 patients
Minor illnesses	
Upper respiratory infections	500
Emotional disorders	300
Gastrointestinal disorders	250
Skin disorders	225
Acute tonsillitis	100
Middle ear infections	75
Ear wax	50
Acute urinary infections	50
Acute major illnesses	
Acute bronchitis and pneumonia	50
Severe depression	12
Acute myocardial infarction	7
Acute strokes	5
All new cancers	5
Chronic illnesses	
Chronic arthritis	100
Chronic mental illness	55
Chronic bronchitis	50
Iron deficiency anemia	40
Chronic heart failure	30
High blood pressure	25
Asthma	25
Peptic ulcer	25
Coronary artery disease	20
Cerebrovascular disease	15
Diabetes	10

Source: Present State and Future Needs of General Practice, 3d ed., Royal College of General Practitioners, London, 1973.

quality to primary care patients with sufficient physician back-up. Lewis et al.[23] evaluated, in one of the first such efforts, an ambulatory clinic in which nurses served as the primary source of care for adults with chronic illness. Patients cared for by the nurses were in a relatively stable phase of their illness, and represented five diagnostic classifications: hypertensive cardiovascular disease; obesity; psychophysiologic reactions (gastrointestinal or musculoskeletal); and arthritis. They found no differences in deaths or severity of disease between patients cared for in nurse clinics and similar patients cared for by physicians. There were, however, significant differences in outcomes as measured by reduction of disability and relative decreases in discomfort and dissatisfaction of patients seen in the nurse clinic.

Similarly, the Burlington randomized trial of the nurse practitioner documented that in a large family practice, the patient care outcomes were similar along all dimensions whether the nurse practitioner was the primary provider or whether the physician was the primary provider.[24] Runyan, in another recent study of clinical outcomes of the use of nurse practitioners, looked at patients with diabetes, hypertension, and cardiac disease cared for by nurse practitioners in health department clinics near their homes.[25] He found that in comparison with a group of patients attending traditional hospital outpatient clinics, that nurse practitioner patients experienced significant reductions in diastolic blood pressure, in blood glucose, and used 50 percent fewer hospital days.

One of the important questions still to be answered regarding the role of nurses in primary care is the extent to which care provided by nurses should serve as a substitute for the care of other providers, or whether nurses should primarily be involved in supplementing care provided by physicians. From a policy perspective, nursing care that substitutes for other sources is more justifiably reimbursable under third parties than is supplemental care, and many believe that third-party reimbursement is essential for the continued growth of nursing in the ambulatory care sector. On the other hand, many nurses present a strong case that if primary care nurses provide medical care, there will still be no one to provide nursing care, and that the current illness-oriented system will be perpetuated. The issue is not so much whether nurses *can* provide care for patients with common problems, but what are the implications of allocating time to those functions. Both positions are probably correct, and the answer lies somewhere in between.

Part of the difficulty in answering the issue of substitution versus complementarity is that nurses have not sufficiently documented the context of nursing care in ambulatory settings, and the relationship between nursing care and patient needs. The studies cited above provide ample evidence that nurses can be effective primary providers as measured by the traditional outcome measures. However, much of primary care is offering reassurance, providing information, and facilitating the development of coping skills. Primary emphasis should be placed on helping people assume more responsibility for their own health. The ways to do this are not nearly so well documented as the procedures for diagnosing a middle ear infection. Do the unique skills of the nurse lend themselves to the development of this neglected area of patient care? I would like to digress a moment to provide an example from my own research that seems to say yes.

In a recent study[26] of men recovering from myocardial infarction, I found that the typical visit to an outpatient clinic or a physician's office consisted of the taking of the patient's vital signs and weight, an electrocardiogram, possible blood work, and a short physical examination. Little interaction occurred that was not relevant to these tasks. Often wives accompanied their husbands on these visits but were rarely included in discussions with the physician. The sites studied were reasonably representative of medical subspecialty clinics in teaching hospitals, and of cardiologists in private practice, but there was no significant input by nurses. Although these patients probably received quite adequate monitoring and management of many of their physical problems, the number of psychosocial problems receiving no attention was staggering. In fact, these problems were perceived by the couples to be more serious than the medical problems that the physicians focused on. There was a high prevalence of depression and unhappiness among both the men and their wives. Three-quarters of these couples experienced serious difficulties dealing with health restrictions such as diet, smoking, and activity limitations. Although 78 percent of the men studied were in at least their second year since the heart attack, 60 percent were still unemployed. Unemployment brought about significant problems not only of a financial nature but also placed great strain on the husband-wife relationship. In addition, many of the men and their wives had incapacitating fears brought about by a lack of information.

Many of the problems that existed in the study population could have been alleviated by a nurse who assumed responsibility and accountability for these patients. Instead of a psychiatry consultation, most of these couples needed a knowledgable person to help them establish new patterns of coping, and to serve as a liaison with other community and social services. They needed a practitioner who could assess physical problems in the context of problems of living and maintaining a reasonable quality of life, and who would provide care on a continuing basis. Most of the care entailed in the routine examination could have been done by nurses while they were communicating about illness-related problems. Thus, the dichotomy between cure and care is many times amplified, and may represent a political issue related to the status of the profession rather than being a viable issue for practitioners.[27]

Of course, chronic illness is not the only important area for nurses in primary care. Increasingly, nurses are defining roles for themselves in all aspects of primary care. Pediatric nurse practitioners have demonstrated their competence and effectiveness in dealing with the well child, and many are increasingly involved in treating common acute illnesses. Family nurse practitioners, working in collaboration with family physicians, are beginning to establish an impressive record measured both in terms of health outcome and patient satisfaction. Although some progress has been made in recent years to improve the quality of primary care provided to women, this realm remains uncharted despite growing dissatisfaction among women in this country that the health care they receive is illness-oriented and unresponsive to their overall needs.

Reimbursement for nursing services are to be a key in the continuing growth of nursing in primary care. For example, the Burlington randomized trial cited earlier concluded that although the care given by nurses was comparable in outcome to that provided by physicians, nurse practitioners were not economically feasible because of current restrictions on reimbursement for nursing services. Attention must be given to the current options of entering into fee-for-service arrangements, of receiving reimbursement from government and private third parties, or of reallocating existing resources to pay for these services. Nurses in hospital settings have never really had to establish that nursing care was worth paying for. However, in the world of primary care, it is increasingly important for nurses to develop methodologies to document the contributions nursing care makes to health.

School health serves as an example of a primary care area that has employed nurses for a long time. However, it can be argued that school nurses have been supported by school systems primarily for legal and bureaucratic reasons, not because school nurses have demonstrated their effectiveness. In fact, we know relatively little about the potential value and feasibility of using the school as a locus for the delivery of primary care to children despite the long history of the school nurse. In addition, we do not even have a clear idea of the health problems of the school-age child. Many of the same comments can be made about public health nurses. Although interesting case studies of the effectiveness of public health nurses with particular patients appear in the literature, the number of systematic evaluations of public health nurses are quite limited. A notable exception is Runyan's study reported earlier.

In the primary care sector, the economic viability of nurses depends primarily upon some variant of fee-for-service to be payed by the consumer or by third-party insurers, or by the allocation of salaried positions supported by public funds. In either case, given the inflation spiral in health care and consumers' growing awareness of out-of-pocket costs and rising taxes, nurses must begin to document their practices. They must be able to define the services rendered and to establish outcome criteria to measure the effectiveness of those services. They must become accountable to the people they serve. Accountability in the hospital setting in some ways is easier to establish because the time frame is shorter and the nursing care tasks are more discrete than in the ambulatory setting. For instance, one can measure from day to day the effectiveness of skin care of the comatose patient. However, even the description of nursing tasks sometimes becomes ambiguous in the ambulatory setting, and evaluation of the nurse's effectiveness may have to take place over many weeks or months. Take, for instance, the mother who frequently brings her child in with vague presenting problems. It takes some time to establish whether the mother's anxiety is really the problem, and if so, how she can be helped. In addition, it would take months to evaluate whether the mother's utilization patterns changed.

I would make the case that ultimately the accountability of nurses in the ambulatory setting depends upon whether a defined population of patients exists. A defined population could consist of a panel of patients in a group practice, the children in a school, all new mothers in a community, the residents of a specific neighborhood, or many other variations. The critical ingredient is that the nurse have the opportunity to assess the health of her patients in ways that do not necessarily require the patient to make a decision that a visit is needed. Our health care system is primarily illness-oriented, even in the ambulatory setting. Thus, most encounters with health professionals are initiated by the patient because of some problem. People have quite different perceptions of illness and only those people who have reached some threshold will seek out the physician or the nurse. Until the health care system has developed the capacity to assess the health of populations and takes specific measures to deliver care to those who may not come but who may be at the greatest risk of serious illness, the system will continue to be illness-oriented.

Accountability in the ambulatory setting means having a reasonable assessment of the health prob-lems of the population to be served. Such an assessment can be made by estimates based upon published statistics, by surveying the population in some way, or by gathering information over time by "intake" interviews, chart audits, or other prac-tice information. The latter method is the least desirable unless there is information on the entire panel of patients. Many evaluations of practices suffer from using information that is only repre-sentative of people who present themselves for care, but says nothing about the people who did not come. There are a number of straightforward techniques that can be used to document the effectiveness of a practitioner. This should not be considered "research" but should be accepted as a normal responsibility of groups of practitioners. Thus, the techniques of practice evaluation should be an integral part of nursing curricula just as other knowledge and skills necessary for the prac-tice of nursing.

IMPLICATIONS FOR NURSING EDUCATION

This paper has attempted to make a case for the increased involvement of nurses in primary care. It has been pointed out that the consumer demands for ambulatory care are high, and that the unique skills of nurses can be quite important in improving care in this area. Further, ambulatory settings appear to offer greater potential for autonomy and joint practice with physicians than has been feasible in most hospital settings, and at a time when there are some projections of an over-supply of nurses, particularly in hospitals. How-ever, in order for nurses to assume greater respon-sibilities in primary care, some significant changes must occur in nursing education.

First, there must be greater efforts to provide learning experiences outside the walls of tertiary care centers with populations representing com-mon health problems. Second, a serious problem facing schools of nursing today is the lack of clinically prepared faculty to serve as role models for students and to provide meaningful clinical experiences. This problem is particularly serious in primary care since skills are now needed in primary care settings that many nurse faculty never learned in their own training. Further, in order to keep skills current, it is necessary to practice. In primary care, this optimally means having responsibility for a panel of patients. Given the heavy teaching loads in most schools of nursing, without reorganization and a commitment on the part of the dean it is almost impossible for faculty members to have enough time to develop a practice. Thus, it is essential that schools of nursing explore ways to provide faculty with practice time in addition to the time spent with students in clinical teaching. This may mean experimenting with ways to reduce teaching loads or of gaining reimbursement for the clinical services delivered by faculty members that can then be devoted to the salary of an additional faculty member to share teaching responsibilities.

Effective practice in most primary care settings includes joint practice with physicians. As mentioned previously, primary care offers a unique opportunity to develop autonomy. However, by "autonomy" it is not meant that nurses should work alone. On the contrary, primary care offers nurses the opportunity to develop autonomy through their professional relationships with physicians and other providers. Joint practice is a relationship to which both participants, as colleagues, bring their unique skills and knowledge to care more effectively for a patient population.[28] There has been considerable discussion in recent years about training physicians and nurses together in the hope that there would be greater appreciation of the unique contributions each could make to health. However, until there are faculty role models of joint collaborative practice, it is unlikely that student nurses and physicians will be able to overcome the traditional barriers associated with their respective roles. Our hopes and dreams for new practitiners must be embodied in the roles of the faculty. If joint practice is a goal for nursing and medicine, there must be faculty engaged in such practice.

NOTES

1 D. E. Rogers, "The Challenge of Primary Care," in J. Knowles (ed.), *Doing Better and Feeling Worse: American Health—Individual Dilemmas and Social Choices, Daedalus,* **106**(1), 1977.

2 C. Lewis, R. Fein, and D. Machanic, *A Right to Health,* Wiley, New York, 1976.

3 U.S. Department of Health, Education, and Welfare, "National Health Expenditures, Calendar Year 1974," in *Research and Statistics Note,* Social Security Administration, HEW Publications No. (SSH) 76-11701, Note No. 5, April 14, 1976.

4 R. Andersen, J. Kravitz, and O. Anderson, "The Public's View of the Crisis in Medical Care: An Impetus for Changing Delivery Systems?," *Economic and Business Bulletin,* **24**(1):44–52, Temple University, Philadelphia, 1972.

5 S. Strickland, *U.S. Health Care: What's Wrong and What's Right,* Universe, New York, 1972.

6 A. Donabedian et. al., *Medical Care Chart Book,* 5th ed., University of Michigan, Ann Arbor, 1972.

7 V. R. Fuchs, *Who Shall Live?*, Basic, New York, 1974.

8 R. Andersen, J. Kravits, and O. W. Anderson, *Equity in Health Services,* Ballinger, Cambridge, Mass., 1975.

9 W. McDermott, "General Medical Care: Identification and Analysis of Alternative Approaches," *Johns Hopkins Medical Journal,* **135**(5):292, 1974.

10 J. J. Alpert and E. Charney, *The Education of Physicians for Primary Care,* U.S. Department of Health, Education, and Welfare Publication No. (HRA) 74-3113, 1973.

11 S. Andreopoulous (ed.), *Primary Care: Where Medicine Falls,* Wiley, New York, 1974.

12 R. H. Ebert, "The Medical School," *Scientific American,* **229**(3):138–148, 1973.

13 N. Milio, *The Care of Health in Communities,* Macmillan, New York, 1975, p. 152.

14 K. L. White, T. F. Williams, and B. G. Greenberg, "The Ecology of Medical Care," *New England Journal of Medicine,* **265**:885–892, 1961.

15 A. Donabedian et al., *Medical Care Chart Book,* 5th ed., University of Michigan, Ann Arbor, 1972, p. 198.

16 *Hospital Statistics,* 1975 ed., table 1, p. 3, American Hospital Association, Chicago.

17 J. P. Newhouse, C. E. Phelps, and W. B. Schwartz, "Policy Options and the Impact of National Health Insurance," *New England Journal of Medicine,* 290:1345-1359, 1974.

18 D. Yett, *An Economic Analysis of the Nurse Shortage,* Lexington Books, Lexington, Mass., 1975.

19 A. V. Roth, "Trends in the Distribution of Nursing Manpower," in D. Hiestand and Miriam Ostow (eds.), *Health Manpower Information for Policy Guidance,* Ballinger, Cambridge, Mass., 1976.

20 V. R. Fuchs, op. cit.

21 *Present State and Future Needs of General Practice,* Royal College of General Practitioners, 3d ed., London, 1973.

22 W. McDermott, op. cit.

23 C. E. Lewis, B. A. Resnick, G. Schmidt, and D. Waxman, "Activities, Events, and Outcomes in Ambulatory Patient Care," *New England Journal of Medicine,* 280:645-649, 1969.

24 W. O. Spitzer et al., "The Burlington Randomized Trial of the Nurse Practitioner," *New England Journal of Medicine,* 290:251-256, 1974.

25 J. Runyan, "The Memphis Chronic Disease Program: Comparisons in Outcome and the Nurse's Expanded Role," *Journal of the American Medical Association,* 213:264-267, 1975.

26 L. H. Aiken, "Chronic Illness and Responsive Ambulatory Care," in D. Mechanic, *The Growth of Bureaucratic Medicine: An Inquiry into the Dynamics of Patient Behavior and the Organization of Medical Care,* Wiley, New York, 1976, pp. 239-251.

27 A. Bliss, "Nurse Practitioner: Victor or Victim of an Ailing Health Care System," *Nurse Practitioner,* pp. 10-14, May-June 1976.

28 I. Mauksch and P. Young, "Nurse-Physician Interaction in a Family Medical Care Center," *Nursing Outlook,* 22:113-119, 1974.

EDITOR'S QUESTIONS FOR DISCUSSION

What present skills of the nurse may be of value in primary care? What new skills will have to be developed? To function in a primary care setting, what should be the level of educational preparation for a nurse? What methods might be used to document type, quality, and accountability of care given by primary care nurses? How is autonomy developed through colleagial relationships? What effect(s) might fee-for-service as third-party reimbursement of nursing services have on the patient and on the professions of nursing and medicine?

Chapter 24

The Nursing Process

Dagmar E. Brodt, R.N., Ph.D.
Associate Professor, College of Nursing
Howard University, Washington, D.C.

Nurses are attempting to define their profession and to explore the unique role of nursing. Dagmar E. Brodt traces the early attempts to answer the question, "What is nursing?" She uses the term *nursing process* to include the broad function of assessing a patient's needs, planning action to meet those needs, implementing the plan, evaluating the patient's response, and reassessment of the patient. Brodt explores each of these steps and suggests that the term *assessment* is less controversial than *nursing diagnosis*. She uses a modified systems approach as a taxonomy of the patient's physiologic needs. The nursing activities are classified into six dimensions of nursing practice, and examples of nursing action appropriate to each dimension are provided. Brodt indicates the parallelism between the steps of the nursing process and the American Nurses Association Standards of Nursing Practice.

The nursing process as we know it today emerged from the intense introspection during the period of time nursing scholars were identifying the role of the nurse. During the early and mid-1960s, nursing leaders were trying to answer questions such as: "What is Nursing?," "What will be the role of the future nurse?," and "Are nurses really needed in today's technological society?" It was during this same period that McCain, Rothberg, Young, and the author among others were striving to describe the notions of nursing diagnosis, nursing assessment, nursing implementation, and nursing intervention. These notions evolved almost simultaneously in such diverse parts of the country as New York, Washington State, California, Michigan, Missouri, and Washington, D.C. The simultaneous evolvement of ideas by diversely located scientists occurs frequently in the scientific world.

Evidently, the groundwork for the development of these ideas had been laid, as it had for the basic elements of the nursing process. The idea of the nursing process was in response to the questions being generated about the role of the nurse.

The nursing process in its most concise form consists of assessing patient need, planning nursing action to meet that need, implementing the planned nursing action, evaluating the patient's response to the nursing action, and reassessing patient need and its reapplication in a cyclic pattern. Basically, the nursing process is an amplification and application of the problem-solving process to the task of nursing care of patients. The effective, comprehensive application of the nursing process will propel the patient to maximum potential recovery, as defined by the pathophysiological status of the patient.

The ANA (American Nurses Association) function studies and the sociological studies of the role of the nurse that were conducted during the decade of the fifties and the early sixties generated the introspective questions previously cited. Gillan (1951), Gordon (1953), and George and Kuehn (1955), who participated in the function studies for the American Nurses Association, identified the frequency with which various nursing procedures were performed and the time spent in their performance. Hughes, Hughes, and Deutscher (1958) summarized the findings of these studies and concluded that hospital nursing care is very unstandardized and that bedside care is no longer the principal occupation of the professional nurse. It comes as no surprise then that Reissman and Rohrer (1957), Bennis, Berkowitz, Malone, and Klein (1961), and Corwin (1961) discovered a conflict between what the nurse conceived as her job and what she actually did. Thorner (1955) and Meyer (1960) found a conflict between the expressive role with patients and the impersonal administrative values. These cited studies are only a small sample of research investigations about the role of the nurse.

In addition to the above evidence nurses began to find an increasing number of allied health personnel functioning in the health area, such as the physician's assistant, surgeon's assistant, dietary assistant, medical social work assistant, and many others. The advent of these health personnel relieved the nurse of some of the traditional responsibilities and further caused the nurse to question the uniqueness of the nurse role and the service contributions of the nurse. The delegation of duties to nursing service formerly performed only by physicians further added to the nurse's confusion as to the identity of the mission that the nurse is expected to embrace.

It is against the backdrop of this evidence from research and the realities of practice in health agencies that the nursing scholar tried to face these realities of nursing practice and began to pose questions such as: "What is nursing?" and "How can we define nursing?" It was then that nursing scholars stated that it was knowing *when* to perform a nursing task as well as *how* to perform it most effectively for a particular patient that was significant to patients and nursing. The number of times a nursing procedure was performed is not in itself significant. It is admittedly much more difficult to measure why an action was taken and whether that action was appropriate, than to measure the occurrence of the action. This realization led to identification of nursing assessment— the first step of the nursing process. Several nursing scholars encouraged the use of the term *nursing diagnosis* to be used for *nursing assessment*. The use of the term nursing diagnosis led to considerable controversy among many nurses, since the act of diagnosis in the medical arena had been the sole prerogative of the physician. However, the term assessment met with little or no objection by nursing; therefore, this term has been identified as the first step of the nursing process.

Nursing assessment of patient need consists of data collection, and analysis of data. These data are collected from interviewing the patient and his family and friends, the laboratory reports, the patient's medical history, the patient's chart, the physician, and the observation of the patient. In order to conduct a comprehensive and systematic data collection for nursing assessment of patient need, a detailed taxonomy of patient need must be employed. Maslow's hierarchy of human needs has application for the psychological realm but has minimum application for the specific pathophysiological response of the patient to illness. In order to systematically identify the needs of the patient, the author has employed for nursing assessment a modified physiological systems approach as a taxonomy of a patient's physiological need. Table 24-1 illustrates this taxonomy and examples of the data to be collected using the taxonomy. Unless systematic data collection is employed during the assessment phase, many important needs will be unrecognized and consequently unmet by appropriate nursing action. The analysis of the data collected leads directly into the second phase of the nursing process—the planning of the

Table 24-1   Patient Need Taxonomy

Areas of need/problem	Examples of need/problem
Patient positioning and movement	Be placed in functional alignment Be assisted with walking or moving with wheelchair or walker Be instructed in use of cane or crutches
Patient cardiopulmonary support	Receive monitoring of vital signs Receive adequate pulmonary ventilation Receive pharmaceuticals for cardiopulmonary function
Patient elimination support	Receive monitoring of elimination function Relief of bladder or bowel distention Receive bowel and bladder retraining (incontinence)
Patient skin integrity promotion	Relief of pressure on the skin Receive protection of skin Relief of dry skin Receive observation of skin temperature and color
Patient nutrition and fluid provision	Receive balanced diet and adequate fluid intake Receive food in appealing manner Receive monitoring of food and fluid intake
Patient psychosocial support	Receive information of routines and procedures Receive permission to express needs and feelings Receive discharge instruction Regain control of self and environment Maintain contact with family

appropriate nursing action to meet the needs identified and analyzed in phase one, assessment of patient need.

The analysis of nursing activities has led to the discovery that they can be classified into six dimensions of nursing practice. The dimensions provide an additional taxonomy to assist in planning the appropriate nursing action to meet the identified patient needs. These dimensions of nursing practice are as follows: (1) the prevention of complications; (2) the preservation of body defenses; (3) the detection of changes in the body's regulatory systems; (4) the reestablishment of the patient with the outside world; (5) the implementation of the physician's prescribed diagnostic and therapeutic activity; and (6) the provision of comfort and safety. All of nursing actions designed to meet patient need can be classified in

one of the cited dimensions of nursing practice.

Table 24-2 provides examples of nursing actions appropriate to each dimension. Even though these dimensions of nursing practice are not discrete and some nursing actions can be placed in more than one category, the use of these dimensions permits increased comprehensiveness in planning patient care and decreases the possibility of overlooking required nursing actions to meet patient need. The matrix that appears in Table 24-3 illustrates the nursing actions in each of the dimensions of nursing practice that can be planned for each area of patient need. The use of a matrix such as this will assist the nurse and the health team members to plan and provide for the diversity of nursing actions required by each individual patient.

The identification of the above-cited dimen-

Table 24-2   Dimensions of Nursing Practice

Dimensions of nursing practice with examples of appropriate nursing action	
1 Prevention of complications	a Observe for urinary retention-suppression
	b Teach patient deep-breathing exercises
	c Align patient's extremities anatomically
	d Turn patient frequently and massage compressed tissue
2 Preservation of body defenses	a Bathe and dry skin thoroughly
	b Position patient for optimum pulmonary ventilation
	c Provide and encourage adequate bowel elimination
	d Cleanse the mouth regularly
3 Detection of changes in body's regulatory system	a Monitor vital signs
	b Monitor intake and output (bowel and bladder)
	c Monitor diaphoresis—or dry flushed skin
	d Monitor neurological signs
4 Reestablishment of patient with the outside world	a Provide newspapers and radio news
	b Discuss current events
	c Arrange for visitors
	d Provide grooming aids and own clothes
5 Implementation of physician's prescribed diagnostic and therapeutic activity	a Instruct patient regarding therapy regimen
	b Administer medications and treatments
	c Observe and report effect of medications and treatments
	d Instruct patient regarding diagnostic tests
6 Provision of comfort and safety	a Install siderails for confused patient
	b Clear walkway of obstruction for ambulating patient
	c Support body with pillows for increased comfort
	d Support patient ambulating for first time

sions of nursing practice resulted from the author's research effort in the development of a tool to evaluate the quality of patient care. Through this effort the author was able to identify to her satisfaction the unique contribution of the registered nurse. Of all the health professionals, only the registered nurse can administer actions in response to patient needs represented by each of the nursing dimensions cited in Table 24-2. These dimensions are helpful in explaining to nonnurses the role of the nurse in the patient care arena.

The third step of the nursing process is to implement the planned nursing actions. Of course, it is incumbent on the nurse to implement the planned nursing actions in a safe manner that pro-duces the least possible discomfort for the patient and that does not violate the therapeutic effect of the nursing actions. Adaptations to the particular patient's limitations will be required. Such adaptations frequently will be dictated by the patient's needs, such as discomfort when turning on right or left side, or a spica cast that prevents him from turning to either side; by a prolapsed rectum requiring adaptations in the enema procedure; or by a 30 percent second-degree body burn requiring adaptations in the bath and dressing procedures. Safety and adaptations are the special requirements for the nurse in implementing the appropriate nursing actions planned in Step 2 of the nursing process.

Table 24-3 Areas of Patient Need

Dimensions of nursing practice	Positioning and movement	Cardiopulmonary support	Skin integrity promotion	Elimination promotion	Nutrition and fluid provision	Psychosocial support
Preservation of body defenses	Turn patients frequently	Position for optimum pulmonary excursions	Bathe patient or infant	Establish regular elimination schedule	Provide balanced diet and encourage fluid intake	Inform the patient what you are going to do for him
Prevention of complications	Position footboard to prevent footdrop	Teach deep breathing exercises	Massage reddened skin areas	Palpate for a distended bladder	Regulate flow of IV fluids	Allow patient to ventilate his feelings
Provision of comfort and safety	Raise siderails	Splint incision while assisting patient to cough	Rub back at bedtime	Provide privacy toiletry warm bedpan	Serve hot foods hot and cold foods cold	Reduce patient's anxiety by orientation to hospital routine
Implementation of physician's prescribed therapeutic and diagnostic activity	Give range of motion exercises	Suction to maintain patient airway	Apply sterile dressing	Administer enema or catheterization	Give IV fluids	Instruct patient in special procedures
Detection of changes in body's regulatory systems	Observe balance in movement	Monitor vital signs	Observe skin temperature and color	Monitor urine and bowel elimination	Monitor food and fluid intake	Observe patient's contact with reality
Reestablishment of patient with outside world	Move the patient so he can visit with other patients	Teach patient to give himself aerosol therapy	Teach patient to change his own dressings	Implement bladder and bowel retraining	Arrange for patient to eat in company of others	Discuss patient's plan after discharge and focus attention on world around him

The last step of the first cycle of the nursing process is to evaluate the effects of the planned and implemented nursing action upon the assessed patient need. Questions must be asked during this evaluation such as: "Did the nursing action relieve the patient's discomfort?," "Is he resting more comfortably?," "Is the decubitus ulcer giving evidence of healing?," "Is the paralyzed foot remaining in alignment?," "Is bladder retraining becoming a reality?," "Is the patient less withdrawn?," "Is he communicating more easily?," and "Does he seem to be in closer contact with reality?" Each identified patient need and planned and implemented nursing action must be evaluated to determine if the need was relieved or attenuated. The data received during this evaluation process become a portion of the data required for the assessment of patient need for the subsequent cycle of the nursing process.

It is significant to point out that Standards of Nursing Practice published by the American Nurses Association in 1973 possess a striking parallelism to the nursing process. The assessment phase encompasses Standards I and II.

ANA Standard I. "The collection of data about the health status of the client/patient is systematic and continuous. The data are accessible, communicated and recorded."

ANA Standard II. "Nursing diagnoses are derived from health status data."

Standards III and IV are included in the planning phase of the nursing process.

ANA Standard III. "The plan of nursing care includes goals derived from the nursing diagnoses."

ANA Standard IV. "The plan of nursing care includes priorities and the prescribed nursing approaches or measures to achieve goals derived from the nursing diagnoses."

The implementation phase of the nursing process is represented by Standards V and VI.

ANA Standard V: "Nursing actions provide for client/patient participation in health promotion, maintenance and restoration."

ANA Standard VI. "Nursing actions assist the client/patient to maximize his health capabilities."

ANA Standards VII and VIII of the 1973 ANA Standards of Nursing Practice comprise the evaluation phase of the nursing process.

ANA Standard VII. "The client's/patient's progress or lack of progress toward good achievement is determined by the client/patient and the nurse."

ANA Standard VIII. "The client's/patient's progress or lack of progress toward goal achievement directs reassessment, reordering of priorities, new goal setting and revision of the plan of nursing care."

These ANA Standards for nursing practice appear to validate the nursing process. The parallelism is apparent.

The nursing process using the taxonomies of patient need and nursing practice has been used successfully as a framework for curriculum development of a new program in nursing. The basic skills and concepts appropriate to each area of patient need were clustered to form a unit of instruction. This organization of instruction assisted the student to establish learning hooks so that he could assimilate and organize the many facets of patient care. Behavioral objectives with corresponding evaluation items were formulated for each unit and subunit. Commercially prepared audiovisual materials were reviewed and those appropriate to the behavioral objectives were purchased and incorporated into the instructional content of the respective units. Behavioral objectives unmet in this manner were transmitted either through instructor-prepared audiovisual presentations or through other forms of instructional presentation forms such as lecture, discussion, seminars, etc. The nursing process and the taxonomies were used in clinical practice, preparation of care plans, and the preparation of care studies. The diagrammatic conceptual framework appears in Figure 24-1. Repeated references to this diagram and the manner in which the nursing process was to be applied were made during the instructional program.

It is possible that at sometime in the future a computer will be programmed for arrays of patient needs and problems to match a range of appropriate nursing actions. By providing to the computer input terminal the need status of the patient, a printout of appropriate nursing actions and expected results would be obtained. Protocols of patient need—nursing action—and expected results from application of the nursing process would be a prototype of the software required for computer readouts.

As a nurse becomes adept in using the nursing process with the taxonomies herein described, it will be found that the nurse will interrelate dimen-

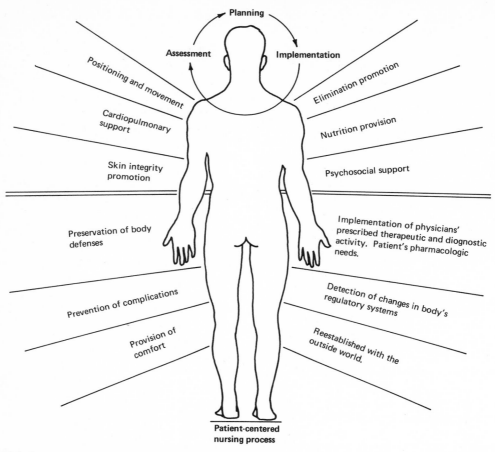

Figure 24-1 Patient need — The reason for nursing care

sions of nursing practice to meet the various areas of patient need almost simultaneously. It is the expert nurse's ability to minister to patient need in this manner that lends uniqueness to her role in the health care arena. The dynamic exquisite application of the nursing process in all of its complexities to the needs of patients will propel patients to recovery and improve the health status of the community.

The application of the nursing process to patient care provides a rational approach to that care. Intuition is replaced by rationality. The nursing process specifies the nursing action appro-

priate to each patient need. It indeed leads to comprehensiveness in patient care, minimizing the unmet patient needs. The application of the nursing process using the appropriate taxonomies should lead to increased satisfaction obtained by the nursing practitioner.

BIBLIOGRAPHY

American Nurses Association: *Standards of Nursing Practice*, Kansas City, Mo., 1973.
Bennis, W. G., N. H. Berkowitz, Mary F. Malone,

and M. W. Klein: *The Role of the Nurse in the Outpatient Department*, American Nursing Foundation, New York, 1961.

Brodt, Dagmar: *Rationale for Nursing Practice*, unpublished paper, 1964.

———: "A Synergistic Theory of Nursing," *American Journal of Nursing*, **69**:1674–1676, 1969.

———, and Ellen H. Anderson: "Validation of a Patient Welfare Instrument," *Nursing Research*, **16**(2):167–169, Spring 1967.

Corwin, R. G.: "The Professional Employee: A Study of Conflict in Nursing Roles," *American Journal of Sociology*, **66**:604–615, 1961.

George, Frances L., and Ruth P. Kuehn: *Pattern of Patient Care: Some Studies of the Utilization of Nursing Service Personnel*, Macmillan, New York, 1955.

Gillan, Ruth I.: "Effective Organization of the Nursing Services Leads to Improved Patient Care," *Modern Hospital*, **51**:49–51, 1951.

Gordon, H. P.: "Who Does What—The Report of a Nursing Activities Study," *American Journal of Nursing*, **53**:564–566, 1953.

Hughes, E. C., Helen Hughes, and I. Deutscher: *Twenty Thousand Nurses Tell Their Story*, Lippincott, Philadelphia, 1958.

McCain, Faye R.: "Nursing by Assessment—Not Intuition," *American Journal of Nursing*, **65**: 82–84, 1965.

Meyer, Genevieve: *Tenderness and Technique*, Institute of Human Relations, University of California, Los Angeles, 1960.

Reissman, L., and J. H. Rohrer: *Change and Dilemma in the Nursing Profession*, Putnam, New York, 1957.

Rothberg, June S.: "Why Nursing Diagnosis?," *American Journal of Nursing*, **67**:1040–1042, 1967.

Thorner, I.: "Nursing: The Functional Significance of an Institutional Pattern," *American Sociological Review*, **20**:531–538, 1955.

Young, Lucie S.: "Needs of the Patient as Seen by the Nurse," *Pennsylvania Medicine*, **71**:51–55, 1968.

Yura, Helen, and Mary Walsh: *The Nursing Process*, Appleton-Century-Crafts, New York, 1973.

EDITOR'S QUESTIONS FOR DISCUSSION

Are there other areas in the taxonomy of patients' needs and dimensions of nursing practice that might be included in the matrix of nursing action? What are the implications for patient care and nursing practice of the use of a computer to program areas of patients' needs to be matched with appropriate nursing actions? How does one individualize patient care in using the nursing process? How might different types of nursing personnel use the nursing process? Is the use of the nursing process a function of a unique role in nursing?

Chapter 25

Nursing Diagnoses
and the Diagnostic Process

Marjory Gordon, R.N., Ph.D., F.A.A.N.
Associate Professor, Department of Nursing
Boston College

Marjory Gordon introduces the controversial subject of nursing diagnosis and proposes a distinction between nursing diagnoses and medical diagnoses. A nursing diagnosis describes a state of the patient rather than focusing on functional needs and the nursing activity that Brodt includes in assessment. A diagnosis is considered as a separate entity within the nursing process. Diagnosis involves a synthesis of assessment data and provides the focus for determining nursing activities. In the definition of a nursing diagnosis Gordon includes the health problem, the cause of the problem, and the signs and symptoms of the problem, but limits the definition to actual or potential health problems that nurses, by virtue of their education and experience, are capable of treating and are licensed to treat. In addition, she suggests that professional domains should not be rigid and absolute.

Diagnoses are shorthand ways of referring to a cluster of signs and symptoms that occur as a clinical entity. For example, rather than describing a patient's cold and clammy skin, pallor, tachycardia, fall in blood pressure, verbal expressions of nervousness, and restlessness three hours after abdominal surgery, the term hemorrhagic shock is used.

Nursing diagnoses describe health problems in which the responsibility for therapeutic decisions can be assumed by a professional nurse. In general, these problems encompass potential or actual disturbances in life processes, patterns, functions, or development, including those occurring secondary to disease.

Traditionally, preventive health care or health maintenance has been a nursing concern. Many high-risk states or potential health problems are amenable to nursing therapy. Within areas of potential or actual disturbances in health, additional diagnostic nomenclature needs to be identified.

According to Bloch in her review of crucial terms in nursing, the word diagnosis, when used in nursing practice, is still considered controversial (1). However, until nurses can name the health problems they treat, nursing will remain a vague entity to legislators, third-party payers, administrators, professional colleagues, and sometimes to other nurses.

This article is reprinted from *The American Journal of Nursing*, vol. 76, no. 8, pp. 1298–1300, August 1976.

Paralleling the development of diagnostic nomenclature is the need for increasing diagnostic skills. The use of nursing diagnoses is inseparable from the use of the diagnostic process.

WHAT IS A DIAGNOSTIC CATEGORY?

As a general guideline, diagnostic categories should be clear, concise, well-defined, and should convey sufficient information to suggest to the knowledgeable nursing practitioner the major elements of a care plan.

Each diagnostic concept, or category, is distinguished by its label and defining cluster of signs and symptoms. Having a specific category permits discrimination among different states-of-the-patient. For example, redness and increased warmth over the coccygeal area are defining characteristics of potential skin breakdown in a patient who has been supine for long periods. When a small ulceration appears, the state-of-the-patient has changed. Now, the appropriate diagnosis is decubitus ulceration.

Diagnostic categories may vary in their levels of abstraction. Acute anxiety is a more specific category than the rape-trauma syndrome described by Burgess and Holstrum, which encompasses a cluster of related problems, each with its own signs and symptoms (2). The degree of abstraction is influenced by such factors as clinical usefulness or therapeutic practicality and by the extent of available knowledge. Dropsy, for example, was once a medical diagnosis. As more became known about dropsy and its etiology, more discriminating categories replaced it.

WHAT ARE THE COMPONENTS?

A diagnostic category as it is now evolving has three components: the state-of-the-patient or health problem, the etiology of the problem, and the signs and symptoms. This format appears most clinically practical at the present stage of nomenclature development.

In writing the first component, the patient's problem, it might, for example, be described as anticipatory anxiety, independence-dependence conflict, or mobility impairment. Qualifying or quantifying adjectives or other specifications are employed to identify stages, phases, or levels of a particular problem. Mobility impairment, for instance, to be of clinical use must specify the level of impairment. Similarly, such terms as acute or chronic may be used to specify stages. The anatomical site may also be specified when this needs to be known.

Considering a diagnostic category as representing a state-of-the-patient helps one focus on describing a patient rather than a nursing activity. Many nurses tend to talk about a patient's health problem in terms of functional concepts like "needs reassurance" or "provide adequate oxygenation," rather than to specify the problem first. One way to shift emphasis is to ask why this person needs reassurance, suctioning, or any other nursing activity. The answer is a description of the patient's state—anticipatory anxiety or potential respiratory obstruction.

The second major component is the etiology of the problem. Differentiation among possible etiologies is extremely important because each may require different therapy. In an ambulatory care setting, for example, noncompliance with drug therapy may result from lack of knowledge, a motivational deficit, or denial of illness. The action taken depends on the probable cause of the patient's problem.

Signs and symptoms are the third component. They define the category; or from a utilization perspective, they are the patient behaviors used to make the diagnosis.

With some diagnoses, it is useful to know the level of compensation the patient and his family have attained. A patient may have a permanent mobility problem, but he has compensated for it by using a cane or other device; or his anxiety may be somewhat lessened by a supportive family. A fully compensated but chronic problem must be recognized, especially when it can influence or be influenced by another health problem. Designating the compensatory level is particularly useful when care is provided over long periods.

The Problem-Etiology-Signs/Symptom (PES) format for nursing diagnoses can be easily adapted to current clinical record-keeping or charting systems. In the problem-oriented system, for example, when there is a sufficient data base, the "problem" diagnosed may be anticipatory anxiety. Under the "assessment" entry may be placed the etiology or suspected etiology, such as impending surgery. The observed signs and symptoms that were used to diagnose the problem would be recorded under the subjective and objective categories of the SOAP format. If nursing care plans are in use, the problem and etiology can be recorded in the "problem" column and the therapy, as usual, in the "methods" column.

NOMENCLATURE OF DIAGNOSTIC CATEGORIES

The content of diagnostic categories as well as their structure must be considered. A number of classification systems are available that list standardized diagnostic nomenclature (3,4). These, however, were developed to classify causes of death, disease, or pathology, and therefore do not meet nursing practice needs. Additional categories have to be identified, standardized, and added to existing nomenclature systems (5). The report of National Conferences on a Classification System of Nursing Diagnoses is an excellent point for clinicians to start using and refining terminology(6).

Rather than delaying using nursing diagnoses until sophisticated labels are developed, terms found to be clinically useful can be employed. Once nurses begin to describe the health problems they treat, discussions about the best way to state a diagnosis will result.

I offer the following definition for reaction and to clarify the concept of a nursing diagnosis so that it can be put into practice:

Nursing diagnoses, or clinical diagnoses made by professional nurses, describe actual or potential health problems which nurses, by virtue of their education and experience, are capable and licensed to treat.

To treat, or the provision of treatment, refers to the initiation of accepted modes of therapy, that is, the management of the problem. This definition thereby excludes health problems for which the accepted mode of therapy is prescription drugs, surgery, radiation, and other treatments that are defined legally as the practice of medicine.

Obviously, the basis for defining nursing diagnoses in this way is to discriminate between medical and nursing diagnostic categories. Current definitions do not give sufficient guidelines for practice, although they do help to clarify the concept. A definition must be open enough to accommodate changes. As knowledge and understanding change, treatments change, producing changes in practice.

The phrase, "capable and licensed to treat," and the definition of treatment are used to exclude medical diagnoses, such as lymphatic leukemia. Nurses are not educated or licensed to initiate the accepted modes of cancer therapy. Some nurses may have the knowledge and skill to make such diagnoses, but legally they cannot *independently* institute currently accepted treatments.

The diagnosis of medical diseases by nurses is merely an intellectual exercise or a *medically dependent* function controlled by protocols. If nurses wish to include this in their practice, they are free to do so, but it is confusing to refer to this activity as nursing diagnosis.

This definition does not negate the fact that nurses identify possible carcinoma in a patient or such secondary pathophysiological complications as hemorrhagic shock, arrhythmias, cardiac arrest, or pulmonary edema. Clearly, a nurse tentatively identifies those conditions before she decides to refer the problem or the patient to a physician or other professional or to institute palliative, emergency therapy. The definition does suggest that identifying medical problems *should not be formally referred to as making nursing diagnoses.*

Underlying the proposed statement on nursing

diagnosis is the assumption that many health problems require a collaborative effort of physician and nurse. With the complexity of human beings and their health problems, professional domains cannot have boundaries that are totally absolute or rigid.

By including the phrase "capable to treat" and the scope of the major responsibility for therapeutic decisions, I am implying several things. First, each nurse needs to assume professional responsibility for evaluating her current knowledge, experience, and capability. Next, formal and continuing education programs should offer nurses opportunities to attain needed competencies. And last, as diagnostic categories are identified, nursing research on therapy and prediction of outcomes must be undertaken.

THE DIAGNOSTIC PROCESS

The process of clinical diagnosis involves collecting, clustering, weighing, and validating information. Isolated signs and symptoms, generally, have no meaning and, therefore, do not suggest a therapeutic approach. For example, a care plan cannot be decided upon with just the symptom "crying at intervals" or "dyspnea." Cues to the state-of-the-patient/client have to be combined, weighed, and, perhaps, observed across time before meaning can be derived. The end product is the placement of the patient in one or more diagnostic categories for purposes of determining therapy for him.

Beginning research on cognitive strategies used by nurses in diagnosing patient problems suggests that diagnosis is much more complex than has been assumed (7). However, as King points out, some similarities do exist between the diagnostic process and the everyday discrimination or identification of things encountered in the environment. The difference lies in the nature of the information that has to be processed in making clinical inferences or diagnoses. According to King,

. . . although diagnosis ordinarily has medical

connotations, this is not essential, for the term involves activities by no means unique to medicine. Although we may think of diagnosis as the identification of disease, such usage is far too narrow. The word means *to distinguish.* It involves the process of deliberate choice or discrimination, the process whereby we say that *this*—whatever it may represent—is an example of *that*—whatever that may happen to be. If I say, *this* is a *rose*, I am making a diagnosis, and so also with *this* is a *yellow warbler* or *this* is *cancer of the breast.* (8)

Some information will be difficult to process. For example, human behavior varies and inferences from behavior to a diagnostic category cannot be made with absolute certainty (9). Even in the more objective pathophysiological categories, inferences from signs and symptoms to states-of-the-patient, or vice versa, are usually probabilistic. The sign, elevated temperature, does not always signify an infection nor does its absence negate an infection. Because of this probabilistic nature of diagnostic concepts, the clinician must learn the most highly reliable and distinguishing signs and symptoms and place most confidence in these in reaching a diagnosis.

Highly reliable clinical cues are the signs and symptoms most highly correlated with a particular state. Most patients having a particular entity will exhibit these signs and symptoms. Only if these factors are present may the category be used appropriately. For example, the most reliable signs of hemorrhagic shock in a normotensive patient are systolic blood pressure below 100 and a potential or observable source of bleeding. Other signs may accompany this state, like cold and clammy skin, tachycardia, and apprehension. Yet, without knowing the blood pressure, these signs are insufficient for making this diagnosis.

Some diagnostic categories cannot be defined by objective, clinical signs and symptoms, especially those describing psychosocial states. Because human behavior is variable, there is a need for subjective validation by the patient. Signs may point to anxiety due to alterations in body image. The probability of this diagnosis increases greatly if the patient has said that he views his body differently than he previously did and that this worries him.

If the uncertainty-geared, probabilistic nature of clinical diagnosis is appreciated, the most reliable cues to the patient's state will be sought. This should increase the clinician's confidence in the diagnosis that is made. Delaying a diagnostic judgment to continue to collect information will not necessarily decrease error. The quality, not necessarily the quantity, of information is important. However, the avoidance of premature closure is equally important. A premature decision leads to precipitous diagnostic judgments without sufficient, reliable information.

Diagnostic categories can also be misused by stereotyping, closing out alternatives, or employing value-laden categories. To avoid this, practitioners must learn the ethical, legal, and professional use of nursing diagnoses.

REFERENCES

1 Bloch, Doris. Some crucial terms in nursing: what do they really mean? *Nurs. Outlook* **22**: 689–694, Nov. 1974.

2 Burgess, A. W., and Holstrum, L. I. Rape trauma syndrome. *Am. J. Psychiatry* **131**:981–986, Sept. 1974.

3 American Psychiatric Association, Committee on Nomenclature and Statistics. *Diagnostic and Statistical Manual of Mental Disorders.* 2d ed. Washington, D.C., The Association, 1968.

4 Huffman, E. K. Disease and operation nomenclatures. In *Medical Record Management,* ed. by E. Price. Berwyn, Ill., Physician's Record Co., 1972.

5 Roy, Sister Callista. Diagnostic classification system for nursing. *Nurs. Outlook* **23**:90–94, Feb. 1975.

6 Gebbie, K. M., and Lavin, M. A. eds. *Classification of Nursing Diagnoses.* Proceedings of the First National Conference, held in St. Louis, October 1–5, 1973. St. Louis, C. V. Mosby Co., 1975.

7 Gordon, M. *Strategies in Probabilistic Concept Attainment: A Study of Nursing Diagnosis.* Boston, Mass., Boston College, 1972. (Doctoral Dissertation)

8 King, L. S. What is a diagnosis? *JAMA* **202**:715, Nov. 20, 1967.

9 Brunswick, E. *Systematic and Representative Design of Psychological Experiments.* Berkeley, Calif., Univ. of California Press, 1947.

EDITOR'S QUESTIONS FOR DISCUSSION

What are some examples of health problems that nurses are capable of treating and are licensed to treat? How did you use a nursing diagnosis to arrive at these examples? Which term best describes this function of nursing—*assessment* or *nursing diagnosis*? Is nursing diagnosis actually a part of nursing assessment or vice versa? Of what importance is it for the nursing profession and nursing practice to define and label these functions?

Chapter 26

Nursing and Medical Diagnoses: A Comparison of Variant and Essential Features

Carol A. Soares, R.N., Ph.D.
Associate Professor, School of Nursing
Boston University

Carol A. Soares delves further into the issue of defining the process of making a nursing diagnosis and comparing it with a medical diagnosis. She provides clear, distinct examples to differentiate the two types of diagnoses. She also analyzes the nursing diagnosis in sociological terms. Soares differs from Gordon in her declaration that the term *state* is insufficiently discriminative to differentiate a nursing diagnosis from other types of diagnoses. A medical diagnosis defines the pathologic state of a patient, which would identify abnormal organ systems (disorders or diseases); in comparison, a nursing diagnosis by use of a holistic model defines altered patterns of human functioning (problems). Soares examines the differences in terms of resultant *actions* for therapy. Soares's taxonomy of patient needs differs from Brodt's, except in the biophysical category. Contrary to Brodt's, her categories of patients' needs in themselves do not suggest which nursing acts to prescribe. The identification of the underlying cause of a problem is a further necessary step that directly affects nursing intervention.

Nursing as a professional discipline comprises practitioners, i.e., nurses, who arrive at similar decisions, i.e., nursing diagnoses, and who perform similar actions, i.e., nursing interventions. Nurses have always collected patient information, made decisions about states of health and/or illness, and performed actions in light of their inferences. However, the process in which nurses have engaged to arrive at nursing diagnoses has been, until recently, a taken-for-granted activity. The selecting of information and the making of decisions about patients by nurses in the United States prior to the sixties had been, for the most part, an unsystematic and intuitive process. Nurses who developed clinical cognitive skills based their intuitive hunches on their past experiences of working closely with master clinicians, nurses, and physicians.

As a discipline emerges from preprofessional status, its members begin to parlay intuitive hunches into rational inferences. The discipline begins to establish a formalized systematic ap-

The author appreciatively acknowledges the dialogic exchange of ideas related to this discussion with colleagues and students of Boston University School of Nursing.

proach to the problem solving within its practice. Currently in nursing, this emergent, organized, problem-solving activity is referred to as the *nursing process.* However, process is not unique to nursing. All disciplines whose practitioners make judgments and act on them use process. Inherent within this latter statement are the two essential features of process: (1) the judgment, and (2) the action. In nursing, these are referred to as *nursing diagnosis* and *nursing care* or *intervention.*

Although several authors have written about nursing diagnosis, the definition of the term is still unclear (Block, 1974, p. 692). Nurses vary in their opinions as to what constitutes the essential features of a nursing diagnosis. Their definitions of a diagnosis vary from stating it is a symptom, a need, or a problem, to a concern and/or a prescription. In addition, other nurses interchange the terms *needs, problems,* and *concerns.*

Part of the problem leading to this confusion in terminology is related to the level of professionalism reflected in the emerging articulation of a conceptual framework for nursing. For example, when nurses offer diagnoses, they address themselves to the *state* of the patient. Is this term particular to nursing? Do not physicians and other health care workers also address themselves to the state of the patient? Thus, the term state in itself is not sufficiently discriminative to differentiate nursing diagnoses from other types of diagnoses. Nursing diagnoses are differentiated from other diagnoses by the particular frame of reference the disciple utilizes to define *the* state of the patient. This frame of reference is referred to as a *conceptual framework.* It includes the specific knowledge that a person needs to have in order to identify and solve the particular problems within the domain of the field.

An analysis of the components of the diagnostic process in the health field should be invariable for all problem-solving professions. The variability in the diagnosis of problems in the health field stems from each individual discipline's viewpoint about the state of the patient. Since the recognized and legitimized diagnostician within the health field is the physician, an analysis of the

essential features of medical diagnosis should reveal the invariable features of diagnosis and shed light on how nursing's perspective of the state of the patient differs from medicine's.

The state of the patient that the physician addresses himself to in a confirmed medical diagnosis can be analyzed as comprising a statement about the pathological state of a person's anatomical structure and/or pathological organ functioning that can be alleviated or corrected by surgery or pharmacodynamics. These statements (diagnoses) are categorized by members of the medical profession and can (potentially) be independently treated by the practitioners of that discipline. The second part of this statement is an important component. It implies that diagnostic categories made by members of a particular discipline can potentially be independently treated by the practitioners of that discipline.

Thus, there are two aspects to a medical diagnosis: (1) the pathological state of the patient, and (2) the implied right of medicine to treat the diagnosed state. The ability and the ethical and legal right to independently perform a treatment, prescription, or intervention is inherent within a diagnostic statement.

If a nurse diagnoses a patient as being in diabetic coma, is she making a *nursing* diagnosis? The implied treatment, the administration of intravenous insulin, is not an *independent* nursing action. It is within the domain of medicine and, in this case, the nurse made a medical diagnosis. Therefore, one aspect of the definition of the state of the patient has to do with the practitioner being able to change or maintain it. The other aspect defines the state the physician is assessing, i.e., disease processes—something that is not normal. The abnormal is diagnosed from the expected criterion of normal.

What normal states does the nurse assess in order to diagnose an abnormal state that can be alleviated and/or corrected by independent nursing intervention? The answer to this question will frame the kinds of categories the nurse will use in defining a nursing diagnosis.

It has already been said that diabetic coma is a

Table 26-1 Medical and Nursing Diagnoses

	Medicine	
Normal criteria	**Abnormal findings**	**Medical diagnosis**
Pancreatic structure and physiological function	Deterioration of beta cells in Islet of Langerhan and inability to produce insulin and metabolize carbohydrates with resulting acidosis	Diabetic coma

	Nursing	
Normal criteria	**Abnormal findings**	**Nursing diagnosis**
Balanced circadian rhythm in rest/wake patterns	Disruption in rest/wake pattern—inability to awaken	Altered state of consciousness

medical diagnosis, not a category of nursing diagnosis. The implied treatment is not an independent nursing intervention. Is altered state of consciousness a nursing category? Since there are nursing actions that nurses can independently perform for patients with altered states of consciousness, it is a nursing category.

The categories *diabetic coma* and *altered state of consciousness* refer back to dysfunctions of two different states of the patient (see Table 26-1). Examining the two diagnoses in terms of implied *actions* distinguishes medical therapy from nursing. Deterioration of beta cells and the inability to produce insulin cannot be treated by *direct* nursing intervention. The nurse assists the physician when she administers insulin. This is a medically delegated task. In these tasks, the nurse functions as a physician's assistant. Altered state of consciousness as a nursing diagnosis of disruptions in rest/wake patterns cuts across many medical diagnoses, e.g., cerebral glioma, cardiovascular accident, diabetic coma, etc. All may present a state of altered consciousness. Nursing actions are in the realm of all those activities the patient would do for himself if he were able, such as breathing, eliminating, eating, moving, attending to personal hygiene, etc. (Henderson, 1966, p. 15 and Wiedenbach, 1964, pp. 14–15). Assisting the patient with

his human functioning is within the domain of nursing and constitutes its independent practice.

The independent practice of nursing is autonomous from medicine. Its dependent practice intersects with medicine. If the crucial aspect of each discipline is its respective diagnoses, nursing and medicine are not competitive but cooperative. Each supports and complements one another.

A comparison of nursing diagnoses with medical diagnoses shows that medicine defines findings that are abnormal organ systems (diseases), whereas nursing diagnoses define altered patterns of human functioning (problems). Persons with a disease, in most cases, also have an altered pattern of human functioning. The nursing and medical therapies for these patients and/or clients will support one another. Conversely, persons who have altered patterns of human functioning *do not* necessarily have a disease process, e.g., persons in an alpha state induced through meditation. The problems of altered human functioning constitute independent nursing practice. However, a persistent altered pattern of human functioning can lead to biophysical pathological dysfunction. Therefore, nursing interventions aimed at reordering patterns of human dysfunctioning can lead to the prevention of biophysical disease, and thus support medicine in an independent manner.

In order to diagnose an altered pattern of human functioning, the nurse initially assesses the patient's needs. The nurse's assessment tool must incorporate *neutral* categories from which the nurse can collect data that point to the absence or presence of healthy patterns of human functioning. The category is neutral; the collected empirical data imply a positive or negative value inference.

The physician's assessment tool, i.e., the physical examination, also includes a list of neutral categories. In this case, the medical perspective of the state of the patient stems from an organic structural approach to health and illness. The neutral categories are conceptualized in terms of body systems, e.g., the gastrointestinal system. Illness inferences about the gastrointestinal system, such as paralytic ileus or bowel obstruction, are interpreted from concrete data.

Interviews with nurses about the empirical evidence they use to make inferences revealed that, in many cases, assessment is a taken-for-granted activity and cannot be easily articulated. Nurses commonly stated, "I had a hunch," or "I've seen this before." Frequently, concrete and inference data are interchanged as being observable, e.g., cyanosis (an inference) and clubbing of the fingers (concrete datum). Cyanosis is not an immediately observable phenomenon. It is a first-order inference made from observing a blue tinge of the skin. The blue color is observable; cyanosis is not. Another example is hemorrhage. In itself it is not a concrete observable datum. In fact, it is a clustering of a number of empirical data, such as blood pressure readings, color and temperature of the skin, hemoglobin and hematocrit laboratory findings, etc.

Differentiation between concrete, first-order, and second-order inference data is not merely an academic exercise. It is to the absence or presence of the concrete data, not inferences, that the nurse must return to evaluate the effectiveness of nursing intervention. In other words, it is precisely the taken-for-granted concrete presenting evidence

(signs) that nurses use to point to first-order concepts (symptoms)[1] which are further delegated into second-order categories (needs). Neither symptoms or needs are empirically observable. They are subjective, positive or negative meanings (values) imposed upon empirical evidence from a preexisting set of categories, such as are used in an assessment tool. Thus, the neutral categories used in an assessment tool are of crucial importance, since they determine what is or is not to be observed.

The particular neutral categories nurses use in assessing wellness are embedded within a particular point of view. Since nursing differs from medicine, which is primarily concerned with the biophysical disease processes assessed through body systems, nursing's perspective is much broader.

A review of major nursing theorists, such as Virginia Henderson (1966), Imogene King (1968), Florence Nightingale (1946), Ida Jean Orlando (1961), Dorothea Orem (1971), Martha Rogers (1970), and Ernestine Wiedenbach (1964), indicates that their theories focus on nursing as promoting health and preventing disease. Health or wellness is an essential feature of nursing. The holistic approach to patient care is stressed in nursing.

In considering individuals as holistic beings, there are several conceptual systems in the literature that can be used to describe needs in terms of neutral categories. An example of one is Abraham Maslow's "hierarchy of needs." Basically, the holistic conceptualization of being incorporates the following systems: (1) biophysical, (2) psychosocial, (3) cognitive-perceptual, and (4) cultural-spiritual. For the purpose of discussing nursing diagnoses, references will be made to holistic being in terms of these four systems. This does not imply that these four systems are the only way to define human beings. The functions of these four systems are as follows:

---

[1] Symptom, here, is not used in the traditional sense—a patient's subjective impression—but as the practitioner's subjective inference of objective evidence.

1 The function of the biophysical system is to sustain life.

2 The function of the psychosocial system is to sustain the individual as a person and to sustain and perpetuate the community.

3 The function of the cognitive-perceptual system is to sustain and create meaning of life for an individual within the world of every-day life.

4 The function of the cultural-spiritual system is to sustain, create, and perpetuate the meaning and purpose of life for the individual and the community within the context of the experienced world and that of the unknown.

Each of the four systems, biophysical, psychosocial, cognitive-perceptual, and cultural-spiritual, can be ordered into a range of bipolar neutral categories that begin to delineate concepts of health. These bipolar categories are as follows:

1 Biophysical: Conservation of energy—expenditure of energy

2 Psychosocial: Individual—society

3 Cognitive-perceptual: Normative (imposed) meaning—constituted (created) meaning

4 Cultural-spiritual: Meaning of lived experience—meaning of unknown experience

For purposes of definition, wellness will be considered to be that which is constituted by a balance between the polarities within and between each of the four systems (see Figure 26-1). All four systems are conceptualized as a spiral, each entwined with the others. An imbalance or need in any one system affects all others. Each set of bipolar categories can be further delineated into the need categories nurses can incorporate in the assessment of the four systems of human functioning. Noninclusive examples[2] of each system's need categories are as follows:

[2] The examples used within this discussion are to be interpreted simply as examples. No implication is being made that these are established categories. Further discrimination of categories could be made. However, for the purpose of discussion, these categories are sufficient.

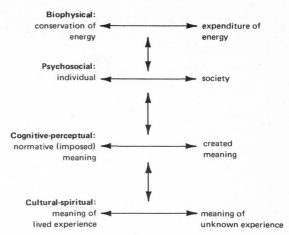

Figure 26-1 Wellness

Biophysical need: something required, either to be supplied, removed, or maintained, in order to create or recreate an energy conservation-expenditure balance

Energy Conservation	Energy Expenditure
Intake	Output
Oxygen, water, food	Elimination—respiratory, urinary, bowel, skin
Recreation	Reproduction
Rest	Activity
Safety	Risk
Comfort	Pain

Psychosocial need: something required, either to be supplied, removed, or maintained, in order to create or recreate balance between the person as an individual being and the person as a part of a larger community

Individual	Society
Solitude	Social interaction
Uniqueness	Belongingness
Independence	Interdependence
Identity—person, male, female	Role—family, work, community
Authority	Subordinate

Cognitive-perceptual need: something required, either to be supplied, removed, or maintained, in order to create or recreate a balance between the imposed and constituted meanings individuals experience in their lives.

Created Meaning	Determined Meaning
Spontaneity	Predictability
Adventure	Security
Creativity	Order
Flexibility	Ritualistic
Responsibility	Dependence

Cultural-spiritual need: something required, either to be supplied, removed, or maintained, in order to create or recreate a balance between the meaning of known and unknown experiences

Meaning of Known Experience	Meaning of Unknown Experience
Participation	Noninvolvement
Commitment	Detachment
Freedom	Stability
Love	Self-fulfillment
Rational	Faith
Immediacy	Hope
Realism	Idealism
Openness	Legalism
Fear	Anxiety

In each of the four broad system categories a need has been defined as something real or imagined that the person requires to be supplied, maintained, or removed in order to maintain the balance within and/or between each system. This need falls within the scope of nursing when the person cannot fulfill the need by himself, but it can be met by the nurse. Nurses do not meet all patients' needs; they do not financially support patients, love them in exclusive relationships, adopt them, etc., although patients may have these needs. The limits of what patient needs nursing may address itself to are still not clearly defined and perhaps can only be so defined by each individual practitioner.

Within each of the four human functioning systems, the need categories in themselves do not suggest which nursing acts to prescribe. Defining needs into bipolar neutral categories is inadequate

for describing the person's need; however, it is the base from which nurses can assess what it is that is needed. In regard to each neutral need category, the value judgment of what is required or necessary for an individual is in terms of the potential nursing actions to be taken. These are implied in the three need modifiers: (1) to increase or to supply something, (2) to maintain or to support something, and (3) to decrease or to remove something. In other words, "circulation," "oxygenation," and "water and electrolyte balance" without modifiers are neutral categories. They do not imply what is required. The addition of the modifier "to increase" to circulation defines what is required. Thus, the inclusion of the modifiers—increase, decrease, and maintain—becomes crucial to stating a need.

A need stated as a modifier and a neutral category, such as the need to decrease pain (or the need to increase comfort[3]), is not a nursing diagnosis. Similarly, cyanosis, edema, and the need to be turned every 2 hours, are not nursing diagnoses. Two are symptoms and the other is a treatment. A nursing diagnosis is a statement about a health problem and its underlying causes. A need in itself is not a problem. All persons have needs but they do not become a matter of concern until the needs can not be easily managed by the individuals. However, a statement describing an unmet need is a step toward defining a problem. The identification of a problem emerges from (1) analysis of the assessed patient's unmet needs, and (2) the potential nursing actions that

---

[3] It should be noted that each set of bipolar categories, by definition, are in opposition to each other. The addition of conflicting modifiers to the opposing categories makes them identical. For example, rest—activity are opposing categories. Adding "increase" and "decrease," conflicting modifiers, so as to read "increase rest" and "decrease activity" results in a synonymous statement. The converse is true; that is, "decrease rest" is synonymous with "increase activity." This suggests that there are yet to be defined normative value categories characterizing the balance between each of the bipolar categories. The isolation of these unidentified value categories should make manifest descriptors for the state of wellness.

can be taken to supply, support, or remove something.[4]

The identification of a list of patient's needs may or may not be a problem. For example:

> Mr. X needs decreased activity
>   decreased circulation
>   decreased respiration

Examination of these needs indicates that there are no opposing neutral categories describing the patient's needs, activity, circulation, and respiration. Similarly, there are no conflicting modifiers (all are "decrease") pointing toward nursing actions. Although Mr. X has these three needs, the nursing action—supply rest—is aimed at meeting all three needs. If the action is carried out, the needs should be met. If the need list were stated as follows:

> Mr. X needs increased activity
>   decreased circulation
>   decreased respiration

then a problem has emerged. There is now a conflict in needs in terms of the modifiers or nursing intervention. How to decrease respiration and circulation, while simultaneously increasing activity, is a problem.[5] A problem statement, then, is a description of a conflict between two or more needs. The conflict can be between (1) the needs, e.g., activity and rest, (2) the modifiers, e.g., to increase activity and decrease circulation, and/or (3) between the potentially implied actions to meet the needs, e.g., isolation precaution and social contact.

The above example of Mr. X's conflicting needs

or problem in itself is not a nursing diagnosis. A statement that identifies a problem (a conflict in needs) *and* the underlying indirect or direct cause or causes associated with producing the conflict, is a nursing diagnosis (fourth-order inference).[6]

One way to write a nursing diagnosis is to connect an identified problem to its underlying cause by using the phrase "due to." Some nurses have expressed concern regarding the legality of making the inference that a particular underlying etiology has a *direct* causal effect on the problem (Mundinger and Jauron, 1975, p. 97). An example is: anxiety due to fear of dying. An alternative way of stating the diagnosis is: anxiety associated with fear of dying. This latter statement incorporating "associated with" implies *indirect* causation and allows the nurse some freedom in stating the underlying etiology.

It is important to define the direct and/or indirect cause of a problem in the nursing diagnosis. The identification of the underlying cause *directly* affects the nursing intervention. For example, a diagnosis of pain isolates a problem but provides insufficient direction for nursing action. However, increased pain due to fear of surgery or noncompliance to therapy due to lack of understanding provides the nurse with more information to determine a preferred course of treatment. Medicating the patient in pain without allowing the patient to express his fears may be an effective treatment. The pain may persist or increase in intensity. In much the same way, treating the non-compliant patient in an authoritarian manner without focusing on the lack of understanding

---

[4] Further distinctions can be made between the modifiers: (1) increase, decrease, maintain and (2) supply, remove, support. The former refer to *patient* needs, whereas the latter elaborate *nursing* interventions.

[5] It should be noted that in this case, this is a *nursing* problem. There are other conflicts of needs that become management problems for the patient, especially in the psychosocial, cognitive-perceptual, and cultural-spiritual systems. Thus, the distinction between nursing and patient problems is made in terms of the person(s) responsible for the management of them.

[6] Writing diagnoses in terms of needs and not patient responses has been identified by Mary O'Neil Mundinger and Grace Dotterer Jauron as one of the "seven deadly sins" committed by beginning nurse diagnosticians. Although Mundinger's and Jauron's observation may be correct, further clarification needs to be made. Arriving at a diagnosis is a time-ordered series of cognitive perceptual events. It is most probable that at assessment time, the nurse diagnostician may only have perceived empirical evidence to make a second-order inference, i.e., a statement of need. The identification of a need is not a diagnostic error, merely a step in the process.

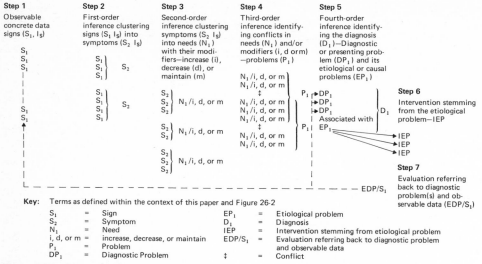

Figure 26-2 Diagnostic Process

may yield some compliance, out of fear, but the underlying cause will not be addressed. The noncompliance will probably reoccur. Therefore, nursing interventions are directly related to and emerge from the identified underlying etiology and not, necessarily, from the immediately perceived problem, e.g., noncompliance with therapy (perceived problem) due to lack of understanding (etiology). In this case, the intervention is a teaching one and not a motivational one.

It should be noted that the underlying cause is another problem or conflict of needs. In other words, a diagnosis is a problem with its underlying cause being another problem or problems. For a schematic representation of the diagnostic process, see Figure 26-2. Most of the examples stated have been conflicts or problems within the biophysical functioning system. These are first-order problems. Second-, third-, and fourth-order problems are conflict of needs within each of the other three human functioning systems. These four orders of problems can be classified into four orders of diagnoses, based on the etiological problem (see Table 26-2). A cognitive-perceptual distinction between first-order diagnoses and second- through fourth-order diagnoses can be made. Since first-order diagnoses consist of biophysical phenomena,

they are arrived at and confirmed by the appearance of concrete, biophysical, objective data. This implies that practitioners dealing with biophysical phenomena can more often than not confirm their subjective inferences (diagnoses) by appealing to objective evidence, whereas second- through fourth-order diagnoses deal with subjective phenomena (psychosocial, cognitive-perceptual, and cultural-spiritual meaning systems). These are arrived at and confirmed by the subjective meaning system of the practitioner. Objectivity in the scientific sense cannot be applied to meanings and values. However, to the extent that members of a discipline can collectively agree upon subjective inferences (diagnoses) about clients' subjective meaning systems, practitioners can attribute some semblance of objectivity to their diagnoses (Soares, 1974). First-order diagnoses for the most part are in the domain of medicine. Although some nurse practitioners appear to be functioning at this level, to date problems with biophysical causation are not within the scope of independent nursing practice.[7] The second- through fourth-

[7]The discriminative criterion for ascertaining whether a first-order diagnosis is a nursing one is precisely the evidence of being able to perform a nursing action to alleviate the problem.

Table 26-2 Classification of Diagnoses

First-order diagnosis	= Problem and etiology within the biophysical system
Second-order diagnosis	= Biophysical problem with psychosocial etiology
Third-order diagnosis	= Biophysical and/or psycho-social problem with cognitive-perceptual etiology
Fourth-order diagnosis	= Biophysical and/or psycho-social and/or cognitive-perceptual problem with cultural-spiritual etiology

order diagnoses are within the domain of nursing. These are the nursing diagnoses. In many instances these subjective diagnoses about subjective meaning systems will be related to objective biophysical problems, thus pointing to collaborative and supportive relationships between nursing and medicine. The relationship between medicine and nursing should become more clear as nursing articulates its diagnoses (Soares, 1974).

Currently, nursing diagnoses are being written in a statement form. This format may be necessary until nurses examine their practice and begin to collect a number of the problem-etiology statements and to analyze them comparatively in order to isolate repetitive patterns of problem-etiologies. Once these repetitive patterns are isolated, nurses can begin to categorize these "syndromes" into diagnostic labels. Some work has begun in the area of collecting diagnoses at the First (Gebbie and Lavin, 1974) and Second National Conference on the Classification of Nursing Diagnoses. The participants at these conferences were nurse practitioners, nurse educators, and nurse-researchers. Examples of the *tentative* diagnoses are: skin integrity, impairment of sleep-rest pattern, ineffective nutrition, alterations in cognitive functioning, and alterations in level of faith.

These categories include: (1) a neutral category that is related to normal human functioning, e.g., skin integrity, and (2) a value modifier that is added to the category, e.g., impairment of. Al-

though these have been identified as nursing diagnoses, they meet the definition of needs as presented within this discussion. Some could be problems or conflicts of needs. However, none of the problems identified are presented with their etiologies. An example of how the classification of nursing diagnoses (which are problems and not diagnoses) could be incorporated into the writing of a diagnostic statement is as follows: alterations in nutrition associated with alterations in cognitive functioning.[8] This then, would be a third-order nursing diagnosis (a biophysical problem with a cognitive-perceptual etiology).

Since diagnoses are problem/problem (etiology) statements, it is debatable whether diagnoses need to be classified as problem/problems. That is, it is feasible that a classification system could incorporate only problem statements without their corresponding etiologies. However, strictly speaking until labels are identified for problem/etiology statements, a classification system would only be classification of *problems* and *not* diagnoses.[9]

The reason for adhering strongly to the necessity of incorporating the etiological problem with the perceived problem, in a diagnostic statement, is related to evaluating the effectiveness of interventions. For example, in the nursing diagnostic statement—noncompliance (perceived problem) due to lack of understanding (etiological problem)—the intervention (teaching) stems from the *causal* problem. However, the evaluation of this diagnosis is not in terms of whether the patient learned, but instead of whether the patient continues to be noncompliant. Given simply the problem, lack of understanding an effective teaching intervention may or may not eliminate the problem of noncompliance. It is quite feasible that the underlying etiology, in this case, may not be lack of understanding. Thus, by not incorporating the perceived diagnostic problem with the etiological problem, the nurse can overlook the effectiveness

[8] However these categories. being tentatively defined need further refinement and empirical testing.
[9] If indeed a diagnosis is a multiple problem statement, than a classification of diagnosis as separate from a classification of problems can be debated.

of interventions on the presenting problem(s).

In summary, nursing, as it emerges from a pre-professional to a professional status, is beginning to systematize its problem-solving (diagnostic) process. Its features of diagnosis are consistent with other health professions' diagnostic processes. These have been described as: (1) the assessment of negative and positive inferences from neutral categories; (2) the hierarchical order of inferences, i.e., first-, second-, third- and fourth-order; (3) fourth-order inferences (diagnoses) implying the identification of the presenting problem and its indirect or direct causation; (4) interventions stemming from the underlying cause; and (5) evaluation referring back to the presence or absence of concrete data pointing to the presenting problem.

The essential features of nursing diagnoses differ from medicine's. The differing conceptual frameworks of medicine and nursing influence the categories describing the particular state of the patient each discipline is examining. Medicine perceives the state of the patient through an organic structural-functioning model, incorporates body system categories, and has systematically classified problem syndromes into diagnostic labels, i.e., diseases. Nursing perceives the state of the patient through a holistic model, incorporates human functioning categories (needs), and has not systematically classified problem/etiological statements into diagnostic labels per se. However, research efforts have begun in the area of nursing diagnoses and nursing process. It is the responsibility of every professional practitioner to examine and critically evaluate his or her practice and, in this way, participate in the articulation and the rationalization of nursing practice.

BIBLIOGRAPHY

Block, Doris: "Some Crucial Terms in Nursing: What Do They Really Mean?," *Nursing Outlook*, **22**:689–694, 1974.

Gebbie, Kristine, and Mary Ann Lavin: "Classifying Nursing Diagnoses," *American Journal of Nursing*, **74**(2):250–253, February 1974.

Henderson, Virginia: *The Nature of Nursing*, Macmillan, New York, 1966.

King, Imogene: "A Conceptual Frame of Reference for Nursing," *Nursing Research*, **17**(1): 27–31, January–February 1968.

Mundinger, Mary O'Neil, and Grace Dotterer Jauron: "Developing a Nursing Diagnosis," *Nursing Outlook*, **23**(2):94–98, February 1975.

Nightingale, Florence: *Notes on Nursing. What It Is and What It Is Not.* (facsimile of 1859 edition), Lippincott, Philadelphia, 1946.

Orem, Dorothea: *Nursing Concepts of Practice*, McGraw-Hill, New York, 1971.

Orlando, Ida Jean: *The Dynamic Nurse-Patient Relationship*, G. P. Putnam's Sons, New York, 1961.

Rogers, Martha: *An Introduction to the Theoretical Basis of Nursing*, F. A. Davis, Philadelphia, 1970.

Soares, Carol A. *Ethnoscience and Phenomenology as Methods for Isolating Categories of Nursing Diagnoses.* Paper presented to Task Force on Modus Operandi Meeting, St. Louis, Missouri, February 8–9, 1974.

Weidenbach, Ernestine: *Clinical Nursing: A Helping Art,* Springer, New York, 1964.

EDITOR'S QUESTIONS FOR DISCUSSION

What diagnostic categories potentially can be treated independently by nurses as the result of a nursing diagnosis? Where does nursing's dependent practice intersect with the practice of medicine? How do a nursing diagnosis and a medical diagnosis support each other? To what extent is a diagnostic category recognized and used in nursing practice to make a nursing diagnosis? To what extent should the process of making a nursing diagnosis be recorded? How can labels be developed for nursing diagnoses? Should a classification of nursing diagnosis be separated from a classification of problems? What would be the value of classifying nursing diagnoses and problems? How can nursing communicate the value of a nursing diagnosis to the medical profession?

Chapter 27

The Why's and What's of Private Practice

Nancy S. Keller, R.N., Ph.D.
General Partner, Nursing Care and Consultation, Ltd.
Tucson, Arizona

The remaining contributions in this section specifically pertain to a new role for nurses, that of the "nurse practitioner." Nancy S. Keller traces the history of the role of the independent nurse practitioner as it evolved from the role of the private-duty nurse. A duality of responsibility and accountability to the physician and to the patient was inherent in the role of the private-duty nurse. Keller outlines the predominant effects on nursing of the transition from private duty to the model of agency employment, predominant among which was a shift of the nurse's loyalty and commitment from the patient to the organization. One of the outcomes of development in nursing education programs, however, has been the adoption of values inherent in the private-duty model of practice—total patient care, continuity of patient care, and frequent interaction with the patient. Routinization and standardization of care in organizations and political and socioeconomic pressures led to the emergence of the primary care nurse and her extended roles. The nurse in independent private practice and in joint practice functions within sets of interdependencies, although she may strive for control and autonomy as a practitioner. Keller suggests that the development of these new roles is based on the inherent values in the role of the original private-duty nurse.

Beginning a private practice of nursing is exciting, challenging, and full of alternating periods of satisfaction, ambiguity, frustration, and loss. Many alternatives seem equally possible in developing new ways to market nursing services and to establish more direct linkages between nurses and clients, but to be faced constantly with such critical administrative decisions leads first to waves of confidence, then to doubt. As soon as one method to attract and maintain a certain clientele is chosen, one can expect to feel regret over competing options that must be postponed or foregone.

This is not to say that all decisions are approached so rationally. A good number of operational decisions are, in fact, explicated *after* one has said, "Yes, we can do that," or "No, that serv-

This is a revision of the original article that appeared under the same title in the *Journal of Nursing Administration*, vol. 5, no. 3, pp. 12–15, March–April 1975.

ice isn't available yet." To be in private practice is to identify with the mythical Killeyloo bird: whenever it took off on a new flight it would always fly backward first—because it couldn't tell where it was going until it had seen where it had been.

The relatively recent social forces that have paved the way for nurses to enter private practice have also influenced the kinds of services offered and accepted through that model of nursing practice. Understanding private practice depends upon understanding the reasons for its emergence as a health care trend.

FORERUNNER: THE PRIVATE-DUTY NURSE

In the days when private duty was the most prevalent nursing practice design, nurses were quite accustomed to the idea of fee-for-service. The fees may well have been realized in the form of room and board, but nonetheless nurses were employed directly by patients, family members, or legal representatives of the patient. Private-duty nurses developed a clientele of satisfied consumers, were recommended to other families and physicians, and consequently received other cases.

If a patient or family considered employing a private-duty nurse, the physician was usually consulted about the actual need for one. Or, if a physician wanted the patient to have a nurse his decision was based—at least as we tend to idealize it—on a rather extensive first-hand knowledge of the patient, his home situation, and a wide range of community resources. Therefore, engaging a nurse for private duty was not a simple matter of establishing communication between nurse and patient. The physician decided how much nursing care was needed and acted as a consultant in locating the best nurse for the case.

Just as important to note is the duality of responsibility and accountability that the private-duty nurse maintained. Nurses were expected to fulfill a variety of roles, many of which are no longer in the province of nursing—housekeeper, companion, babysitter. So, while the physician's orders dictated some of the nurse's work, so did

the patient's nonmedical needs. The patient could be as grateful for having employed a good cook and bath-giver as for having employed someone who understood what to do about his signs and symptoms. Patients could better evaluate the nurse's work performed in those familiar nonmedical roles, and probably assigned greater value to those performances when judging whether the nurse had earned her fee or not. And, since the patient (or some representative of his) was paying her fee, the private-duty nurse undoubtedly felt as obligated to the priorities of the home's management as to those determined by the illness.

But while the nurse was being evaluated by the patient in terms of one set of priorities, she was also being evaluated by the physician in terms of another. Thus, the private-duty nurse had two "employers"—one who paid for a variety of services including comfort measures, and another who depended on her to be the doctor's eyes and ears between his visits to the home or, later, to the hospital. It is a moot point whether the nurse felt more attached to the patient because of her direct contact with him, or to the physician who helped her find more cases and who taught her, over time, to be an ever better assistant in the medical management of her cases. She was responsible and accountable to both.

THE MOVE TO INSTITUTIONS AND AGENCY EMPLOYMENT

With rapid developments in medical technology, the medical model demonstrated obviously effective attacks on dread diseases. Physicians emerged as the rightful leaders of the health team. At the same time, they extended their locus of decision making and influence to include the modern hospital, since medicine can be more efficiently practiced in complex centers that bring patients, technology, and health workers together. The outcome was to make the patient more dependent on medical practitioners for organized cure activities than on nurses for care activities.

Patients today have stronger relationships with physicians than with nurses, even though most practicing nurses are employed by complex organizations to care for or direct the care of patients. Contributing to this is the fact that the patient-physician relationship is likely to occur *first* in time and is probably more *constant* over time. The decisions involved in diagnosing disease and in prescribing and managing its treatment are of primary importance; such medical decisions then initiate sets of organizational routines and role expectations for other health workers and agencies. The patient's contacts with other people and agencies usually occur after the physician-in-charge has "triggered" the appropriate, patient-specific set of extended relationships. Some patients "doctor hop," but most seem loyal to a family physician who, even while sending his patients for consultations with specialists, remains in charge of the total plan of treatment. In sum, particular patients and physicians "belong" to each other before admission to a hospital and their relationship is apt to remain intact throughout and after the hospitalization.

Not so with patients and nurses. By and large, patients no longer have their own nurses; rather, organizations salary nurses to care for groups of patients. Individual nursing personnel have become interchangeable by virtue of their status as agency employees. The patient may not be cared for by the same nurse or even by the same staff of nurses while hospitalized. And, although a patient may have some constancy of nursing care planning by the same head nurse or team leader during his hospital stay, he may see so little of the nurse that his subjective feeling of constancy comes from his relationships with nonprofessional staff.*

*Even nursing care provided in the home does not afford nurse and patient the constancy that characterizes the physician-patient relationship because the actual focus for stability is the client-agency relationship. The patient is seen (or not seen) for the agency's and the patient's reasons; the agency then either assigns a nurse to the case according to some criteria, or refers the patient to a setting such as a clinic where nursing expertise is to be found. Of course, the model of private duty has changed also. With registries and shortened hours of duty, that model of nursing practice has become more formally organized with personnel who are interchangeable in meeting the demands of certain types of cases.

When nurses begin agency employment today they are entering an arena in which groups of patients are managed primarily by groups of physicians, groups of policies and procedures, or both. This context is further complicated by the groups of other health workers, bureaucrats, and functionaries necessary to make the system of delivery of services reliable and efficient. This situation in health care delivery developed slowly, it is true, but keeping in mind that when nurses initially made the move into institutions, they came equipped with (1) on-the-job training that complemented the medical model; (2) a history of being utilized as physician surrogate to keep the treatment plan "going" in the physical absence of the doctor; and (3) internalized societal expectations that nurses would institute and supervise care and comfort activities, one can see that as the delivery system became more complex, it was a logical step for institution employers to charge nursing personnel with the job of coordinating organizational routines and adapting them to unique sets of physician-patient preferences. Inherent in the coordinator role is a liaison function. Not surprisingly, the nurse began to spend a great deal of time transmitting information to the multiple groups involved—explaining the doctor's orders to patients, explaining patients' complaints to doctors and hospital administrators, explaining patients' behavior to coworkers, and the like. Over time, the hospital employed numerous others to do the work that nurses used to do, and although this has supplied status to nurses within the organizational hierarchy, it has simultaneously disrupted a formerly held direct linkage with consumers of nursing care. The hospital—not the patient, or the physician, but the organization—has become the evaluator of nursing care. And while nurses may now assess the need for nursing care, they no longer deliver it directly.

It's reasonable to expect that the salary-provider will have some power over the nature and evaluation of the tasks performed by its employees. And it is predictable that the focus of the employee's loyalty will be influenced by economic factors. But as nurses have committed themselves to hospital goals of delivering safe and improved patient care via the coordinator role, the unintended consequence has been a disrupted nurse-patient relationship in comparison with that enjoyed by the private-duty nurse. In fact, the issue of greatest import in the evolution from private duty to agency employment as the predominant model of nursing practice is the nurse's shift of loyalty and commitment from the patient to the organization.

DEVELOPMENTS IN NURSING EDUCATION

Add to this picture the historical changes in nursing education. Having rejected the word "training" as less acceptable than "education," we moved away from apprenticeships and on-the-job training (the system by which the early private-duty nurse was educated) in order to prepare nurses to provide care based on theoretical principles. Ironically though, the early private-duty practice model seems to provide a better fit with current programs of baccalaureate and higher degree education in nursing—if we assume that the private-duty nurse had, at best, the opportunity to individualize her care when working fee-for-service for the patient in his home. Since the nurse had only one case at a time, the private-duty model was the epitome of one-to-one interaction. Providing highly individualized nursing care within the framework of one-to-one interaction still permeates philosophies of nursing held by our educational institutions, and perpetuates curricula that are incongruent with what happens in the agency-employment model. One outcome is a continuous flow of graduates who adhere to the values and look for the job satisfactions inherent in the private-duty model of practice—total patient care, continuity of nursing care, constant attention to particular patient needs, and frequent interactions. Another outcome is a continuous need for inservice education programs to socialize new graduates to the realities of the organizational approach to health care delivery.

Programs of nursing education and departments of nursing service have earnestly tried to find ways to bring the forementioned values of a professionalized nursing to fruition. Nursing education's need to define nursing for the sake of students and curriculum planning coincided with nursing service's need to be able to better utilize the skills of the graduate nurse. Nursing education's attempt to separate independent from dependent nursing functions in order to define nursing resulted in a new category of nursing personnel, the clinical specialist, and nursing service tacitly agreed to try the role in practice. Both had high hopes that the clinical specialist, at least, would be able to provide the highly individualized care still touted in philosophies of nursing and would be able to do this in a more autonomous, independent fashion than head or staff nurses. But these hopes did not materialize as envisioned.

The relative lack of success of the clinical specialist role is related to an organizational fact of life; that is, the organization's primary mode of survival is routinization, *not* individualization. Thus, a professional whose intent is to identify individual patient needs is bound to confront system resistance to meeting those needs unless those needs can be shown to pertain to most or all patients. Unfortunately, in the process of identifying general patient needs, the concept of unique needs often disappears into the background. And, many clinical specialists suddenly found themselves busy with identifying and meeting generalized needs of staff, particularly the learning needs of new personnel, rather than patient needs.

RECENT POLITICAL AND SOCIOECONOMIC PRESSURES

A more recent frustration to nurses who want to fashion a plan of care that is tailor-made for the individual patient is the mounting pressure to standardize nursing care. Standardization is frequently viewed as the ultimate contradiction to "total patient care," but we might as well make ready for continuing pressures from government, insurance companies, and representatives from the medical community to standardize. Issues of the cost and availability of health care services have accelerated the movement toward defining explicit criteria for "quality" care for all, and other forms of regulation of health services will no doubt also emerge around these issues.

Three additional trends in the health care field have developed in response to these issues, and they are probably here to stay: (1) the utilization of health workers other than physicians to minimize the cost and time spent for educational preparation; (2) attempts to stabilize and distribute health care costs over time by capitalizing on early detection of illness and prevention of disability; and (3) the continued search for new ways to organize manpower, care, and technology into systems that will meet consumer needs—health maintenance organizations and neighborhood health centers are good examples of this effort.

So, even though organizational and economic forces have always plagued nursing's efforts to devise and implement a model of practice reflective of the profession's ideals, we are now faced with political and socioeconomic forces that are apt to culminate in an even more bureaucratized health care system that, by definition, further curtails the realization of individualized and total patient care. Yet hope springs eternal. In the midst of pressures to routinize and standardize care there have appeared other unplanned, emergent "experiments" in nursing practice: primary care, extended role or nurse practitioner, joint practice, and independent (private) practice.

Primary care has at least two meanings. For hospital nursing it represents an avenue for increasing the ratio of professional nurses to patients and for placing the accountability for patient care planning on the most comprehensively prepared unit personnel—the RN. The work pattern is changed so that RNs are expected to have more direct contact with patients and the nonprofessional staff are assigned duties in a more accurately applied sense of the term *nurse assistants*. The primary care model seems to be a reversal of the team concept, that is, a flow of information from those working with the patients to the team leader. The team leader would make certain decisions and assist the team members with completion of assignments; the team was responsible for constructing and implementing the care plan.

The primary care nurse can be that former team leader, but practicing in the new model of care she is theoretically more proximal to the patient's needs that in turn require her judgment; the plan that the primary care nurse and patient construct becomes the basis for deploying other staff to implement the directives. The hospital nurse practicing in the primary care model will no longer attempt to make care plans from the syntheses of information from a myriad of coworkers but instead will exercise judgment based on data collected from her own interactions with the patients.

The implications for this newer model of practice in hospitals evolve from the necessary organizational changes that will place more status on the nurse-patient relationship than on nurse-coworker relationships. The model is likely to gain nursing administration's blessing since it operationalizes management by objectives to the patient care level and presents a less complicated method of locating accountability and quality control for patient care.

Nursing education, on the other hand, will have to assess the demand for primary care nurses and will have to address the challenge of moving from a focus of problem solving to that of planning. Primary care nurses will need to know as much about the planning process as they presently know about problem solving. Unfortunately, this dilemma is the crux of the development of the model of practice itself. Short-term planning for hospitalized patients may indeed be no more than problem solving for short-term benefits.

Until we can demonstrate and document the differences among functional, team, and primary care models of patient care we cannot expect a widespread revolution and reform of nursing practice in hospitals. We may expect some further development of the primary care model in chronic care centers and/or nursing homes, but the general hospital as a set of organizational factors does not provide the best fit for planning modalities of thought and action.

Primary care, however, has another meaning. As it was first introduced into health care terminology reference was made to time and place of entry into the health care delivery system. The dimensions underlying classifications of primary, secondary, and tertiary were applicable to disease and severity of illness. Nursing, it seemed, could conduct certain screening and assessment procedures at the primary (first contact) point for the nonacutely ill. More acute patient problems would need the resources available from physicians and acute care centers.

Inequities in accessibility to health care and the economics of delivering the care made preparation of physicians' assistants a popular option for managing those primary contacts with patients. So when the medical community confronted the accessibility and economic problems with the physician assistant, the nursing community countered with the nurse practitioner.

THE NURSE PRACTITIONER AND EXTENDED ROLE

Practice in the extended role may well provide the nurse practitioner with more legitimate influence over a patient's entry into and passage through the health care system and more independence to make certain decisions that are valued by patients. It even seems that nursing's search for some set of independent functions is satisfied when a nurse practitioner's role capabilities are reviewed. Clients or patients are given the opportunity to appreciate the number of nurse activities that are not dependent on "we will have to ask your doctor." The implication is one of public confirmation of a nurse as health care provider in charge of her or his own work.

But, in fact, nurses' dependence on the physician and his orders has been replaced by reliance on pieces of discrete medical knowledge, and the nurse's capability to be more independent in practice is directly related to the acquisition of medical knowledge and skill. Nonetheless, practice in the extended role has been commonly labeled as "independent" practice of nursing.

The astute nurse might wonder: "independent from what?," certainly not from the medical model or from ultimate reliance on medical direction or protocols. Neither are they independent from legal interpretation of the interface between medicine and nursing.

The change in nurse practice acts necessitated by the development of the nurse practitioner role is a prime factor that affects those who work in the extended role. As an example, the key phrase "under the supervision/direction of a licensed physician" is being omitted from or relocated within statements of law that regulate nursing practice. Omitting the phrase frees the whole set of nursing functions from obligatory medical supervision and relocating it places the restriction upon the activities of the nurse practitioner. Whether the phrase is omitted or relocated is not as important as the interpretations of the nurse practitioner role as handed down by attorneys who work in the state's legal hierarchy. Even then, however, the permission to exercise legal autonomy does not imply an independent, i.e., self-determined, self-reliant practitioner who is relatively free from influence and persuasion by others.

Nurse practitioners are not independent from agency pressures either. The vast majority of nurse practitioners is employed by clinics, health departments, health maintenance organizations, or physicians; all are thereby directed by other than nursing goals. While some practitioners indicate that the new role brings more satisfaction because they can finally find out more about the patient's "total needs" as opposed to only his medical needs, others voice their displeasure with organizational or medical expectations that they screen an ever increasing number of cases that, in turn, limits the time and thought that can go toward solving the problems of any single case.

Independent practice is a misnomer. A professional always works within sets of interdependencies, influences and counterinfluences, persuasions and counterpersuasions. Both private practice and joint practice highlight the interdependency.

Private practice indicates simply that nursing is conducted under the auspices of nurses in solo or group association and that the business of that practice belongs to that nurse or those nurses—not to the public, to another profession, or to the government. The responsibilities and delegations of authority are administered within the bounds of said ownership much as any private-duty nurse administers her own practice. The nurse or group enjoys legal autonomy, direct linkage with the client, and capacity for controlling one's own work—the very hallmark of professionalism.

Nurses in private practice can use the skills of as many physicians or other health care professionals as cases require; some utilize the clients' physicians as medical back-up, others have contractual agreements with specific physicians for consultation and referral. The nurses work in cooperation with several physicians at a time with the intent of widening the circle of collaboration as the clientele grows in volume and diversity of problems.

Joint practice, like private practice, recognizes interdependence and emphasizes colleagueship. Instead of negotiating for work rights and status over additional tasks of physical diagnosis and management of chronic disability as an alternative to physician assistants, this model of practice seeks to form alliance at the professional-to-professional level rather than at the paraprofessional level, that is, nurse practitioners and hospital primary care nurses following doctors' orders or protocols for diagnosis and treatment.

Joint practices are alliances made with specific physicians or specific health care professionals for the treatment and care of a clientele. Nurses in joint practice work in tandem with a consistent set of professionals as the clientele changes. This model of practice may well lead to a new level of physician appreciation of nursing skills and to collaborative models of medical practice. The nursing community, however, will not learn via this model which, if any, nurse specific skills are valuable to the general public *and* in sufficient demand to warrant full-time effort (whether fee-for-service or salaried). Private practice, on the other hand, can test the marketability of nursing services to the general public.

Tracing the development of the private-duty model into modern staff nursing in hospitals and community health agencies seems linear in progression. Add the recent changes in health care, technology, and finances and we see the emergence of not just a single new experimental model in nursing practice, but four such models. There may be more models prompted by the same set of forces or, at best, some combination of the best of these four models—a testable model that will deserve the support of the health care and nursing communities.

Each of the new models of practice enables nurses to be in a better position to inform, instruct, counsel, and otherwise directly influence the patient/client. Each model adds a particular, and potentially significant, perspective to the idea of extension of care. Primary care in hospitals extends nursing beyond decision making, problem identification, and goal setting into areas of evaluation of action and planning. The nurse practitioner movement seems to be an attempt to achieve a balance of extending nursing via an extension of medical knowledge and technology. Joint practice extends a totality of perspective about health care and about consumer needs: that is, if no one health care professional can respond to the needs of the client/patient, then a team of professionals can practice health care instead of medicine, nursing, pharmacy, and soon. Private practice can be a powerful client extender making nursing play a truer advocacy role for the person who is trying to make sense of the services and information delivered by the system of health care.

A common dimension that unites all these models of practice is the search for control *and* autonomy as a practitioner. To be in control and command of necessary resources is to enable one to be an initiator of action rather than a responder to someone's directive. These models also indicate the serious search for a structural way of supporting nursing practice that is consonant with philosophies and beliefs of the *practitioner*, not the educator or the administrator or the researcher.

The social value of occupations/professions is to be found in practice, not in teaching others to practice or in the environment in which others practice. One thing seems certain. Something is happening in nursing practice today that may ultimately bring status to the practice of nursing. The trends in practice as exemplified by the newer models of practice are emerging—without plan, without formulas or tactics for success, some without official endorsement or blessing. Nonetheless, we find growing enthusiasm and pride in practice and in devising structures that permit a greater degree of satisfaction with one's work of performing the art, if not the science, of nursing.

BIBLIOGRAPHY

Browning, Mary H., and Edith P. Lewis (eds.): *The Expanded Role of the Nurse*, American Journal of Nursing Company, New York, 1973.

Bullough, Bonnie, and V. L. Bullough: *The Emergence of Modern Nursing*, 2d ed., Macmillan, New York, 1969.

Davis, Fred (ed.): *The Nursing Profession: Five Sociological Essays*, Wiley, New York, 1966.

Davis, Marcella Z., Marlene Kramer, and Anselm L. Strauss (eds.): *Nurses in Practice, A Perspective on Work Environments*, Mosby, St. Louis, 1975.

Freidson, Eliot: "Dominant Professions, Bureaucracy, and Client Services," in W. R. Rosengren and Mark Lefton (eds.), *Organization and Clients: Essays in the Sociology of Service*, Merrill, Columbus, Ohio, 1970, pp. 71–92.

Hall, Richard H. (ed.): *The Formal Organization*, Basic, New York, 1972.

Keller, Nancy S.: "The Nurse's Role: Is It Expanding or Shrinking?," *Nursing Outlook*, 21:236, April 1973.

Marram, Gwen D., Margaret W. Schlegel, and Em O. Bevis: *Primary Nursing, A Model for Individualized Care*, Mosby, St. Louis, 1974.

EDITOR'S QUESTIONS FOR DISCUSSION

In actual practice, how does primary care differ from team nursing? What is the difference between using nursing knowledge and medical knowledge in a joint or independent practice role? In joint or independent practice, on what type of role should the nurse focus—a nursing role or an extension of this role into a medical one? What values have stimulated nurses to develop roles in independent practice? What should be the educational preparation and qualifications of the nurse in joint or independent practice? What is the difference between the role of a physician's assistant and that of a nurse in joint or independent practice? What might be the difference in the expectations of patients regarding nurses in joint or independent practice versus nurses in hospitals or ambulatory care settings?

Chapter 28

Putting the Health in Health Care

Dorothy M. Talbot, R.N., Ph.D.
Professor and Chairperson, Department of Public Health Nursing
University of North Carolina

Dorothy M. Talbot provides insight into the mechanisms of social change, such as the evolution of the nurse practitioner role. She describes the development of this role in terms of "diffusion theory," the assumption of which is that social change comes from the diffusion of ideas. She proposes that the nurse practitioner role stems from dissatisfaction with the status quo and with traditional knowledge as applied to health problems and predicts future changes in nurse practice, such as the self-monitoring of patients by means of biofeedback mechanisms. The gradual acceptance of change is part of cultural lag. Factors that hinder and promote changes are discussed, and guidelines for implementing changes are outlined.

In the autumn of 1974 the Golf Hall of Fame was opened in Pinehurst, North Carolina, with President Gerald R. Ford on hand to honor the inductees and tee off for a round with current greats of the game. The previous year the first members of the newly established Academy of Nursing were also selected. If the Academy of Nursing was inaugurated with less fanfare, it may nonetheless be linked to the game of golf by more than this coincidence in time. For nursing, like golf, can test, indeed can make or break, champions.

Certainly, there are hazards. There are varying distances to be covered. The rough is always waiting at the edge of the fairway. And it takes a varied, well-balanced game to win. Do you attack the course, or let it play you? Do you use a wedge in the sandtrap, or a 5-iron? Do you try to hit over the trees, or aim for the opening between low

limbs? Similar strategies are required in nursing. Do you confront the issues in nursing, weigh the alternatives for action, choose what appears to be the most effective alternative, and then act, or do you exist from one crisis situation to another? Do you try to avoid conflict completely, or aim to accept its existence while being alert for opportunities to tactfully resolve it?

Knowledge, stamina, and practice come into play over the long course, as does an awareness of one's own limits, strengths, and weaknesses. And always there are those elements beyond our control that may take their toll and effect the outcome despite all one's skills and experience—the wind, the rain, and the thunderstorms that bring their lightning. These elements can be likened to the disagreements, power struggles, lack of understanding, and the social and economic elements

This article is a revised version of two articles, "Cultural Lag and Occupational Health," *Occupational Health Nursing*, vol. 23, no. 10, October 1975, and "Social Change and Occupational Health," *Occupational Health Nursing*, vol. 22, no. 4, April 1974.

that are not only a part of nursing, but also of life itself.

Yet for all the hazards and challenges, the sand-traps and water holes, there are joys and rewards—not the least of which is the fact that it is a long, leisurely game, played over a sprawling course, with beauty spots and scenic vistas. Further, much as the changing terrain of a championship golf course offers new delights to be seen and enjoyed, so too the social change of our time—especially as it relates to nursing—should be seen and enjoyed, even welcomed. For change is not only inevitable, it also offers opportunities that should be reached out for and embraced.

A recent book told us "grow or die" (Lockland, 1973). And that is the message of nature. It is also a lesson that nations have learned (or failed to learn) down through history. All life is dynamic. Death comes when there is no growth. In moving water there is light and health, in stagnant water darkness and death. The bubbling trout stream has only water in common with the Louisiana bayou.

Today, however, there is not only change, there is rapid-fire change. Change hits us again, again, and again, with machine gun rapidity. *Future Shock* has not only become a best-selling book of classic proportion, its title has gone into the lexicon as a quick-fix expression for uncommonly fast development.

Science, entertainment, fashion, education—all have seen their kaleidoscopic quick changes in our time. View for example, transportation, which has greatly changed. For something like 2,000 years, down through the centuries that saw the rise and fall of civilizations, the discovery of the New World, and the expansion of our young nation to the Pacific, man traveled on a beast of burden, when he did not walk. The Bible tells us that Christ sent his disciples for a colt that he rode into Jerusalem on Palm Sunday, and legend tells us that Wyatt Earp rode a horse to that gunfight at the O.K. Corral. Well into our own century, the new automobile owner who ventured out on the road heard not just his fellow drivers' horns but the cry: "Get a horse!" Today men blast off from

the earth, encircle the moon, and land. So too, change has affected nursing.

One of the few things we still have in common with our ancestors, as it were, is a resistance to change. It is understandable. It is natural. It has even been codified in cliches, mottos, and truisms. "Look before you leap," grandmother said, and great-grandmother, and great-great-grandmother. "Fools rush in where angels fear to tread." There is no end to the words that make our resistance to change seem all right—even right. "What's wrong with the old way?" "What was good enough for them is good enough for me," "Maintaining the status quo," "Biding your time," "Steering an even course"—these are all brakes on change.

"Thou Shalt Not" may be best known for its place in Biblical history and the Ten Commandments, but former Supreme Court Justice William O. Douglas relates it to our own time and natural resistance to change, telling us that "Thou Shalt Not" has been used by each age to shackle the mind and put severe restraints on the freedom of inquiry (1962, p. 2). The curious man, the dissenter, the innovator has been burned, booed, or exiled for questioning contemporary dogma. Douglas also states that there has been a trend to conformity, a desire to maintain the status quo in this country since World War II (1962, p. 2). He ascribes this to the fact that we have had a surplus of everything; amid this affluence, and its corresponding fear of losing what we have, conservatism has flowered.

In the field of nursing, Justice Douglas might well have related his remarks to the period following World War I. For 50 years after the Frontier Nursing Service "invented" the expanded nursing practice concept, we are still hearing that the nurse's primary work is that of carrying out the physician's orders. This narrow viewpoint has not—and will not—be accepted by the nursing profession. We are well aware that over two-thirds of all professional nurses work in acute care settings, with the carrying out of physicians' orders a major nursing responsibility. But we should all be equally aware that, like the lowly turtle, we lurch forward only if we first stick our necks out and chance the consequences.

To best understand how we may do this, the following pages will offer a definition and overview of social change, as an introduction to a discussion of diffusion theory, touch on the concept of cultural lag, and conclude with guidelines for implementation. Where—and what—will nursing be in the year 1996? It is our choice. We may direct, or be directed. What safeguards do we want in the technetronic age we are now entering? There are no rules; no precedents yet exist.

Growth, it should be recognized, is accomplished through two forces: the first is genetic in origin, the second, ectogenetic. In nursing, the genetic force stems from the nurturing instinct to care for the helpless, representative activities of which are bathing, feeding, and protecting. The ectogenetic force stems from society and the entire health care system, representative activities of which are examining, diagnosing, and treating. The former will not change. The latter changes constantly.

Social change may be described as that which affects the way societies live and are organized. Such change may be cataclysmic. For example, the recent earthquakes in Peru, Guatemala, and Italy: the way people live, and the kinds of group interaction, will be different there in the years to come. Social change is micro in nature, also, The nurse practitioner movement is changing the structure and process of nursing practice. No longer is "a nurse is a nurse is a nurse." There are now various levels of nurses, and the type of practice differs from level to level.

This writer subscribes to the idea that growth, or death, is inevitable, that society is transformed as it grows. And that this is nowhere more true than in modern nursing. This article describes these changes in nursing in terms of "diffusion theory," which is only one of many theories of change. *Diffusion* is the process by which material and/or ideas permeate in all directions.

Take the word "viable" or "mainstream," even "detente." Each was used by a prominent person, or persons, in regard to a current event. The word was picked up in the reportage of the event, repeated in wire dispatches and on TV network news programs, used in commentary and columns, until the word was diffused throughout the nation—even the world—and became part of our every-day language. "Ecology" was a word to be found in spelling bees one day and a national movement the next.

The late Senator Everett M. Dirkson in answering a reporter's question as to why he was taking a certain position on a crucial national issue replied, "There is nothing so powerful as an idea whose time has come." He might have added, *or one that catches on.* The renowned Egyptologist, G. Elliot Smith, put it a bit differently (LaPiere, 1965, pp. 23-24). He believed there is nothing so powerful as a dominant center. Citing the spurt in cultural development in the Nile Valley, he notes that the new and improved ideas were then diffused to all peoples of the world. Such a single theory, however, overlooks the fact that people, independently, develop their own ideas. As we shall see, the timing may be so close and the claim so strong that court cases and long years of litigation are required to determine the legal (if not the true) inventor.

Diffusion theory is based on the assumption that social change comes from the diffusion of ideas or material things. It is a particularistic theory utilized in this article to describe the diffusion of a single idea—the spread of the nurse practitioner movement. Diffusion theory also rests on a tripod, the three legs of which are:

1 The innovators, who produce something new—an organization, a new vaccine, or a new method for delivering health services
2 The advocates, who then sell the idea
3 The adopters, who finally pick it up and use the innovation

The innovators, the advocates, and the adopters—each represents a distinct type with a decided set of personality traits (LaPiere, 1965, pp. 103-211).

The changing role of the nurse practitioner

illustrates diffusion theory in our profession. During World War I, nurses began expanding their practice by working with the wounded. In 1923, the Frontier Nursing Service invented the expanded nursing practice concept, introducing nurses from England who had the knowledge and the skill for providing more health services than other nurses were prepared to give here in the United States. They, together with supportive physicians, invented and refined the idea that nurses could make diagnoses of disease or injury; could provide primary care; could administer to the chronically ill; could minister to the healthy, pregnant woman and the well to "moderately ill" child—always under guidelines provided by physicians. First on horseback and later by jeep, nurses for half a century have provided the mountain people of Kentucky with services only *now* being diffused throughout the United States by nurse practitioners. This expanded role has evolved very slowly, although it received fresh impetus in the early 1950s when the Canadian Bell Telephone Company began teaching nurses how to conduct complete, preemployment physical examinations, and when "clinical nurse specialists" were being taught how to give care to the ill in intensive care units by utilizing tools and knowledge previously used only by physicians.

The rest is history. In 1965, the pediatric nurse practitioner program was initiated at the University of Colorado. Ten years later, the Nurse Training Act of 1975 was enacted into law, providing for the education and utilization of many types of nurse practitioners. Today, there is almost universal adoption of the "invention." To be considered permanent and not merely a fad, this change, as with all others, must span a generation. It takes this long for the new to become the norm. Evidence that this invention is becoming the norm is the fact that nursing schools today are teaching students the "expanded skills." These students are being socialized into this new role, although it is one that the majority of professional nurses in this country are not yet prepared to assume.

It has been said, and is applicable here, that it takes 50 years for change to occur. The "S" hypothesis states that little change occurs at first; then suddenly there is rapid change; this, in turn, is followed by a leveling-off period (Talbot, 1974). It should be noted that not all people accept the new. Today change can be directed and controlled as never before. One can predict alternative futures and choose. Just as golfers have to choose between clubs when traveling the course, nurses have to choose between options in their career. Changes in the health care field are accruing exponentially.

Science is causing man to live longer, so much so that the great goal of modern nursing should be to make this longer life more worth living. Only 5 to 10 percent of the population at any one time have illness needs. Health is man's most precious possession. Our work is to help clients keep it. That is the mission of nursing; in my opinion, there is no other. How we do it however, changes, often quickly, and often as a result of previous "pioneer" work.

Lavinia Dock, for example, in an article published in 1903 entitled "Sanitary Inspection: A New Field for Nurses," stated that a nurse's training prepared her to do sanitary inspections (1903). She believed that a nurse was uniquely qualified to look into every nook and cranny, turn out every closet, and bring to her nose every whiff of suspicious air. A short 6 years later, she is quoted as saying to a group of nurses who were complaining because they were being called on less and less as a result of people's improved hygiene and sanitation, "you must be directed" into lines of preventive work (February 1909).

The changes we must cope with come not only from our previous efforts but also from social or cultural developments. Of the latter, there are also two kinds: material and nonmaterial. Examples of cultural material change are rather obvious—tools, medicines, machinery, those things that have been invented over a period of time. Nonmaterial items are less apparent—customs, behaviors, and attitudes, developments such as caring for the sick outside the home, in health centers, hospitals, and nursing homes. These, too, were invented and are referred to as social inventions.

Why do these changes occur? Usually, social changes such as the nurse practitioner role stem from dissatisfaction with the status quo. John Dewey, in 1930, said that conflict "shocks us out of sheep-like passivity, and sets us noting and contriving" (Coser, 1957). The nurse practitioner invention resulted from conflict between vested interests. On the one hand certain physicians were afraid they would lose their power, wealth, and status. On the other hand nurses were tired of their handmaiden role. The nurse practitioner movement also stemmed from the accumulated knowledge that traditional ways of handling health problems would no longer suffice, due to advances in knowledge, increased technological complexity, burgeoning demands, rising costs, and insufficient manpower. Running through all this was the gleaming bright thread that reflected the evolving philosophy of the times—that health is a right for all, not a privilege for just a few. If vested interests had to be fought, the time was right.

Suddenly a change initiated years ago has been adopted by the elite. Some nurse practitioners and physicians have become adopters. As a result, their type of collaborative practice is slowly becoming the norm. Those of us who have not been trained for this type of practice are affected, each in his or her own way, by the type of personality with which we are endowed, and the traits that will make us an innovator, an advocate, or an adopter.

It is perhaps easiest to fall into the category of "the affected." For while some welcome the change and are doing all that is possible to facilitate the development of neophytes into this type of nurse, others, not wanting to lose what they have gained in the world in the way of status and security, resist. Sociologists throughout the past century have been developing a theory of social change, so that now it may be said these professionals see it as a process that occurs as a result of a power struggle, an adaption to new technologies and man's powerful instinct to grow.

Today there is intense interest in the Third World concept, i.e., that of a postindustrial society where consumption is the problem, not production. The movement is being carried forward by the youth culture and countercultures, and is a reaction against the status quo, against the affluency of power, and against the complacency with "what is." Not that all resistance to change is bad; in fact it serves its purpose by giving stability to society. The cornerstone of the social system is consensus. And the power struggle resembles the old milling process that sorted the wheat from the chaff.

EFFECT OF CHANGE ON NURSING

A century ago, man learned about the germ theory of disease and about the effects of poor nutrition and environmental hygiene on health. Our nursing forebears, Florence Nightingale, Lillian Wald, Isabel Hampton Robb, to name a few, began to make use of these social inventions by incorporating them into nursing practice and to make the environment more conducive to health by teaching health care practices such as dental hygiene and by instructing mothers and school children about nutrition. Gradually this new way of practicing nursing was taught, until teaching or counseling individuals and groups in these basic facts regarding the promotion of health and the prevention of disease has become the accepted norm.

Today, thanks to new social inventions, our practice is changing again. New techniques are being incorporated, from making electrocardiograms to instructing clients in the use of chemical and other fertility-control measures. Assisting clients to care for themselves while wearing cardiac pacemakers, taking more detailed health histories, subjecting our records to peer audit, and utilizing more outreach health workers—all are inventions of recent date.

In the future, our practice will change again as social and technological changes occur. On the horizon is *cloning*, a process by which exact replicas of humans may be reproduced now that the secret of DNA is known. Patients will monitor themselves with many biofeedback mechanisms. Genetic and abortion counseling will become one of our major responsibilities now that amniocentesis reveals abnormal chromosones in the fetus. John Platt even suggests that there will be automated biochemical tests that will identify 200 compounds in our breath, sputum, urine, blood, and vaginal smears within 5 minutes (1972).

We will administer medications at different times, as we learn more about our biophysical and circadian rhythms. Already it is known that the drug, aldomet, given at the same time of day, every day, affects individuals' blood pressures differently at different times, although the dose is the same. We all have different biologic time clocks.

Larger numbers of people will be living to over 100 years of age. Our work force will become reduced as the population decreases; nonetheless, the smaller group of young people will support the rest. Job obsolescence will occur even more rapidly than it does today with the result that people will retire sooner. And many more hours of leisure will be available to all ages as we go to shorter work weeks. Nursing's work will be to put quality into that life that science is providing.

There will be drastic changes in our health care systems. Prepaid systems of care will make preventive work even more important, and national health insurance is no longer a debatable issue. The only question remaining is just when will it begin, and what will be its scope. People will demand more personalized, dignified, human attention in illness care, particularly as they approach death. Man's need for the human touch, for caring, are the two universal considerations in nursing. Life is not worth living if no one cares.

We will assume more responsibility for primary health care and will serve as gate-keepers to the health care system. Nurses will be making the first assessment of the health condition, will handle the preventive aspects of care, and will assume increasingly greater responsibility for the care of the chronically ill and disabled. Nursing's work is and always will be health care. We must not only help people retain health we must, once it is threatened, help them to attain it as quickly as possible, or help them to live a more worthwhile life with their handicap. Sometimes health care means helping people to die peacefully.

CULTURAL LAG

Inventions are not diffused through society at even rates. Maladjustments occur, a phenomenon termed *cultural lag.* Cultural lag may be defined as the period of delay and maladjustment that occurs while adaptation to change is occurring at different rates.

An example of cultural lag may be illustrated by the concept of the nurse practitioner. The material condition of the culture would be the type of health service available to the population. The nonmaterial condition would be the type of nursing practice. 1923 could be the date for Time 1 in Figure 28-1. This is when the Frontier Nursing Service began practicing nursing as an expanded role, thus embracing the medical skills of diagnosis, prescription, and treatment. Maladjustment in the world of health care services marked this period. Vested interests advocated the status quo. Doctors did not want the changes; nurses were far from unanimous in agreeing that this was for them; and patients wanted freedom from uncertainty, preferring the status quo of having physicians treat their ills. Nevertheless, the idea continued to be diffused. The year 1965 could be the date for Time 2. Again, approximately one-half century had passed before the material condition of health services and the nonmaterial condition of nursing practice began to become compatible. During the intervening years, there was turbulence and stress (see Figure 28-1).

Sociologists tell us that the periods just before and just after a social invention are turbulent. Thus, we are in a period of turbulence today, with the nurse practitioner movement not being fully accepted by those with vested interests. Some doctors, for example, see their roles as diagnosti-

Cultural components	Norm	Innovation	Advocacy	Early adopters	Mass adoption	Norm
Nursing practice						
Health services	Traditional	Very little change	Rapid change			Traditional
	1900	1923*	1965†	1976	2000	

*1923 is date when Frontier Service Nurses began practicing an expanded role.

†1965 is date when the Pediatric Nurse Practitioner Program was started at the University of Colorado.

Figure 28-1 Diffusion and cultural lag theories applied to the expanded nurse role movement.

cians threatened. Some nurses fear it, for this means their practice is obsolete. Clients are uncertain. But the change is occurring, and wihin a generation this new type of nursing practice will no doubt be the norm. Nurses entering graduate school today want to learn the expanded role. They represent those within the profession who recognize that change is occurring, who are trying to do something about it, and who want to keep up and grow. They welcome the change, realizing that more and more people can be cared for. Four factors explain social change: (1) an invention; (2) an accumulation of inventions from previous years; (3) a diffusion of the invention; and (4) a subsequent adjustment to the change. Today's status quo was yesterday's conflict.

SHAPING CHANGE

Stability and progress in the field of nursing are subordinate to the larger world problems of population, industrialization, pollution, food production, and resource consumption. If these are not addressed decisively, and soon, nursing will regress. Nor can we leave it to others; our profession must address itself to these larger issues now. We must recognize those factors shaping nursing practice that are beyond our control. But we must also

recognize the factors that are within our control. I shall describe three of each.

Factors that hinder nurses in shaping the future are an individual's normal resistance to change, woman's traditionally passive role, and lack of know-how in guiding change toward the desired goal. The first factor is a result of one's basic fear or insecurity. The new is not familiar. Only secure people gamble with uncertain futures. One way to identify nurses with this trait is to hear the words, "But, this is the way we have always done it." Such resistance is to be expected, and should be taken into account when change is contemplated. Obsolescence will take care of those of us who cannot or will not change. Eric Hoffer says that to adopt the role of the pioneer and the avant-garde is to place oneself in a situation where ineptness and awkwardness are acceptable, and even unavoidable, for experience and knowledge count for little in tackling the new (1963).

An individual on the verge of change is a "marginal" person and becomes anxious while trying to decide his or her identity. The nurse practitioner is such a marginal person, no longer a nurse in the traditional sense and not yet a doctor. Marginal people are cultural hybrids; they live in the cultural life and traditions of people, never quite willing to break with the past, yet not quite accepted, because of prejudice in the new society in which he or she is seeking a place. In fact, this very non-acceptance is often a deterrent used against them, as Hughes tells us when he notes that "people of the statuses threatened by marginal people generally favor ... putting them back into their traditional places. Measures of repression and exclusion are used to this end" (1959, p. 61).

How can people be changed so that they neither restrict the freedom nor limit the potentialities of growth for others? We may turn to the body of knowledge in the field of group dynamics. We know that how much self-confidence, how energetic and productive one is, what one aspires to, is determined by one's group membership. There are several principles one uses to achieve satisfaction and productivity in the new role.

The first is that those people who are to be changed and those who are to exert influence for change must have a strong sense of belonging to the same group. The second is that members of that group must share the same perceptions of the need for the new role. The third is that changes in one part of the group will produce strain in other parts, which can only be reduced by eliminating the change or bringing about readjustments in the related parts, and the fourth is that, in attempting change, one involves three levels of personnel—the target group, the group below, and the group above—in all aspects of the plan, from its inception.

Utilizing the idea of the nurse practitioner to overcome resistance to the change, the nurse practitioner, the various other types of nurses, and the physicians must all have a strong sense of belonging to the same group, that of health care providers. All those in the system must share the same perceptions of the need for the nurse practitioner. All will need to understand, and then act upon that understanding, that the practice of all three types of providers will be changed. Most of all, as the change is considered, all three levels of persons must be involved in the plan from its inception—physicians, nurse practitioner, and nurse (both professional and practical). These four principles are means for social interventions, mechanisms

developed through research. Without them and preparation for the change, there can only be conflict and confusion.

A second major factor that hinders us in shaping change is woman's traditionally passive role. Nursing is still primarily a woman's occupation, although change is taking place in this realm, too. Philosopher Dena Justin has written a delightful article describing how women became passive (1973). She tells us that once a great mother goddess reigned and women played the dominant role in society. This goddess reigned over the sky, earth, and underworld, revealing herself in the ever-occurring productivity of the earth, in the ever-recurring rhythm of the moon and seas, and in woman. Woman shared with her the magic of procreation and nurture and the menstrual cycle that coincided with the lunar cycle. The theory was revised around 3000 B.C., which dovetails with Egyptologist G. Elliot Smith's theory of social change. One of the ideas diffused to all peoples of the world was that of man as the prime mover of the universe. Man, through Holy Writ, established the dominant male principle and subordinated to him woman in economic and social spheres. Eve was taken from Adam's rib; matriarchy became patriarchy. Until our own generation, the passivity of women and their second place in the scheme of things was expected female behavior by the majority of both sexes. Only now is equal opportunity a matter of both legislation and ethos.

The third factor mitigating against change is the lack of knowledge of how to guide it. Social engineering is an invention of this century. In Figure 28-2 there is a list of principles one may use to plan for effective changes. These are means for instigating change based on social research.

Change is accepted more easily when reasons for it are understood, when administration approves and accepts the idea, and when all who are involved and affected by the change have a part in planning for it.

Three factors that promote change are a strong professional association, application of principles founded upon research of change, and assertive

Involvement

Involve all who are to be affected by the change in the planning for it from the very beginning. Together, discuss what could be changed and what strategies should be used to effect it. People will usually adopt innovations that they perceive will be beneficial to themselves.

Motivation

One needs to understand that feelings and emotions govern behavior in order to motivate people. To do this, advocates of change create an openness of communications, a trust, and a reduction of status barriers. Motivation involves honesty in recognizing one's own feelings as well as in caring for and respecting those of others. It means knowing and practicing the art of a helping relationship.

Planning

This is the sine qua non for effecting permanent and productive change. Planning means considering the inputs and constraints that are "givens"; it means considering inputs that should be sought. It means communicating and arranging the physical, social, and emotional environment so that all needed resources are available.

Legitimation

For change to be permanent, it must be sanctioned by society and legitimized. For the expanded nurse role to be sanctioned, all who will be affected by it must see the new role as a desirable and legitimate one. The idea of expanded nursing practice must be sold to the power structure in the occupational setting and in the community, both medical and nonmedical, for it to be accepted.

Education

To implement change, one reeducates, using principles of "people" and "thing" technology. "People" technology refers to techniques one uses in relation to the behavior of man. "Thing" technology refers to techniques involved in implementing ideas. In order for administrators to educate those who will be involved in the movement, knowledge of both human behavior and the functions and responsibilities of the expanded nursing role is vital.

Management

Practice is required in striking a balance between the two aspects of management, that of maximizing freedom for those at the grass-roots level and enforcing agency policy and authority. This is the art of management. Nurse administrators use techniques for changing people's attitudes; they also use strategies of power. How to be flexible with power is the most important aspect of management.

Expectations

In implementing change, one holds many expectations. One expects resistance; one expects only a few adopters in the beginning; one expects problems. There will always be some who will not accept the new. There will always be problems when change is introduced. According to the theory of cultural lag, problems occur when change is implemented before people's customs and environment are adapted in order to accommodate the change.

Nurturance

One must nurture those who change, the adopters. They have much resistance to overcome, from patients, nurse colleagues, and physicians. They need support, both emotional and administrative. The best way to obtain early adopters is to locate those dissatisfied with the status quo, those who want to change. These are often the young and most highly educated, those desiring status and prestige, and those willing to take risks; they have less to lose in their professional lifetimes.

Trust

Trust is the key to effectively changing people's ways of doing things. Trust people to do what is right for themselves. Be trustworthy; administrators have power.

Figure 28-2 Guidelines for implementing change.

action. The first, a strong professional association, promotes change through political clout. Through power, which comes when nurses speak collectively, forcefully, and knowledgably, comes change, in the desired direction. The second factor is the application of the principles related to planned change. Practice makes perfect. However, principles of overcoming resistance to change have been founded on research, and can only be utilized if they are known well by all those involved. The third factor, assertive action—vocal participation in the arena where decisions about nursing are made—is a powerful facilitator of change. Where are we as plans for national health insurance are being made? Are we talking with our legislators? If not, why not?

Let me not end, however, with the notion that as nurses we need to be militant. Society has trained us to believe that people, especially men, are driven by the idea that winning is the only thing. But that leads us to forget that man's basic nature is one of love and cooperation.

Games of many cultures have no competitive aspect to them at all. For example, the Tangu people of New Guinea have a game called "Take Tak" that consists of throwing a spinning top into massed lots of stakes placed in the ground. Two teams try to touch as many stakes as possible with the top. The object of the game, however, is not to win, but to tie. The game goes on until a draw is reached.

Cooperation is basic to man's nature. If we will cooperate with other health professionals, especially physicians, in taking on primary care assessment, in teaching the prevention of disease and disability, in managing the chronically ill and disabled, the healthy pregnant woman, the well child, and those with minor ills, we will find a more satisfying role for ourselves. Diagnosis, treatment, and cure of disease and management of the acutely ill and disabled—these are the work of the physician. It is predominantly in the primary care segment that our roles are blurred, that there is conflict and confusion. Figure 28-3 depicts my concept of modern nursing and medical services.

You will note that the pyramid method of caring for those with health needs, with the physician at the top, is history; whereas the "pie" division of labor is 1976 (see Figure 28-3).

There is much work for us all. In the realm of primary health care services, we have traveled a long way from that of our ancestors, the *feldshers*, who began as medical officers in the Tsar's army in the 17th, 18th, and 19th centuries by delivering medical and preventive care to soldiers. We have come a long way, too, from the nurses who practiced in previous centuries, who fed, bathed, and encouraged the ill and who taught people how to better care for the health of themselves and their loved ones. By expanding our skills we are able to contribute even more to the improvement of health care delivery. It is a big task, but we are equal to it.

Almost any revolution in history—political, literary, industrial, scientific, or social—began with one, then two, then three, or four, or five who believed. We have a choice. Choice is a matter of commitment. Commitment is indicated by behavior—not what we *say* we do, but what we *do*—today, tomorrow, and through the days that follow. For that is how the future is made.

SUMMARY

Nursing can *shape* its future. It need not be shaped by the ubiquitous changes in today's world. Taking on both health care services and the primary care of individuals with health needs as our wedge of the pie, but leaving diagnosis, treatment, cure of disease and disability to physicians and their extenders—physicians' assistants, modern nurses may practice an expanded role, in a cooperative manner, with other health disciplines, all the while having the patient as the focus of concern.

Yesterday's nurse followed Nightingale's precepts. She had a clear sense of her own identity and that of others. Today's nurse is working in the midst of a period of cultural lag. She is caught up in a period of unrest, uncertainty—and, yes, excitement—as the concept of the nurse practitioner and

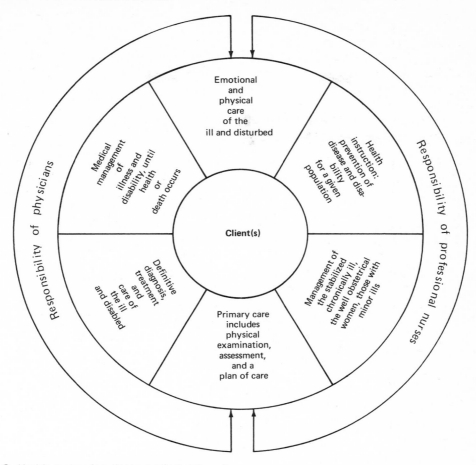

Figure 28-3 Health services for clients: medical and nursing

the expanded nursing role move toward full acceptance. Tomorrow's nurse will settle into the status quo. She will practice at the new level, or become obsolete. What will the new level be? The details will unfold with the decades. But there is no doubt that nurses are moving rapidly into new areas of caring for the health of people.

Health is now considered a right for each of us. Keeping healthy means knowing what behavior, what lifestyle must be followed. Just as today's nurse helps the victim of a heart attack adjust to a new regimen and yesterday's nurse took his blood pressure, tomorrow's nurse will help one choose an appropriate lifestyle early in life in order to avoid the heart attack.

Nurses have always considered teaching and counseling part of their role. Today good health and prevention of disease is the sine qua non for a progressive nation and its people. If this represents a revolution—or evolution—in nursing in our time, it should be remembered that Florence Nightingale's ideas are only 100 years old, that nursing as a profession did not exist, as such, in the centuries prior to this one, and that we have already come through one revolution/evolution. Will nursing complete its evolution and exist in the expanded role so many of us foresee for it in the 21st century? I believe it will, if we want it to.

Like water, the complacent nurse follows the easier course—downhill. She or he draws false strength from looking back. Let us not be complacent. As we have seen, it is hard to change. There are myriad ways, and reasons to resist. Even education means change: education for tomorrow's nursing practice will take effort, and not be easy. Grow or die. We will be transformed either way. We should also know, though—and never forget—that the word "improvement" begins with "I."

BIBLIOGRAPHY

Coser, Lewis A.: "Social Conflict and the Theory of Social Change," *British Journal of Sociology*, 8:198, September 1957.

Dock, Lavinia: "Sanitary Inspection: A New Field for Nurses," *American Journal of Nursing*, 3: 529–532, 1903.

———: "The Changing Outlook of Nursing," *American Journal of Nursing*, 9(4):504–507, February 1909.

Douglas, William O.: *Freedom of the Mind. Reading for an Age of Change*, American Library Association, New York, 1962.

Hoffer, Eric: *The Ordeal of Change*, Harper & Row, New York, 1963.

Hughes, Everett C.: "Social Change and Status Protest: An Essay on the Marginal Man," *Phylon*, 1:58–65, First Quarter, 1959.

Justin, Dena: "The Downfall of Woman," *Intellectual Digest*, pp. 90–91, October 1973.

LaPiere, Richard T.: *Social Change*, McGraw Hill, New York, 1965.

Lockland, George T.: *Grow or Die: The Unifying Principle of Transformation*, Dell, New York, 1973.

Platt, John R.: "The World Transformation and What Must Be Done," in *Social Change and Human Behavior*, National Institute of Mental Health, Rockville, Md., 1972.

Talbot, Dorothy M.: "Social Change and Occupational Health Nursing," *Occupational Health Nursing*, 22:9, April 1974.

———: "Cultural Lag and Occupational Health Nursing," *Occupational Health Nursing*, 23: 11–15, October 1975.

EDITOR'S QUESTIONS FOR DISCUSSION

How might resistance to the acceptance of the roles of nurse practitioner and independent nurse practitioner be overcome by some professionals in nursing and medicine? How might nursing facilitate the acceptance of new roles in nursing? What underlying factors contribute to the development of new roles in nursing? How are new roles in nursing legitimated? Who have been the innovators, advocates, and adopters of the nurse practitioner role? Is the nurse practitioner a "marginal" person to nursing? How can changes in nursing be directed? What factors might effect future changes in nursing?

Chapter 29

The Expanded Role of the Nurse: Current Status and Future Prospects

Jean Hofmann Tomich, R.N., Ph.D.
Associate Professor of Health Administration
University of Missouri at Kansas City

Jean Hofmann Tomich describes the current status of new roles in nursing, prescribes a unique theoretical framework for nursing, and presents a means of applying theory to practice. She differentiates the domains of nursing and medicine. Tomich reveals inconsistencies in terminology for new roles in nursing and indicates what types of programs initiated these roles. The proposed fee-for-service is viewed as a self-defeating action for nursing. She prefers the development of a model different from that for medicine, based on the *social* activity of nursing. The *social* meaning, relationship, and consequence of activity are defined as the domain of nursing. The philosophy of David Bakan, which provides a basis for understanding social meanings of disease, death, suffering, and pain, is articulated as the foundation for defining nursing roles. Diagnostic categories in nursing are viewed as ill-founded replications of the medical world.

INTRODUCTION

This chapter is addressed to the problem of relating the phenomenon of the expanded role of the nurse as a set of challenges to the health care system of today. The introduction further defines the problem, locates the problem in a conceptual framework, and relates it to the larger societal issue of professional-client relationships. The rest of the chapter is divided into three parts: part 1, entitled "Current Status of New Roles," provides a description of the current status of new roles in nursing, defining them in relation to customary roles and nursing practices; part 2, entitled "The Leading Edge," provides a theoretical framework consistent with the wellness-perspective and the patient-need emphasis of nursing, as a substantive

base for recognition of nursing autonomy in the division of labor in the work of healing; and part 3, "Implications for the Future of Nursing," describes some means of applying the theory to practice, specifying some nursing techniques appropriate to the social nature of the work of healing that may legitimize and provide credibility for the nursing enterprise.

A central thesis of this paper is that the primary task in the movement toward professional autonomy by nurses is to clearly and definitively differentiate the arena of nursing from the arena of medicine, that adoption of any other strategy will inevitably short-circuit that objective.

The sociological concept of roles denotes reciprocal relationships; thus, nursing roles must be considered in the context of a defining role set, namely in relation to the roles of the physician and of the patient. The relevance of the problem concerns modifications in the role of nurses and how those modifications affect relationships among nurses, physicians, and patients. Such relationships are shaped, in large part, by the framework for social interaction imposed by the health care system. Central to that system is a "division of labor surrounding the highly professionalized activity of healing . . . ordered by the politically dominant profession," namely the medical profession (Freidson, 1971, p. 48). On the other hand, as Freidson points out, there are few traditional tasks of healing, once considered the prerogative of the physician, that are not also performed by other personnel organized around the work of healing. What distinguishes medicine from other health occupations or professions is the primacy of the physician in the division of labor, not only in the technical areas but also in the location and social organization, and the economic aspects of the work of healing.

The dominance of the physician, legitimized by the state and supported by members of society, is vulnerable to challenges by the state and by the people. The emergence of new roles in nursing may be considered as a set of challenges to the primacy of the physician. Parallel challenges to health professionals by the consuming public are organized around client-rights, the right to health care, the right to make decisions regarding one's own body, and the right to die. Indeed, the problem fits a larger perspective—an essentially universal contemporary challenge by the lay public of secrecy, including that implied by esoteric knowledge, and of the hierarchical power and authority of the "expert." An increasingly knowledgable and sophisticated consuming public is beginning to agree with George Bernard Shaw that "every profession is a conspiracy against the laity."

CURRENT STATUS OF NEW ROLES

The generalized concept of the expanded role of the nurse, under which rubric most new and emerging roles are subsumed, points to the necessity for elaborating relationships inherent in the descriptive term "expanded" and providing a base for considering features and characteristics of such roles. The current status of expanded roles is considered against the backdrop of customary roles as a movement by nurses toward an offensive rather than a defensive stance relative to health system role-set relationships.

The proliferation of formal programs of education and training for expanded roles is a phenomenon of the past decade, with the numbers of programs for nurses increasing from 170 to 350 (106 percent) (Roth, 1975, p. 23). That the expanded role of the nurse is not a unitary concept is evidenced by the multiplicity of labels assigned to products of such programs. For example, an official directory of programs in existence during 1974–75 differentiates programs leading to an academic degree from those awarding a certificate (ANA, p. iii, 1975). However, there is little consistency in the terminology applied to products of either type of program. Most products of certificate programs are labeled "nurse practitioner," with prefixes designating areas of specialization. "Ambulatory child health care nurse" and "nurse midwife" label other products of certification programs. On the other hand, graduates of master's degree programs may be titled clinical nurse specialist, clinical specialist, nurse associate, nurse clinician, specialist, nurse practitioner, nurse specialist, or simply nurse (community health, public health, school, maternal-child) or nurse midwife. The overlapping of labels (titles) adds to confusion in attempts at definition. Length of programs run from 4 weeks to 2 calendar years, adding differential preparation as another ambiguous variable.

The report of an evaluation study of the use of expanded roles of health workers in the United States prepared for the National Science Foundation states the philosophy underlying the introduction of such personnel is that "physician support personnel can assume a large portion of preventitive, acute, and restorative care, thereby freeing physicians to care for more seriously ill patients" (Cohen, 1974, p. 1). Findings of the study have led to expectations for impressive gains in physician productivity. The major objective of the study was to review and evaluate existing research on the costs and benefits of introducing new health practitioners, i.e., such personnel as physician assistants and nurse practitioners, assuming their impact to be similar. The fallacy of that basic assumption invalidates the findings. According to Cohen, limitations in research designs in general, and studies conducted by persons with vested interests in outcomes, as well as the failure to differentiate types of roles, impose serious qualifications on results (Cohen, 1974, pp. 123-127). These criticisms appear to apply with equal force to this study. Thus, the major conclusions of the study were that:

> There is a paucity of valid and useful policy related empirical findings both on the impact of health workers in new and expanded roles, and on the effects of factors influencing their efficient use which represent comprehensive evaluation of both costs and benefits of new health practitioners. Rather, the studies we have reviewed offer perspectives and raise hypotheses which need to be tested. (Cohen, 1974, pp. xxi–xxii)

All in all, the results of the study are not illuminating but present evidence of needed documentation of the "expanded role." Prospective studies, comparative studies, controlled experiments, and longitudinal studies conducted by outside investigators are needed.

A recent survey of pediatric nurse practitioners yielded the most definitive data to date on an expanded nurse role (Bishop and Roth, 1975). As of 1974, 2,300 pediatric nurse practitioners were identified and enumerated, 85 percent of whom were actively employed in nursing. Of the total 85 percent of employed pediatric nurse practitioners, 41.7 percent were prepared in a baccalaureate degree program; 34.6 percent in a diploma program; and 19.2 percent in a master's degree program or higher (Bishop and Roth, 1975, p. 15). Forty-two percent of the pediatric practitioners

were employed in public/community health centers; 21 percent in hospitals or clinics; and 19.2 percent in physician's offices (Bishop and Roth, 1975, p. 21). In terms of distribution in the United States: 19.2 percent were employed in the East North Central Region, 18.7 percent in the Pacific, 13.7 percent in the Middle Atlantic, and approximately 9 percent in the New England, South Atlantic, East South Central, and Mountain areas. Areas of 5 percent or less representation were the West South Central and West North Central (Bishop and Roth, 1975, p. 18).

Other classifications of new or emerging nursing roles include the nurse-researcher, defined as "doctorally prepared nurses" who hold a Ph.D. degree—basically acknowledged as a research degree.[1] Legitimization of this role is inherent in the Ph.D. degree. The registered nurse consultant in the intermediate care facility serving older adults is a new role that has achieved legitimization via Title 45—Public Welfare.[2] Popular recognition of emerging roles is evidenced by an article in the *Wall Street Journal* referring to "supernurses."[3]

There is no reporting of data on the number of nurses functioning in expanded roles, and no consensus on estimates nor quality of service provided. This may be, in part, a consequence of varieties of titles, sources, and types of preparation, functioning in their role, as well as lack of legitimization.[4] The American Nurses Association (ANA)

---

[1] From the vertical files of ANA. Between 1,100 and 1,200 nurses hold doctoral degrees in academic fields, about half of whom hold the Ph.D. As of this writing, fifteen doctoral programs in nursing are underway in university settings.

[2] *Federal Register*, vol. 39, no. 12, sec. 249.12 (a) (9) (i), Jan. 17, 1974, p. 2225.

[3] Joann S. Lublin, "'Supernurses Provide Care for Thousands, Helping Doctors Cope," *Wall Street Journal*, vol. 54, no. 183, pp. 1, 13, 1976.

[4] The author has had practicing physicians introduce office nurses as "clinicians" trained by their employers. Indeed, this has been a long tradition among general practitioners in small towns and rural areas based on expediency and perpetuated by the fact that it works. One perspective accounting for the emergence of certification programs for expanded roles is the legitimization of an already existing category in the nurse labor pool.

has attempted to correct this state of affairs by requesting the congress of the ANA for a definition of nursing practice to clarify the situation. As an initial step in approximating uniformity of identification for practitioners, employers, and consumers, in May 1974, definitions were stated as follows:

> *Practitioners* of professional nursing are registered nurses who provide direct care to clients utilizing the nursing process in arriving at decisions. They work in a collegial and collaborative relationship with other health professionals to determine health care needs and assume responsibility for nursing care. In the course of their practice they assess the effectiveness of actions taken, identify and carry out systematic investigations of clinical problems, and engage in periodic review of their own contributions to health care and those of their progressional peers.
>
> *Nurse Practitioners* have advanced skills in the assessment of the physical and psychosocial health-illness status of individuals, families or groups in a variety of settings through health and development history taking and physical examination. They are prepared for these special skills by formal continuing education which adheres to ANA approved guidelines, or in baccalaureate nursing programs.
>
> *Nurse Clinicians* have well-developed competencies in utilizing a broad range of cues. These cues are used for prescribing and implementing both direct and indirect nursing care and for articulating nursing therapies with other planned therapies. Nurse clinicians demonstrate expertise in nursing practice and insure ongoing development of expertise through clinical experience and continuing education. General minimal preparation for this role is the baccalaureate degree.
>
> *Clinical Nurse Specialists* are primarily clinicians with a high degree of knowledge, skill and competence in a specialized area of nursing. These are made directly available to the public through the provision of nursing care to clients and indirectly available through guidance and planning of care with other nursing personnel. Clinical nurse specialists hold a master's degree

in nursing, preferably with an emphasis in clinical nursing.[5]

The difficulty and acknowledged transitional nature of the task notwithstanding, these and other attempts at definition suffer from frequent failures to specify a substantive core of nursing differentiating the work of nursing from medicine and the work of other professional health workers.[6]

The focus of medicine as a consulting profession is on the diagnosis and treatment of disease. Thus, physicians approach the work of healing from the perspective of pathological conditions. By contrast, nursing approaches the work of healing from the perspective of patient needs with the emphasis on care rather than cure, on health or wellness rather than illness. What nursing has not yet effected is a basic, generic focus differentiating the nursing arena from the medical arena. This issue will be dealt with in detail in a later section of this paper.

Official definitions frequently seem to be written in response to requests for clarification or as attempts to impose some order on the consequences of unplanned change.[7] For example, the professional nurse, in the official description, is a registered nurse who may hold a 2-year associate arts degree, a 3-year diploma, or a 4- or 5-year baccalaureate degree, or have advanced preparation at the master's and doctoral levels as well as

[5]Congress for Nursing Practice, "DEFINITION: Nurse Practitioner, Nurse Clinician and Clinical Nurse Specialists," provided to the author from American Nurses Association files.

[6]Ongoing efforts are being made in this area, e.g., efforts to develop an integrated policy for primary care; to develop professional standards of care; and to develop quality assurance programs.

[7]See "Nurses, In the Extended Role, Are Not Physician Assistants," undated ANA vertical file. See also M. G. Lesnik and B. E. Anderson, "Nursing Practice and the Law." From ANA files, "The American Nurses' Association Views and Emerging Physicians Assistant," December 17, 1973, (revised); The National Joint Practice Commission, June 18, 1973; and Statement on Certification of Nurses and Physicians, February 8, 1974.

certification in areas of specialization. In the context of participation in the nursing labor force, only 18 percent of employed nurses have baccalaureate or higher degree preparation (Heistand and Ostow, 1976, pp. 61–73). Three of the official definitions of practice cited, with the single exception of the basic undifferentiated registered nurse practitioners, require a baccalaureate or higher degree for practice.

Roth raises questions regarding the distribution of skills as well as the geographic maldistribution of nursing manpower. The supply of nursing manpower on a national level currently approximates projected levels of need, displaying an increase from 298 per 100,000 population in 1962 to 380 in 1972. Geographic maldistribution is evident in the range: from 235 in the East South Central to 596 in New England in 1972 (Roth in Heistand and Ostow, 1976, p. 65). Even with an increase of 33 percent in total supply during the decade, the gap between the highest and lowest regional ratios increased from 305 to 361. As projected requirements in numbers are met for customary positions, there is some concern about the supply of qualified nurses to fill teaching, supervisory, and administrative positions and to assume expanded roles (Roth in Heistand and Ostow, 1976, pp. 61–73). The budgeted unfulfilled nurse faculty positions for 1972 were approximately 4 percent for diploma, associate degree programs and 5 percent for baccalaureate or higher degree programs (Bishop and Roth, 1975, p. 10).

Approximately two-thirds of all registered nurses work in hospitals, with nursing homes and physicians' offices running a poor second at approximately 7 percent each (Bishop and Roth, 1975, p. 70). As Scott and Levine (1976, pp. 25–46) also point out, most (approximately 81 percent, using Roth's estimate) nursing services are currently delivered within complex organizations with their formal bureaucratic structures that require an array of supervisory and administrative nursing personnel. These care patterns are largely consequences of the privacy of medicine in the location and social organization of

health care and, if appropriately challenged, are subject to change in the future.

Claims related to supply, demand, utilization, and distribution of personnel, as well as claims implicit in practice definitions, must be validated in terms of substantiation of a central focus of nursing. The role of the nurse and the "turf" of nursing must be clearly and definitely differentiated from the role of the physician and the turf of medicine. Definitions of nursing must be consistent with both the positive health perspective and the emphasis on patient needs. That focus constitutes the substance of the next section. The expanded role of the nurse may be viewed as the leading edge into the future of nursing.

THE LEADING EDGE

The concern is with ways in which the expanded role of the nurse may be directed in order to contribute to the development of nursing in the future. The specific task at hand is to move in the direction of specifying a central core for nursing, which differentiates nursing practice from medical practice, provides grounds for recognition of nursing as self-governing, and establishes a base of credibility for nursing. Identifying and articulating barriers impeding progress in that direction appears to be an appropriate approach.

Adoption of the medical model by nursing constitutes the single most salient and most self-defeating barrier to achievement of full status for nursing in the work of healing. Self-government and self-direction are prerequisites to full stature in the division of health labor. To rely on the medical model implies lack of self-government and self-direction.

A tendency to develop nursing from the medical model reflects a passé overdependency, insecurity in conceptions of the unique service nursing can provide, and lack of risk-taking in leadership. The ability to take risks, after careful reflection, is necessary for nursing to meet the challenges of the future.

The American physician-based health care

system, itself, may be ineffective in three ways: (1) clinical damage to clients may outweigh potential benefits; (2) the system enhances political conditions that may render society unhealthy; and (3) the system tends to mystify the role of the patient in health care processes. Illich conceptualizes *iatrogenesis* as the major obstacle to a healthy life, and differentiates types of iatrogenesis as follows:

> *Clinical iatrogenesis* results when organic coping capacity is replaced by heteronomous management;
>
> *Social iatrogenesis* in which the environment is deprived of those conditions that endow individuals, families and neighborhoods with control over their own internal states and over their milieu; and
>
> *Cultural iatrogenesis* in which the medical enterprise saps the will of people to suffer their reality . . . to accept as inevitable and often irremedial pain and impairment, decline, and death. (Illich, 1976, pp. 127–128)

Such criticisms suggest the opportunity for nursing to forcefully reiterate its focus on health, emphasize patient needs across settings, and increasingly seek noninstitutional settings for practice of expanded roles. The distribution of pediatric nurse practitioners indicates there are patterns of practice clearly departing from those of nursing in general, with 21 percent of pediatric nurse practitioners in hospital settings compared to 65 percent for nursing in general, and most of the pediatric nurse practitioners—42 percent—functioning in ambulatory care settings (Bishop and Roth, 1975, p. 21). That departure, however, is not sufficiently different from the pattern currently under fire. It would behoove nursing to not try and control both supply and demand of personnel, but to concentrate now and in the future on the redistribution of both skills and supply in underserved areas.

The recent emphasis on the development of diagnostic categories in nursing could be an ill-founded replication of the medical model. Classification is, on one level necessary for theory building, relatively open while categories based on empirically sound data are necessary if errors in practice as consequences of rigid classificatory schemes are to be avoided.

There are other self-defeating actions that nursing has taken. For example, a number of official statements by the American Nurses Association supporting the notion of reimbursement for nurses on a fee-for-service basis reflect a relatively uncritical adoption of a medical position that is related to the escalation of health care costs and that may work to the detriment of nursing. Another example of a self-defeating position is the statement made by an official ANA document that with the decreases in employment in industry and agriculture, it is important to expand employment opportunities in the health services (from the vertical files of ANA). Apparently this document was formulated without considering the impact of escalating labor costs on the costs of health care. The statement would seem to reflect a pretentious position. This constitutes an example of generating social distance from the client population analogous to that inherent in institutionalization of health care with the control of environment solely in professional hands. A pattern such as this is singularly destructive to professional-client relations.

The central question that needs to be addressed is why nursing adopts a medical model reminiscent of outmoded professional relationships? Specification of a central core of nursing, articulated universally and applied consistently, may move nursing from the defensive position implicit in adoption of the medical model, thereby focusing attention on the nature of the nursing role.

Freidson (1971, pp. 341–343) defines four dimensions of the content of work: (1) basic assumptions and theoretical concepts; (2) selective attention; (3) a body of knowledge; and (4) techniques of management. In medicine, the etiological notion of disease constitutes a basic assumption underlying the theoretical concept of the germ theory: selective attention is implicit in the notion of pathology that leads to diagnostic categories (as well as nondisease categories) underlying a moral theory of normality. Medicine consists of a large and complex body of knowledge about empirical chemical, physical, and other conditions or states designated as illnesses, about procedures for dealing with those states or conditions, and techniques of management, i.e., rules determining how knowledge and techniques are applied. It is the latter, techniques of management, that I wish to address. There are inevitable overlappings in the other dimensions of the content of work, by virtue of the commonality of the *object* of physician and nursing activity, namely the patient. It is in the area of application of *applied* knowledge of the sciences that the core of nursing may be identified and substantiated. This is the area in which the client has primary interest, and for which nursing is ideally fitted.

Although nursing cannot claim it as its exclusive domain, the core activity of nursing itself is social. Nursing has *social meaning*, is embodied in *social relationships*, and has *social consequences* for the members of that relationship (Freidson, 1971, p. 341).

This, then is the turf that nursing might further develop as its own, and thus clearly and distinctly differentiate nursing from medicine. The distinction between nursing and medicine has been implicit in such statements as those that the nurse is at the bedside of the patient around the clock while the physician is a transient in hospital settings. The quality of social interaction, the articulation of social and psychological principles in the core of basic, continuing, and inservice education efforts are imperative if nursing is to be validated in practice and recognized by the client population as well as by its professional peers. At psychological and social levels, the exchange of social meanings and the fostering of social relationships can promote healing and extend life. Such social consequences are predicated on the notion of involving clients in decisions about their care, working to reduce the threat of separation/estrangement as a

stress factor, and openly sharing information about every aspect of the health problem, including prognosis and treatment alternatives. Although nursing currently has made advances in "psychosocial aspects of nursing," the tenuous hold on the concept is evident in the afterthought way in which it is identified and in the tendency to ascribe such aspects to psychiatric nursing. Psychiatric nursing may distort normative interactive principles into pathological principles with the almost inevitable concentration on medical notions of etiology and pathology. Providing nursing with an alternative theoretical approach to health and illness may help to resolve these problems and provide a set of guidelines consistent with the nursing emphasis on health and client needs and also support claims to expertise peculiar to nursing. This concern will be addressed in the final section of the paper, providing a base for establishing credibility of nursing practices in the future.

IMPLICATIONS FOR THE FUTURE OF NURSING: MOVEMENT TOWARD INTERDEPENDENCY AND EQUALITY

Even with the emergence of the expanded role of the nurse, given the existing locus of power and organizational aspects of the health care system, new roles, in and of themselves, are not going to lead to greater autonomy, legitimacy, and credibility for nurses.

It is critical that nurses *define* their own roles, and there is evidence that this is being initiated.

In contrast to the medical model there is a philosophy articulated by David Bakan (1971), which could and should be the basis for the definition of nursing roles. Bakan synthesizes some aspects of post-Darwinian theory and the theorizing of Freud and Selye, and utilizes that synthesis in a profound effort to understand the conditions of human mortality.

Bakan (1971, pp. 61–73) presents the case for viewing disease, death, pain, and suffering as natural conditions, i.e., biologically inherent in human growth. Given disease, death, pain, and suffering as internal, the locus of management of such processes is likewise within the human being and may be mobilized by increasing understanding (particularly self-understanding) and increasing communication at all levels, from the cellular to the societal.

Rather than a contest between physician and agent of disease fought out with the patient's body as the battleground, management of processes associated with disease, death, pain, and suffering is aimed at providing conditions that *allow* the patient to engage in a natural process of self-healing. Bakan states as a premise that disease is a natural condition, as inevitable as death, and warns against believing in physical immortality.

Biologically inherent *defensive reactions*, according to Bakan, constitute the nucleus of disease, i.e., the *automatic* defensive reactions to the perceived threat of danger, whether physiological or psychological are, paradoxically, both self-injurious and self-preserving, and, simultaneously, homeostatic. Management of disease involves resolution of the paradox of "tearing asunder and joining" implicit in the defensive reactions to threat (Bakan, 1971, pp. 22–31).

The way to overcome the injuriousness is to overcome the *automaticity* of the reaction and convert that reaction to a genuine defense in order to restore a sense of unity—of wholeness. This may be accomplished by bringing the process into conscious awareness, by recognition and acknowledgment that the process is a struggle within the self and that surrender to natural healing processes is more appropriate and effective than battle or struggle. The process is accomplished through contact and communication with at least one other human being in the larger social body. As Bakan (1971, pp. 46–53) points out, the human organism is at once strongly individualistic and strongly social; there are some degrees of freedom at both the psychological and the societal levels that enable the patient to maintain health by an increase in understanding and via communication, and thus

extend life. Bakan views pain as the psychic manifestation of disease or disorder. A cry of pain that tends to evoke helping responses in others may be viewed as a signal of organic disunity and a demand for returning to unity. Pain is inversely related to well-being and can be overwhelming in its demands for the attention of the ego. Pain may be eliminated by stimulation of ego functions and by other means, e.g., by auditory stimuli, by exercises in the direction of attention, such as yoga or self-hypnosis, or simply by engaging in activities that require high concentration. Pain, physical or psychological, places a demand on the conscious ego to work to bring the diseased part back into the unity of the organism. According to Bakan, beyond all the alternatives associated with its management, pain is a harbinger of death. An understanding of the pain-annihilation complex is essential to the management of pain (Bakan, 1971, pp. 79–85). Thus, the healing arts, including nursing, may be viewed as a collective response to that demand, announced by pain.

Bakan's explanation of disease, death, pain, and suffering and the emergence of the expanded role of the nurse provide a base for carving out an area of health care as the province of nursing, and for suggesting some techniques appropriate to the management of these areas. The theory provides a basis for understanding social meanings of disease, death, suffering, and pain, promotes understandings of the importance and nature of associated social relationships, and establishes a base for predicting social consequences of relationships between nurses and patients. It seems patently clear that nursing has an essential management role in the areas of pain, suffering, dying, grief, mourning, psychosomatic illnesses, and teaching the public about processes associated with stages across the life cycle (growth and development, decline, disease, and death).

Through processes of sharing information and engaging in open and honest communication, the nurse may be instrumental in shielding the patient from being overwhelmed by the perception of threat; the nurse may also provide the conditions that allow the conversion of self-injurious reactions to self-preserving ones. To her customary set of techniques and procedures, the nurse in the expanded role might add the teaching of progressive relaxation and precision techniques. The latter are particularly applicable in working with patients who have chronic diseases. This would provide an alternative to more typical professionally directed monitoring techniques. The central objective of such efforts would be to serve patients by teaching them to self-administer techniques of survival.

Working within such a scheme would render unnecessary any tendency to defensively proclaim professionalism and any tendency to put perpetuation of the profession ahead of service to the community. Our ubiquitous educational programs, formal and informal, attest to the fact that the work of teaching is never done. It could be profitably brought to bear on the shared work of healing. Ultimately the goal is for the primary orientation of the nurse to be toward the patient but not in conflict with the physician. In the ideal-typical health care system, nurses and physicians would be viewed as interdependent partners and colleagues dedicated to doing whatever (and only what) is necessary for the patient.

BIBLIOGRAPHY

American Nurses Association: *Facts about Nursing, 1972-73,* American Nurses Association, Kansas City, Mo., 1974.

American Nurses' Association, Inc., and U.S. Department of Health, Education, and Welfare: *A Directory of Programs Preparing Registered Nurses for Expanded Roles, 1974-75,* DHEW Publication Publication No. (HRA)76-31, DHEW, Washington, D.C., May 1975.

Bakan, David: *Disease, Pain and Sacrifice: Toward a Psychology of Suffering,* Beacon, Chicago, 1971.

Bishop, Barbara E., and Aleda V. Roth: *Pediatric Nurse Practitioners—Their Practice Today,* American Nurses Association, Chicago, May 1975.

Buytendijk, F. J. J.: *Pain,* translated by Eda O'Shiel, University of Chicago Press, Chicago, 1962.

Cohen, Eva D. et. al.: *An Evaluation of Policy Related Research on New and Expanded Roles of Health Workers; Final Report,* Yale University School of Medicine, New Haven, Conn., October 1974.

Freud, Sigmund: *Group Psychology and the Analysis of the Ego,* translated by J. Strachey, Hogarth, London, 1949.

———: *Beyond the Pleasure Principle,* translated by J. Strachey, Liveright, New York, 1950.

———: "Further Remarks on the Defense-Psychoses," in *Collected Papers,* translated by J. Rickman, Hogarth, London, 1950.

Freidson, Eliot: *Profession of Medicine: A Study of the Sociology of Applied Knowledge,* Dodd, Mead, New York, 1971.

Heistand, Dale L., and Miriam Ostow (eds.): *Health Manpower Information for Policy Guidance,* Ballinger, Cambridge, Mass., 1976.

Illich, Ivan: *Medical Nemesis: The Expropriation of Health,* Pantheon, New York, 1976.

Life and Death in Medicine, A Scientific American Book, Freeman, San Francisco, 1973.

Lublin, Joann S.: "'Supernurses' Provide Care for Thousands, Helping Doctors Cope," *Wall Street Journal,* vol. 54, no. 183, pp. 1, 13, 1976.

Roth, Aleda N.: *Trends in the Distribution of Nursing Manpower,* paper presented to the Conference on Current Information on Health Manpower, April 16–18, 1975. Denver, Colorado, American Nurses Association, Chicago, revised June 1975.

Scott, Jessie M., and Eugene Levine: "Nursing Manpower Analysis: Its Past, Present and Future," in Dale L. Heistand and Miriam Ostow (eds.), *Health Manpower Information for Policy Guidance,* Ballinger, Cambridge, Mass., 1976, pp. 25–46.

Selye, Hans: *The Physiology and Pathology of Exposure to Stress: A Treatise Based on the Concepts of the General Adaptation Syndrome and the Diseases of Adaptation,* Acta, Montreal, 1950.

———: *The Stress of Life*, McGraw-Hill, New York, 1956.

———: *Stress Without Distress*, Lippincott, New York, 1974.

EDITOR'S QUESTIONS FOR DISCUSSION

What are the advantages and disadvantages of using the medical model, based on diagnosis and treatment of disease, for nursing? What models might be more effective for nursing? (See Collita, *Nursing Outlook*, Nov. 1976.) Can one define the social *meaning* of nursing activity as being the domain of nursing without including the *action* involved? Are the two essential to each other in defining the nursing role? What are the implications of Bakan's philosophy for intervention in patient care? What type of intervention does his philosophy propose for nursing?

Chapter 30

The Law and the
Expanding Nursing Role

Bonnie Bullough, R.N., Ph.D.
Professor of Nursing
California State University at Long Beach

To discuss the expanding role of the nurse without citing the legal implications of changing nursing practice for nursing and the other health professions would be inappropriate. Members of the nursing and medical professions, because of their vested interests, anxiously await public acceptance of the nurse's expanded role via legislation, since establishment of new professional roles requires this legitimation before the changes can be fully implemented. Bonnie Bullough predicts what future changes in legislation might take place. She traces the major phases in nursing licensure from 1900 to 1975. Thirty states have now revised their nurse practice acts to facilitate role expansion for registered nurses. No single pattern has emerged, but four approaches are identified. The key factors are the extent to which a nursing diagnosis is differentiated from a medical one and the extent to which physicians delegate practice activities to nurses through their medical practice acts. Bullough explores the psychological barriers of nurses and the attitudes of physicians to the formation of the state nurse practice acts. Changes in the law are facilitating the development of an autonomous, independent practice in nursing. However, legislation has not solved the problems of continuing education needed for continued competence, requirements of educational programs, or accreditation of the expanded nurse role.

INTRODUCTION

The role of the registered nurse is in a period of rapid change as many nurses shed their traditional caution and take on an expanded role in both acute and primary settings. Various factors have contributed to the need for this role expansion, including the shortage of primary care physicians created by the shift away from primary to a specialty orientation in medicine, the growing consumer demand for adequate health care, and, in some cases, such as the coronary and intensive care units, the improved technology which has afforded new opportunities for skilled nurses to save the lives of a significant number of patients.

Although these factors have been present for

Address reprint requests to Professor Bullough, Department of Nursing, California State University, Long Beach, CA 90840.
This article, submitted January 26, 1974, was revised, updated and accepted for publication December 19, 1975.
Reprinted from the *American Journal of Public Health*, vol. 66, no. 3, pp. 248–254, March 1976.

more than a decade and are a part of the complex group of problems which are now being called the crisis in health care, nurses have moved rather slowly to fill the gap in the medical care system. In fact, the movement was so slow that for a time in the late 1960s it looked as if a handful of ex-corpsmen physician's assistants would have to carry the burden alone of filling the vacuum in the health care delivery system, because nurses at that time faced severe psychological barriers as well as legal ones.

While this paper will focus primarily on the changes now taking place on the legal front, it will also comment on the psychological barriers because the two factors are so intertwined. Traditionally, the physician-nurse relationship has been one of superordination-subordination to the point that, when the need for some type of middle medical worker emerged, many physicians simply did not think of nurses as being capable of independent or cooperative decision making, turning instead to physician's assistants. The mind set of the physicians, however, was only part of the problem; the more important psychological barrier was the feelings which nurses held about themselves. Many nurses experienced difficulty in seeing themselves as decision makers in the diagnostic and treatment process. They had, of course, been making diagnostic decisions for years but had protected themselves with elaborate games which cast the physician in a decision-making role even when the decision had been made by nurses.[1] While some nurses enjoyed these feminine games, others were afraid of formal responsibilities, and these latter often expressed their fears in terms of the legal consequences which they felt might follow if they took on a more responsible role in patient care. There was yet another group of nurses, including many of the major theoreticians of nursing in the decade of the sixties, who felt that nursing should travel a separate road from medicine and focus on the attendant social and psychological problems of illness rather than the presenting complaint of the patient.[2]

Added to these psychological barriers were some very tangible barriers in the form of the state nurse practice acts. In order to understand the interaction of these two barriers, the author will trace the history of nursing licensure in this country. Divided into three major phrases, the goals of the nurses who sought legislation in each of these periods will be discussed as well as how the types of laws which were passed in response to these efforts differed.[3]

The first phase coincided with the beginning of the 20th century when nurses actively campaigned for state laws to register trained nurses. This effort was necessary to bring some order into a chaotic educational system and to differentiate the trained nurse from the untrained. Following the example of, and stimulated by the publicity given Florence Nightingale in England, a few American hospitals opened training schools in the 1870s. Students quickly demonstrated themselves to be a lucrative source of cheap labor, and a period of rampant growth in hospital training schools followed— in 1880 there were 15 nursing schools, and in 1910 there were more than 1,000.[4] Since the hospitals were staffed primarily by their students, graduate nurses were forced to seek employment as private-duty nurses, and as such they competed with untrained workers and correspondence school graduates.

In 1894 and 1896 two national organizations, which eventually became the National League for Nursing and the American Nurses Association, were organized. Primary objectives of these two groups were to establish some control over the profession and to stem the untrammeled growth of substandard nursing schools.[5] State licensure seemed to be a reasonable mechanism for achieving these goals. Physicians were already registered in all of the states then in the Union. In obtaining state medical practice acts, the American Medical Association and its constituent state organizations had already fought a major court battle, and the United States Supreme Court had ruled that occupational licensure was a legitimate function of the police powers of the states.[6]

Thus, the model was available and the way

cleared for nurses to seek licensure. However, the fact that medical licensure predated that of nursing, as well as most other health occupations, also had other implications. Medicine was in a monopoly position and could claim unlimited function for physicians. All subsequent licensing acts for other health workers were essentially amendments to the medical practice acts.

To facilitate the registration campaign in the states, the nursing organization moved to set up constituent state groups, and the local membership did the necessary work of lobbying through the registration acts.[7] The nurses in North Carolina were the first to succeed[8]—a nurse registration act was passed in March of 1903; three other registration acts were passed that same year in New Jersey, New York, and Virginia. The North Carolina act allowed for licensure by waiver for the rest of that year, but, starting in 1904, only those persons who were certified by the board could be designated as Registered Nurses, use the initials "RN", and be listed on an official registry kept by the county clerk.[9]

One by one, the other states followed and by 1923 all of the states then in the Union had nurse licensure laws on their books.[10] Although state governments had the constitutional right to pass these acts, it did not mean that the legislation was ordinarily planned or initiated by members of the legislatures. Rather, the first steps were usually taken by nurses who contacted supportive representatives for assistance. Programs of local, state, and national nurses' associations often featured "how to" seminars to help nurses with the lobbying process.[11] This pattern is not unusual; although the professions often speak of public control by means of state licensure, the members of these occupations have always participated significantly in the process of licensure.[12]

None of the original registration acts included a definition of nursing in terms of the scope of practice of the profession; at that point in time they could be more accurately called nurse registration acts rather than nurse practice acts. The term "registered nurse" was defined as someone who had completed an acceptable nursing program and passed a board examination, rather than someone who engaged in a specific type of practice. This placed emphasis on the educational process, and early reform efforts tended to be focused on upgrading the educational background of registered nurses. Some of the laws became quite elaborate in their requirements for specific theoretical or clinical content.

The second phase in the development of nursing licensure began in 1938 when the first mandatory practice act was passed in New York. This law established two levels of nurses, registered and practical, and restricted nursing functions to members of these two groups.[13] This event marked the beginning of a new thrust for the efforts of nurse activists. Although there was still some concern about the fact that 19 states still did not require high school graduation for registration and 17 states still included one or more physicians on their boards,[14] the primary goal for reform became mandatory licensure.[15]

While mandatory licensure can be thought of as a long-range aspiration from the beginning of the century when abortive attempts were made to restrict the title "nurse," the goal did not seem realistic until the New York nurses broke the barrier. Their efforts, and those of nurses in several states which followed their precedent, were facilitated by the development of licensure for practical nurses. Employment patterns for nurses were changing in this period from private duty to hospital nursing, and hospital administrators argued with some justification that all nursing functions did not require the standard three-year training period which was by then the norm. The development of the practical nurse as the basic bedside practitioner allowed registered nurses to argue more successfully for licensure for all practitioners.

Besides being linked with the stratification of the nursing role, mandatory licensure included another interesting implication. In order to pass a mandatory act of any kind, it was necessary to spell out the scope of practice of the occupation which was being protected against encroachment.

The older nursing laws merely made it illegal for an unauthorized person to use the title "registered nurse," but it was not illegal for such a person to practice nursing. Once the new mandatory laws made it illegal for an unauthorized person to practice nursing, a definition of the scope of practice had to be written into these laws so that violations of the mandatory provisions could be identified. Eventually the definition even came to be thought of as a goal in and of itself. Nurses and the legal advisors of the day advocated that the scope of practice be defined in nurse practice acts.[16]

The process of defining nursing and passing mandatory nurse practice acts was facilitated in 1955 when the Board of Directors of the American Nurses Association (ANA) adopted a model definition of nursing. Professional practice was defined as:

> ... the performance, for compensation, of any acts in the observation, care and counsel of the ill, injured or infirm or in the maintenance of health or prevention of illness of others, or in the supervision and teaching of other personnel or the administration of medications and treatments as prescribed by a licensed physician or a licensed dentist; requiring substantial specialized judgment and skill and based on knowledge and application of principles of biological, physical and social science. The foregoing shall not be deemed to include any acts of diagnosis or prescription of therapeutic or corrective measures.[17]

This definition becomes the new model for changing nurse practice acts, so that, by 1967, 15 states had incorporated the language of this model into their state laws, and six states had used the model with only slight modifications.[18] A notable aspect of this model act, as well as the other similar definitions of practice, is the disclaimer which clearly spells out the fact that nursing did not include any acts of diagnosis or the prescription of therapeutic measures. Before the era of mandatory licensure, nurse registration acts did not define

nursing, with the result that they did not include any such disclaimer. Moreover, some of the definitions passed before the ANA model act was formulated used other language which did not forbid diagnosis and treatment.

Actually, by 1955, when the model act was issued by the ANA, nurses were a fairly well-educated group of workers. While there were still a few states which did not require high school graduation for licensure, this had become a dead issue, because the schools themselves, aided by standards developed by the National League for Nursing, had moved to uphold the standard. A trend to move educational programs into colleges and universities was developing and although only about 15 percent of the schools were collegiate,[19] the movement was already a significant factor in motivating the diploma schools to improve their programs and move away from the old apprenticeship model. National pool examinations had been developed to upgrade state board examinations and to facilitate the movement of nurses between jurisdictions.[20] With this educational background nurses were, in 1955, observing patients, collecting data about their conditions, and acting on those decisions to deliver nursing care. They were in short, making diagnostic and therapeutic decisions, and the disclaimers in the scope of practice statements which were enacted in this period were out of date at the time they were written.

Various coping mechanisms evolved to attempt to deal with the restrictions in the nursing and medical practice acts. One of these mechanisms was the joint statement. Since the California medical practice act reserved to physicians the right to pierce the skin, representatives of the California Nurses' Association met with representatives of the medical and hospital associations in 1957 to draw up a statement supporting nurses doing vena punctures.[21] Following this precedent, similar statements were issued by joint committees in Ohio and Pennsylvania. In 1966, the Michigan Heart Association passed a resolution favoring the use of defibrillators by coronary care nurses,[22] and in 1968 the Hawaii nursing, medical, and hospital associations approved nurses doing cardio-pulmonary resuscitation.[23] The nurse practice acts in all four of these last mentioned states forbid nurses performing medical diagnoses or treatments. The joint statements were given further support when permanent state joint practice commissions were set up in response to recommendations by the National Commission for the Study of Nursing and Nursing Education.[24] These joint practice commissions are now drafting statements supporting extended functions for nurses.

While it is clear that these various types of statements do not have the force of law, they seemed to lend some support to nurses whose functions fell outside the boundaries of the statutes. It is possible they may have prevented some legal sanctions against them; in 1967 the California Nurses' Association reported that not one single nurse, following criteria set up under one of the statements, had been indicted.[25] Of course, the truth of the matter is that nurses have not ordinarily been sued or cited for exceeding their scope of practice unless negligence was in some way involved.

Nurses are, however, law abiding citizens. The fact that there have been few nurses punished for exceeding the scope of practice statements in their state nursing acts did not really satisfy them. The clear prohibitions in the majority of the state acts against nurses diagnosing and treating were, therefore, a significant barrier to the development of expanded roles. This was in spite of the fact that a special committee, appointed by the Secretary of the Department of Health, Education, and Welfare, issued a report in 1971 stating that its members saw no legal obstacles to role extension for nurses.[26] The statement lacked credibility as the Attorneys General of Arizona[27] and California[28] issued statements that it was illegal for nurses in their states to diagnose or treat patients. In this climate of opinion it was not surprising that some educational institutions, agencies, and nurses, adopted a wait and see attitude about role expansion.

This state of confusion, however, ushered in the third phase in nursing licensure, and events are now moving so fast they have taken on an almost revolutionary character. As indicated in Table 30-1, there are 30 states which have enacted amendments to their nurse practice acts in the last five years to facilitate nurses taking on diagnostic and treatment functions. One state, Virginia, amended its medical practice act to assign regulatory responsibility for nurses with expanded functions to the Board of Medicine.[29] There are ten other jurisdictions out of the 54 in the table which do not include a prohibition against diagnosis and treatment in their nurse practice act, although new legislation may still be needed in some of these states because of prohibitions in the medical practice acts. There are still 13 jurisdictions which have statutory prohibitions against nurses diagnosing and treating patients; these acts are clearly in need of revision, and bills are being drafted in several of the states to make the necessary changes.

The first state to revise its nurse practice act in this new direction was Idaho; in 1971 the legislature inserted the following clause after the prohibition against diagnosis and treatment:

> . . . except as may be authorized by rules and and regulations jointly promulgated by the Idaho state board of medicine and the Idaho board of nursing which shall be implemented by the Idaho board of nursing.[30]

Following passage of the amendment, the combined boards met and developed regulations. Nurses seeking to expand their activities to include acts of medical diagnosis or treatment in Idaho are required to submit evidence to their agency that they have obtained the necessary special education. Committees of nurses and physicians or dentists in the facilities must then draw up standardized policies and procedures to guide the new nursing functions. Certain special rules have also been made to supplement the agency protocols. For example, nurses who give anesthesia must be certified by the American Association of Nurse Anesthetists, and nurses who write prescriptions

Table 30-1   The State Nurse Practice Acts and the Legitimization of Diagnosis and Treatment by Nurses (as of year-end 1975)

State	Year last amended	Amended since 1971 to facilitate role expansion	Diagnosis and treatment prohibited under all circumstances
Alabama	1965		Yes
Alaska	1974	*	
Arizona	1973	*	
Arkansas	1971		Yes
California	1974	*	
Colorado	1974	*	
Connecticut	1975	*	
Delaware	1970		Yes
Florida	1975	*	
Georgia	1956		
Hawaii	1965		Yes
Idaho	1971	*	
Illinois	1975	*	
Indiana	1974	*	
Iowa	1975		
Kansas	1968		Yes
Kentucky	1966		Yes
Louisiana	1966		Yes
Maine	1974	*	
Maryland	1974	*	
Massachusetts	1971		
Michigan	1967		Yes
Minnesota	1974	*	
Mississippi	1974	*	
Missouri	1955		
Montana	1975	*	
Nebraska	1975	*	
Nevada	1973	*	
New Hampshire	1974	*	
New Jersey	1974	*	
New Mexico	1975	*	
New York	1972	*	
North Carolina	1974	*	
North Dakota	1971		
Ohio	1967		Yes
Oklahoma	1967		Yes
Oregon	1973	*	
Pennsylvania	1973	*	
Rhode Island	1956		
South Carolina	1975	*	

Table 30-1 The State Nurse Practice Acts and the Legitimization of Diagnosis and Treatment by Nurses (as of year-end 1975) (continued)

State	Year last amended	Amended since 1971 to facilitate role expansion	Diagnosis and treatment prohibited under all circumstances
South Dakota	1972	*	
Tennessee	1972	*	
Texas	1967		Yes
Utah	1975	*	
Vermont	1974	*	
Virginia	1970		
Washington	1973	*	
West Virginia	1965		
Wisconsin	1971		
Wyoming	1975	*	
Washington, D.C.	1967		
Guam	1962		Yes
Puerto Rico	1965		Yes
Virgin Islands	—		

Notes

54 acts were analyzed in the table.

30 jurisdictions have added provisions to their nurse practice acts which facilitate role expansion, and Virginia has revised its medical practice act.

10 jurisdictions have not added new provisions, but the nurse practice act does not prohibit diagnosis and treatment.

13 jurisdictions still prohibit the nurse from diagnosing and treating.

for controlled substances must be registered with the U.S. Bureau of Narcotics and Dangerous Drugs.[31]

The Idaho pattern for role expansion, using guidelines drawn up by joint action of the Boards of Medicine and Nursing, was subsequently adopted in Alaska,[32] Florida,[33] Indiana,[34] Nebraska,[35] New Hampshire,[36] North Carolina,[37] Pennsylvania,[38] and Wyoming.[39] The Mississippi statute calls for regulations by the Boards of Health and Nursing[40] and Maine includes the Osteopathy Board as a third voice.[41] In Arizona,[42] Maryland,[43] New Mexico,[44] Nevada,[45] Oregon,[46] Utah,[47] and Washington,[48] the Boards of Nursing carry the regulatory function alone. However, no one pattern has emerged for the shape of the regulations;

the Boards are selecting a variety of approaches. For example, the Maine Boards certify training programs for nurse associates.[49] Arizona approves programs and certifies nurse practitioners and midwives.[50] Washington supplements the registered nurses license with advanced registered nurse and specialized registered nurse categories.[51] North Carolina has a process for approving nurses who carry out medical functions,[52] and Nevada has defined an independent level of nursing practice, suggesting that those nurses who want to include medical diagnosis or prescriptions in their practice would have written agreements with physicians.[53]

The second approach to opening up the nursing role was first used by New York in 1972 when it adopted the following definition of professional nursing:

> The practice of the profession of nursing as a registered professional nurse is defined as diagnosing and treating human responses to actual or potential health problems through such services as case-finding, health teaching, health counseling, and provision of care supportive to or restorative of life and well-being and executing medical regimens prescribed by a licensed or otherwise legally authorized physician or dentist. A nursing regimen shall not vary any existing medical regimen.[54]

This basic approach also seems reasonable and may eventually emerge as the dominant one as nurses become more confident and the public becomes more aware of their abilities. Nineteen other states have expanded their definition of the registered nursing role or have differentiated a nursing diagnosis from a medical one so nurses are allowed to diagnose and treat but not perform a medical diagnosis or carry out medical treatments. Fortunately these laws do not clearly operationalize any behavioral differences between the two so that a nursing diagnosis appears from these statutes to mean a diagnosis performed by a nurse. The other states that have in some way expanded their basic definitions of nursing are Arizona, California,[55] Colorado,[56] Connecticut,[57] Florida, Illinois,[58] Maryland, Minnesota,[59] Montana,[60] Nebraska, New Jersey,[61] New Mexico, Oregon, Pennsylvania, Tennessee,[62] Utah, Vermont,[63] Washington, and Wyoming. Some of these states are also using board regulations to spell out the new nursing functions while others are simply relying on the broader definitions.

California uses a variety of approaches; in addition to an expanded definition of nursing and board rules which will apply only to nurses who work in unlicensed facilities such as private physician offices, the 1974 Act also mandates the use of standardized protocols to structure new nursing responsibilities. Since standardized procedures were also called for by the joint boards in Idaho

and the nursing board in Tennessee,[64] this approach can be thought as a third mechanism for role expansion. It is a useful mechanism because it helps keep patient care policy making at the local level where nurses and physicians in collaborative roles have face-to-face contact.

The fourth pattern of legislation is exemplified by the nurse practice acts of Maine, North Carolina, and South Dakota,[65] which allow individual physicians to delegate more responsibilities for diagnosis and treatment to registered nurses. The Maine statute indicates that the practice of professional nursing includes:

> . . . diagnosis or prescription of therapeutic or corrective measures when such services are delegated by a physician to a registered nurse who has completed the necessary additional educational program.[66]

Even before the current phase in nursing licensure, there were state medical practice acts, including those of Arizona, Colorado, Florida, Kansas, and Oklahoma, which gave physicians broad powers to delegate medical acts to other health workers.[67] More recently, 14 other states have added delegatory provisions to their medical practice acts. Some of these delegatory statements allow the physicians to decide to whom they will delegate, while others specify physicians' assistants and/or nurses.[68] While this approach may well be reasonable for physicians' assistants who are unlicensed (except in Colorado) and need some immediate legitimization, it leaves nurses with less autonomy and less motivation for intellectual growth than the other approaches.

SUMMARY AND CONCLUSIONS

Nursing has moved through two major phases in licensure. From 1900 to 1938 the basic acts registering nurses were passed and amended to raise educational standards. Starting in 1938 the goal became mandatory licensure for all those who nursed for hire. This move was linked with the stratification of the nursing role to include both practical and registered nurses. The third phase in licensure started in 1971 with the Idaho revision of the nurse practice act; 30 states have now revised their laws to facilitate role expansion for nurses.

The rapid changes which have occurred on the legal front will undoubtedly act as a stimulus to the development of nurse practitioners. Moreover, some of the other obstacles to role expansion seem to be lessening. The Women's Liberation Movement came along at the right time for nurses. As the norms of the society change to allow more autonomy for all women, nurses are encouraged to take on more responsibility for decision making in the patient care process, and they feel foolish about participating in some of the more blatant forms of the doctor-nurse game. The men who are coming into nursing in somewhat increased numbers feel particularly foolish in those games, so a bit of long needed honesty seems to be creeping into relationships with physicians. The nurse practitioners are also making their peace with the theorists of nursing who felt that the only proper focus was on the psychosocial aspect of care. It now seems apparent that one of the reasons nurse practitioners deliver such good primary care is because of their dual focus and their backgrounds in both the biological and behavioral sciences. With all of these changes it seems safe to predict an impending rapid increase in the number of nurses working in expanded roles in acute, primary, and long-term care of patients.

This does not mean that all of the problems on the legal front are solved. Nurses and health care planners in those states which have not yet joined the current movement may need to prepare for a legislative campaign and, as experience accumulates, even the new acts will need revision to make them more workable. It is also important to realize that these changes in the laws which have occurred are merely facilitating. They have not solved the problems of continuing education which is surely needed for continued competence;

educational programs for specialists and practitioners are not accredited in any systematic way; and the individual practitioner is certified in only a few states. While these may well be professional rather than legislative responsibilities, it is clear that there are many issues related to the law which are yet to be addressed.

NOTES

1 Stein, L., The doctor-nurse game, Archives of General Psychiatry 16:699–703, 1967.
2 Kreuter, F. R., What is good nursing care?, Nursing Outlook 5:302–304, 1957; Johnson, D., A Philosophy of Nursing, Nursing Outlook 7:198–200, 1959; Rogers, M., Reveille in Nursing, Philadelphia: F. A. Davis, 1964; American Nurses Association's First Position Paper on Education for Nursing, American Journal of Nursing 65:106–111, 1965.
3 For a more detailed coverage see The Law and the Expanding Nursing Role, Bonnie Bullough, Ed. New York: Appleton-Century-Crofts, 1975.
4 Dock, L. I., A History of Nursing, Vol. III, New York: G. P. Putnam's Sons, 1912, p. 141.
5 Roberts, M. M., American Nursing: History and Interpretation, New York: Macmillan, 1961, pp. 20–30; Bullough, V. and B. Bullough, The Emergence of Modern Nursing, New York: Macmillan, 1969, pp. 149–153.
6 United States Reports: Cases Adjudged in the Supreme Courts 129, 1888, Dent v. West Virginia, p. 114–128.
7 West, R. M., History of Nursing in Pennsylvania, Pennsylvania State Nurses' Association, 1933, pp. 41–58.
8 Robinson, V., White Caps: The Story of Nursing, Philadelphia: J. B. Lippincott, 1946, pp. 282–83.
9 Lesnik, M. J. and B. E. Anderson, Legal Aspects of Nursing, Philadelphia: J. B. Lippincott, 1947, pp. 312–314.
10 Ibid., 306–7.
11 The Biennial, American Journal of Nursing 34: 603–627, 1934; West, op. cit., pp. 97–108.
12 United States Dept. of Health, Education, and Welfare. Report on Licensure and Related

Health Personnel Credentialing, Pub. #72-11, U.S. Government Printing Office, Washington, DC, June 1971.

13 Editorial, American Journal of Nursing 39: 275–277, 1939; Trained attendants and practical nurses, American Journal of Nursing 44:7–8, 1944.

14 Statutory status of six professions, Research Bulletin of the National Educational Association 16:184–223, 1938.

15 Editorial, *op. cit.*; Jamieson, E. M. and M. Sewell, Trends in Nursing History, Philadelphia: W. B. Saunders, 1944, pp. 533–34.

16 Jacobsen, M., Nursing laws and what every nurse should know about them, American Journal of Nursing 40:1221–1226, 1940; Lesnik, *op. cit.*, p. 47.

17 A.N.A. board approves a definition of nursing practice, American Journal of Nursing 55: 1474, 1955.

18 Fogotson, E. H., R. Roemer, R. W. Newman, and J. L. Cook, Licensure of other medical personnel, Report of the National Advisory Commission on Health Manpower, Vol. II, Washington, DC: U.S. Government Printing Office, 1967, pp. 407–492.

19 Facts About Nursing: A Statistical Summary 1955–56, New York: American Nurses Association, p. 76.

20 Anderson, B. E., The Facilitation of Interstate Movement of Registered Nurses, Philadelphia: J. B. Lippincott, 1950.

21 Barbee, G. G., Special procedures: I.V.s, blood transfusions and skin testing, Proceedings: Institute on Medico-Legal Aspects of Nursing Practice, Santa Monica, CA: California Nurses' Association, 1961, pp. 41–44.

22 Sarner, H., The Nurse and the Law, Philadelphia: W. B. Saunders, 1968, pp. 89–90.

23 Hershey, N., Legal issues in nursing practice. *In* Professional Nursing: Foundations, Perspectives and Relationships. E. K. Spalding and L. E. Notter, Eds. Philadelphia: J. B. Lippincott, 1970, pp. 110–127.

24 National Commission for the Study of Nursing and Nursing Education, An Abstract for Action. New York: McGraw-Hill, 1970.

25 Willie, S. H., The Nurse's Guide to the Law, New York: McGraw-Hill, 1970.

26 Extending the Scope of Nursing Practice: A Report of the Secretary's Committee to Study Extended Roles for Nurses, November, 1971.

27 Arizona Attorney General Opinion, No. 71-30, August 6, 1971. Cited in A. M. Sadler, Jr. and B. L. Sadler, Recent developments in the law relating to physician's assistants, Vanderbilt Law Review 24:1205, November, 1971. See also Amendment of the Arizona nursing practice law broadens definition of professional nursing, American Journal of Nursing 72: 1203, 1972.

28 California Attorney General Opinion, No. CV 72/187, February 15, 1973 and an Indexed letter from the California Attorney General, October 4, 1972.

29 Virginia Code, Section 54-275.

30 Idaho Code, Section 54-1413. (Note: State nurse practice acts are cited once only unless there is a direct quotation.)

31 Minimum Standards, Rules and Regulations for Nurse Practitioners (Expanding Role) and Guidelines for Nurses Writing Prescriptions. Jointly promulgated by the Idaho State Board of Nursing and the Idaho State Board of Medicine as authorized by Section 54-1413 (e), Idaho Code.

32 Alaska Statutes, Section 08.68.410.

33 Florida Statutes, Section 464.021.

34 Indiana Code, Section 25-23-1-1.

35 Nebraska Revised Statutes, 71-1,132.05.

36 New Hampshire Revised Statutes, 326-A:2.

37 The joint committee of the two boards is established in the medical practice act; North Carolina General Statutes, Section 90-18(14); the nurse practice act is also revised: North Carolina General Statutes, Section 90-158.

38 Pennsylvania Statutes, Title 63, Section 212.

39 Wyoming Statutes, Section 33-279.1.

40 Mississippi Code, Section 73-15-5.

41 Maine Revised Statutes, Title 32, Chapter 31, Section 2102.

42 Arizona Revised Statutes, 32.1601.

43 Maryland Code, Article 43, Section 291.

44 New Mexico, Article 2, 67-2-3.

45 Nevada Revised Statutes, Chapter 632.010.

46 Oregon Revised Statutes, Title 32, Chapter 31, Section 2102.

47 Utah Code Annotated, Section 58-31-4.

48 Washington Revised Code, Section 18.88.030.

49 Board of Nursing, Board of Registration in Medicine, and Board of Osteopathic Examination and Registration. Standards for Nurse Associate Programs: State of Maine, September, 1974.

50 Arizona State Board of Nursing. Rules and Regulations, October, 1974, Article 5.

51 Washington Board of Nursing. Rules/Regulations, February, 1975 WAC 308-120-190 through WAC 308-120-250.

52 North Carolina Board of Medical Examiners and North Carolina Board of Nursing. Rules and Regulations for Registered Nurses Performing Medical Acts, March 14, 1975.

53 Nevada State Board of Nursing. Minimum Requirements for Schools of Professional and Practical Nursing and Licensure of Registered and Practical Nurses, July 10, 1975.

54 New York State Education Law, Title 8, Article 139, Section 6902.

55 California Business and Professions Code, Section 2725.

56 Colorado Revised Statutes, Chapter 97, Article 1, 2.

57 Connecticut General Statutes, Section 20-88.

58 Illinois Revised Statutes, Chapter 91, Par. 35.35.

59 Minnesota Statutes, Chapter 148, Section 171.

60 Montana Revised Codes, Title 66-1222.

61 New Jersey Public Law 1974, Chapter 109, September 30, 1974, C. 45:11-23.

62 Tennessee Code Annotated, Section 63-740.

63 Vermont Statutes, Title 26, Chapter 24, Section 1552.

64 Rules and Regulations of the Tennessee Board of Nursing Concerning Licensure and Education of Registered Nurses. Nursing *RN*, 34–39.

65 South Dakota Session Laws, Chapter 101, Section 27.09.

66 Maine Revised Statutes, Title 32, Chapter 31, Section 2102.

67 Fish, M. S., Nursing vis-a-vis medicine: a proposal for legislation, Licensure and Credentialing: Proceedings, ANA Conference, Council of State Boards of Nursing, Detroit, 1972. Copyright, A.N.A., 1974, pp. 14–22.

68 Educational programs for the physician's assistant, American Medical Association, September, 1973, p. 9.

EDITOR'S QUESTIONS FOR DISCUSSION

What socioeconomic and political pressures have facilitated the changes in nurse practice laws? What are the implications of defining nursing roles by legislation? What accounts for the different approaches to the legislation of nursing practice? What factors will increase or decrease the number of nurses in the role of nurse practitioner? What may health care planners and health services agencies do to effect an expanded role for nurses? What appears to have been the function of physicians in the development of the nurse practitioner role? What are the implications for nursing of changes made in nursing practice via changes made in medical practice law?

Part Six

Interdisciplinary Professional Relationships

The relationships between medicine and nursing should be explored, particularly since historically these two professions have been regarded as functioning conjointly as the basic health team. Role differentiation, transfer of functions, and leveling of statuses are all part of social change, an ubiquitous element in the social structure of professions. Changes in roles evolve as a result of discontent within a profession and also because of external influences such as advanced technology, increased costs of delivering care, and expanded knowledge. Basic to any culture are the rules, norms, and values that govern relationships. In the following chapters we see that the norms and values governing the physician-nurse relationship are changing. The current emphasis is on developing interdependent relationships between nursing and medicine. The basic relationship is becoming one of equality and reciprocity.

Chapter 31

Problems in Interprofessional Relations

Shirley A. Smoyak, R.N., Ph.D., F.A.A.N.
Professor and Chairperson, Graduate Psychiatric Nursing
Rutgers, The State University of New Jersey, New Brunswick, N.J.

Shirley A. Smoyak traces the conflicts between medicine and nursing to the historical development of the role of women. Technologic and scientific developments provoked further divisions. When the effect of the growing gulf between the two professions was realized, efforts were made to communicate. As a result, the National Joint Practice Commission was organized in 1971. Much discussion followed concerning the restructuring of the professional division of labor in health care and the territorial rights of nursing and medicine. Five impediments to full collaboration between medicine and nursing are identified by Smoyak. She defines joint practice and shared responsibility and discusses the corresponding implications for nursing and medicine.

In the beginning, when life was simple, there were no physicians and no nurses. The inevitable crises in health were handled by families—more accurately, they were handled by women in families. This division of labor was influenced greatly by the fact that 90 percent of societal groups were hunters. In hunting societies men were in charge of procuring the food, usually animal meat (a full-time occupation) which women stored or dried. When cooking foods rather than eating them raw became fashionable, women added this to their tasks.

Newborns, infants, older children, and sick and debilitated adults all came within women's bailiwick. Much of a woman's adult life was spent in bearing, nursing, and rearing children. When she was finished with that, there were usually very few years left before death. These categories of people—infants, the ill, the crippled, the aged—were associated with women and were classed as their problem or their responsibility. The sick and infirm also threatened the lives of entire hunting societies and usually were treated with a mixture of suspicion, disdain, and hostility. When hunting groups moved their camps across long distances, these people often were left behind. If women stayed behind to care for them, both perished, since the procurer of food was absent. Only the healthiest infants survived this kind of life. Survival of the fittest was the order of things.

Women's history, thus, is colored by this early association with the helpless and the less-than-fit. Men recognized that women were more useful to

Presented in a panel, Sources of the Problem, as part of the 1976 Annual Health Conference of the New York Academy of Medicine, *Issues in Primary Care*, held April 22 and 23, 1976.
Reprinted from the *Bulletin of the New York Academy of Medicine*, **53**(1):51–59, January–February 1977.

society if they properly fulfilled their functions of bearing, nursing, and rearing children, but they were ambivalent when women extended their caring to the other groups. The sick and the old were a drain on scarce food supplies; in times when food was not plentiful, these people were not merely a drain on resources but an actual threat to the survival of the group. Death was welcomed. If they could, in hard times the aged or crippled sometimes walked away from the camp to invite death.

Women's status in ancient societies was less than that of men because of this association. Those who do demeaning work—who clean up the messes of others—are treated with little respect. The people who appreciated these comforting, caring efforts historically had little status, hence their respect was unimportant.

When agrarian patterns of living emerged, farming allowed a better support system and sharing of food, which permitted survival of the ill and debilitated. As less time was spent in the procurement and processing of food, more time could be spent in developing humane qualities.

Our complex, urbanized, industrialized society has come full circle. Nowadays entire groups of occupations and professions are occupied with what formerly was women's work—caring for the helpless and sick. How ironic that this women's work, once the lowliest kind of labor, now is accorded such high value and high status—when men perform it. Obstetricians rank higher than midwives on our social scale.

This historical perspective lends understanding to problems in interprofessional relations. Women and men, physicians and nurses, find it useful to consider their present in the light of their past. The relative influence of genes and chromosomes versus attitudes, cultural styles, and systems of belief needs further study.

Medicine and nursing are the oldest of the health professions. The long history of their working together is starred by documented instances of outstanding collaborative effort, but it also is marred by other instances of interprofessional and interpersonal conflict.

Before the discord, disharmony, and distrust which are so evident now between medicine and nursing, there was a period of very little animosity—in fact, "colleagueship" would accurately describe the relation. That was roughly a century ago, before advanced technology and the development of knowledge in all aspects of the health field. A century ago physicians had no antibiotics, no tranquilizers, no suites of operating rooms. Intensive care units and coronary care units are recent inventions. In the old days physicians could do little more than nurse their patients. Nurses allowed this and were not dismayed by territorial invasion. Disparity in economic compensation between the two professions was not a big issue then. The disparity in skills was not so great either.

New discoveries, new technologies, and new sciences emerging in this century encouraged a broadening gulf between the two professions. Men were free to study and learn; women were not. Men went to universities and women nursed babies. Medicine developed with leaps and bounds; nursing barely crept along.

When nursing did emerge in the late 1940s from its version of the dark ages, nurses challenged the established order. Physicians had become comfortably fixed in their views of nurses as subservient, nice-but-not-too-bright individuals who were useful to have around so long as they knew their place, people who were available to do whatever anyone else in the health-care delivery system forgot or did not want to do or classified as demeaning. Those were the dark days before the dawn.

In the 1960s organized medicine and nursing began to say publicly that the discords, distresses, and dysfunctions needed repair. Hostilities and miscommunication between the two professions were further straining the already limping system of health care delivery. The new order of the day included collaboration, colleagueship, and realigned roles. At conferences and in the literature there was much talk of team effort. The American Medical Association (AMA) and the American Nurses Association (ANA) jointly supported three national conferences on issues of practice and health care delivery in 1964, 1965, and 1967. Although much collaborative effort was expended on relations between the work of the physician and that of the nurse, there were no further large-scale interorganizational efforts until 1971, when the AMA and ANA agreed to form the National Joint Practice Commission (NJPC).

Before the NJPC began its work there were some scattered conferences wherein the collaboration of nurses and physicians functioning as a team was discussed and analyzed. A basic definition of team describes two or more persons with diverse skills associated together. Horses or mules working as teams do not have diverse skills, but human teams in other than the tug-of-war or all-do-one sport such as swimming are characterized by their diversity.

The structure of a team includes several persons and diverse skills. But what about its functions? A classification here includes: (1) the work to be done by the team and (2) how the team is organized to do the work. What are the rules of organization? Who is in charge? Who does what under what conditions? How are violations (both commissions and omissions) handled? When work is analyzed as a specific dimension there are two major possibilities:

Type I—When work is highly specific (that is, when persons who do the work undergo a highly specialized, technical training) there are few clashes or conflicts of role among the workers. In baseball a pitcher throws and a catcher catches. In surgery a surgeon operates and gives orders to others; they support him and comply with his commands. Both are instances of highly differentiated function. There are no territorial or jurisdictional disputes.

Type II—When work is such that two or more persons from different backgrounds (or professions, disciplines, or roles) can do it equally well, there are many conflicts. In baseball a center fielder and right fielder are equally competent to catch a fly ball. In practice, many balls are missed, slipping between these positions. A pediatric nurse-practitioner and a pediatrician are equally competent to take care of healthy babies. Many babies also are missed.

Under the latter condition methods of allocating work undergo a dramatic shift—from assignment based on skill to assignment based on negotiations about time available (the time of day, day of the week), proclivity for the task (liking or satisfaction), costs, numbers of professionals available in each category (the people-power distribution issue), supply-and-demand requirements, seniority or status of members in a system (both professionals and patients), locus of the care (home, hospital, or highway), the nature of the requirement for care (emergency, acute, or chronic), and the patient's view of himself or herself (participation in decisions about his or her care or a passive role in which the patient is acted upon by others).

These jurisdictional issues must be faced. Nowadays there are more and more persons in Type II work. The jurisdiction of nursing practice always has comprised the nurturing, caring, helping to cope, comforting, counseling, supporting activities in health care delivery. However, when nurses today do what only physicians did previously, conflict is generated.

The boundary battles begin when teams or potential teams are faced with pragmatic questions. How may a nurse know or discover what a patient needs in the area of nursing care? This "how-to-know?" is a very important question. May she or should she use her eyes only? How shall she report what she sees? Must her observations always be attenuated or clouded by words such as "appears," "seems," and "perhaps?" Or should she say, "The patient is bleeding?" May she use her hands? For what? To soothe a fevered brow? To palpate an enlarged liver? How shall the nurse know what patients need? May she use an instrument? A thermometer? Stethoscope? Otoscope? Ah—back to looking! Must she use her eyes only? Or may she visualize the retina? The eardrum? If she looks with the aid of instruments, may she interpret? How about acting on the basis of the interpretation?

Interpretation, of course, is simply a process of

naming. What is it that the nurse may or should name? Naming requires conceptual activity. Is the nurse an automaton? A person with a functioning brain? Do only physicians think? Is cerebral activity masculine? There is no God-given, overriding law or principle by which nurses and physicians can determine who does what. Expanding knowledge and increased technology require a reordering of the professional division of labor.

There is one more dimension to the jurisdictional battle. Who owns a body? The physician? The registered nurse? The patient? Who has a right to what information? What does the right to know really mean?

Perhaps if enough questions are asked, some answers will emerge. A Chinese philosopher would assure us that within all questions their answers reside. Also, within answers there is of course some element of questioning.

The NJPC has been asking many questions since its inception. After four years of work some definitions and statements of philosophy have been made, providing an approach to answers. Sources of the difficulty have been identified. During the course of the NJPC's discussions and proceedings over the years, several major impediments to full collaboration between medicine and nursing have been identified. There are five such areas.

1 *Most nurses are employed in hospitals.* The larger the hospital, the more likely that it suffers from bureaucratic problems and difficulties which are well-documented by organizational sociologists. Thus, a nurse who has been educated to give enlightened, tender, judicious care finds her energies depleted by her struggles against the bureaucracy. Often, however, rather than recognizing that she is a victim of an organizational illness, she tends to reduce her anxiety by placing blame on physicians. Physicians, who are not trapped in the same way by organizational demands, respond with anger and reciprocal blame.

2 *Poor communication causes trouble.* Misinterpretations, lack of follow-through, failure to write things down—all contribute to mishaps.

3 *Excessive demands on both professionals* because of increased patient loads and decreased budgets. Rather than teaming up to fight these system or organizational troubles, RNs and M.D.s fight with each other.

4 *Unjustified inequalities in payment and compensation.* This will be discussed later (see the third paragraph before the end of the article).

5 *The continuation of male-dominance and chauvinism.* Chauvinism is deadly. It produces anger, game-playing, and superficial interaction in offensive and defensive styles.

The NJPC, having identified these trouble spots, moved unanimously in 1975 to adopt this definition of joint practice: *"Joint practice is nurses and physicians collaborating as colleagues to provide patient care."**

Joint practice produces action which results in the attainment of mutual goals. Patients bring nurses and physicians together. Problems of patient care provide the impetus for professional interaction.

Joint practice is not synonymous with overlapping functions of nurses and physicians or areas of commonality between the two. Rather, in a joint practice two different professionals find themselves articulating their work as they put their separate talents together toward a common goal. The content of these separate talents changes from time to time. Functions formerly performed only under the jurisdiction of medicine now are commonly performed by nurses. That is not to say that nurses are becoming physicians. The more useful perspective is that the expansion of knowledge requires a reordering, within systems, of the division of labor. When doctors and nurses discuss this reordering openly and make decisions collectively, they are in joint practice.

Joint practice means the combined action of medicine and nursing, with the focus on the prevention of illness, restoration of health, and care of the sick and dying. By definition it excludes unilateral, isolated, or independent actions of professionals as a generalized style. While a nurse or a physician may be seen as acting individually in

*Available as a leaflet from NJPC, 35 E. Wacker Drive, Suite 1748, Chicago, Ill. 60601.

certain instances, a nurse and a physician are in joint practice if they have mutual concern for patients and families and have acted upon this concern to produce a concerted, synchronized effort. Joint practice eliminates duplication of effort, unnecessary conflict, and energy-depleting discord.

Combined action has several distinct, pragmatic outcomes: In some instances the same tasks may be performed equally well by nurses or physicians. Who does the task is determined by the situation—such as the geographic variables, clinical settings, pressures from other sectors, the time of day, and the other exigencies mentioned earlier. In other instances the special skill of either the physician or the nurse is needed. The diversity of the academic and clinical backgrounds produces different skills and competencies. Thus, the concerted efforts of nurses and physicians sometimes consist of engaging in very similar activities and at other times of performing very different tasks in a synchronized manner.

Medicine and nursing are two distinct professions, both with their complexities, specialists, and changing dimensions of clinical practice. While their areas of expertness are separate (usually, physicians are concerned primarily with identification of disease and strategies for treatment and cure, while, in general, nurses are concerned primarily with nurturing, caring, helping to cope, comforting, counseling, and life-supporting activities of the care of patients) the two professions have mutual and overlapping concerns and responsibilities for patients.

Nurses and physicians work best as colleagues where there is:

1 Mutual agreement on a goal
2 Equality in status and personal interactions
3 A shared base of scientific and professional knowledge with complementary diversity in skills, expertise, and practices
4 Mutual trust and respect for each other's competence

The nature of the structural and economic arrangements in joint practices varies widely. In the least complex arrangement, a nurse and a physician share responsibility for all or a part of the care of a particular population of patients. There may or may not be a formal contract between the two. The nurse may be a hospital employee while the physician may be engaged in fee-for-service practice. In other arrangements nurses and physicians in various numbers and with varied specialized skills have formally regularized their joint practice in such patterns as corporations, partnerships, institutional contracts, and the like. These are readily identifiable to others as a constant team or joint practice, with a specific group of patients, caseload, or population. In some instances other professionals may be members of the practice group also.

Shared responsibility has a definite meaning. Sharing means equality in the making of decisions about the needs and problems of patients. Contributions from nurses about the care required may be largely sociocultural and contributions from physicians may be largely physiological, but each would be valued equally. Sharing also means the equitable distribution of monetary and other rewards, based on a system which is mutually agreed upon by nurses and physicians. Responsibility for the patient must be ongoing, whatever the arrangement or setting. Obligations for care cannot be relinquished by either of the parties until transferred to a different practice.

How the patient pays for his or her care affects the manner in which the professionals are paid and the amount they are paid. In prepayment plans nurses are employees, but in a slightly different manner from doctors; nurses receive no incentive bonuses while doctors do. In clinics run by foundations or by governments, both may be employees and receive no incentive bonuses. Differences in pay may fairly reflect differences in education and training, but often they do not. In some academic settings, where nurses and physicians both hold academic appointments, the differences in income may be narrower and the payment of nurses may approximate distributive justice. Nurses and physicians in joint private practice are struggling to arrange fee-for-service costs which

Professional Consciousness-Raising Questionnaire for Realigned Roles of M.D.s and R.N.s*

Tasks	1850 R.N.	1850 M.D.	1900 R.N.	1900 M.D.	1925 R.N.	1925 M.D.	1950 R.N.	1950 M.D.	1975 R.N.	1975 M.D.
	m s	m s	m s	m s	m s	m s	m s	m s	m s	m s
1 Read a thermometer										
2 Tell the reading to the patient										
3 Confirm a pregnancy										
4 Prescribe a diet for a pregnant woman										
5 Physically assess a newborn child										
6 Use a stethoscope with a sphygmomanometer to determine blood pressure										
7 Use a stethoscope to listen to heart										
8 Use a stethoscope to listen to lungs										
9 Draw blood from a finger										
10 Draw blood from a vein										
11 Administer fluids IV										
12 Administer drugs IV										
13 Counsel family with school-phobic child										
14 Counsel family with adolescent pregnant out of wedlock										
15 Administer oxygen										
16 Intubate										
17 Defibrillate an arrhythmia										

*Assume that the R.N. or M.D. is technically competent to do the task.
m = may, s = should, IV = intravenously

are based on which service is provided rather than on who provides it.

Joint practice may mean that a doctor and a nurse or a group of doctors, nurses, and sometimes other health workers have formed a partnership for their practice. A partnership, however, is not a joint practice if there is no collective decision making and open discussion of who performs what tasks under what conditions. Combined action of involved professionals is the guiding framework of a joint practice. Directed action as the usual order is not joint practice, nor is using either profession as a consultant to the other.

A professional consciousness-raising questionnaire is offered as the ending of this chapter—and as a potential beginning for those readers who have not explored interprofessional issues at length. Try filling in the chart by placing m (may) or s (should) in the appropriate columns to indicate who performed the listed tasks in the various years. Assume the nurse or physician to be technically competent to do the task.

EDITOR'S QUESTIONS FOR DISCUSSION

What effect have territorial disputes over role functioning between medicine and nursing had on the patient? What evidence exists today of collaboration between nursing and medicine in health care? How is the task environment defined for nursing and medicine? What process is involved in the negotiation of role boundaries? How does one encourage other members of the two professions to accept the recommendations of the National Joint Practice Commission?

Chapter 32

Nurse-Physician Relationships: Problems and Solutions

Robert A. Hoekelman, M.D.
Professor of Pediatrics, Health Services, and Nursing
Strong Memorial Hospital and Medical Center
University of Rochester, Rochester, N.Y.

Because this chapter is focused on professional relationships between medicine and nursing, to include a contribution by a physician is appropriate. Hoekelman's affirmations of nurse-physician collaboration are indicative of the attempts by those in the field of medicine to strengthen the existing relationships between physicians and nurses. He defines six problems that exist between medicine and nursing: basic dishonesty in their relationships, sexism, difference in educational preparation, variable income, social status difference, and lack of understanding of each other's roles. Hoekelman proposes some solutions to these problems.

Nursing and medicine, as the two major health professions, have the greatest potential to improve the quality and quantity of health care delivered in this country through their collaborative efforts. That potential, however, is not being realized. Collaboration between the two professions and collegial relationships, as colleagues, among their members are proposed by innovative, idealistic educators, administrators, and organizers in nursing. There are precious few supporters of this line of thinking in medicine or, indeed, among the rank and file of nurses. In order to understand why this is so, we must understand past and present interrelationships between the two professions. We need to define the problems that exist. Then perhaps we can determine whether solutions can be found to those problems so that collaboration and collegiality can occur.

Stein states that "the relationship between the doctor and the nurse is a very special one. There are few professions where the degree of mutual respect and cooperation between co-workers is as intense as that between the doctor and nurse."[1] This would seem so to the casual observer. The mutual respect, however, is not always there, and the cooperation is often only obtained by playing "the doctor-nurse game."

The game is played to allow the nurse to share in the medical decision making concerning patient care without seeming to, and without concomitantly sharing in the responsibility for those decisions. According to the rules of the game, the

Adapted from a commencement address delivered to graduates of the pediatric and medical nurse associate training programs, Rush-Presbyterian–St. Luke's Medical Center, Chicago, Illinois, June 26, 1974.

This article is a revision of the original article that appeared in the *American Journal of Nursing*, vol. 75, no. 7, July 7, 1975.

decisions and the responsibility for those decisions must remain with the physician. Decisions concerning nursing care and responsibility for those decisions lie with the nurse. The doctor does not take part in them.

The single most important rule of the game is that open disagreement between the players must be avoided at all costs. The reward for playing the game well is the winning of the respect and cooperation of the other discipline. The penalties for playing poorly are the loss of that respect and cooperation. More important, however, are the penalties to both players for playing the game in the first place. For nurses, these penalties are the suppression of initiative and intellect and the opportunity for self pride; for physicians, the penalty is self-deception; and for both, it is dishonesty.

Why is the game played in the first place? Stein says that the physician does so because he fears he will commit errors of judgment in managing his patient. He copes with that fear by developing the belief that he is omnipotent and omniscient, and therefore incapable of making mistakes. He does not always recognize this, and if he does, never admits it to others. This posture on the physician's part does not allow him to show he does not know all the answers. Thus, he engages in the game so he will not have to make such an admission. The physician finds himself in this position primarily because of his experiences in medical school and house officer training and because nurses have sanctioned this behavior, perhaps for the patient's peace of mind and benefit, but also, in large part, for their own.

The first problem, then, that must be overcome in nurse-physician interactions is the basic dishonesty nurses and physicians have demonstrated in their relationships with each other and with themselves. The solution is for physicians and nurses to be honest with each other, recognize realistically the contribution each profession can make to patient care, and then allow these contributions to be made and properly rewarded.

The second basic problem in nurse-physician relationships arises because most physicians are men and most nurses women. This leads to what Schutt calls the "male-female syndrome,"[2] referred to by some as "sexism." This relationship is a prime example of the male's exploitation of the female.

The Women's Liberation Movement has fertile soil in nursing. Wilma Scott Heide, former president of the National Organization for Women, has stated, "The very welfare and future of nursing may be dependent on the fulfillment of the objectives of the feminist movement."[3] She sees the problems of nursing as symptoms of the oppression of women, and feels that if there is to be any significant strategy for change in nursing, nurses will simply have to understand how the male-oriented, male-dominated society has determined the nature of their private and public lives. As males, and therefore persons who operate from a position of strength (in the opinion of Mrs. Heide), many physicians consider themselves supporters of the Women's Liberation Movement. Nevertheless, we would have to agree with Sandler who says, "the intent to discriminate or not to discriminate is irrelevant. The effect of the practice is what counts. Even the pure of heart may often act in a discriminatory manner."[4]

The gains the Women's Liberation Movement makes in its fight against male domination and female suppression, in general, will probably do more to solve that problem within our professions than anything we can do, such as increasing the number of women physicians, increasing the number of male nurses, or changing the name of nurse, as Silver has suggested, to "health care practitioner" in order to attract more men into the profession.[5]

To solve this problem not only will medicine have to give more than lip service to the support of the general liberation of females, but also nursing will have to assert itself by accentuating its liberated femininity and by changing its role from one of submission to one of equality with men, irrespective of the hierarchal relationships in the work situations of doctors and nurses.

The third problem affecting nurse-physician relationships is the difference in their educational preparation in terms of time and content. People with more educational experiences and credentials tend to dominate those with less. This is done in both overt and subtle ways. The title "doctor," in itself is an ever-present reminder of the differential. However, physicians are not alone in this attitude. Even within the nursing profession, educational level differentials create discord.

The solution to this problem is not simple. We do, however, see trends toward decreasing the years required for obtaining the M.D. degree and increasing the years and scope of education for some nurses at the preparatory level. These trends will close the educational gap in some cases, but will not in the majority. The resolution of the education-credentials problem lies in recognizing, accepting, and rewarding the individual in greater measure for what he or she does competently and not just for the years spent in preparation to acquire that competence.

Economics presents a fourth problem to good physician-nurse relationships, and this relates, in part, to both the "male-female syndrome" and the "educational gap." Men, in general, earn more than women. Income is, in general, positively correlated with educational levels attained. However, within occupational categories, the male usually wins out over the female in terms of salary and and promotions. Male physicians earn more than female physicians. Male educators, at almost all levels, earn more than female educators. Scheffler and Stinson reported that in 1972 male physician's assistants had earnings averaging $10,284 annually while female physician's assistants averaged only $8,084 annually.[6] Furthermore, in all of these areas, the income gap widens as experience accumulates. To compound the money problem, doctors are usually employers of nurses, or, if not, often act as their supervisors in situations where they are mutually employed.

Until society recognizes the worth of the services rendered by nurses as fully as it has recognized and accepted the worth of the services rendered by physicians, this problem will remain. Nursing, however, must push for that recognition

and medicine must support increased remuneration for nursing services rendered. An improved salary structure would attract and retain greater numbers in the nursing profession and improve patient care.

Nursing must control its own profession and medicine must relinquish its present administrative controls over nursing. Collaborative efforts and colleagueship cannot be accomplished without these changes since neither can effectively exist in the presence of hierarchal differentials between the professions. There are some signs of such alteration with the emergence of independent nursing practice and with physicians and nurses working in team relationships with others under systems not controlled or administered by physicians.

The "social status gulf" (classism) between physicians and nurses is the fifth problem that affects nurse-physician relationships. As long as the educational, economic problems already outlined remain, medicine will continue to enjoy a higher social standing within the community, and this will hamper relationships between physicians and nurses.

Nursing, unlike medicine, has not been and still is not a profession into which parents of higher societal levels have pushed their children. Therefore, many nurses and physicians come from different social levels, which affects their professional interactions. Since social standing correlates highly with the level of education attained and the amount of money one earns, nurses will improve their social standing by obtaining more education and earning more money. We may, however, move more rapidly toward equalization in the social-standing sphere by reducing the educational requirements to obtain the M.D. degree and reducing the income levels physicians attain, while raising both for nurses.

Finally, the sixth and most important problem in nurse-physician relationships is the basic lack of understanding each discipline has for the other's role in the provision of health care. Physicians, for the most part, do not know what is meant by the "expanded role of the nurse" because they do not even know of the restricted role, except the one that, traditionally, nurses have performed as physicians' helpers. Similarly, many nurses do not understand what the "expanded role" concept means, and particularly how it relates to the physician's role in health care.

We will not solve the problem of misconception of roles until we have an adequate number of nurse-physician team models that can demonstrate their superiority in the provision of care over traditional models. Barbara Bates astutely points out that "people standing in isolation cannot be colleagues."[7] The key to accomplishing this goal is the increase of exposure each discipline has to the other during their formative educational years and throughout their professional training. Interdisciplinary educational efforts to date have been few and far between, sporadic and unsustained, simplistic and unstudied. Medical and nursing students who learn together should gain an understanding of and respect for each other's professional role that will remain with them and create a positive force for collaborative functioning throughout their careers.

The elimination of the barriers to constructive nurse-physician relationships will take a good deal of time and effort. There is little evidence today that predicts meaningful change in the immediate future, but the seeds of revolution, or better, of evolution, have been planted and are being nurtured.

One of the recommendations of the National Commission for the Study of Nursing and Nursing Education was that "a National Joint Practice Commission (NJPC), with state counterpart committees, be established between medicine and nursing to discuss and make recommendations concerning the congruent roles of the physician and the nurse in providing quality health care."[8] The NJPC was formed in 1971 by joint action of the American Medical Association and the American Nurses Association. Its broad goal is to improve the delivery of health care in the United States through the joint practice of nurses, physicians, and other health workers. One of its seven

major objectives is "to address the traditional problems which affect nurse-physician relationships in order to establish enhanced role functioning."[9] It is hoped that the NJPC and its counterpart state and local joint practice committees will become a guiding force for positive changes in nurse-physician relationships.

Pessimism over the prospects for eliminating the barriers to constructive nurse-physician relationships is well founded. Although we have seen, over the past decade, indications of collaboration and collegial relationships between nurses and physicians emerging, these have represented only a small segment of the total health care scene.

Looking at the developments in the expanded role of the nurse in primary care as an example, there are approximately 40 training programs for pediatric nurse practitioners (PNPs) throughout the country.[10] These programs are capable of producing 500 PNPs annually to add to the over 3,000 who have completed training since the first program was established in 1965. Comparable figures for medical nurse practitioner, family nurse practitioner, and other primary care nurse practitioner programs are not available. However, at this time we can estimate that in regard to the number of nurses prepared to practice in an expanded role in primary care we are speaking of less than 1 percent of the nurses in practice (6,000 of 850,000). In considering the annual yield of primary care practitioner training programs in relation to the number of graduates of diploma and baccalaureate programs we are at the 3 percent level (1,500 versus 45,000). It, of course, cannot be presumed that all graduates of those nurse practitioner training programs are practicing or, if so, are practicing in collaboration, as colleagues with physicians.

More disturbing is the realization that many of the nurse practitioner programs are going out of existence because of lack of funds. The cost of training nurse practitioners is extremely high, approximately $5,000 per graduate. The public and private funding sources that have provided seed monies and supported programs for evaluation purposes will not continue to do so. Programs will then need to rely on tuitions from students. Who can afford such tuitions? Not the individual nurse, particularly when you add to tuition the costs of travel, books, equipment, room, board, baby sitters, and loss of income while in training. The potential employer of the nurse could well underwrite tuition and other expenses since economic studies indicate the nurse practitioner can more than earn her way in primary care settings.[11, 12] One wonders, however, how many employers would be willing to underwrite the full costs of such training if required to.

The future holds the prospect of moving nurse-practitioner training out of the continuing education area into the basic undergraduate nurse training programs where costs of training could be supported by categorical funds. Such prospects are exciting to contemplate, but, realistically speaking, in light of all the other changes that are taking place in basic nursing education, do not offer immediate solutions.

What then will we tell nurses who have completed nurse practitioner training—those who are prepared to practice in an expanded role? What does the future hold for them and those who will follow them? Many nurse practitioners will make important individual contributions to patient care and will make inroads in the area of collaborative and collegial nurse-physician functioning. They will be the models that others will emulate. However, their efforts will not be enough. Two catalysts are needed to bring about the changes in nurse-physician relationships described above and to create a demand for nurses functioning in expanded roles. The first catalyst is one that will remove the economic and educational barriers currently keeping those in need of health care from obtaining that care. Some form of national health insurance that will remove the economic barrier to health care coupled with extensive education of the public at an early age to their health needs and a means of meeting those needs will create a tremendous demand for health services. Then physicians and administrators of health care systems will ask, "Where are the nurse practitioners?" This catalyst will be a slow-acting one. Even where public-supported health care systems have been enacted and implemented, it will take several years before their effect, in terms of increasing the total demand for health services, will be felt and many more years before our professional educational system will respond to those demands.[13, 14]

The second catalyst is even slower in its action. That is the catalyst of the demonstration (with models of collaboration and collegial relationships between physicians and nurses) that interprofessional functioning in the provision of health care is superior, in terms of efficiency, efficacy, quality, and satisfaction to all concerned, to the efforts of individuals. When we see this demonstration, over time, we will be ready to accept those models and our medical and nursing students will be taught to emulate them.

As a variety of nurse-physician teams practice together they will acquire the potential to overcome the barriers to constructive nurse-physician relationships, and those who follow them, even though a generation or more later, will be able to provide, without constraint, the kind of health care our population needs.

REFERENCES

1 Stein, L.I.: "The Doctor-Nurse Game," *Archives of General Psychiatry*, **16**:699–703, 1967.

2 Schutt, B.C.: "Child Health Care in the '70s," in *The Joint ANA-AAP Guidelines: For the Good of the Child*, American Nurses Association, New York, 1972, p. 8.

3 Heide, W.S.: "Nursing and Women's Liberation: A Parallel," *American Journal of Nursing*, **72**:824–827, 1973.

4 Sandler, B.: *Some Little-Noticed Rulings with Enormous Import. The Academic Women*, Association of American Colleges, Washington, D.C., May 29, 1973 (leaflet).

5 Silver, H.K.: "A Blueprint for Pediatric Health Manpower for the 1970's," *Journal of Pediatrics*, **82**:149–156, 1973.

6 Scheffler, R.M., and O.D. Stinson: "Physician's
Assistants: A Report on Earnings," *P A Journal,* 3:11-18, 1973.
7 Bates, B.: *Nurse-Physician Dyad: Collegial or
Competitive? Three Challenges to the Nursing
Profession,* American Nurses Association, Kansas City, 1972.
8 National Commission for the Study of Nursing
and Nursing Education: "Summary Report
and Recommendations," *American Journal of
Nursing,* 70:279-294, 1970.
9 Lysaught, J.P.: *Action in Nursing,* McGraw-Hill, New York, 1974, p. 720.
10 Taunton, R.L., and J.M. Soptick: *Characteristics of Short-Term Continuing Education Programs Existing September 1974–June 1975,*
American Nurses Association, Kansas City,
Mo., 1976.
11 Schiff, D.W., C.H. Fraser, and H.C. Walters:
"The Pediatric Nurse Practitioner in the Office
of Pediatricians in Private Practice," *Pediatrics,*
44:62-68, 1969.
12 Yankauer, A., S. Tripp, P. Andrews, and J.P.
Connelly: "The Costs of Training and the Income Generation Potential of Pediatric Nurse
Practitioners," *Pediatrics,* 49:878-887, 1972.
13 Entertive, P.E., V. Salter, A.D. McDonald, and
J.C. McDonald: "The Distribution of Medical
Services Before and After "Free" Medical
Care—the Quebec Experience," *New England
Journal of Medicine,* 289:1174-1178, 1973.
14 Roghman, K.J., P.J. Haggerty, and R. Lorenz:
"Anticipated and Actual Effects of Medicaid
on the Medical-Care Pattern of Children," *New
England Journal of Medicine,* 285:1053-1057,
1971.

EDITOR'S QUESTIONS FOR DISCUSSION

What effect has the Women's Movement had on relationships between physicians and nurses? In the past, how has the nurse shared in the *medical* decision making concerning patient care but not shared in the responsibility for that decision making? What future trends can be predicted concerning decision making and responsibility? How are the decreasing differences between educational programs for medicine and nursing likely to influence the physician-nurse relationship? How can nursing encourage society to recognize the monetary worth of its services? How will an improved salary structure for nursing influence patient care? What relationship exists among ascribed status, educational preparation, and the ability to provide a specialized task or function? Is status assigned because of educational prerequisites or because of difficulty of the task performed? Is the social status of nursing likely to change? What factors influence the social status of nursing? How can communication be facilitated between physicians and nurses? Should the social status of nursing and medicine be equalized and, if so, to what extent?

Chapter 33

Interdisciplinary Stresses of Extended Nursing Roles

Lois Monteiro, R.N., Ph.D.
Assistant Professor of Community Health and Sociology
Brown University, Providence, Rhode Island

Lois Monteiro reviews the interdisciplinary issues that are critical to the physician-nurse relationship. Primarily, the issue of territory is examined and some underlying factors are enumerated: discrepancies between role perceptions and expectations of physicians and nurses; the question of responsibility for the patient; economic, diagnostic, and treatment infringement on medical actions; and competition for patients. Monteiro suggests that socialization of physicians and nurses into collaborative roles in an educational environment rather than in an on-the-job setting may reduce conflict. Joint clinical experiences during a time of professional socialization, as well as the use of action-research models, may assist a new socialization process for collaborative roles. Intradisciplinary conflict is also indicated by the lack of acceptance of the role of nurse practitioner. The opinion that the nurse practitioner has accepted a role of medicine and diminished the role of nursing is a minority one.

As one of the conclusions of its report, the Department of Health, Education, and Welfare Secretary's Committee to Study Extended Roles for Nurses stated that:

> An extension of nursing practice will be realized only as physicians and nurses collaborate to achieve this objective. Expanded roles for nurses will require major adjustments in the orientation and practice of both professions. . . . A determined and continuing effort should be made to attain a high degree of flexibility in the interprofessional relationships of physicians and nurses (*Nursing Outlook*, January 1972, p. 48).

This emphasis on the importance of interpersonal relationships between nurses and physician practi-

tioners underlined the interdisciplinary support necessary for the implementation of the nurse's expanded role and recognized one of the key areas for possible failures of the new nursing role. The experience of nurse practitioners, and of educators developing such programs, has shown that the committee's concerns were justified, and the growing literature on the nurse practitioner shows the extent to which interdisciplinary issues have hampered the establishment of individual nurse practices. For example, of fifty-eight articles included in a selected bibliography of articles on the nurse practitioner that appeared in the decade 1965–1975 (Devlin, 1975), about 45 percent mentioned interdisciplinary conflicts or tensions involved in the nurse practitioner role. This study will review the interdisciplinary issues that have received the greatest attention in the literature, and in particular will examine the stresses that have arisen around the disruption that the extended role presents for traditional nurse-physician-patient relationships. In addition to the role definitions issue, questions of accountability, costs, reimbursements, and certification of the practitioners have also raised issues of an interdisciplinary nature.

The issue of territory, that is, of which activities belong to which discipline, has received the major part of the attention to interdisciplinary tensions in the nurse practitioner literature. The basic question that underlies the issue is whether the nurse, in primary care to patients, supplements, substitutes for, or replaces the physician as the provider of services to these patients. Articles in the nursing literature emphasize that the nurse's role complements rather than usurps the physicians role, e.g., "the nurse practitioner is not practicing medicine, she is practicing nursing. And to practice in this way she has developed an appropriate—and for most nurses, new—concept of herself and her nursing identity" (Lewis, 1974). Articles written by physicians have tended to consider the nurse practitioner in the context of a physician's assistant, who works in concert with but under the supervision of the physician. In this conceptual view nurse practitioners and physician's assistants (e.g., Medex graduates) are seen as interchangeable entities (Barnett, 1974; Wakerlin, 1972), and although these practitioners are practicing on medical territory they are seen to assist the physician and to act at his discretion and thus are not in competition or conflict with the discipline. Nurse-writers have viewed the nurse practitioner not only as a complement to physicians but also as different from (and by implication more competent than) physician's assistants (Rothberg, 1973). This distinction has been most cogently spelled out by Ingeborg Mauksch (1975 p. 1842).

A physician's assistant serves as an extension of the physician's identity. This functionary has no more knowledge than the physician and performs no task which the physician could not do had he the time and inclination . . . has no distinct body of knowledge or sphere of practice . . . is a "doctor stretcher," a dependent practitioner. . . .

The nurse practitioner performs nursing complementing at times the physician's doctoring. She is licensed in her own right. . . . She bases her practice on a body of nursing knowledge which is distinct. . . . Her nursing actions do include implementation of a physician's therapeutic regimen but by far the larger part of the role consists of the development of a therapeutic relationship with her clients and the application of the nursing process. . . . The nurse practitioner practices interdependently with the physician. . . .

Since social interaction is based on shared expectations for behavior of the actors in any situation, these discrepancies in the role perceptions and expectations of these two major acting groups predispose the disciplines of nursing and medicine to conflict regarding the basic issue of what in fact the nurse practitioner does.

One author, writing for a medical journal, has described this territorial dispute in dramatic terms:

It may be helpful to visualize primary health care as territories shaped in two overlapping circles, with traditional nursing on the left and medicine on the right . . . the physician can wander freely in both countries. The nurse, in contrast, cannot legally cross the border to roam in the land of medicine. . . . The role of the nurse can now be seen as an expansion into or even an invasion into the diagnostic and therapeutic domain of medicine. . . . Many individual physicians and much of organized medicine have mobilized their forces to fight back. . . . Where the turf is occupied by paying patients, however, medicine has put up its most vigorous fight, as if defending its oil fields. The most lasting and productive peace has probably been negotiated in territories that are so large, and are filled with so many patients, that neither doctor nor nurse is threatened by the other (Bates, 1975, p. 703).

In using the metaphor of territory and warfare to describe the situation, this author may somewhat overstate the extent of the conflict between physicians and nurses on the subject; but she does point out the most salient issues, (1) economic infringement and (2) infringement on the physician's exclusive hold on diagnosis and treatment as legitimate medical actions. Physicians' feeling of total responsibility for their patients, which critics call their sense of "ownership" of their patients, further feeds into the issue of territorial disputes.

In a study of the use of nurse practitioners in the Health Insurance Plan of New York, Galton et al. were surprised at the length of time required to settle these territorial disputes. As they note;

> The activities of our nurses have been largely supplemental to those of the family physicians with whom they are working. These supplemental activities are, of course, valuable . . . however the movement toward a team for the care of patients in which certain complementary roles would have evolved . . . has been slower than was initially projected. It is clear that we were overly optimistic.

Rather than the simple matter that they had expected the introduction of nurse practitioners would be, these administrators found that physician "anxiety about 'losing' their patients to the nurses" made even those physicians who volunteered to participate in the project cautious about moving forward into new areas of nurse practitioner responsibility (Galton et al., 1973, p. 117).

This sense of the loss of the patient to other health professionals may, as one physician has suggested, be a subtle guilt feeling that arises when the sharing of the patient is viewed as abandonment of the patient. Thus, becoming involved in a professional effort with a nurse practitioner as her colleague may involve a psychological risk to the physician (Bates, 1974, p. 11):

> Most physicians enjoy their patient contact. . . . To share a patient relationship with a nurse may be painful, especially if the doctor knows the patient well, has established a warm relationship, and perceives the patient as his own private patient. Sometimes he simply cannot relinquish the patient.

However, a different, and less prevalent, point of view on the territorial issue puts it in more economic terms, e.g., "some physicians do see nurse practitioners as competitors and as threats, particularly family nurse practitioners, who may go into private practice" and when these nurse practitioners begin to act beyond the role of physician's assistant, "the doctors fear competition" (Judge, 1974, p. 32). This attitude is also reflected to some extent in the belief that physicians view nurse practitioners as a temporary solution to a national shortage of physician primary care providers, but if the supply of physicians were to increase the nurse practitioner would no longer be needed (Judge, 1974, p. 32).

Despite the emphasis on the territorial issue as a potential problem, the findings from nurse practitioner experiences also show that physician acceptance can be achieved. In a controlled study of the medical clinics of Peter Bent Brigham Hospital in Boston, researchers concluded that "nurses can be integrated into direct patient care in a large teaching hospital internal medicine clinic *without difficulty*" (my italics). As evidence of this acceptance the authors showed that two-thirds of the 115 physicians involved in the clinic referred one or more patients to the nurse practitioner during the 3 months of the study period (Spector et al., 1975, p. 1236). A survey of 3,000 Missouri physicians found that 45 percent of solo practitioners and 62 percent of group practitioners felt that physician assistants (the survey did not specify nurse practitioners) might meet a need not adequately met by current office assistants. Of these favorable physicians, 84 percent indicated some willingness to hire a physician's assistant (Wakerlin, 1972, p. 830).

Of the various methods that have been suggested to eliminate the territorial conflict, to help change role expectations, and to improve working relationships, the most frequently mentioned pertains to a change in the system of educating physicians and nurses. The Committee to Study Extended Roles for Nurses recommended that "collaborative efforts involving schools of medicine and nursing should be encouraged to undertake programs to demonstrate effective functional inter-action of physicians and nurses in the provision of health services" (1972, p. 48). Resocialization of nurses into nurse practitioners, and the socializa-tion of doctors and nurses into collaborative roles could no doubt be accomplished in an educational rather than an on-the-job setting; however, such educational programs have been slow to develop. In terms of practical realities the probability of joint education programs occurring is likely to be small, although, as one report stated, "the evolu-tion of the health care team will be significantly accelerated if both nurses and physicians share in educational and clinical experiences specifically designed to meet this objective (Galton et al., 1973, p. 119). While the authors admit that "this is not an original observation, but it does bear re-peating," they note that nevertheless, "neither medical nor nursing education has, for the most part, succeeded in implementing such programs" (Galton et al., 1973, p. 119).

One faculty group at the University of Califor-nia at San Francisco attempted to develop profes-sional role definitions through such a program of student-level interaction of nurses and doctors rather than isolated education of each of these dis-ciplines. A hospital primary care clinic was staffed by teams of medical and nursing students working with a shared caseload of six families per team. The patient problems encountered in such a learn-ing situation provided, according to the faculty, ample experience to convince the participants that "one discipline cannot meet all the patient needs," and it was concluded that such joint clinical exper-iences during a time of professional socialization can teach nurses and physicians to work together more effectively (Rosenaur and Fuller, 1973, p. 162). However, since the evaluation did not in-clude the study of the behaviors of the students in work situations after their education was com-pleted we do not know the extent to which such joint learning influences later interdisciplinary interaction of the practicing professionals.

Over time, on-the-job interaction in supervised preceptorships also gradually solves the territorial and role expectation problems of individual practi-tioners, but not without risk. As the director of one nurse practitioner program warns:

> The greatest problem with which nurse-prac-titioner students must deal during the pre-ceptorship was touched upon earlier: helping the physician learn about nursing. This is difficult because of the pressures in the situa-tion to become like the physician. . . . Generally speaking, physicians do not understand either the capabilities or the role of a nurse practitioner . . . [and are] likely to exert tremendous pres-sure on the nurse practitioner to assume a de-pendent, illness-oriented, physician's assistant role. . . . Since the faculty continues to exer-cise some supervision over the nurse during her preceptorship, however, they can support her in her efforts to function as a nurse practitioner until the nature of the role is finally demon-strated to the physician (Malkemes, 1974, pp. 91–92).

The new, and often insecure, nurse practitioner must demonstrate by her actions what she per-ceives her role and her legitimate functions to be. As these are tested in practice, shared expectations of the partners grow and new role definitions are formulated. Even in the best of settings these can be difficult weeks or months, e.g., a nurse practi-tioner who joined a new group practice, and was involved as early as the planning and development stages, nevertheless wrote that "I realized there might be some misunderstanding of the definition of nursing. I didn't realize its extent. Defining nursing to physicians involves tackling hidden atti-tudes and misconceptions. . . . I refrained from aggressive and impatient behavior in the early months of the practice. . . . As my role became more clearly defined, I began to contribute more" (Brown, 1974, p. 111). Sometimes, despite the continued and determined effort to define roles through actions, some nurse practitioners still face a lack of understanding; "Some physicians simply refused to alter their relationship with them [nurse practitioners]. Certain physicians were unwilling to share patients or information" (Linn and Lewis, 1976, p. 784).

Allowing the fledgling nurse practitioners to

ventilate their feelings about their new role through the means of regularly scheduled "rap sessions" to discuss stressful aspects of the role has been successful in providing these practitioners with social support and in reinforcing their abilities to cope with the diverse expectations (Linn and Lewis, 1976, p. 782). The talking out and sharing of problems was done in an all-nurse group, however, so it had no effect on the attitudes of the other disciplines.

Wise et al. have suggested that shared expectations can be developed through an action-research model that they have used in an actual multidisciplinary team situation in a medical center setting. This group-oriented program allowed each team member to express his or her view on such items as the team's goals, working structure, and participation of members. These were first expressed privately to the researcher and then fed back anonymously to all other team members. Group discussion sessions with all members were then built on the anonymous commentaries, and from these the teams developed statements of priorities and shared objectives. As Wise notes, "it is naive to bring together a highly diverse group of people and to expect that, by calling them a team, they will in fact behave as a team" (1974, p. 546). From his point of view the team itself must spend some time working on its own functioning process, must "treat itself as a patient—periodically diagnosing its own state of health" (1974, p. 542).

Occasionally it is the nonphysicians in the setting who refuse to acknowledge the new role, as in the story of "an angry nurse practitioner" who tried for more than 18 months to obtain privileges to visit her groups' patients in the hospital (O'Shaughnessey, 1976, p. 1165), and who, despite frustration at the series of barriers to her request, remained firm in her resolve. "I am adamant in maintaining that I am a nursing professional, and that the skills I have to offer my patient are nursing skills, not the practice of medicine. I refuse to try to gain access to my patients through [a means] . . . which does not acknowledge me as a professional." The means that had been offered

was for the hospital to contract with her physician partner to allow her hospital privileges by specifying her as a "physician's employee." The practitioner viewed herself as a colleague, not an employee of her partner. In this case, although the physician with whom this nurse practitioner was associated in a "team approach to health care" was supportive of her position and understanding of her role, other medical staff and the hospital's board and its administrator were not, and these persons were able to prevent her from carrying out in-hospital nurse practitioner activities that both she and her physician partner had agreed on as legitimate.

We have concentrated on medicine-nursing interdisciplinary issues regarding nurse practitioners, but intradisciplinary conflict among nurses about the nurse practitioner's role, although relatively slight, cannot be overlooked. Martha Rogers (Mauksch and Rogers, 1975), one of the most vocal internal critics, called nursing a "house divided" over the practitioner issue, and strongly attacked the "blatant perfidy spawned by such terms as pediatric associate, nurse practitioner, family health practitioner, primary care practitioner, geriatric practitioner, physician extender, and other equally weird and wonderful cover-ups designed to provide succor and profit for the nation's shamans" (1975, p. 1834). In quoting the title of a newspaper story "A Nurse Is a Nurse—Unless She Is a Practitioner," Rogers quipped, "They should have added 'And Then She's a Physician's Assistant—Not a Nurse.' " What Rogers feels is the issue is that nursing is a profession in its own right, and that to take over some of medicine's roles is to diminish that nursing role that she views as social commitment, and the promotion and maintenance of health, along with the care of the sick. Finally, in addition to disparaging the role, she also hints that the medical profession's "real intent behind this con game" is to diminish the number and power of professionally educated nurses "and to force these nurses to practice at a lower level in medicine." Her words are strong, as are her convictions on the matter, but hers is definitely a minority opinion.

However, in spite of such intraprofessional criticism, extended nursing roles can be expected to continue to grow, although there may be program refinements and a move toward a standardized plan for the preparation of such practitioners. This will be accelerated by the need and the pressures to develop criteria by which the quality of services of nurse practitioners can be certified. Such certification for a level of competency will be required for reimbursement of these practitioners under federally funded programs such as Medicare. In this way the third-party payers will, in effect, define the limits of the role by specifying the services for which they agree to pay nurse practitioners.

Interdisciplinary conflicts can be expected to continue, but there is at least some evidence of a move toward better relationships between the care providers. There are well-integrated interdisciplinary health care teams in existence, as for example the Brookside Park Center in Jamaica Plains, Boston, an interdisciplinary low-income client center at which the director is a nurse with a Master of Public Health degree. This center has been cited for providing innovative and sophisticated care. In addition, a regional DHEW (Department of Health, Education and Welfare) Conference on health manpower has proposed that rather than developing more new primary care practitioners (either physician assistants or nurse practitioners) the agency should support continuing education programs on team functioning that would allow physicians, nurses, and physicians assistants already in working situations the opportunity to explore ways to improve their work relationships and to improve the effectiveness of the team in providing better care for patients. Such developments will go far to solve the interdisciplinary stress created as nursing expands its area of practice.

BIBLIOGRAPHY

Barnard, Martha U., and Edward C. Defoe: "Nurse Practitioner," *Journal of the Kansas Medical Society,* **75**:173–179, May 1974.

Barnett, Margery: "Nurses Learn to Share Physicians' Case Load," *Medical Tribune,* **15**:1, March 6, 1974.

Bates, Barbara: "New Nursing Roles: Implications for Medicine," *Hospital Practice,* **9**:11–12, April 1974.

——: "Physician and Nurse Practitioner: Conflict and Reward," *Annals of Internal Medicine,* **82**:702–706, May 1975.

Brown, Kathleen Cavanah: "The Nurse Practitioner in a Private Group Practice," *Nursing Outlook,* **22**:108–113, February 1974.

Darnell, Richard E.: "The Promotion of Interest in the Role of the Physician Associate as a Potential Career Opportunity for Nurses: An Alternative Strategy," *Social Science and Medicine,* **7**:495–505, July 1973.

Devlin, Mary M.: *Selected Bibliography with Abstracts on Joint Practice,* National Joint Practice Commission (AMA), Chicago, May 1975.

Galton, Robert et al.: "Observations on the Participation of Nurses and Doctors in Chronic Care," *Bulletin of the New York Academy of Medicine,* **49**:112–119, February 1973.

Henriques, Charles C., Vincent G. Virgadamo, and Mildred D. Kahane: "Performance of Adult Health Appraisal Examinations Utilizing Nurse Practitioners-Physician Teams and Paramedical Personnel," *American Journal of Public Health,* **64**:47–53, January 1974.

Januska, Charlotte, Carol Dawn Davis, Ruth N. Knollmueller, and Patience Wilson: "Development of a Family Nurse Practitioner Curriculum," *Nursing Outlook,* **22**:103–108, February 1974.

Judge, Diane: "The Coming Battle Over Nurse Practitioners," *Modern Healthcare,* **1**:29–36, April 1974.

Klinkhoff, Alice, and Barbara Fraser: "The Visible Nurse: 'The Thing I Hate Most Is Being Ignored,'" *McGill Medical Journal,* **44**:10–12, Fall 1975.

Levin, Arthur: "More Than Nurses," *Professional Life,* **6**:35, June 1974.

Lewis, Edith P.: "A Role by Any Name," *Nursing Outlook,* **22**:89, February 1974.

Linn, Lawrence S., and Mary Ann Lewis: "Rap Sessions for Nurse Practitioner Students," *American Journal of Nursing,* **76**:782–784, May 1976.

Malkemes, Lois C.: "Resocialization: A Model for Nurse Practitioner Preparation," *Nursing Outlook*, 22:90-94, February 1974.

Mauksch, Ingeborg, and Martha E. Rogers: "Nursing Is Coming of Age... Through the Practitioner Movement" PRO, I. Mauksch; CON, M. Rogers; *American Journal of Nursing*, 75:1834-1843, October 1975.

—— and Paul R. Young: "Nurse Physician Interaction in a Family Medical Care Center," *Nursing Outlook*, 22:113-118, February 1974.

McGivern, Diane: "Baccalaureate Preparation of the Nurse Practitioner," *Nursing Outlook*, 22:94-98, February 1974.

Moore, Ann C.: "Nurse Practitioner: Reflections on the Role," *Nursing Outlook*, 22:124-127, February 1974.

O'Brien, Margaret, Margery Manly, and Margaret C. Heagarty: "Expanding the Public Health Nurse's Role in Child Care," *Nursing Outlook*, 23:369-373, June 1975.

O'Shaughnessey, Camie: "Diary of an Angry Nurse Practitioner," *American Journal of Nursing*, vol 76, no. 7, July 1976, pp. 1165-1168.

Pomerantz, Rhoda S.: "The Nurse in an Expanded Role," *Journal of Chronic Diseases,* 28:561-563, 1975.

Rosenaur, Janet A., and Dorothy J. Fuller: "Teaching Strategies for Interdisciplinary Education," *Nursing Outlook*, 21:159-162, March 1973.

Rothberg, June S.: "Nurse and Physician's Assistant: Issues and Relationships," *Nursing Outlook,* 21:154-158, March 1973.

Spector, Reynold et al.: "Medical Care by Nurses in an Internal Medicine Clinic—Analysis of Quality and Its Cost," *JAMA*, 232:1234-1237, June 23, 1975.

United States Department of Health, Education, and Welfare: Report of the Secretary's Committee to Study Extended Roles for Nurses: "Extending the Scope of Nursing Practice," *Nursing Outlook,* 20:46-52, January 1972.

Wakerlin, George E., William Stoneman, III, and Arthur E. Rikli: "Physician's Assistants—Nurse Associates: An Overview," *Missouri Medicine,* 69:779-785, October 1972.

Wise, Harold, Irwin Rubin, and Richard Beckard: "Making Health Teams Work," *American Journal of Diseases of Children*, 127:537-542, April 1974.

EDITOR'S QUESTIONS FOR DISCUSSION

Does the nurse who provides primary care supplement, substitute for, or replace the physician or the provider of services? What is the relationship between the nurse's self-concept and others' expectations of her? What evidence is there of the application of nursing knowledge in the delivery of primary care? How can the nurse practitioner reduce the threat to some physicians as well as to other nurses of her role? How might joint learning influence later interdisciplinary actions? What should be the specific functions of a nurse practitioner?

Chapter 34

Credentialling, Power Relationships, and Interdisciplinary Pressures

Donna F. VerSteeg, R.N., Ph.D.
Assistant Professor, School of Nursing
University of California at Los Angeles

Accreditation is also an issue involved in interdisciplinary relationships because it legitimates the domains of professionals. Donna F. VerSteeg discusses the power relationships that are part of this process. Requiring credentials is a means of ensuring technical and moral competence in a professional, for the purpose of protecting the patient. The state acts on behalf of the patient in the accrediting procedure. VerSteeg emphasizes the importance of responsibility and accountability of professionals in supervising others. She outlines the concerns of the state, the patient, the student, and the practicing professional and suggests that compromise is needed to appease all of their concerns. Corporate responsibility presumably cannot promote quality or responsible service; the obligation lies in the individual provider. She suggests that nursing and medicine should unite to ensure the credibility of expertise.

There was a long-distance bicycle rider out on the plains of Texas one summer. It was very hot and he had lost his water canteen and was beginning to wonder if he was going to make it to the next town. He was really feeling desperate when a little sportscar pulled up beside him. The driver asked if he needed help. They talked a little bit and the driver finally said: "Well, I can give you a ride to the next town, but there is no way I can carry your bike. There is one thing we can do. I have a safety helmet, a rope, and a whistle I can loan you. You take the helmet and the whistle and we'll tie the rope on the bicycle frame so that I can tow you into town. If I go too fast you just blow on the whistle to slow me down."

The cyclist was desperate so he agreed to this arrangement and they started off down the highway. For a while things went very well. If the car began to go too fast, the cyclist would blow his whistle and the driver would slow down again. They had been proceeding in this fashion for about 30 minutes when another sportscar came by, racing its motor and challenging the first car to a race. Without thinking, the driver of the first car speeded up and the race was on.

In the last scene of our drama we see a police car parked by the side of the road. The patrolman grabs for his radio and calls headquarters.

"Sergeant, I need help quick!"

"Why, what's wrong?"

This article was originally prepared for presentation to the American Congress of Rehabilitation Medicine, November 20, 1974, San Francisco, California.

"Two cars just went by here doing at least 85 and I don't know what to do."

"What do you mean, you don't know? Stop them, and write out some tickets."

"I was going to Sarge, but there's already some yo-yo chasing them on a bicycle!"

The point to this story is that we sometimes tie ourselves into relationships that we later regret. This is particularly true when the parties involved are poorly matched in terms of their relative power. It sometimes results in situations that are dangerous for everyone involved.

Any time the mechanism of credentialling is involved, we can be certain that we are standing on somebody's professional turf. When the credentialling relationship exists between two groups that have very disparate power, we can expect that power difference to be perpetuated. In some areas involving the public health and safety, the method of credentialling used may not be adequate. A whistle and a bike are just not effective substitutes for a siren, a black-and-white, and the full majesty of the law.

We must consider also that when we speak of "profession," we are using a variety of definitions. These have to do with length of education, special bodies of knowledge, autonomous practice, etc.

Ultimately, what we are talking about are levels of *technical* and *moral competence*. Only the professional is considered to be *fully* morally and technically competent. Those whom the professional supervises are considered to be *less* competent morally or *less* competent technically or both. Thus, we can have highly dedicated workers or highly skilled workers, but only professionals are both highly dedicated *and* highly skilled and therefore competent to be fully responsible, fully accountable for their own practice.

When a worker operates at a *supervised* level, the responsibility and accountability rest with the professional who does the supervising. This is fine if the professional is able and willing to perform this function. We are beginning to realize that this assumption is faulty, particularly in the case of complex organizations.

More and more we find instances where the responsible professional is placed in a bureaucratic position where it is impossible for him or her to exercise the supervision upon which this concept depends. Faced with an impossible task, the professional resorts to what Dalton (1958) refers to as "illegal working arrangements." The worker is allowed to work *without* supervision providing he does not tell anybody. This situation is like the Prohibition era—lamentable, but very real. We end up with bathtub gin medicine being practiced across the country. If you, as a consumer, have contact with one of the better producers, everything is fine. If you happen to get involved with a bad batch or an unscrupulous runner, you may be in deep trouble.

What does this have to do with credentialling? A great deal. When we provide someone with a credential, we are giving warranty that this individual is what he or she claims to be—that he or she is competent to provide such and such a service at such and such a level, with such and such a degree of autonomy. Our licensed vocational nurse statute in this state defines what such an individual is entitled and competent to do—*under the supervision or direction of a registered nurse or a licensed physician and surgeon in the State of California*. When we go out and look at what LVNs do, however, we find them practicing in situations in which their supervising professionals have effectively abdicated control, not responsibility in the sense of status, of authority, or of pay scale, but in the sense of actually overseeing the work that is done. This is not only poor practice, it is also unfair both to the worker and to the consumer.

Regardless of what we say as to the hidden reasons of turf protection, practice monopoly, or whatever you want to call it, the ultimate authority that legitimates whatever credentialling mechanism we use is the consumer. In the health business, the consumer is the patient.

The consumer *is* the state. The state, speaking for the consumer, has certain concerns:

1 *Safe* practice by its licensees (not excellence, but safety)

2 Efficient and economical use of its educational facilities

3 The amelioration of conflict between professional groups (some of which have more political clout than others)

4 The largest effect for the least dollars that it spends on maintaining and restoring the public health and welfare

The consumer as an individual has additional concerns. He is concerned with:

1 Paying the taxes to support the state, paying the fees that support the professional, and, very likely, paying through the use of his own warm body for the education of students to learn their occupational skills

2 The fair distribution of the resources of care (kidney dialysis machines, immunization programs, rehabilitation facilities)

3 Access to professionals to provide the care that he requires in a manner that he feels comfortable with (given his particular subculture) and in which he can place his warrented trust

4 Being certain that the care he is given by students is of good quality because it is properly and expertly supervised by competent professionals

What about these students? They too are consumers of an educational process. They too have concerns:

1 To have access to educational opportunities based on the student's *demonstrated potential* rather than his finances, ethnic identity, sex, or prior educational access.

2 To have access to faculties and eventually employment opportunities that facilitate his development in an occupation that meets his expectations.

Finally, there is the professional. The professional is (or should be) concerned with:

1 Delivery of the *best* care he or she knows how to give (This is different from *safe* care)

2 Maintenance of the credibility (and therefore, respect and effectiveness) of professional expertise

3 Protection from limitations on effective practice that are arbitrary and serve no necessary purpose in relation to the needs and concerns of the other interests we have mentioned

It is impossible for all of these groups—the state, the consumer, the student, and the practicing professional—to achieve all of their concerns. There will have to be compromise. The question is not whether to compromise, but at which point and on what basis the compromise will be achieved. The time for interdisciplinary warfare is past. Either we make a just peace among ourselves, and join to face the common danger, or we will cease to exist.

In the delivery of health care, corporate responsibility will not insure quality service. It will not even insure safe service. Corporate responsibility has not even resulted in safe automobiles without a lot of outside pressure, and some pretty embarrassing statistics. People services must depend upon the individual responsibility and accountability of the provider. This means, by definition, that the individual provider must be prepared to provide responsible, accountable service.

It means also that the system—educational, practice, or governmental—must face up to its responsibilities in terms of what to do with those individuals who fail. Do we brand them as outcasts? Rarely. The investment is too great and not only in terms of time, money, and energy spent to educate and train. There is also the painful knowledge that all of us—*all of us*—make mistakes. The determination of that fine line beyond which mistakes can no longer be tolerated is emotionally costly. Do we cool them out? Sometimes. An unqualified and unqualifiable individual can sometimes be conned into going away—up, down, or sideways—thus removing the problem. Do we recycle? This technique of keeping individuals in a program until they qualify (or go away) is perhaps the most easily accepted by the profession, and one of the more costly. Do we ignore the problem, satisfying our consciences by being certain that our own clients are not referred to the failure but leaving the naive at his or her mercy? Many professions have practiced this method. It is the prime reason for the lack of credibility of professional expertise today.

Or, finally, do we credential, by one means or another, and educate the public to use this means to select a qualified provider. This would seem, on the face of it, to be the most desirable, and it is if it is effectively carried out. If it is not, for reasons of incompetence, greed, or lack of authority, it is worse than any of the others because it promises what it cannot deliver.

You can do many good things *with* a bicycle that are creative, innovative, and of considerable value to society. There are some things, however, that you cannot do *on* a bicycle. For these, you need a V-8 engine and a siren. The difficulty is deciding which is which.

BIBLIOGRAPHY

Dalton, Melvin: *Men Who Manage,* Wiley, New York, 1958.

VerSteeg, Donna L.F.: "The Physicians' Assistant: Interorganizational Influence on the Creation of a New Occupation," Ph.D. dissertation, University of California, Los Angeles, 1973.

EDITOR'S QUESTIONS FOR DISCUSSION

How can licensing or accreditation be enforced to prevent violations? To what extent does a professional have an obligation to report incompetency in another professional? What should be done to ensure competency after a professional is licensed? Should there be mandatory, legislated requirements to ensure competency? What might these requirements be? To what extent should accreditation be standardized? What factors have influenced the decreased credibility of professionals? What are the implications concerning accreditation for increasing specialization in nursing?

Part Seven

The Future of Nursing

We have knowledge of the past in nursing and health care delivery, the present status of nursing has been assessed, and a look into the future of nursing would be valuable. Planning is essential in health care in order to make the most efficient use of our resources and to develop what is needed to meet possible future demands. The following section treats issues that must be considered if the needs of patients are to be met. Some resolutions for problems in nursing and health care delivery are offered and some predictions are made. Because these issues are controversial, you may disagree with the proposed resolutions and projected predictions.

Chapter 35

The Future Health Delivery System and the Utilization of Nurses Prepared in Formal Educational Programs

Myrtle K. Aydelotte, R.N., Ph.D., F.A.A.N.
Executive Director, American Nurses Association*
Kansas City, Missouri

Utilization of nursing personnel is a key issue at present and will continue to be important in the future. Myrtle K. Aydelotte deals with this problem by making a plea for nursing to consider what the profession can do effectively at a cost acceptable to society. She classifies three types of centers for the future delivery of health care: primary, intermediary, and tertiary. Nursing functions within each type of center are outlined and an analysis of these functions indicates the types of nursing roles needed. She insists that basic, major differences in nursing performance are inevitable among the graduates of dissimilar educational programs. The basic knowledge acquired by the graduate from each type of nursing program is described, and a scheme for utilization of graduates from each of these programs for each of the three types of health centers is devised.

One of the major problems confronting individuals in the health professional education and clinical leadership practice is the vagueness with which the future health delivery system is conceptualized. Although we have read a great deal about the deficiencies of the present system, its inefficiency, its insensitivity, and its failures to deliver what the clients want, and although there are a number of individuals writing and speaking on the question, we really have no distinct and tested comprehensive models of delivery. The failure of comprehensive planning groups to produce acceptable descriptions for use has begun to be recognized. Hopefully, a position paper will be forthcoming outlining the total problem of planning and proposing ways of mounting the lack of conceptual models.[1]

The problem of nursing education and the utilization of graduates must be divided into two questions:

[1] Private conversation with Dr. Paul Densen, Professor of Community Health; Director, Harvard Center for Community Health and Medical Care, Harvard University, Boston, Massachusetts.

*This article was originally prepared for presentation at the University of Nebraska School of Nursing, January 11, 1973, while the author was Director and Professor, University of Iowa Hospital and clinics, Iowa City, Iowa, and has been revised for this edition. This chapter is *not* to be interpreted as a policy statement of the American Nurses Association.

1 What is the utilization of the graduates of the proposed curricula in the present-day delivery system?

2 What will be utilization patterns of future graduates in the future system as that system might be predicted?

Before these two questions are answered, however, major concerns about present nursing curricular planning and the lack of insight among most nursing educators about the outcomes of present-day educational programs must be expressed. These statements may be harsh, but seedlings of unreality exist in the planning of current educational programs. These concerns revolve around the purpose nursing chooses to serve. To what do we give our attention and what do we achieve? Are our accomplishments worth the investment of money and time?

THE PURPOSE OF NURSING

The major issue confronting the leadership group in nursing today concerns its purpose and, although we claim that we are informed about what society wants, the validity of our interpretation of what society wants can be questioned.

Nursing is only one of the many health professions operating under a social mandate. The recent publicity about failure to deliver care, the legislative action taken in some of the states, the amount and kind of financial support provided nursing, all these speak to the point that society is disillusioned about nursing, or, perhaps, it has not been convinced that what we offer cannot be offered by someone else. The reaction of society to nursing's responsiveness is found in the amount of dollars and cents it has been willing to invest in the purchase of its services, in the education of nurses, in its acceptance of nurses as a power force, and in its endorsement of certain trends in practice and education. You will agree that the support has not been overwhelming.

What kind of charge has society given to the health professions? In the writings today, one theme appears again and again and is basic to many of the proposals for change. The "right to health" has evolved as a natural right—an outgrowth of philosophical certainty and conviction that individuals must be guaranteed the opportunity to seek health. This right has developed from our basic need to delay the harsh reality of death, and, with the growth in medical and scientific technology and with guarantors of payment of services, the right to health is being structured in our society to accommodate this need.[2] Therefore, our society expects us to meet the charge to provide services that are basic to health.

What are these services? They are not new, but it may help to review them. Society wants the following: food, a diet that is nutritious for the individual and that, in his opinion, is sufficient to enable him to live as he wishes to live; shelter, a place for him to live his own lifestyle; clothing, to keep him warm or cool, and again in his own lifestyle; recreation; a state of being in which he feels competent; and a means of obtaining his own living. What is new in the discussion of these basic needs is the growing awareness of the need for the professionals to practice *that which is relevant* to the client, rather than that which enhances the image of the professional. It is becoming apparent that each profession, "out of the universe of all possible health needs ... carves its own role, identifying those needs to which it will address its knowledge, skill and efforts."[3] Nursing has not stated what kinds of services it can offer to the various groups of clients and how much these services will cost. Furthermore, we have not made clients aware of the options that we can offer them and have not predicted for them what the results will be for each option and the cost. We

[2] For a comprehensive discussion of this topic, see Robert Lanon White, *Right to Health: The Evolution of an Idea*, Graduate Program in Hospital and Health Administration, University of Iowa, Health Care Research Series, no. 18, 1971.

[3] Barbara Bates, "Nurse Physician Dyad: Collegial or Competitive?," in *Three Challenges to the Nursing Profession,* selected papers from the ANA Convention, 1972, p. 5.

have assumed, and perhaps incorrectly so, that what we have to offer is marketable and effective, and for the common good. We have also assumed that we hold a special place in the patient's world. I believe that such thinking is naive and the assumption invalid. It is imperative that nursing come to terms with itself and delineate, in precise terms, that to which it will attend. This decision should be based upon consideration of what it can do effectively at a cost that society will tolerate. It is urgent that nursing accomplish this essential goal.

Members of society are challenging the right of professionals to jealously guard the knowledge they have garnered as their own. There is evidence that some of the tasks and judgments previously considered professional can be exercised by non-professionals. Further, there is some evidence that professionals do not assume the accountability that has been given to them. For these reasons, today's acceptance of professionals is not firm.

Society has assigned to nursing the primary task of assessing patient wants and needs; designing and executing care practices to meet these needs; and the further function of instructing patients and others in the maintenance of health, the avoidance of malady, and the extension of care. From society's standpoint, it wants individual nurses who are sensitive to patient's needs and have a thorough knowledge of technology and a clear grasp of the behavioral and physical sciences as a base for decision making in patient care.[4]

MODEL OF HEALTH CARE DELIVERY SYSTEM

Discussions of health care delivery systems include reference to three types of units, each relating to the other. It appears that each center interdigitates with the other and all operate as one universe, with the academic health center serving as the source of knowledge, new therapy and procedures, and personnel—the energy point, upon which the others rest.

Society has as its major concern today primary care delivery. This is the major unmet health care need. Primary health care is defined as that care, provided by a health professional, at the first contact.[5] The initiation of the first contact may arise for a variety of reasons, none of which are really more significant than the other. The question confronting the patient or client is "What do I do next?" Primary care delivery is characterized, then, not by geographic placement, or type of need, but by first entry into the total system.

Pelligrino provides four characteristics of the primary care delivery:

1 It is accessible to every individual.
2 It is provided in quality.
3 It is available within 20 to 30 minutes.
4 It is available 7 days a week, 24 hours a day.

If we view primary care delivery, in this sense, we come to the conclusion that the health delivery system is not a longitudinal arrangement of a simple collective of health workers to one of a highly complex collective of specialized health workers, but a dynamic interconnection of communications about services, knowledge, and practices. Primary care centers may be found within intermediary care centers and tertiary care centers, and first access to care could be made at any point in the system. The movement of an individual client within the system might pass over other units, depending upon the nature of the problem of the client. The total system is highly articulated and integrated. From the point of entry, the ordering of the client's care rests upon the consideration of where he can be treated most effectively, with the least amount of effort on his part, and at the least cost to society.

[4] National Commission for the Study of Nursing and Nursing Education, *An Abstract for Action,* McGraw-Hill, New York, 1970, pp. 96–98.

[5] Acknowledgment is given to Dr. Edward Pelligrino's lecture on January 5, 1973, University of Iowa Medical Center, and Department of Family Practice, College of Medicine, for clarification of these ideas about primary care delivery.

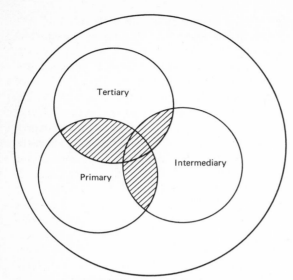

Figure 35-1 Scheme of health delivery system

Instead of the usual portrayal of the health delivery system as either that of a pyramid or satellite, it can be viewed as a series of concentric, overlapping circles, encompassed within one field.

The overlapping and shaded areas represent those functions that occur in all centers: (1) initial entry to the system; and (2) emergency services for maintenance of life until the patient can be moved to a center where special facilities and personnel are provided in greater numbers or in more effective arrangements to care for him. The external boundary is the knowledge field upon which all in the delivery system rests. This knowledge field is generated by the tertiary center, which, by its very nature, provides the intellectual leadership required. The tertiary center, in which a health center hospital is located, is in an academic environment where research is conducted, where the new knowledge, the new technology and procedures, and new programs of care and delivery are identified and reduced into simpler language to be used by the practitioner. The tertiary center must assume the responsibility for feeding and nourishing the total health care system.

The system may be thought of as a consortium of health institutions, agencies, and health care practitioners, the concern of which is the design and conduct of health care programs for a specific population. The classification of these constituents into the three types of centers is based upon the major purposes each serves in the care program and the nature of the environment, the scientific and technical services, which each must provide to accomplish those purposes.

The major purpose of the center classified as primary care center is to provide: (1) entry into the system; (2) emergency care; (3) health maintenance; (4) long-term and chronic care; and (5) treatment of temporary malfunctioning that does not require hospitalization. The intermediary centers exist to provide: (1) the treatment of malfunctioning that is temporary but requires hospitalization of such a nature that highly skilled services and high risk intervention is not required; (2) the evaluation of long-term and chronic illness, to determine whether a change in intervention is required, when the evaluation requires hospitalization; and (3) the provision of counseling and therapy that cannot be provided within the primary care center because of cost of services, equipment, or the infrequency with which it must be provided. The tertiary center's major purposes are related to the treatment of malfunctioning in which very highly skilled personnel and equipment are required: (1) the treatment of the esoteric illnesses of patients that occur infrequently; and (2) the provision of manpower, new programs, new knowledge, and demonstrations of delivery for the total health delivery system. It is in the tertiary center that program planning originates, where health teaching and maintenance plans are tested, where new technology arises, and where the total group of health professionals can find assistance, understanding, support, and counsel. In order to establish such a relationship, the academic health center must assume its responsibility for leadership and account for itself. This means that it remains sensitive to the realities of the situation outside the center, promotes confidence through feasible approaches to the problems of the others, and that it makes itself available at all times to demands from the outside. In order to serve this role, the senior personnel of the health center must exert itself to remain attuned to the external environment.

The personnel functioning within the total health delivery system draws upon knowledge from the academic disciplines. The classifications of knowledge for health care functioning are: normal functioning of individuals; malfunctioning of individuals; technology and procedures related to normal functioning and malfunctioning; specific therapy and intervention for correction of malfunctioning; economics; and the community and family institutions. The health disciplines will extract from these bodies of knowledge that which is pertinent to its practice, but all use generalizations from all of the above. The problems of educating today's practitioners are that of identifying the most up-to-date knowledge in the practice discipline so that it can be taught to the student; that of enabling the student to learn how to add to his own knowledge as future knowledge is synthesized and added to the total knowledge base; and how to make current knowledge relevant to what the student intends to do as a practitioner.

In each of the centers there will be a mix of professionals and paraprofessionals to achieve the purpose of the center. Hopefully, the mix in all centers will be such that a well-balanced health program can be offered. Certain conditions will be necessary to achieve balance. First, the available manpower in all centers must be sufficient in amount to assure that the workload can be tolerated without strain and frustration. Second, the program of care must be carefully developed so that interdigitation of care to individual patients is feasible and evaluation of effect assured. Third, the great sense of the practitioners being isolated and trapped in a center is avoided. Somehow, we must overcome the feelings of geographic and social isolation that occur among personnel regardless of type of setting.

NURSING UTILIZATION

A careful analysis of what nursing will attend to in each of these centers is required. A few general statements can be made from what was proposed in the preceding discussion. First of all, in all centers there must be individuals prepared to provide access to the delivery system and emergency care. The skills of interviewing and clinical assessment at entry can be readily taught to individuals of reasonable intelligence. What can not be readily taught, simply because we have not identified it, is the content to which the interview is directed and the reasons for which the clinical assessment has been made. We must honestly state that we do not know how some of the content will be used. Furthermore, we are terribly clumsy in getting the information. The task confronting nursing on assessment is that of preparing nurses how to rapidly, expertly, and readily obtain data from the patient or client for use by all health professionals. We can no longer spend, because society will not tolerate it, hours of time in assessment. We neither have evidence that health professionals use the data, nor know that use of some of it makes a difference to the patient.

Second, in all centers, there must be individuals prepared to render emergency treatment. The nature and extent of emergencies can be identified, if we study the subject, and we can teach it. The challenge is to keep the knowledge and skill requested to act in emergencies current and up-to-date. There is no time in emergencies for delay and for refreshing our knowledge base and skills.

These two matters, initial assessment at point of entry and initial emergency treatment, must be taught to *all* health professionals, not only nurses. This is common knowledge that we should all possess. There is a minimum knowledge and skill base that can be identified, if we attend to it.

The nursing services within each of the health care centers relate to the purpose of each center. A scheme outlining these major functions is described in Table 35-1.

Careful, studious analysis of these functions and the specific populations to be served could lead us to identify the knowledge and skills required for the personnel in each. We could then classify what type of nurse would be needed. Thorough structural analysis of these functions needs to be done.

Table 35–1 Outline of Scheme of Nursing Functions Within a Health Care Delivery System

Type of center	Grouping of functions
All centers	1 Enabling access to health delivery system 2 Providing emergency care 3 Administration of nursing program
Primary	1 Providing and evaluating health counseling relating to well-infant and child care, school health, control of communicable diseases, physical and mental fitness, sex education, and prevention of occupational illness. 2 Providing and evaluating the care of women, including antepartum care, home delivery of the uncomplicated patient, follow-up care of the postpartum patient, detection of cancer of the breast and cervix, and family planning. 3 Participating in the evaluation of individuals for their health status and performing diagnostic procedures not requiring highly costly specialized equipment. 4 Provision of and evaluation of clinic and home care for the patient with the simple episodic illness and the follow-up care for the chronically ill and long-term patient including rehabilitative measures that do not necessitate specialized equipment.
Intermediary	1 Participating in the evaluation of individuals entering the center and performing diagnostic measures requiring specialized equipment and skills. 2 Planning, implementing, and evaluating programs of nursing care for the patients who are ill and requiring hospitalization, but do not require highly specialized procedures and equipment. 3 Planning, implementing, and evaluating programs of nursing care for patients who are extremely ill, but cannot be transported to the tertiary center at the moment because of the seriousness of their condition. 4 Planning, implementing, and evaluating instructions to patients who are hospitalized and arranging for necessary follow-up upon discharge. 5 Planning, implementing, and evaluating continuing educational programs for nursing personnel in both the primary and intermediary centers. The content of these programs has been identified, structured, and programmed for transmission to practitioners.
Tertiary	1 Planning, implementing, and evaluating programs of nursing care for critically ill patients, or the patients whose malfunctioning requires highly life-threatening interventions, or on whom a newly developed intervention is being used. 2 Planning, implementing, and evaluating programs of care for patients who come for diagnostic or treatment measures requiring highly specialized knowledge, skill, and equipment. 3 Preparation of teaching materials to be used for patients and clients, relating to health maintenance or self-care, and testing the materials for effectiveness, economy, and feasibility. 4 Exploration, design, and testing new procedures, approaches, and methods of delivery care to patients and ways of preventing illness. 5 Planning, implementing, and evaluating educational programs to prepare nursing personnel. 6 Planning, implementing, and evaluating programs of continuing educational programs for nursing personnel in the total health delivery system. 7 Conduct of research to identify new knowledge and the translation of that new knowledge into practice and delivery systems. 8 Conduct of political and social maneuvers to keep the public informed of needs of nurses in all parts of the system and to keep nurses aware of political and social changes in attitudes and in mandate.

However, there are some brief statements about the individuals and how they function that can be made. First of all, I would like to comment on the relation of one so-called level of nursing personnel to another. We can no longer tolerate a system of education for the preparation of nurses based on the *degree* of difference of the same dimension. There must be a basic, major difference in educational outcomes—we must be able to state that the nurse with an associate degree is different from the nurse with a baccalaureate degree, and that a nurse with a master's degree is different still. If education makes no difference in what the person *can* do, then why the investment of time and energy in further educational effort?

Second, we are overlooking the difficulty inherent in the teaching of the behavioral sciences and their translation into nursing practice, a difficulty that affects the patient's behavior. There is much concern about compliance with medical and nursing orders, counsel and advice, and therapy, but professionals fail to recognize that there are options from which the patient or client may choose. Our responsibility is to reduce our knowledge of health practice to options for the patient or client and let him choose, knowing what outcomes are related to each option. The nurse-patient-client relationship, and how it is taught, has become vastly overrated, smacks of sentimentality, and, in many respects, violates the principle of privacy. The reason we fail to examine the effect of nurse-patient interaction is that it is a source of great satisfaction to the nurse. We fail to determine whether a change in patient behavior really results from the interaction alone. Therefore, since this area of knowledge, the behavioral sciences, is a very difficult one to teach and to translate, we must give more attention to it.

Third, one of the major failings of professionals is their inability to reduce their knowledge to concrete terms that can be understood by the client or patient and to prove that what they provide is useful. As professionals, we should also be able to study groups of patients, identify their specific care requirements, order these into a logical and feasible framework, design criteria for evaluating their care, perform the care, and evaluate the results. The primary expectation we must have in order to provide what society expects of us is that we must be able to do this kind of study, this kind of conceptualization, this kind of evaluation, and do what is feasible, real, and practical. If we do not have graduates who can do such things, we will have an unmarketable product.

Four, in order for the future delivery systems to work, we must instill in graduates of all kinds the sense of service and accountability. Nurses have been exploited, underpaid, and discriminated against in many ways. But, on the other hand, we have not met our obligations. We can not think of responsibility as ending at the end of the 8-hour day, or the 40-hour week. We must in some way restore the principle of accountability.

The associate degree nurse is a nurse prepared to render nursing care to specific groups of patients in organized health delivery systems. She is prepared to function in planned programs of care. This means that where the knowledge base and its translation is clearly identified and well tested, and the kinds of decisions she has to make are predictable, she can operate effectively and efficiently. The professional, on the other hand, deals with ambiguity, with the identification and reduction to practice of ill-defined knowledge, and with the more nebulous areas of concern. The scheme given in Table 35-2 best illustrates this.

If we study this scheme with relation to nursing practice we can see where the associate degree can function. She can function in settings where the clinical nursing requirements for service have been well identified, well programmed, and where the data with which she must deal are circumscribed and specific. She can function where policies, procedures, and decisions are programmed, or where she will have direct access to someone who can assist her. The nursing care of the majority of patients in the health delivery system in all settings can be met by persons prepared in these programs. What she cannot do, because she has not been taught to do it in her formal program, but may be

Table 35-2 State of Knowledge and Skill by Educational Program and its Relationship to Nursing Practice

Associate	Master's or professional degree
1 Well-structured knowledge with distinct boundaries	1 Knowledge being developed, identified, and synthesized
2 Generalizations developed	2 Generalizations not developed
3 Language precise	3 Language imprecise
4 Procedures developed for practice	4 Procedures emerging and being tested
5 Predictions established	5 Predictions uncertain, being tested
6 Programmed decisions	6 Unprogrammed decisions based on data uncertain
7 Knowledge easily communicated	7 Knowledge not easily communicated

able to, if encouraged to continue new formal education, is to manage and educate other personnel, develop and coordinate new programs, establish policy and procedures, conduct research, and provide professional nursing leadership.

The associate degree graduate's role, therefore, is to provide and evaluate direct care to groups of patients. What she does for patients will vary because the needs differ in different settings. In addition to the general background, the educational program should provide her with an introduction to one clinical nursing specialty area where she can learn to function comfortably with a large group of patients.

It is easier to visualize how postbaccalaureate-, master's-, and doctoral-level persons may function than how the baccalaureate degree graduate may function. Individuals with advanced preparation must assume the tasks of nursing leadership—the design of new nursing programs, their conduct, and evaluation; the direction of personnel; the coordination of nursing with other disciplines; and the development of policy and direction. This

is not to say that they are in administrative positions, although a number must be, but they *are* accountable for studying groups of patients to determine care requirements and for establishing the conditions that make it possible for nursing to contribute to the total programs of care. A number of them may be assuming senior practice roles, where extensive clinical knowledge is required, or where the variables are many and elusive. For example, the involvement of change in family interactions, community situations, and the complex social interactions require individuals with much preparation.

Just where the baccalaureate degree graduate fits in is more difficult to envision. She cannot be used purely for bedside care, as a general practitioner, as we have been proposing over these years. Neither can she be seen as a change agent. Let us not delude ourselves. She has neither the background, and she cannot acquire it in the time allowed, nor the maturity that commands or affects change. For years we have said she is a change agent. What change has she brought about? Further, until major changes occur in the attitude of women themselves toward employment, the less than master's degree education group will continue to be an unstable work force, characterized by high turnover and lack of commitment. How can we place the future of the nursing care of our population in the hands of this group?

In thinking about the baccalaureate degree graduate in future health delivery systems, I believe she may best fit in as a beginning nurse clinician in a specific clinical nursing field, where she will function in meeting special needs of patients, in planning programs for patients and nursing staff, and in evaluating effectiveness of care and the like. With increased maturity and experience, and with continuing education, she can move, if she demonstrates ability through performance, into leadership positions and become a professional in nursing practice.

In order to function in this role, her preparation must be vastly different than that currently being offered in many of the colleges of nursing.

Table 35-3 Scheme of Deployment of Graduates of Nursing Programs

Type of center	Type of graduates needed to meet functions
Primary	1 Master clinicians or practitioners—nursing administration leadership in midwifery, long-term illness, and chronic illness, and infant and child care 2 Baccalaureate degree graduates in beginning master clinician roles 3 Associate degree graduates for evaluation and diagnostic procedures and execution of care in various programs
Intermediate	1 Master clinicians in nursing administration and nursing specialties 2 Baccalaureate degree graduates in beginning master clinician roles 3 Associate degree graduates for evaluation and diagnostic procedures and execution of care in various programs
Tertiary	1 Doctorally prepared clinical specialized nurses in administration, education, and specialities 2 Master clinicians in nursing specialities 3 Associate degree graduates for evaluation and diagnostic procedures and execution of care in various programs

First of all, she must be able to conceptualize and describe the nursing care of groups of patients in precise terms, drawing upon pertinent data, and develop generalizations about the data. The nursing intervention she proposes must be realistic and feasible within the constraints of the system. Her predictions must allow for error. Options for the patient and the staff to consider are needed. What is proposed is a far different type of nurse than we have seen. What is being identified is a baccalaureate degree graduate who possesses pertinent, delineated knowledge, tested for its effectiveness, and one who not only possesses manipulative and assessment skills, but who also is able to synthesize knowledge and reduce it or translate it into action that is reality-oriented. This graduate is not only process-oriented in the usual sense of the term, i.e., interested in assessment, planning, design, execution, and testing, but she has also been introduced to scientific inquiry and investigative skills, and this has provided the guide for building the logic of her nursing practice.

The combinations of individuals in the different settings will depend upon what needs of the particular population are served by the center. For example, the care needs of a newly developing suburb may be fewer than those of a town in rural southern Iowa where an elderly population exists along with a small young one.

Specifics of role functioning are being avoided since tailoring to individual populations must be done. However, Table 35-3 indicates a perception of the deployment of graduates.

Nurses can perform much that they are not doing and eliminate a lot that they are doing. Our problem is to make up our minds about what we will attend to. The public wants nurses who are kind and considerate, but above all they want competence—competence over a large range of technology and practice, competence of knowledge, and competence in the skills of identifying, synthesizing, and testing knowledge.

The public will no longer tolerate either territorial disputes among the professions, or obsolete, ineffective, and costly practice. Professionals cannot afford to do something that a paraprofessional can do as well. Our responsibility is to see that care is given and given well. To do this, our graduates must be well prepared and we must demonstrate that additional education makes a difference in function, and does not simply offer more of the same with a small improvement.

EDITOR'S QUESTIONS FOR DISCUSSION

What nursing functions outlined by Aydelotte should be assigned to master clinicians and baccalaureate and associate degree graduates in primary and intermediate centers? What functions in tertiary centers should be the domain of nurses with a doctoral degree, a master's degree, or an associate degree? What role do you believe the baccalaureate degree graduate should have in tertiary care? How does one become an "agent of change" in a nursing role? Do you believe that the associate degree graduate is prepared to evaluate the direct care given to patients? How might the performance of graduates from various educational backgrounds be measured? What preliminary steps will be required by nursing before educational outcomes can be measured?

Chapter 36

Alternatives in the Role Expression of Nurses That May Affect the Future of the Nursing Profession

Luther Christman, R.N., Ph.D., F.A.A.N.
Dean, College of Nursing
Rush University, Chicago, Illinois

Luther Christman identifies the variables that perhaps will be the most influential for the future of the health professions and outlines the conditions existing within the nursing profession that have impeded the development of the nursing role. He believes that the nurse practitioner programs will have predictable effects on the future of nursing. Demands by patients for assurance of quality may lead to professional interdependence. New nursing models that will contain elements of equity and parity are envisioned. The knowledge gap between nurses and physicians has diminished and many skills are corporately shared. Primarily because of economic reasons, he predicts that future education for all health professions will be in health university centers. Christman perceives the development of a pattern wherein nurse faculty members will assume a teaching-practice-research role. He sees nurses as being the main health resource for primary care.

When one speculates about the future, one should do so with caution. A careful person cannot go too far astray, however, if he draws his conclusions from the main trends in society that are agreed upon by most observers. The variables that are important for the future of the professions are easily identified. The extensive and continuous expansion of knowledge; the vast build-up of technology; the steady rise of the level of general education of the population; the ready means of rapid communication available through the media; the numerous, activist-type movements (Women's, Black, physically handicapped, Chicano, American Indian, and Gay Liberation) that are giving a restless, anti-establishment theme to many traditional areas of society; the heavy demands on professional services caused by the sharp increase in the size of the population; the spread of affluency that has given many more persons the ability to purchase desired services; the pressure of large numbers of applicants trying to enter professional schools; the real possibility of mandatory continued study throughout the entire career of each professional person; and the imminent possibility of national entitlement to health care are collectively acting to create a milieu for the professional that is seething with change.

In order to make even tentative guesses about the future, one should first draw some base line of time and outline a set of conditions for comparative purposes. Until almost the last decade, the state of affairs within the profession of nursing lead to a widening of the gap in professional competence between registered nurses and the members of the other leading health professions. This condition existed primarily because (1) the largest percentage of nurses were not prepared at the university level and thus lacked the depth and breadth of education necessary to keep pace with their more advantaged fellow workers who had such education; (2) most of the schools of nursing were of the small, neighborhood type that were relatively unaffected by the major changes on university campuses and, in addition, were rife with inbreeding; (3) most nurses were not equipped to investigate (or perhaps even identify) clinical problems; (4) the faculty members of all types of schools of nursing were not active practitioners and as a consequence had little effect on the improvement of general nursing practice; (5) the base for recruitment of nurses qualified to enter areas of clinical specialization at the graduate level was very small, thus the means of generating clinical leadership was limited; (6) most faculty members, even in university schools of nursing, were not prepared at the doctoral level and were unable to act as influential disseminators of new knowledge; (7) most curricula reflected the lack of scientific sophistication; (8) most of the nursing service departments of hospitals and agencies were highly stylized in form and the modus operandi was a ritualized type of care that tolerated but little innovation; (9) most nursing actions were physician dependent in their general nature; (10) quality control was limited mostly to dos and don'ts rather than to scientific assessment; and (11) the extrinsic reward system for nurses was not sufficient to inspire the development of care patterns.

DEVELOPMENTS OF CONSIDERABLE INFLUENCE

There are developments under way in the nursing profession, in professional education in general, and in society at large, that have the potential for strongly influencing the future of the nursing profession. One of these, the so-called nurse-practitioner program, has all the ingredients for having a tremendous effect on the future role of nursing practice. It has the capability of changing the behavior pattern of nurses from that of a semi-professional format to that of a self-directing, highly expressive, applied scientist role. Nurses with the rudiments of these kinds of skills have been in existence for a long time. However, they were hidden or silent because they were functioning in physicians' offices and were taught diagnostic and management skills by their physician employer. The use of these skills by nurses was down played. A collusion of silence was almost mandated by the necessity to conform to practice laws. Furthermore, this teaching pattern was not an organized effort and there was a wide variation in the range of skills that was transmitted.

Physician and nurse educators at the University of Colorado and at the University of Kansas began a more formalized and a more scientific training endeavor and this form of nurse preparation obtained considerable visibility. The reaction within the two professions to this venture was mixed. Both physicians and nurses were divided as to its desirability. It finally took hold after a number of years of uncertain existence.

The acceptance of the program took place for a number of reasons. Some physicians and nurses were enthusiastic; they were fully aware of its potential for helping to provide access to health care, and pushed its acceptance. Other physicians and nurses were more politically oriented and saw the nurse practitioner as a more acceptable alternative (to them) than the physician assistant programs. A major impetus to increasing the numbers of nurse practitioners came about when Congress underwrote the funding of training programs through the Division of Nursing, Department of Health, Education, and Welfare (DHEW), and a fairly large critical mass of nurses with this type of preparation came into being. The loosening of physician and nurse practice acts contributed to the acceleration of its acceptance. The action to legitimize the use of this form of knowledge and skills by nurses first came into existence through the legislatures of the more rural states, with Idaho taking the lead. Changes in practice laws continue to take place even in the heavily populated states where there is a richer assortment of physicians. Legal interpretations of practice laws as well as new actions by state legislatures will reduce the legal impediments to new ways of working together. Because the practice acts have been amended with the cooperation of both nurses and physicians, it is predictable that future amendments will be enacted as nurses acquire the needed skills in greater depth. The National Joint Practice Commission of physicians and nurses helped to speed the pace of action by the substantial effort of its members to bring physician and nurse cooperation to new and higher levels of mutual helpfulness.

The issue of quality assurance as a consumer movement is bound to change professional orientations. The combined pressure of consumer advocate groups, the focus on legal liability, the increasing scope of government through a system of laws and regulations, and the requirements of voluntary regulatory agencies, such as the Joint Commission on the Accreditation of Hospitals, will all converge on individual performance as well as organizational arrangements to insure an acceptable level of quality performance. Territorial imperatives will undergo continuous erosion and will be replaced by multidisciplinary efforts designed to facilitate the actions of others and to serve as a check and balance system to protect patients. In all probability, each hospital will have a joint practice committee composed of representatives of each profession. This organizational device will be needed to reduce the impediments to the use of new knowledge and skills, to aid in making them available to patients, and to develop cybernetic models to establish a basis for overcoming deficits and shortfalls in practice. Out of this form of interaction the interdependence among professional persons will likely emerge as a state of balance of power based on individual competence.

The inequality of competencies within each profession will tend to give all multidisciplinary efforts a form of open-systems model. This prototype will come about because there is as much variation in competency within each profession as among professions. Thus, no one profession can bring about closure of the system.

A better informed public that is the result of better general education and an omnipresent media will be able to discern more clearly between mediocre and good quality care. This state of greater awareness will produce more surveillance and monitoring than the health professions have experienced heretofore. The heat of the controversies as to how science will be used for the public good will bring about adaptive changes within the educational and care systems. One of these adaptations will be the designing of care so that role complementation instead of role conflict will be a major motif of work arrangements. The rights, obligations, and accountability for each of the different types of participants will be harmoniously balanced.

Shared power or shared responsibility (based on competence levels) also will be a major ingredient.[1] Under the notion of shared power, whoever is closest physically and/or psychologically to the patient at the time a need is evident or expressed, and has the skill to supply the need, can act to fulfill that need without first genuflecting through a hierarchy of other professional persons. Decision making will be decentralized as much as possible to permit most of the operational decisions to be made at the direct-action level. The major constraint against the misuse of this right to act will be personal accountability, because each person will have to assume that onerous responsibility. There is enough organizational theory available to build in a system of

---

[1] For a more complete discussion of this notion, see L. Christman, "Community Resources—The Role of the Other Professionals," *Medical College of Virginia Quarterly*, 5(3):143–146, 1969, and "Community Context," in Harry Gottesfield (ed.), *Controversies in Community Mental Health*, Behavioral Publications, New York, 1972.

perfect accountability so that each practitioner will be as visible as a goldfish in a bowl. In addition, computer-managed record systems will clearly document all errors of omission and commission and will help serve as a record of individual performance.

The new designs of care will have as their main concern the demand systems of patients instead of being built around one or another of the health professions. Any other configuration will be less effective and will alienate both patients and health workers. New models will contain not only the main elements of equity but also of parity. Nurses have long had equity, that is, a stake in the health care endeavor, but they have lacked parity. Parity connotes equality and is crucial to having much influence on the decision-making power. Organizationally, there will be much more symmetry and balance. Symmetry and balance will provide not only equity, but also movement toward a consideration of parity. Parity breeds commitment. For example, the medical staffs are organized as autonomous units and report to the boards of trust of the hospital. It is conceivable that nursing staffs will be organized in a similar fashion.[2] This will make nurses highly accountable to patients, will call for much self-policing of practice, and will make nurses legally liable for after-the-event sanctions. In turn, it will give nurses much more opportunity for self-direction and control of practice privileges. Models such as this arrangement will aid in distinguishing the ultimate social worth of each of the health professions.

The concept of the measurement of the effectiveness of each of the professions is an exciting and challenging one. Nurses are now closer to having measurement devices that will either refute or affirm their claims about the value of their services. Nurses are beginning to inch toward a more autonomous role. Wherever the so-called primary nursing care model is used instead of team or functional nursing, nurses are getting experience that will enable them to move into a full autonomous model. Primary nursing offers an opportunity for self-supervision, with all its difficulties and rewards. It helps demonstrate that aides and licensed practical nurses are dispensable; it permits nurses to learn how to cope with a great deal more accountability; it provides a better format for peer review; it offers a more effective base for developing quality measurements; and it gives nurses and patients an opportunity to cultivate a relationship similar to that which should emerge between the patient and the autonomous nurse on an autonomous nursing staff.

No matter what final form(s) national health insurance may take, basic educational requirements for practice are understood. The development of clinical graduate programs has laid a foundation for expansion of scientific training and for speculation about the future. Due to this graduate education, the differences in knowledge and skill systems between nurses and physicians are shrinking, even if somewhat unevenly. This decrease in the knowledge gap means that there is an increasing amount of knowledge and skills shared jointly by doctors and nurses. For example, a science does not change its theory with the teacher, and its content does not change with the learner, be it nurse, physician, pharmacist, or physiologist. The particular role expression of the knowledge, however, may have some effect on its use as does the depth of the study. If nurses desire to be viewed favorably, by the other clinical professions that sometimes are used as reference groups, they will have to accumulate a body of knowledge that compares favorably to the others. Nurses will have to develop a highly visible clinical research effort that is apparent, not only to members of their own profession, but to members of kindred professions as well. A sign of this achieved stature will be when nurse-researchers are sought

[2] For a more complete discussion, see L. Christman, "An Autonomous Nursing Staff," a paper presented under the auspices of the National Joint Practice Commission at the American Nurses Association Convention, June 9, 1976 in Atlantic City, N.J.

out regularly as coprincipal investigators by members of other disciplines.

EDUCATIONAL METAMORPHOSIS

Educational processes will take on new structures out of economic necessity. The high cost of funding the various individual health professions with separate support does not appear to have had the expected outcome for society in terms of cost effectiveness. In the future, all of the students of the health professions will be educated in health universities or in the appropriate subpart of major universities. The education will occur in complete schools, that is, schools that are composed of undergraduate, graduate, and continuing education components, and research enterprises geared to improving the care processes. All schools not of this type of educational cluster will be either phased out or moved into this educational complex. This would mean no more "free standing" medical or nursing schools. We may end up with about 125 such health university centers.

The overhead saved by this approach is very considerable, as can be estimated from the large reduction in the number of schools of nursing alone. The sharing of the use of instructional media and learning centers will contribute to cost effectiveness. Other cost-saving elements can be identified. Furthermore, the sharing of many courses, especially in the fundamental sciences (behavioral and physical), adds to this saving.

There are many more benefits to this approach. Shared classes bring into being shared knowledge systems and this leads to the development of a meta language to facilitate communication while at the same time plateauing costs. Having a better means of communicating with each other will eventually lead to better ways of working with each other in the care system. The use of common science pathways have as a logical concomitant the designing of common clinical experiences wherever possible. The reality shock of working together after graduation will be minimized. The

federal government could catalyze the formation of this approach to professional training by withholding funding for those components of the health professions that refrain from participating in this form of training.

Health universities will develop consortia with nontertiary health care agencies in order to provide appropriate education for the effective management of this large portion of the care spectrum. These consortia also should enable regions and areas to develop balanced manpower systems because the demand for different kinds of professional personnel, and the specialists within each group, could be estimated more accurately. The factors of disease control, health maintenance, better nutrition, and population control will always be combining and recombining to change the focus of attention on health care.

The shift in attitude toward the delivery of care and orientations about career patterns that may develop as a product of the democratization of the health professions is not clearly predictable. The impact of fairly steady change on the composition of the previously white, male-dominated health professions has not been fully chronicled. It may be that many of the males who now find their paths blocked to a professional career in the traditional fields may turn to the predominantly women's professions for career alternatives. Women nurses and dietitians may find that their female-dominated professions will be experiencing the same disruption of sex-linkage that is occurring in the formerly male-dominated professions. The outcomes should be salutary for all, because the disruptive aspects of male-female relations, in nursing specifically, which are noticeable in present interaction patterns, will be minimized.

NURSING SPECIFICALLY

Much of what may be the outcome for nurses is wrapped in the broader blanket of the future for all of the health professions. However, a few specifics are called for. Some of the clumsy role socialization of nursing students stems from a lack of imagery about expert practice due to the withdrawal from practice of most nurse faculty members. The nurses on faculties of schools of nursing behave more like liberal arts faculty members than their faculty counterparts in the schools of medicine, dentistry, clinical psychology, and podiatry. Most nursing students have to model their behaviors and cues for career development on less well prepared nurses, because they are unable to study and emulate their teachers. As the pressure for professional behavior builds up in the nursing profession, it can be expected that nurse faculty members will become more similar in their behavior to other clinical faculty types and will enact the full professional role of service, education, consultation, and research. This move to full professionalization will probably accelerate when the majority of nurse faculty members are prepared at the doctoral level.

If centers of excellence in nursing are to come into existence, the teaching-practice-research role will have to form the basic lifestyle. Centers of excellence will have as their characteristics (1) the development of high quality practice and care; (2) the cultivation of a learning milieu for students; (3) substantial amounts of clinical research and demonstration projects; (4) the development of outreach projects to enable nurses in less-favored settings to improve care programs; and (5) the designing of new ways to promote interdisciplinary collaboration in patient care.

Probably one of the most startling possibilities of the future is that of the management by nurses of most of the primary or first encounter care. There is some doubt that even the strong effort being undertaken to prepare primary physicians will have a lasting effect. If physicians coalesce around secondary and tertiary care it seems apparent that nurses would be the prime health resource to manage this aspect of care. Several indicators would support this notion: (1) nurses are as numerous as all the other health profes-

sionals combined; (2) nurses are dispersed throughout the population more than any other group; (3) the increase in clinical graduate programs provides a steadily enlarging base from which to select candidates for more advanced training; (4) nurses, for the most part, have an ideological orientation to health maintenance; (5) many married women nurses could set up a practice in their own neighborhood without much inconvenience if they could obtain the appropriate education; (6) the evolution of the clinical doctoral degree in nursing can furnish excellently prepared nurses who could manage this area of care with a great deal of sophistication; and (7) the vast technology can be used to provide telemetry back-up of all sorts and permit closed-circuit television consultation with physicians in secondary and tertiary care hospitals.

In addition to the increasing competency of nurses, there may be another source of highly qualified persons who could enter the nursing profession and enrich it further. Many persons with Ph.D.s in the fundamental sciences are finding their career pathways limited. With a well-conceived postdoctoral program, these persons could become first-rate clinicians and pass the state board examinations to function as registered nurses. They would provide a new force within the profession because they entered it in such a nontraditional manner.

Many collegiate schools of nursing are enrolling a high percentage of students with earned liberal arts degrees. This may be a harbinger of the future. If this population of students continues to build, it well may mean that the entry into nursing practice will start at the graduate level. Given this base, the level of scientific sophistication within the nursing profession would escalate rapidly.

The future of nursing does not exist in a vacuum but is closely keyed to the developments in the health field in general. The degree of variance from this bonding depends greatly on how diligently large numbers of nurses prepare themselves for graduate clinical education, especially in the programs where physical assessment and clinical management of skills are taught. There are indications that nursing, the slumbering giant of the health professions, is about to discard the pedestrian pace of the past and move with the giant steps that are needed to become a front-running profession.

EDITOR'S QUESTIONS FOR DISCUSSION

What effect(s) might a form of national health insurance have on the role of the nurse, interdisciplinary relationships, and nursing education? What might be some of the effects of placing all health education programs in university centers in terms of the identity and expectations of the nurse and in terms of interdisciplinary relationships? Where might nurse faculty members develop their practice? What obstacles might be encountered by the nurse developing her role in primary care and how might they be resolved? What might be the role and expectations of a person who has a doctoral degree and subsequently completes a postdoctoral program for nursing practice? Is it likely that this might be a future development? Is it probable that eventually entry into nursing practice will be at the graduate level? What socioeconomic and political changes would be necessary before these possibilities could become reality?

Chapter 37

Nursing: A Future to Shape

Margaret D. Sovie, R.N., Ph.D.
Associate Dean for Practice, School of Nursing
University of Rochester, Rochester, New York

Margaret D. Sovie emphasizes the responsibility of nursing to determine its own future through planned change. Four factors are identified as having the greatest impact on the future: the Women's Movement, consumerism, health planning, and the knowledge explosion. The increased number of nurses with doctorates is seen as an outcome of the Women's Movement. The active participation in and evaluation of health care planning by the patient is advocated. The National Health Planning and Resources Development Act is discussed in relationship to nursing. Continuing education for nurses is seen as essential for effective practice and for dealing with the knowledge explosion. Within the nursing profession, collaboration is needed among members in education, research, and practice. Interprofessional cooperation also is important for developing new practice models. The three characteristics of a maturing profession are identified.

Shaping the future of nursing is the responsibility and challenge facing the profession as we ready ourselves for the twenty-first century. The next two decades can mark the coming of age of nursing. These years can be the era in which nurses unequivocally demonstrate their central position in health care and fully assume the responsibility of a profession accountable to its clients and the society it serves.

Realizing this future requires concerted planning and careful management. It means maximizing nursing's assets and minimizing its liabilities. This coming of age can result from the interaction of the multiple forces operating within the profession and in society at large that have created a supportive milieu for nursing's continued growth and development. As planners of the future, nurses must help promote the coalescence of these multiple forces and use the resulting dynamic energies to attain carefully determined goals and objec-

tives. In its efforts to shape the future and realize planned change, nursing must remain flexible and prepared to respond to the unexpected. As in every tomorrow, there are uncertainties and unknowns. These are the characteristics of the future. Nursing's structure must be such that it fosters intellectual creativity and facilitates a readiness to respond to the unanticipated problems that will certainly emerge as society moves into the next century.

The first part of this chapter describes the impact of selected forces in society on the nursing profession and the health care industry. These forces can be classified as the energizers for planning for the future in nursing. The second part focuses on the journey of the future that is already in progress. Current trends and role innovations that are shaping the future are described to support the thesis that nursing, as a profession, is consciously and deliberately inventing its own future through the delicately orchestrated efforts of its practitioners and its professional associations.

SELECTED SOCIETAL FORCES ACTING ON NURSING'S FUTURE

By design, a limited number of societal forces are delineated. This list can be expanded by every reader. However, four factors have been selected that I believe have the greatest impact on and serve as major driving forces in helping nursing shape its own future. These societal forces are: (1) the Women's Movement; (2) consumerism; (3) health planning and policy making; and (4) the knowledge explosion and the learning society.

The Women's Movement

The impact of the Women's Movement is finally being realized. For almost 200 years, pioneering women have been trying to assume their rightful place as equal members in society. The ferment that was created over these many years did not result in significant societal changes (with one exception) until the last decade. The one major exception occurred in 1920 when the Nineteenth Amendment to the Constitution became law—women finally had won the right to vote. It then took the next half-century for women to fully realize that power and position would not be shared with them until they exercised the power of collectivity and began to use the democratic political process to have their rights guaranteed. Women leaders, such as Betty Friedan and Simone De Beauvoir, helped raise the consciousness and activity of women. They began to flex their political muscles. The objective was to move from a male-dominated society to one in which women could enjoy equal rights and benefits with men, as well as share power in determining events of which they were a part. Cleland reminds us of the recent nature of some significant changes:

It was not until 1970, when Bernice Sandler utilized Executive Order 11246 as amended in relation to federal contractors, that the law was first used to protect professional women against sex discrimination. The Equal Employment Opportunity Act of 1972 extended coverage of the Civil Rights Act of 1964 to women in educational institutions and to employees of state and local governments. In that same year the Equal Pay Act of 1963 was amended to extend that law's coverage to women professionals, this act then being called the Higher Education Act of 1972.[1]

Sex discrimination is of such a long-standing nature that deliberate, conscious efforts have to be directed at overcoming the handicaps of sex-role stereotypes. The Women's Movement is helping nursing to achieve this goal.

Data are now available to document that society's investment in the education of professional women is sound. In fact, the more education a woman has, the more likely she is to work. Sandler reports that 91 percent of the women with doctorates work.[2] This premise should be capitalized upon by nursing in its efforts to move entry requirements for the profession to the baccalaureate level. Concurrently, efforts to improve and expand graduate education opportunities in nursing must be maintained.

One may speculate that the societal pressures that were exerted to keep nursing education out of institutions of higher education and within the confines of hospitals were the result of unconscious sex discrimination. The courage exhibited by nursing leaders since the mid-century has overcome this resistance. The majority of nursing programs are now centered in institutions of higher education and the focus is now on more education as an essential requirement for entry into the profession.

The New York State Nurses Association has once again stepped out front and declared in its "1985 Resolution" that a baccalaureate degree in nursing should be the minimal requirement for entry into professional nursing. At this writing, four other state nurses associations have declared similar positions. In addition, the National Student Nurses Association has endorsed the concept with passage of a supporting resolution at its April 1976 convention in Kansas City.[3] The movement can only gain momentum.

When one considers the history of sexual discrimination in our country in all areas, including higher education, it is understandable that nursing, a predominantly female profession, has a limited number of professionals prepared at the doctoral level. Pitel and Vian's "Analysis of Nurse-Doctorates" shows a growth rate exceeding 100 percent in the number of nurses who have achieved doctoral degrees in the period from 1969 to 1973 (504 nurses in 1969 to 1,020 in 1973). In a half-century marked by sexual discrimination, this is a remarkable accomplishment for nurses (the first known doctoral degree was awarded to a nurse in 1927). However, nursing has lagged behind other so-called women's professions and the 1973 total represented only .12 percent of the total employed nurse population in the United States. The demand for nurse doctorates far exceeds the supply and the future rests on a careful expansion of this population. Most nurse doctorates (80 percent) are employed as faculty.[4] One challenge for the future is the preparation of more nurses at the doctoral level and a more equitable distribution of the best-prepared nurses throughout the profession. New doctoral programs for nursing are being implemented and the public and other professionals will, in the future, have the opportunity hopefully to view an increasing number of nurse doctorates in a variety of settings.[5] This force is certainly a major contributor to nursing's coming of age, and a direct outcome of the Women's Liberation Movement.

The protracted development of nursing as a profession is directly related to its traditional heritage as a "woman's profession." The leadership crisis, so articulately addressed by Leininger, is symptomatic of this heritage.[6] Nurses are now cognizant of these past societal conditionings and collectively are acting to exert their power. They have organized for political action; collective bargaining is becoming commonplace; conditions of employment as well as essentials for implementing standards of care are negotiated;

achievable goals are delineated; strategies outlined; and timetables set. Nurses are learning that a profession undergoing rapid change requires creative courage. As stated by May: "Creativity itself requires limits, for, the creative act arises out of the struggle of human beings with and against that which limits them."[7]

Nursing, as a predominantly woman's profession, is struggling with a history of submission and male domination. It is learning to reach for and obtain power, authority, and control over its own destiny—it is a profession that is coming of age.

Consumerism

The era of the bicentennial in the United States may well be remembered as the era of consumerism. Better-educated publics who have personally experienced the Civil Rights Movement of the sixties are demanding their rights in every area. For our purposes, consumerism will be limited to the realm of health care and health services. Health is increasingly being viewed by Americans as their right. No longer will citizens accept lack of adequate health care as an area beyond their influence. No longer will they yield total control of their personal well-being to physicians, nurses, or any other health professionals. United States citizens are demanding their rightful role in a new partnership for health. They are demanding quality, personalized care at reasonable costs. Today's consumer of health care wants answers to his questions. He wants to know what is wrong and participate in making decisions about his treatment, once the alternatives and implications are presented and understood. He wants to learn how to regain control of his health and maintain it at a level he decides is essential for realizing the quality of life he elects or determines is acceptable. In other words, today's recipient of health care services does not want to relinquish control of his own destiny to any other human being if it can be avoided. This is certainly a remarkably different situation than the one that formerly existed where the patient was docile and accepted without question whatever the health professional decided for him.

Despite the fact that health care services have never been better, clients want more. They want to have the best, at costs they can afford, and to have their health care rendered in a humane, respectful way that preserves their individual integrity and dignity.

The "patient's bill of rights" is one direct outcome of consumerism in health care. The American Hospital Association's 1973 statements of patient's rights have served as the basis for the enactment of laws in many states, designed to protect the rights of patients as human beings. I personally regret that outside forces became necessary to guarantee what every health professional should be committed to—providing the best possible care in the most humane, personalized way.

However, if the enactment of laws or adoption of the patient's bill of rights helps realize the desired objective, then the end justifies the means. Quinn and Somers have speculated that several positive outcomes may result from this whole consumerism movement:

(1) The health status of the American people will improve significantly; (2) pressures on, and criticism of, the health professions will decline substantially; (3) there will be more opportunity for nurses and other non-physician members of the health team to practice to their fullest potential and to gain understanding, acceptance, and respect in so doing; and (4) the hospital, now so widely criticized as an inordinately expensive "technological emporium" may yet emerge as a cherished community health center.[8]

Nursing has, from its early beginnings, considered patient/client advocacy a major responsibility. Concern for the dignity and rights of the individual has been a central element in the caring phenomenon that traditionally has been assumed as a major function by the nurse.

The interaction of today's professionalism, which includes a code of ethics,[9] standards for nursing practice, and the concept of accountability to the client, with the consumerism movement, has had noticeable results. Nurses are act-

ing as models for advocacy roles and encouraging the patient's self-determination by his active participation in goal setting and the evaluation of health care outcomes.

Consumerism has also had national impact beyond that already mentioned. It has directly influenced federal legislation in the areas of health planning and resource developments.

Health Planning and Policy Making

Federal legislation in the area of health planning and health care services has had serious impact on the entire American health scene. The implementation of the Medicare and Medicaid programs in the sixties emphasized and accelerated the urgency of seeking solutions to the problems of health planning, administration, quality, and cost control.

In 1972, amendments to the Social Security Act PL 92-603, Section 249F, called for the establishment of Professional Standards Review Organizations (PSROs) to monitor health care services provided under Medicare, Medicaid, and Maternal and Child Health Services.

In 1973, the Health Maintenance Organization Act was passed in an effort to encourage construction of a more efficient and effective health service delivery system.[10]

Accessibility to quality care at reasonable costs continues as a major concern. The economics of meeting the basic health needs of every citizen can bankrupt this society unless new methods and systems of health care delivery are successfully implemented. Every member of the health care partnership, including the client, must be actively fulfilling his individual responsibilities if we are to successfully solve the problems. Health care services now consume approximately nine percent of the gross national product.

Public Law 93-641, the National Health Planning and Resources Development Act of 1974, is the most recent attempt to promote accessibility to quality care at reasonable costs. This act provides for the designation of Health Systems Agencies (HSAs) to serve designated areas in the country.

The act delineates the specific purposes of the HSAs as:

1 Improve the health of the residents of the area

2 Increase the accessibility (including overcoming geographic, architectural, and transportation barriers), acceptability, continuity, and quality of the health services provided those residents

3 Restrain increases in the cost of providing health services

4 Prevent unnecessary duplication of health resources[11]

The role of consumers in health care planning and policy making has been recognized with the provision that the composition of the governing boards of HSAs must include a majority (but not more than 60 percent) of consumers. The remainder shall include representatives from designated health provider categories.

The act calls for the establishment of federal guidelines to assist HSAs in addressing ten national health priorities:

1 The provision of primary care services for medically underserved populations, especially those located in rural or economically deprived areas

2 The development of multi-institutional systems for coordination or consolidation of institutional health services (including obstetric, pediatric, emergency medical, intensive and coronary care, and radiation therapy services)

3 The development of medical group practices (especially those whose services are appropriately coordinated or integrated with institutional health services), health maintenance organizations, and other organized systems for the provision of health care

4 The training and increased utilization of physician's assistants, especially nurse clinicians

5 The development of multi-institutional arrangements for the sharing of support services necessary to all health service institutions

6 The promotion of activities to achieve needed improvements in the quality of health services, including needs identified by the review activities of the Professional Standards Review Organization

7 The development by health service institutions of the capacity to provide various levels of care (including intensive, acute, general, and extended care) on a geographically integrated basis

8 The promotion of activities for the prevention of disease, including studies of nutritional and environmental factors affecting health and the provision of preventive health care services

9 The adoption of uniform cost accounting, simplified reimbursement and utilization reporting systems, and improved management procedures for health service institutions

10 The development of effective methods of educating the general public concerning proper personal (including preventive) health care and methods for effective use of available health services[12]

Realization of these ten priorities demands a major effort on the part of nurses working in collaboration with physicians, other health professionals, the political bodies, and the consumer groups.

Nurses have exercised their professional responsibilities since the inception of PL 93-641. They have been active participants in the task forces established to create the HSAs and currently occupy seats on the boards of directors of already established HSAs. Nursing is demonstrating its long-standing commitment to meeting the health needs of the population not only in the delivery sites, but, as importantly, in the planning and policy-making bodies established to meet national health priorities.

Before HSAs have reached maturity, a national health insurance program will undoubtedly be legislated. Both the National League for Nursing (NLN) and the American Nurses Association (ANA) have taken positions in support of a carefully designed system that will utilize nurses and all other health professionals at their highest level of expertise. It is imperative that the legislation that eventually will be enacted carefully specifies fair and equitable payment to all professionals and institutions for services rendered. Nurses must become increasingly active in the political arena and must maintain their vigilance and pressure to assure that payments for nursing services are as clearly identified as payment for the services of the other health professionals.[13, 14, 15] Their collective voices should be heard since nurses constitute the single largest health professional group and are central to meeting the national priority of providing accessibility to comprehensive health care services at reasonable costs for all the people.

The nursing profession, through its official organization, has recognized the critical importance of political involvement in the nation's health affairs. In 1974, N-CAP (Nurses' Coalition for Action in Politics) was officially organized as the political arm of the ANA. Its purpose is to promote the improvement of the health care of the people. N-CAPs functions are:

1 Encouraging and stimulating nurses and others to take a more active and effective part in governmental affairs
2 Educating nurses about government, the important political issues, and the records of officeholders and candidates
3 Assisting nurses to organize for more effective political action on state and national levels
4 Raising funds for political education, nonpartisan registration, and get-out-the-vote drives
5 Soliciting individual voluntary contributions for the political fund[16]

N-CAP has recently released its analysis of the voting records of U.S. senators and representatives on three key nursing and health issues acted upon by the 94th Congress.[17] This immediate implementation of their functions should certainly assist the million plus nurses in making their voting decisions during the next election. Nurses are thinking in terms of the future and N-CAP is one objective method in use by nursing to shape the future of health care for the nation through active engagement in the political process at the local, state, and national level.

The Knowledge Explosion and the Learning Society

The twentieth century, particularly from its midpoint on, will be noted in history as that period in which man became acclimated to change as a way of life. The ability to cope with continuous change is being facilitated by a new value structure regarding education. The first 50 years were punctuated by an emphasis on developing educational opportunities to provide general access from K-12. Then, this expanded to K-14 with the community college movement. Now, the prevailing notion is that learning and education cannot be bound into a specific period of one's lifetime. Learning is now viewed as a continuous, life-long process. The rate of creation and diffusion of new knowledge has accelerated and caused a more rapid rate of obsolescence of existing knowledge and skills. Continuing education has become essential to successfully meeting the demands of every-day living and central to maintaining competence in one's professional career.

> The need for continuing education emerges from the phenomena of change; change in what's known about man and how he functions in health and illness; change in the ways in which people meet the challenge to survive in a dynamic age; and change in the objectives, organization, and financing of health services. Professional roles are altered as society changes and as new knowledge and technologies emerge. The individual who wishes to avoid obsolescence cannot leave to chance his acquisition of new knowledge or his ability to adapt to changing demands. He must meet the challenge of change actively.[18]

Continuing education in nursing is considered essential to the effectiveness of nursing practice. Its primary objective is to improve the health care provided to the individual citizen by increasing the knowledge, skills, and abilities of the practicing nurse. A second major objective is to stimulate and encourage practitioners to become life-long learners. This characteristic is a basic requirement in every profession. Houle outlined four major needs that continuing education can help the practicing professional meet. He needs to: keep up with the new knowledge related to his profession; continue his study of the basic disciplines that support his profession; establish his mastery of the new conceptions of his profession; and grow as a person as well as a professional.[19]

A better educated public, aware of its rights and seeking quality services for dollars rendered, is cognizant of the knowledge explosion and the danger of professional obsolescence. Professional societies and associations are equally aware of their accountability and responsibility for assuring the competence of its members. Consequently, continuing education requirements are being delineated for society membership; certification programs have been established; and in some states legislation has been enacted that has made continuing education a requirement for reregistration and relicensure in specific professions. Mandatory continuing education is viewed by many as the only successful control mechanism to protect the public from professional obsolescence. Certainly, continuing education must be a way of life for every practicing professional.

Scientific knowledge will continue to expand at an explosive rate. A companion to it is rapid technological change. These two forces demand that today's professional student must learn how to learn. This factor has already had impact upon the nature of basic preparatory, graduate, and postgraduate education programs in nursing as well as the activities in continuing education. The processes of scientific inquiry and problem solving have become essential ingredients in all higher educational programs. Nursing's activities in curriculum design and implementation could well serve as models for other disciplines. Change has been intense and the programs and educational system are responding appropriately. Every nurse is or will be a life-long learner if she or he expects to remain active in the profession.

The Women's Movement; consumerism; nation-al health planning and policy making; and the knowledge explosion in a learning society are interacting with each other and with the nursing profession. They are the driving forces that the nursing leadership is orchestrating, along with internal professional forces, in a conscious effort to shape the future of the profession.

NURSING—A MATURING PROFESSION

The orchestration of these forces is designed to help the nursing profession grow and develop to more effectively deliver health care to all citizens. Nursing must now add the role of initiator to its role of responder. It must take an active role in shaping health care institutions serving society, as well as in shaping health policy. It must initiate more effective intra- and interprofessional collaboration in problem resolution, with the client as an integral partner in the process.

Intraprofessional Collaboration

Intraprofessional collaboration is the first order of business as we shape the future of nursing. This profession, as every profession, has three essential components—education, research, and practice. As we move into that uncertain tomorrow, there must be a closer relationship among these components. Professional nurses must teach, practice, and participate in research. Nursing's full potential in the health sciences and services will not be totally realized until we have an effective interplay and interdependence among these three components. Without the latter, we experience lack of coordination and suffer dis-ease or less than optimal functioning in all the parts.

Intraprofessional collaboration demands our concentrated attention. The separatism of nursing education and nursing practice is finally beginning to be relegated to history. Perhaps this past separatism was a necessary step in the process of the "becoming" of the science of nursing and the nursing profession. Historically, it was the demand for nursing services that spawned nursing education programs. As we all know, these early educational programs for nurses followed the apprenticeship model and education was totally dependent upon service. Education suffered when patient service demands escalated. Consequently, for its own protection and continuing development, nursing education moved from its dependent role in the service settings, and gradually over time, as it matured, took its position in institutions of higher education. Each partner, education, and service, developed its own identity and the accompanying security and self-esteem of independence. This process of staged development—dependency to independency—leads, with continuing maturation, to interdependency. The nursing profession has now developed its science and practice to the level where interdependency is needed to help realize its full potential. This interdependency is not limited to within nursing, but includes interdependent relationships, functioning, and study with medicine and the other health disciplines. Research from all these areas continues to expand our scientific knowledge. As a profession we have begun to realize the many benefits that careful research has brought to the growth and development of the science of nursing and its practice. Now our challenge is to create models in nursing that will facilitate the interdependent functioning of these three essential components: education, research, and practice.

The development of appropriate models will take creative courage, which May defines as "the discovering of new forms, new symbols, new patterns on which a new society can be built." May's premise is that every profession requires some creative courage, and that those professions experiencing radical change require courageous persons to appreciate and direct the change. He maintains that the need for creative courage is in direct proportion to the degree of change the profession is undergoing.[20]

Certainly the nursing profession is experiencing a period of intense change. Expanded role practice, quality assurance programs, the evolvement of primary nursing, a variety of clinical spe-

cialty programs, and the rapid change of practice acts across the United States are obvious indicators of change.

Nursing is demonstrating that it has a great deal to contribute to the improvement of health care. Professional creativity and courage is indeed evident. Nursing is assuming the responsibility to shape its own future through planned change.

Trends of a Maturing Profession

Nursing is a profession that is experiencing the trends of a maturing profession. These trends, as identified by Schein, are:

1 They become more convergent in their knowledge base and standards of practice.

2 They become more highly differentiated and specialized.

3 They become more bureaucratized and rigid with respect to the career alternatives they allow.[21]

Trend 1. Convergence, as defined by Kuhn, is a high degree of consensus on the paradigms to be used in the analysis of phenomena and high consensus as to what constitutes the relevant knowledge base for practice. The convergent basic disciplines include anatomy, biochemistry, physics, and mathematics. The divergent disciplines include sociology, psychology, and anthropology.[22]

Nursing is a profession based on both convergent and divergent disciplines. Its practitioners must draw on the appropriate knowledge base to make clinical judgments and patient care decisions. Nurses, as other professionals, must be prepared to handle warranted uncertainty. Training for uncertainty is an important part of the development of today's health professionals. They must maintain their self-confidence when there is not one definite solution to the problem. They must make decisions and be accountable for the outcomes even when they have incomplete data. They must be able to gain the patient's trust and confidence even when they are uncertain.[23] When dealing with an individual in a changing health condition, with both internal and external variables compounding outcomes, there will always be unique and unpredictable elements that require highly divergent management skills.

Trend 2. Nursing, as other maturing professions, has developed specialty areas of practice. In fact, the last decade has witnessed the development of the role of the clinical nurse specialist (CNS) and the creation of specific standards of practice for nursing in each of the specialty areas. The clinical nurse specialist is a practitioner prepared at the graduate level with a concentration in a specific area of clinical nursing. The American Nurses Association has recently released a rather comprehensive descriptive statement on the practice of the CNS.[24]

Trend 3. The third trend of a maturing profession, increasing bureaucratization, is also apparent in the nursing profession.

> As a profession matures, it not only acquires a greater base of convergent knowledge, making greater consensus possible among professionals, but it also tends to protect its boundaries or its areas of jurisdiction by creating professional associations which, through peer-group control, define educational requirements, standards of entry and ethical standards for practitioners.[25]

The American Nurses Association published, in 1975, *Standards for Nursing Education,* marking a "major milestone in the association's assumption of its responsibility for the nature and quality of the education of those who engage in the practice of nursing."[26] These standards encompass basic, graduate, and continuing education in nursing. This profession has also had a code of ethics since 1950—in fact the ANA was the first national nursing organization in the world to create and formally adopt a code of ethics. The International Code of Nursing Ethics evolved from the ANA code and was adopted in 1953 by the International Council of Nurses.[27]

Role Innovations

Nursing, while maturing, remains relatively flexible and has built in mechanisms to facilitate change

through role innovation. As a profession, it has recognized its obligation to keep itself responsive to the demands made by a rapidly changing, complex society. It has recognized that the profession evolves through role innovators. In its preface to the *Standards of Nursing Education,* the commission specifically identifies the need to support innovation and testing of new roles in nursing.

The nurse practitioner programs, which were pioneered by Ford and Silver in Colorado in 1965, have had tremendous influence on the profession of nursing and have significantly contributed to shaping the future of the profession. Dr. Loretta Ford, in testimony to the House Committee on Interstate and Foreign Commerce's health subcommittee in Washington early in 1976, stated:

> Early publications record the fact that the nurse practitioner evolved to provide quality health care to children in ambulatory settings and, if successful, to investigate ways to influence collegiate nursing curriculums to prepare professional nurses for this model of practice. The physician shortage of the early sixties provided the *opportunity* to try out new roles for nurses.[28]

Complementing the work of these early role innovators was the timely Report of the Secretary's Committee to Study Extended Roles for Nurses, *Extending the Scope of Nursing Practice.*

> We believe that the future of nursing must encompass a substantially larger place within the community of the health professions. Moreover, we believe that extending the scope of nursing practice is essential if this nation is to achieve the goal of equal access to health services for all its citizens. . . . There is growing recognition of the importance of physician-nurse collaboration in extending health care services to meet increasing demand. The nurse is a provider of personal health care services, working interdependently with physicians and others to keep people well and to care for them when they are sick. The role of the nurse cannot remain static; it must change along with that of all health professionals, which means

that the knowledge and skills of nurses need to be broadened....[29]

In this brief period of a decade, nursing has demonstrated its ability to respond to necessary change. There are now over 100 programs that prepare nurse practitioners and approximately 5,000 nurses functioning in expanded roles.[28] The American Nurses Association has initiated a program of accrediting programs that prepare nurses for expanded role functions to assure the quality of the programs and the practitioners. The scope of current practice of the nurse practitioner/clinician has been delineated as

> ...[one that] assesses the physical and psychosocial status of clients by means of interview, health history, physical examination and diagnostic tests. The nurse practitioner/clinician interprets the data, develops and implements therapeutic plans, and follows through on the continuum of care of the client. The practitioner/clinician implements these plans through independent action, appropriate referrals, health counseling, and collaboration with other health care providers. All aspects of the therapeutic plan and the continuum of care are documented in the client's record....[24]

Nursing has demonstrated its maturity as a profession. It has sufficient autonomy and confidence as an independent profession to engage in successful collaborative relationships with physicians and other health professionals.

The nurse practitioner movement began in the continuing education arena. Nurse practitioners have demonstrated their effectiveness in delivering quality health care with cost effectiveness. Patient/client acceptance has been excellent. Physicians have been generally supportive and many have been willing to change their own role as nursing's role has changed. Now, the profession is ready to integrate the concept of expanded role practice into the mainstream of professional nursing education. Currently, experimentation is under way with some programs integrating the concept into the baccalaureate program and an increasing

number incorporating the necessary education and training into graduate programs. I personally believe that as the future unfolds, nurse practitioner preparation will settle into graduate nursing education, with some basic elements integrated into undergraduate nursing programs. The nurse practitioner model requires a carefully developed professional background on which to build if the practitioner is to realize the complete mastery of essential competencies. My projection is that within another decade, nurse practitioners/clinicians will be prepared at the graduate level exclusively and some new practice model or concept will be explored in the continuing education arena.

Interprofessional Collaboration

Collaborative practice models, with nursing and medicine as the primary professions, will continue to receive increasing attention. Joint practice is defined as nurses and physicians collaborating as colleagues to provide patient care. The National Joint Practice Commission (NJPC) is an interprofessional organization to improve health care established by action of the American Medical Association and the American Nurses Association. This commission, established in 1972, consists of equal numbers of practicing nurses and physicians. "It is examining the roles and functions of both professions and defining new roles and relationships; recommending changes in professional education to support new roles; removing sources of professional differences; and assisting in the development and support of state joint practice committees."[30] Nursing and medicine have taken concrete steps in planning for the future of health care through collaborative interdependent action. The bonds of colleagueship between these two professions are young and need to be carefully nourished in order to reach flexible permanence. This is a challenge for each professional group.

As nursing matures as a profession, its practice acts are undergoing revision throughout the United States. The National Joint Practice Commission has extended its support to the professional nursing associations in their leadership activities relating to needed changes in practice acts.

The NJPC prepared and used a statement on medical and nurse practice acts to assist in this effort:

> The accumulation of knowledge and the expansion of techniques and skills able to be utilized in the care of individuals and in the prevention, treatment and cure of disease has necessitated or resulted in a realignment and readjustment of nurse and physician roles.
>
> In view of their growing interdependence it becomes increasingly evident that successful or effective delivery of health care cannot be achieved through unilateral determination of functions by either medicine or nursing.
>
> Practice acts which now serve as conditions for licensure and continuing licensure in each profession must be examined to ensure the legality of these realignments and readjustments for the protection of both the public and the professionals involved. . . .[31]

Virginia Hall's survey of statutory regulations of nursing practice provides an excellent study tool for states that are in the process of appropriately revising practice acts to reflect what nursing's and medicine's role is and should be in the delivery of health care.[32]

It is important to emphasize that the delivery of comprehensive health services, in primary, acute, and long-term settings, involves the dependent, independent, and interdependent coordinated functioning of many different health professionals. Medicine and nursing have been emphasized since they are primary partners along with the client.

Nursing Research

The emergence of new types of practice teams; greater numbers of practicing nurses prepared at baccalaureate and graduate levels; expanding quality assurance and peer review programs; and increased clinical research activity should result in more convergency in practice. Continuing evaluation of both practice and education will highlight areas needing further study and research. Nursing research will expand the base of scientific knowledge and nurture both education and practice. O'Connell and Duffey recently completed a 5-year overview of nursing research as published in *Nursing Research*. A four-part classification system was devised to categorize those studies that related to practice:

1 Research relevant to nursing specialties
2 Research relevant to nursing procedures and techniques
3 Research relevant to specific aspects of nursing care
4 Research relevant to the state or condition of the patient

During this 5-year period, only 26 percent of the studies reviewed were in nursing practice. Physical nursing care was the area least studied. This obviously deserves future attention.

An important observation made by these two investigators was that no single case study approach was used in any of the published research.[33] One may speculate that this too will change in the future as more and more nurses build panels of patients for continuing care; as primary nursing experiences are documented and studied; and as more nurse/physician practice teams begin to critically evaluate their practices.

Research in nursing must be demystified and a greater number of nurses recruited for active participation. We must shape the future to facilitate the formation of research teams with common interests that can collaboratively study selected problems. Simultaneously we must continue to expand our support for individual investigators.

The practice and education models that will serve the future most effectively will have to be carefully investigated. Dr. Loretta Ford's unification model at the University of Rochester warrants careful evaluation and research, as does Dr. Luther Christman's at Rush University in Chicago, to cite but two examples.

The areas demanding research are infinite. As the future unfolds, we will see the key nursing positions occupied by nurses prepared at the doctoral level. They will provide leadership and give direction to the education, research, and practice components of the profession. When we reach this juncture, we will be able to realize the much needed continuous generation of research studies in all areas of nursing and assume our role as an active partner with other disciplines in research relating to a variety of health care problems and issues.

A Future to Shape

Nursing is building and projecting its identity as a primary health profession. It is coming of age and shaping its future one day at a time. Nursing leaders are keeping their vision toward a constantly expanding horizon and, in concert with the members of the profession, are directing the events that will provide the mold for its future.

The theme of the American Nurses Association bicentennial year convention was "A Past to Remember/A Future to Shape." Every indicator reveals that nursing is now a maturing profession. It is a profession dedicated to excellence and continuous self-renewal. The shaping of its future is in good hands.

NOTES

1 Virginia S. Cleland, "To End Sex Discrimination," *Nursing Clinics of North America*, 9(3): 567, September 1974.
2 Bernice Sandler, "Equity for Women in Higher Education," in Dyckman W. Vermilye (ed.), *The Expanded Campus, Current Issues in Higher Education*, Jossey-Bass, San Francisco, 1972, p. 81.
3 *Report,* Official Newsletter of the New York State Nurses Association, vol. 7, no. 4–5, April–May 1976.
4 Martha Pitel and John Vian, "Analysis of Nurse-Doctorates," *Nursing Research*, 24(5): 340–351, September–October 1975.
5 Madeleine Leininger, "Doctoral Programs for Nurses: Trends, Questions and Projected Plans," *Nursing Research*, 25(3):201–210, May–June 1976.
6 Madeleine Leininger, "The Leadership Crises in Nursing: A Critical Problem and Challenge," *Journal of Nursing Administration*, 4(2):20–34, March–April 1974.
7 Rollo May, *The Courage to Create*, Norton, New York, 1975, p. 113.
8 Nancy Quinn and Anne R. Somers, "The Patient's Bill of Rights, A Significant Aspect of the Consumer Revolution," *Nursing Outlook*, 22(4):244, April 1974.
9 Lucie Young Kelly, "The Patient's Right to Know," *Nursing Outlook*, 24(1):26–32, January 1976.
10 James J. McCormack, "Current Public Policy and Medical Care Evaluation" in Madeleine Leininger (ed.), *Barriers and Facilitators to Quality Health Care, Health Care Dimensions*, Davis, Philadelphia, 1975, pp. 47–59.
11 Department of Health, Education, and Welfare, "Guidelines for Applications for Health Systems Agency Designation and Grant under National Health Planning and Resources Act of 1974, PL 93-641," November 1975.
12 Dorothy Jean Novello, "The National Health Planning and Resources Development Act, What It Is and How It Works," *Nursing Outlook*, 24(6):354–358, June 1976.
13 "Goals for a National Health Insurance Program," National League for Nursing, New York, February 1974.
14 Eileen M. Jacobi, "Executive Director's Report," in *ANA Convention '76 House of Delegates Reports 1974–76*, American Nurses Association, Kansas City, 1976, pp. 15–17.
15 "ANA Views the Current Proposals for National Health Insurance," American Nurses Association, Kansas City, March 1976.
16 *ANA Convention '76, House of Delegates Reports 1974–76*, "N-CAP (Nurses' Coalition for Action in Politics)," American Nurses Association, Kansas City, pp. 106–107.
17 "ANA's Political Branch Rates Congressmen on Nursing-Health Votes," *RN*, 39(7):7, July 1976.

18 Frieda Smith Curtis et al., *Continuing Education in Nursing*, Western Interstate Commission for Higher Education, Boulder, Colo., 1969, p. 1.

19 Cyril O. Houle, "The Role of Continuing Education in Current Professional Development," *American Library Association Bulletin*, 61(31):259–267, March 1967.

20 May, op. cit., pp. 21–22.

21 Edgar H. Schein, *Professional Education, Some New Directions*, Carnegie Commission on Higher Education, McGraw-Hill, 1972, p. 43.

22 Ibid., p. 44.

23 Ibid., p. 45.

24 "The Scope of Nursing Practice," American Nurses Association, Kansas City, May 1976, pp. 1–7.

25 Schein, op. cit., p. 48.

26 Commission on Nursing Education, *Standards for Nursing Education*, American Nurses Association, Kansas City, 1975.

27 Kathleen M. Sward, "The Code for Nurses: A Guide for Ethical Nursing Practice," *Journal, NYSNA*, 6(4):27, December 1975.

28 "Nurse Enlightens Congress on Nurse Practitioner," *American Journal of Nursing*, 76(4): 533, April 1976.

29 Department of Health, Education, and Welfare, *Extending the Scope of Nursing Practice, A Report of the Secretary's Committee to Study Extended Roles for Nurses*, November 1971, p. 4.

30 National Joint Practice Commission Program brochure, American Nurses Association Convention '76.

31 National Joint Practice Commission, "Statement on Medical and Nurse Practice Acts," in Virginia C. Hall, *Statutory Regulation of the Scope of Nursing Practice—A Critical Survey*, National Joint Practice Commission, Chicago, 1975, pp. 1–2.

32 Virginia C. Hall, *Statutory Regulation of the Scope of Nursing Practice—A Critical Survey*, National Joint Practice Commission, Chicago, 1975.

33 Kathleen O'Connell and Margery Duffey, "Research in Nursing Practice, Its Nature and Direction," *Image*, 8(1):6–12, February 1976.

EDITOR'S QUESTIONS FOR DISCUSSION

What is the role of the patient and the nurse in health care planning? How effective has the patient been in regulating health care policies? Should patients have specific qualifications in order to be involved in federal processes of health planning? Why has nursing not been active politically in defining health policy and health planning? What are the implications for nursing roles in federal health planning? What effect(s) might increased specialization and bureaucracy in nursing have on the profession and on patient care? Can the cost effectiveness of the role of nurse practitioner in primary care be validly demonstrated? What other types of models for nursing practice might be proposed in organizational and primary care settings?

Chapter 38

Futurology of Nursing:
Goals and Challenges for Tomorrow

Madeleine Leininger, R.N., Ph.D., L.H.D., F.A.A.N.
Dean and Professor of Nursing
Adjunct Professor of Anthropology
University of Utah, Salt Lake City

Madeleine Leininger is a strong proponent of socializing nurses to be nurse-futurists. She states five requirements of a nurse-futurist, which are basically characteristics of effective leaders: the ability to take risks, to analyze the past and present astutely, to predict goals, to fend off intimidation, and to evaluate predictions. Leininger makes specific predictions for progress by the year 2000 that have implications for nursing: the escalation of technology and new specialty roles; new or different communication modes; developed transcultural nursing care practices; advances in aerospace and oceanic nursing; marketing and contracting of nursing care services; control of common conditions such as colds, cancer, and stress; and new modes of health care delivery, health centers, and multidisciplinary practices. She agrees with Christman on the development of university health science centers and discusses the need for future nursing leadership. She predicts that nursing practice will be divided between generalists and specialists and describes the possible types of nursing education programs that will be seen by 1980. Leininger further agrees with Christman that, in the future, a nurse may need a master's degree to enter professional practice. Great advances in nursing research are projected. She issues an enthusiastic challenge to nurses to plan comprehensively for the future.

Tomorrow is already here, and today is not yet finished. This maxim of the author is quite familiar to us Americans as we struggle to keep pace with new technologies, different ideologies, and the many other changes that are occurring in our daily lives. Responding to today's imperatives and being confronted by tomorrow's realities are an integral part of being a human being. Indeed, the history of mankind for nearly 1 million years is a record of people meeting the changes and challenges of the present and future in different places and time periods. Most human beings have a remarkable capacity to adapt and thrive. The nursing profession, in a comparable manner, has

Concepts of this paper were originally presented in June 1974 at the American Nurses Association Convention in San Francisco, California. Ideas from this paper were also used by the ANA Board of Directors' meeting in September 1975 to study future directions in nursing.

been faced with societal changes for many years; its leaders have been trying to respond to today's needs and changes and have had little time to plan tomorrow's nursing world. Helping nurses and the nursing profession plan for and respond to changing societal health expectations is a tremendous challenge and goal.

The goal of this chapter is to help nurses think about tomorrow or more precisely, about the future of nursing by the year 2000. It is to help nurses realize the importance and the value of futuristic thinking, planning and activating modalities so that nursing may become a futuristic profession and make its unique contributions to the future. As a nurse-educator and cultural anthropologist, the author will share some of her ideas about what the immediate and distant future holds for us, along with some of the challenges that nursing practitioners, educators, and researchers will probably face. It is the author's contention that nurses and the nursing profession will have a better chance for survival and growth if they are futuristic and become actively involved in shaping tomorrow's world of nursing, than if they are reactive and continue to dwell on the past.

FUTURISTIC THINKING AND GOALS: ESSENTIAL FEATURES OF A VIABLE PROFESSION

To be viable, to be relevant, and to survive, any profession must be futuristic in its orientations and goals. Nursing, as the largest health profession, with slightly more than 1 million nurses in the United States and probably a total of 4 million in the world, must give serious thought to its future. Although it is difficult to conceptualize the world of nursing in the year 2000 and beyond, nevertheless it is essential to think about how we believe nursing should be in light of societal changes. A core of professional nurses who are sufficiently liberated in their thinking about nursing's future is needed to help us project our ideas from the present into the future. This is one of the most urgent, but difficult, tasks for

nursing. Unfortunately, very little time and attention have been given to the future of nursing since there is a limited number of self-declared futurists in the field.

To look creatively, boldly, and predictively into the future is difficult. Indeed, it is a risky, uncertain activity to predict, plan for, and establish goals for nursing's future. Without question, only knowledgeable, visionary, and bold leaders would venture the exploration of the unknown or of the only partially known.

Since, in my opinion, futuristic goals and plans are essential for any profession to survive and grow, I believe that we must socialize a core of nurses to be futurists. At present, there are far too few nurse-futurists and too many present-oriented nurse-realists. Currently, we also have many action-oriented nurses, and only a few contemplative nurses deliberating about tomorrow's changing world. Reflecting on the past is difficult for many nurses. However, knowledge of the past gives us important clues for our thinking about the future. We must, however, not use the past for absolute predictions, but rather as a knowledge base to learn and think about the future. Nurse-futurists, therefore, must be free to chart new and different courses as we face the different forces that will influence our world of tomorrow. Most importantly, we must teach nurses in our educational programs to think about tomorrow and we must encourage nurses to be futurists.

To be a nurse-futurist, I contend there are five major requirements. First, a futurist must be a risk-taker, or a person who is willing to make bold and uncertain predictions about that which is barely known, or that which does not have a definite form. Second, a futurist must be an astute analyst of the past and present. He or she must, however, be sufficiently removed from today's realities to be able to construct a new reality for the future (Heneley and Yates, 1974). Third, a futurist must not only be able to abstract from past and present events and experiences, but must also be able to predict, logically and explicitly, goals and directions for the future on the basis of limited or non-verified data. Fourth, a futurist must not be intimidated by popular thinking or by the opinion of the majority. Rather, he or she must be ready to present new and imaginitive ideas that no one or only a minority may espouse. Fifth, a futurist must be willing to stand behind his or her hunches or predictions until proven to be mistaken. Indeed, futurists need opportunities to try out their ideas, for if they do not make predictions about the unknown, we shall remain fixed to the present and never discover possibilities and new realities.

When one thinks about the future, one realizes that there are dangers inherent in making predictions about it. A nurse-futurist must be a risk-taker in order to speculate about future events and conditions. In addition, a futurist must be a logical, fearless, and independent thinker, a prophet, dreamer, a cultural historian, a memory-retainer, and a person with a strong sense of identity who will not be threatened by predictions and their consequences upon others. A futurist must also be able to work with structures that are not clearly defined, synthesize ideas and conditions, formulate rare predictions, and accept criticism if those predictions do not come true.

Santayana speaks of the importance of expectations in foreseeing the future. He states: "A creature without memory cannot discover the past; one without expectation cannot conceive a future" (1968, p. 4). Moreover, the ways in which a person anticipates the future vary considerably, as noted in Loren Eiseley's (1964, p. 64) exquisite book, *The Unexpected Universe*: "We of this modern time know other things of dreams, but we also know that they can be interior teachers and healers as well as anticipators of disaster. It has been said that the great art is the night thought of man." So, whether by means of dreams or of experiences, predicting and planning for the immediate and distant future are all necessary for professional growth and survival, and for the development of futurists, especially nurse-futurists.

Traditionally, prophets and prophetesses in our society have been looked upon as nonscientific and of questionable worth. This opinion has been influenced by our belief in science, and by our reliance on concrete phenomena. Most people feel uncomfortable contemplating the unknown or living with hunches or only partially known realities because it leaves them subject to the criticism of being nonscientific, strange, or a "know-it-all." There is also the concern that if a futurist's predictions do not come true, the futurist's credibility will be lost. And if the predictions are accurate, people will often say, "Well, that was inevitable and already known so it was no prediction." Thus a futurist's credibility is subject to a high degree of question and doubt.

In recent years, there have been signs of increased interest in the art and science of predicting the future. This appears related to people's disillusionment with science and to their interest in extrasensory perception, astrology, magic, witchcraft, divination, and to the general development of the occult arts. People are becoming more interested in and intrigued with the unknown from a humanistic and intellectually curious viewpoint. Hence, it is timely to emphasize futurology in nursing and in other health fields, and to deal with uncertainties in nursing and health care. Anticipating future developments and trying to determine their form and meaning helps prepare us to adapt or adjust to what is ahead of us. Futurists who are experienced and skilled in the art of prediction can serve as and help us deal with many uncertainties.

The rationale for the existence of futurists in nursing is not only the necessity of anticipating the future, but also that of considering what forces will affect nursing by the year 2000 and beyond. Today, we are beginning to experience overpopulation. We have limited environmental resources as well as limited space. However, we do have a great deal of technological resources. These and other factors make us realize how necessary it is to look ahead and plan. Since we know that there will be greater competition for money, space, time, and certain human health resources than ever before in the history of mankind, we need to consider solutions to these changing circumstances and to plan for tomorrow's world accordingly. These factors will influence the lives of nurses and of other health care providers as well as recipients of their care.

As nurses, we need to realize that we are living in a world where societal realities are forcing us to be futurists. Usually, one finds that organizations, associations, professions, and individuals that are concerned with the future plan and set up priorities for the future, and they tend to be successful in their efforts. Unquestionably, we are living in a world where planned changes, planned schedules, and planned activities are becoming extremely important, and so one hears of planned parenting, planned living arrangements, planned environments, planned enrollments, planned education, and so on. Almost everything from birth to death is now being planned, and will continue to be in the future. When sudden changes occur within a planned framework, there tends to be less anxiety than when sudden changes occur within an unplanned framework.

Thus, we need a sizeable core of skilled nurse-futurists to help anticipate our world of tomorrow and to plan for it accordingly. We need nurse-futurists with a broad range of knowledge and experiences who cannot only tell us what to anticipate, but who can also give us strategies for making our future successful. As the nursing profession grows, and sets its own goals, its members will rely upon wise nurse-futurists who will become respected for their predictions. These predictions must take into account multiple societal forces, political and economic factors, technological developments, cultural values, and many other variables that influence the future of nursing. Most importantly, we must begin to prepare nurses in our education and service programs to be futurists by assisting them to make bold predictions, and by standing by them and helping them gain respect for their efforts. To date, I know of no programs or settings in nursing that are deliberately preparing nurse-futurists, but there is evidence that a few nurse-leaders have

the ability to be futurists and are attempting to function in this role.

LOOKING TOWARD THE YEAR 2000

Heightened Technology and New Specialty Roles

Looking into the future, we become aware of a number of cultural, technological, political, and social forces that are shaping our destiny as we approach the year 2000. In my opinion, the most significant force is the marked and increased use of technology in nursing and health care services. A wide variety of new devices and equipment will continue to be used, even beyond the year 2000, and will revolutionize nursing care with both positive and negative effects. Nurses will become increasingly dependent upon complex equipment in their care of acutely and chronically ill people.

In the future, many aspects of physiological care will necessitate computerized or automated machines and equipment (Spicer, 1952). Push-button and automated nursing care will be well established in urban, suburban, and rural health care facilities. At times, nurses will feel as if they are nurse-engineers and will question their professional role. Biophysiological instrumentation will intrigue, perplex, and challenge the professional nurse and many nursing and health care assistants. When machines work well, nurses will be happy, but when they suddenly and unexpectedly fail (especially at critical times) many nurses will feel frustrated, angry, and helpless.

By the year 2000, we will have a great variety of monitoring and maintenance machines by which to give health care to clients and families. Nursing care assessments, treatments, and practically all care modalities will be dependent upon improved and refined technological equipment and devices. Large and small mobile and stationary machines will be used regularly inside and outside the hospital setting. Many nurses will be using machines to give nursing care to people in homes, schools, nursing clinics, business premises, and rural satellite settings. Nurses will instruct clients and their families through advanced educational equipment and will help people to use such machines to maintain their health. Home care, self-care, group care, and even community care will be emphasized. The professional nurse must begin immediately to be prepared to use such technology to help prevent illness and maintain health. The nurse must also acquire contemporary teaching-learning principles in order to be effective in helping people use such equipment.

Most important, the professional nurse, with nursing and technological assistants, will be expected to use and monitor many machines effectively. The nurse will need to know when machines are not functioning properly and to be able to diagnose major difficulties affecting client care. Electrical, nuclear, and general engineers will be available through a two-way communication method to repair and maintain the machines. Nevertheless, there will be times when these engineers are not available, and so the nurse will have to rely upon her scientific knowledge of physics and bioinstrumentation to safeguard client care. Therefore, the nurse of tomorrow will need to have considerably more knowledge of bioengineering, biophysics, physics, and nuclear and electrical engineering principles than she possesses today. Consequently, a variety of new courses will appear in our schools of nursing in the next two decades. All basic and advanced nursing education programs will emphasize technological nursing care, the effects of such care, and ways to combine technology with humanized care. Courses in physics, mathematics, communication operations, electrical and nuclear engineering, system management, and computer science will also become part of nursing education programs by 1985. Such courses will help nurses to use technological devices and a great variety of bioengineering instruments intelligently to give nursing care. More multidisciplinary technology and bioengineering courses will be offered in universities for all health professionals.

In the health care delivery world, business corporations will increasingly see the profit to be gained from the use of complex equipment in health care. Indeed, a number of business firms will own, operate, and maintain machines in practically all health care settings. As a consequence, nurses will need to become more business-oriented in order to communicate and deal with business people and agencies so as to establish and assure the quality of client care.

With the marked increase in the use of machines and technological devices in client care will come more signs of *dehumanization* in nursing, medical, and general health care practices. While the consumer of health care will be intrigued with technological devices, he or she will still expect personalized and humanistic care and treatment. Treating clients like robots, computer objects, or other automated response subjects will become more prevalent, and will be of great concern to sensitive and humanistic nurses and physicians. While some nurses will try to provide humanistic care, it will be exceedingly difficult to resist this dehumanization or to integrate technological and personalized care. Because of those strong humanists in health fields, I predict that *rehumanization care clinics* will be established to provide the personalized care and interpersonal communication so essential to human growth and life maintenance. Individuals, especially workers and their families, in industrial settings will especially need rehumanization clinics and health services for they will increasingly suffer from the "machine syndrome" and from that routinization experienced in places where machines and technological equipment prevail. Nurses in psychosocial and transcultural nursing should plan now to monitor and provide such rehumanization health services.

While technology will intrigue some nurses, it will be devoid of interest to others. Antipathy for machine nursing care practices will be found, as well as the desire to integrate humanistic care with technological care. Nurses who learn to master a combined scientific-humanistic techno-care approach will be few in number and will be frequently sought out by others for help. By 1980, biophysiological nurse experts will be in great demand to guide nurses in instrumentation care, but there will be a shortage of these nurses until the year 2000. As a consequence, technical bioengineers, specialists, and technologists will invade the nursing arena, and nurses will find themselves spending time helping technicians understand people and their health problems.

In addition to such technological developments in the health field, the use of artificial organ transplants will be widespread by 1985. The lungs, liver, stomach, colon, urinary bladder, heart, and practically all organs will be replaceable, possibly even the brain. Artificial limb and tissue transplants will increase noticeably. This trend will be related to the increase in car and chemical accidents, and in catastrophic accidents related to bombings, shootings, and violent acts. Hence, artificial limbs that are light, flexible, and functional will replace natural limbs. Nurses will be expected to teach clients how to use and maintain artificial limbs and new body parts, and to ensure the optimal maintenance of these artificial parts. The nurse's role in health teaching and in collaboration with physician organ specialists and technicians will increase significantly. A core of nurse specialists prepared in artificial and human organ transplant nursing will soon be needed to cope with this rapidly growing trend in our society. Accordingly, a new nursing field that specializes in artificial organs and limbs with bioinstrumentation will open up. Bioinstrumentational nursing, emergency nursing, and long-term technohumanistic nursing will also combine with many other speciality nursing areas.

Natural disasters such as earthquakes, tornadoes, hurricanes, floods, and cyclones will increasingly occur with devastating effects despite our attempts to control them. But, of even greater concern will be the increasing number of chemical (gases and other explosives), electrical, nuclear, and technological accidents that will destroy buildings and cause many deaths. This growing number of chemical, electrical, nuclear, and technological accidents will cause more nurses to enter burn, trauma, and emerging accident nursing specializations. The capacity of all health disciplines to meet such mass accidents and disasters will be challenged. The problem of how to organize people and services to function in regional and local disaster areas will perplex health personnel. To date, the behavior of health personnel under stress has been barely examined, but it will be more widely studied in the future. Social scientists will play an increasingly significant role in helping health personnel face large-scale organizational and community-based disasters. At these disaster sites, there will be a need for fast tissue and organ transplants to save lives and for the effective organization and utilization of nurses, physicians, and technicians to work together in a coordinated manner. Handling chemical and electrical burns and dealing with the emotional problems of people who have witnessed mass mutilations and fatal accidents will necessitate a new level of knowledge and skill on the part of professional nurses. Combined specialty areas related to cardiovascular, neurological, endocrinological, burn, accident, and artificial and human organ transplant nursing will emerge due to such mass accidents and natural disasters.

New or Different Communication Modes in Nursing and Health Care

Accompanying the growth of technology will be new modes and systems of communication by which to provide health and nursing care. New modes of technological communication will greatly change nursing, medical, pharmaceutical, and dental practices, for such modes will bring clients and health providers into close and continuous contact with each other. Multiple-way audiovisual communication modes will enable the nurse to keep in constant contact with clients, families, social groups, and multidisciplinary health care members. As a consequence, indirect nursing care through audiomedia technology will be far more common than the direct care practices of today. This shift from direct to indirect nursing care practices will be of great concern to nurses and will be debated at local and national meetings. It will also affect reimbursement for nursing services since communication technicians will receive payments for their part in facilitating nursing care.

The use of audiovisual devices to give health care to people in distant lands will also be common by 1980. Health and nursing care beamed via satellite to people at home and abroad will be a reality by the year 2000. With such modern telecommunications, nurses will need to learn new languages in order to function in transcultural nursing situations. New types of health and nursing care services never even dreamed of by many nurses will soon be in practice.

Through transcultural telecommunication, health care providers will be directly challenged about their beliefs, values, health care practices, and ethnocentrism. This will give rise to culture shock and to conflicts related to the economic, legal, social, and political differences that exist between people of different cultures. Free mass-media health care versus controlled media health care will be a major international and professional issue and will prompt lively debates among international health providers and recipients. Transcultural health counseling, teaching, and supervision related to preventive and restorative care will be monitored by professional nurses trained in transcultural nursing and in modern techno-communication modes. There will be remote satellite communication units, substations, and other such units in different parts of the world. Health communication and technological and transcultural care will be closely linked in practice and education.

Without question, the nursing profession will not be ready to handle new kinds of national and international multicommunication modalities as they relate to nursing care. This situation will remain of major concern to nurse educators and practitioners, and there is limited relief in sight before 1990.

Transcultural Nursing Care Practices

As communication becomes more complex and sophisticated, nurses will begin to fully realize the need for preparation in transcultural nursing care practices. A significant number of nurses will need to master the languages and communication forms of different countries and cultures in order to practice transcultural nursing care. They will also need to be aware of the impact of the nurse's modes of communication and beliefs on other cultures, for at present only a few nurses have been prepared in transcultural nursing.

Transcontinental communication via satellite and nursing care stations will be established in different parts of the United States and the world. Population shifts will bring diverse and strange cultural groups in close proximity to one another. With these trends will come many new and provocative ideas about human beings, health care, folk health care practices, popular medicines, and nursing care practices. As I already have stated, we will see new theories in nursing, new teaching and service practices, and new modes of education—all as a consequence of transcultural nursing and health care (Leininger, 1976a, p. 4; 1975).

In the future, nurses will play an increasing role in working with cultural groups and communities in remote places in the world. Because of their lack of preparation in anthropological concepts, nurses will experience marked culture shock and face serious cultural conflicts and problems that will necessitate different nursing care approaches. In the immediate future, nurses will appreciate and realize the importance of comparative health care systems, comparative nursing practices and theories, and comparative methods by which to help people. In addition, a core of knowledge and skills related to ethnonursing and transcultural theory will be recognized as legitimate and essential to the evolving subfield of transcultural nursing.

As the initiator of the transcultural nursing movement nearly 25 years ago, I anticipated this trend and provided leadership in the encouragement and preparation of nearly forty nurse-anthropologists (Leininger, 1976b, p. 4). Transcultural nursing courses, programs, and departments have been established in several schools of nursing and the nature, purpose, and goals of this evolving and future field have been articulated. The need for transcultural nursing courses and programs will increase significantly in the United States and elsewhere, and transcultural nursing will become one of the most stimulating and challenging subfields in nursing. Substantive anthropological and sociological knowledge and research will be needed to advance the work in international nursing practices, to reduce present ethnocentric tendencies, and modify nonscientific approaches. Some nurses are now focusing on only four major ethnic groups on the basis of color rather than on the nearly 2,000 cultural groups in the world. Nurses actively involved in transcultural nursing will need to use some sort of lingua franca in order to communicate and provide assistance to people in other cultures.

Aerospace and Oceanic Nursing

During the next two decades, *aerospace nursing* will emerge as a legitimate and clearly defined subfield of great interest to nurses. Presently, this area is not well developed and its focus is primarily on aerospace medicine and medical practices. There will be a readjustment of the focus of aerospace nursing with the major emphasis on nursing theories and practices. The roles and positions of nurses in the provision of direct and indirect (even computerized) care to people in outer space will be developed. Problems unknown today, such as those related to the nursing care of people living in space colonies, will be studied and will be the major challenge for the leaders of the future. Indeed, nurses will be making trips to planets and will be expected to do nursing and general health care assessments of people living in outer space. They will learn how to modify the threatening aspects of space environments in order to help people survive. Advanced knowledge of ecology (especially ecological nursing), physics, geography, physical anthropology, and paleontology will be helpful to aerospace nurses. These nurses

will need to study and classify the types of diverse outer-space environments in which people will learn to maintain health and avoid illness. Testing the environment and appraising the survival ability of groups will be within the knowledge and skill domain of the aerospace nurse.

Hydronursing or *oceanic nursing* will be a new and stimulating area of study and practice for nurses. Because of the paucity of nursing knowledge, this subfield will not be fully developed until the turn of this century. In the future, providing expert and specific kinds of nursing care to people in nuclear submarines and ships, hydrofoils, ocean-liners, deep-sea underwater crafts (in search of food, minerals, and oil), and many other types of ocean-bound vehicles will become important as people become more and more dependent upon our oceans for food, energy, oil, and minerals (and other such industrial by-products). Our oceans will become an important resource for travel, agricultural needs (e.g. water for irrigating fields), and for many other important needs. The hydronurse specialist will be dealing with special nursing care problems related to serious water accidents and conditions such as deep-water bends, hyperwater body infusions, seasickness, disequilibrium conditions, gastrointestinal food disturbances, skin disorders, and many other presently unknown sea conditions.

Both hydronurse and aerospace nurse-scientists, practitioners, and educators should begin soon to identify the content of these nursing subfields and the position of nurses in them in order to be able to provide care to people in water and outer-space life modalities. Nurses will need to work closely with physical, behavioral, and environmental scientists to develop theories relevant to the exciting new areas of hydro- and aerospace nursing.

Marketing of Nursing Care Services

In the immediate future, nurses will become active in the marketing and contracting of nursing care services to clients and consumers. Whether or not this is perceived as desirable, nursing care services will have to be sold in our culture and will need to meet production expectations by being cost-effective and cost-contained. This trend fits in with our competitive free market system and our cultural norms. Indeed, all health disciplines will have to "sell" their services in overt or covert ways. This trend is already becoming evident, and it will be difficult for some nurses to accept it as part of professional practice.

At present, few nurses are either sophisticated or knowledgeable about cost management and about ways to politically, economically, and psychologically sell nursing. Contracting for nursing services with people (individuals and agencies), recommending nursing care services, and making nursing marketable in many other ways are, indeed, new and strange concepts to most nurses. Although they may be quite distasteful to some, such concepts are nevertheless compatible with the economical, political, and social lifestyle of the United States. To preserve the professional values of nursing, e.g., its identity as a humanitarian service without illegal profit motives and behaviors, frauds, and negative marketing practices, ethically oriented nurses will be needed. Profit motives, cost-effectiveness, cost-benefits, and contracts for nursing will have ethical implications and will be affected by supply and demand. Nursing services will compete with other types of health services offered by professional and nonprofessional groups. The idea that nursing could and should be salable as a cost-effective and desirable public service product in our society will be difficult for nurses who are not prepared in business and political-economic concepts to comprehend and accept. We must, however, prepare a core of nurse leaders to be astute business managers, economists, and political analysts so that in the future nursing care services will be marketed with a humanistic and profit-equal goal.

Common Conditions Such as Colds, Cancer, and Cardiovascular and Mental Stresses

By the year 2000, common colds and most infectious conditions will be under control as a result of vaccines and the public's knowledge of basic im-

munological prevention modes. The nurse will no doubt play a significant role in preventing such common infections by routinely providing health counseling, administering vaccines, and monitoring health care from nursing clinics and satellite health information stations. By the end of this century, cancer should not be the great enigma it is now, for our knowledge of viruses, cell growths, chemical inoculations, nutrition, and lifestyle factors that affect cancer will be fairly extensive, and most probably we will have at our disposal the means to prevent common cancer types. The professional nurse should play a significant role in cancer detection, prevention, and care.

Because our fast pace of living in this country will aggravate cardiovascular and emotional conditions, we will need to develop new kinds of educational programs to prevent heart, circulatory, and mental illnesses. In the future, we will have different ways to assess, label, and classify mental conditions. Indeed, it will be found that many more types of environmental factors precipitate and aggravate temporary mental conditions (Leininger, 1971). Freudian psychological principles and treatment modes will be replaced by new theories concerning situational and transitional daily life stressors. Thus, many standard theories in psychiatric nursing will be replaced by new ones largely based upon the psychocultural, socioenvironmental, and humanistic needs of people. In general, the nurse should play an active role in the prevention of mental illness, strokes, heart disease, and other cardio-vascular and respiratory conditions all contingent upon advanced study and research in nursing and general health care practices.

New Modes of Health Care Delivery, Health Centers, and Multidisciplinary Practices

By the end of this century, a variety of health care delivery practices will be available in this country and abroad. Several new types of health care services are already beginning to emerge, and others, such as the open-care system and self-care, will soon be in use (Leininger, 1973a; 1973b).

Health care systems in the future must be more responsive to societal changes and the changing needs of population groups by taking into account political, legal, economic, cultural, and environmental factors. Health care will be conceptualized as care to *whole populations or community groups* instead of as care to individuals, families, and small social groups, which is the dominant concept at present. The health needs of communities seen as functional, structural, and cultural groups are barely understood by nurses and other health professionals, but will become a major focus of study in the future.

Health care delivery systems of tomorrow will be *consumer-based*. They will have multiple, open-entry modes rather than the present closed types of health care services (Leininger, 1973*b*). Furthermore, the *prevention of illness* and the *maintenance of health care* according to different cultural and socioeconomic group needs, will be given increased emphasis in the near future. The heart of the health care system of the future will be the *health maintenance* system along with its *restorative and preventive subsystems* (Leininger, 1973*b*, p. 173). The nurse should play a significant role in these systems, but the degree of nurse participation depends upon how actively nurses assume a leadership role and their preparation.

Another challenge to nursing in the future is the quick, effective, and economical provision of services to people. In order to meet this challenge, our extensive multidisciplinary resources and assets in the health field as well as the skills of physical and social scientists must be fully utilized. While the medical profession will try to control and regulate all health care services for economic, political, and legal reasons, the nursing profession will become more politically and legally active and will gradually gain control of those health care areas that logically belong to nursing. In fact, it could well be nurses who facilitate a true partnership among health professions and between health professions and consumers, because of their traditional caring role and because they are the largest health group. Nurses can facili-

tate the establishment of an open health care system and provide for economic rewards to all providers. As soon as our health system becomes *a shared interdisciplinary responsibility*, our present health care delivery modes will change and the public will see that other health professionals are giving care and are deserving of public recognition and financial reward.

Nurses who suffer from the "physician-dependency syndrome" will have a hard time adjusting to this new concept of interdisciplinary equality and colleagueship in health care. However, nurses will adjust in the near future. They will need to function as partners with other health care professionals, to make independent and interdependent nursing judgments, and to receive direct financial payments for their services. Nurses will use the Women's Movement, with its emphasis on equal opportunity, as a means to obtain collegial and collaborative multidisciplinary health care practices.

Health care of tomorrow will not only become more consumer-oriented, but will also be directed and regulated primarily by consumers instead of by health professionals. This trend will be difficult for many nurses, physicians, and other health professionals to accept. Nurses will have to adapt to consumers' perceptions of health statuses and what they believe will keep them well and functioning. It will be important for nurses to be sensitive to consumers and to work closely with them in order to get *their* viewpoints and study *their* particular health and nursing care needs.

With many new reorganized health care systems on the horizon, the professional nurse will need to explicate her or his central role in such services as: (1) emergency and long-term ambulatory care; (2) self-care consumer clinics; (3) primary and tertiary health care services; (4) nursing counseling health education clinics; (5) sociocultural adaptation care clinics; (6) clinics to prevent chronic conditions; (7) family and social health care clinics and other types of special and generalized health care services as described by the author (Leininger, 1973*b*). The central focus of nursing will be *caring* and we will have explicated and tested caring components and behaviors by 1990. Physicians will continue to emphasize *curing*. They will show less interest in primary care after 1985 because of economic and prestige factors, and too little time to offer this service.

A variety of *health service agencies* will emerge as political and economic control units in the United States. The nurse will struggle valiantly to gain and share power in order to make nursing decisions and policies affecting health service and area agencies. New national legislation bills will greatly assist the nurse to share in health policies and decisions by 1980.

By 1980, national health and insurance programs will be established as well as competing private health care programs with support monies. National health insurance programs will arrive on the American scene before nurses are ready to regulate and control their service reimbursements and role responsibilities through other health disciplines. International health insurance programs will also be established. The phasing out of traditional health systems and the establishment of new types of care systems will require considerable effort and creative thought by nurses and other health providers.

University *health science centers* will continue to develop and will become megacenters for professional health care services and education. They will provide new models for multidisciplinary education. Some centers will be handicapped by physicians such as surgeons, neurologists, and internists who have very limited knowledge of social organizations and large group behavior and who serve as leaders of these centers (Leininger, 1974*a*). Gradually, university officials will realize that doctorally prepared nurses can effectively deal with the large and complex social organizations and cultural systems that will characterize future health centers. The fact that this will not occur until late in this century is due especially to the lack of female nurse leaders. In addition, engineers, ecologists, political scientists, communication specialists, sociologists, anthropologists, demo-graphers, and many other professionals interested in health problems will pursue an active leadership and decision-making role in university health science centers. Their contributions will be valuable and should enhance the present insights and skills of the traditional health professions. However, it will be a struggle for these scientists to be fully accepted by the traditional health professionals who will view them as outsiders.

Health science centers will be located primarily in urban areas, but will gradually be reorganized to have outreach rural and suburban satellite education and service centers. Clients and their families who come to urban health science centers will expect a high quality of *specialized* health care and treatment. Rural satellite centers will focus upon *primary and generalized health care* maintenance services. Practically all professional and academic disciplines that are part of large university health science centers will require master's degree or doctoral preparation by 1985. Their members will be expected to combine their teaching, research, practice, consultant, and scholarship roles with other health, social, and behavioral science contributions. Only well-qualified nurses prepared in master's and doctoral programs will be able to function effectively in these complex and specialized urban health centers. Nurse specialists and a few nurse generalists will be expected to work together with multidisciplinary health personnel in teaching, research, practice, and consultation. The superior quality of nursing and health care reinforced by peer review and explicit high standards will be greatly emphasized. Nursing research will greatly help to explicate nursing's contributions to health care services. Only strong and knowledgeable nursing deans and service administrators will be able to survive in these university health science centers (Leininger, 1974*b*, pp. 28–30).

By the year 2000, traditional health disciplines will have gone through an identity crisis. Valuable lessons will have been learned through efforts to develop multidisciplinary work groups that are truly collaborative and collegial. Models for different multidisciplinary groups will have been identified and tested in different learning and service settings. However, professional identity struggles and interprofessional competition will still occur, along with some multigroup cooperation. The concept of *team work* will be replaced by *multigroup collaboration* or a similar term denoting participation but not signifying finely attuned team ties or other idealistic team practices.

Nurses will be stimulated by multidisciplinary health education and service practices, but they will be constantly challenged about the unique domains of nursing's practice areas for which they have responsibility and legitimate control. The need for nursing research and well-prepared nurses in multidisciplinary work will be obvious. Not all nurses will be able to retain their professional role in multidisciplinary work. With the goal of attaining and retaining a true collegial relationship with other health and social science disciplines at stake, nurses will realize the importance of being able to deal with competition, power, prestige symbols, interprofessional identity, and financial rewards.

LEADERSHIP NEEDS FOR THE FUTURE

The critical need for well-prepared nurse leaders with graduate degrees will remain acute for another decade. Nursing leaders who are independent in their thinking, creative in their ideas and action, committed to professional goals, not afraid to take risks, and skilled in collaborative efforts will continue to be sought after in a great variety of service and education settings.

With the increased numbers and kinds of health education and service centers, nurses will need to be politically astute, highly knowledgeable, and skilled leaders and managers in order to establish and maintain nursing's essential position in the health field (Leininger, 1974a, pp. 28-34). Nursing leaders must not only be skilled in handling interpersonal relationships, but they must also be strategists and planners in order to regulate and maintain resources and to fully utilize those nursing skills related to specialized and generalized

education and service settings. Finding intelligent, creative, and skilled nurses to develop new health care services will be a major challenge for nursing leaders. The shortage of well-prepared leaders in university administration and nursing service positions, and at the state, regional, federal, and international health service levels will remain acute until 1985.

Although there are indications that the two worlds of nursing education and nursing service are beginning to come together for the common professional goals, the anti-intellectualism and fear of nurses who are bright, capable, and well-prepared on the part of those nurses who are less well educated will make this unity difficult. If we could get our well-prepared nurses into key leadership positions, now and in the future, many nursing care problems would soon be alleviated. The schism between the "clinical camp" and the "educational camp" will continue to exist and to impede nursing's full impact in service and education arenas. Well-prepared nursing leaders with interests in both camps will be necessary to reduce this artificial barrier and to support the full utilization of nurses who have baccalaureate, master's and doctoral degrees in nursing services.

Business, hospital, and medical administrative managers will attempt to replace nursing and nursing service deans during the next decade through university health science centers. It is imperative that nursing retain its leadership role in the control, development, and maintenance of professional nursing education and service programs. Nursing leaders, especially administrators, will continue to cope with sex discrimination problems, inadequate budgets, insufficient space for facilities, limited nursing research programs, and the dominance of medicine. Indeed, power and political control stresses between nursing and medicine will continue during the next two decades as nursing leaders attempt to regulate their areas of independent and interdependent professional activities and goals. Of special interest to nurses will be a major split between "hard core" physicians, e.g., surgeons and medical internists, and "soft core" physicians, e.g., those in community medicine. The latter group will align itself with nursing in order to facilitate interprofessional health care and educational projects. This linkage between the two groups will help nursing and medicine to develop common health care practices.

Legal battles between nurses and physicians will become more prevalent as each group struggles to define its practice turf and rights. The grey areas of the working turf will remain and will serve as a common ground for collaborative practices. Although true collaborative practices are desired, this goal will be realized in only a few nursing and medical arenas. Effective nursing leadership at local, state, and national levels will be necessary to retain nursing's desired position and to cope with medicine's power and political clout. We will see more legal suits in the future as physicians charge that nurses are practicing medicine, and, hopefully, as nurses charge that physicians are practicing nursing. During the next decade strong and knowledgeable nursing leaders will be needed to overcome power inequalities between nursing and medicine. Furthermore, as physicians are appointed to upper-level administrative positions in universities and to key state and federal positions in new health planning systems, the struggle of nurses for positions and power will become even more acute than it is today. Thus, there is a need for extremely well prepared high-level nurse leaders and administrators.

PREDICTING TOMORROW'S NURSING SERVICE

Nursing, as the largest health profession, must begin now to plan for nursing services for the year 2000. I contend that nursing, by virtue of its large numbers and evolving quality-based nursing and health care practices, will make a significant difference in the health services of the future. There is no doubt that the nursing profession can and should have a major impact upon health care in this country and elsewhere. However, this will occur only if nursing leaders and followers decide *what*

directions they want to take and *why*. The profession must take a stand on its areas of accountability, such as the provision and maintenance of primary and tertiary care, especially care to the young and elderly, and it must implement its decisions. Conceptual models such as the author's Open Client-Centered Model, the CONPUT Model of the Washington State Nurses Association, and the models described by nurse leaders in the American Academy of Nursing offer promise for the future (Leininger, 1973a; Committee on Nursing Preparation and Utilization, 1973; American Academy of Nursing, 1975). We need a core of futuristic thinkers and planners in nursing to work on these plans and strategies now rather than later. A taxonomy of nursing practitioners in service and education, which is now being developed, will help bring order to this field (Committee on Taxonomy, 1976).

Nursing services with intraprofessional referral systems will be much needed in the future so that nurses can deal with nursing problems themselves instead of referring them to physicians as medical problems. Such referral systems will draw on the expertise of nurse-generalists and nurse-specialists in practice and education. While there will always be some difference between the goals of nursing service and nursing education, hopefully, this gap will narrow so that students will have richer educational experiences and graduates of nursing programs will be more effectively utilized than they are today.

In the future, the four traditional areas of nursing will no longer be the major or only areas of generalized and specialized training. Instead, by the year 2000 there will be many new specialty areas in nursing. The Committee on Taxonomy's taxonomy of nursing practice has already revealed nearly fifty new specialty areas (Committee on Taxonomy, 1976). These include thanatological, oncological, burn, aerospace, transcultural, cardiovascular, respiratory, family, oceanic, primary, and secondary and long-term nursing specialty subfields, as well as many others. The combination of two or more subfields of nursing (generalist approach) and the in-depth and breadth practice in *one* subfield (specialist nursing) will occur, as well as a variety of functional research and administrative roles.

In the future, nursing practices will be classified under the general categories of *nurse-generalists* and *nurse-specialists*, with subfield specialties. I believe that out of the total population of nurses two-thirds should be nurse-generalists, i.e., primary care, long-term care, and family care nurses, and one-third should be nurse-specialists by the next decade. Both specialized and generalized educational preparation will be essential to develop the profession and to serve people with a holistic care approach. Nursing must not prepare too many specialists, as medicine has done, because nursing will need more generalists than specialists in the future. Nurses will assume a major responsibility for primary, tertiary, and family care practices, which will make a visible and significant public impact. It will also bring economic gains and professional and personal satisfactions to nurses. The present demand for highly competent primary care, family care, and long-term care nurse-generalists will continue for the next three decades.

By the year 2000, practically all nurse practice laws will have been changed to reflect considerably more independent nursing roles and responsibilities than exist at present. Nurse practice laws will, in time, reflect differences in nursing positions based upon educational preparation, role expectations and responsibilities, and professional competencies determined by societal needs, rigorous tests, and performance. The nurse's position and salary will be based upon these combined factors. The process of legislating nurse practice laws will make the public more aware of nursing's significant role in health care than ever before in the history of nursing.

By the year 1980, consumers will expect the nursing profession to demonstrate the *unique* features of their services, how they complement the services of other health professions, and how effectively their services are meeting general socie-

tal needs. Most important, concepts such as cost-effectiveness, productivity, accountability, and legal *defensive nursing practices* will soon be well known to the majority of nursing practitioners.

Nursing service providers and nursing educators will be confronted with the task of supplying competent nurses to meet our population's health needs in relation to costs and resource requirements. This will be a major task but an essential one for improving and maintaining this country's ongoing health needs. The ratio of nurses to consumers will be based upon research studies, prediction models, and other factors such as the role expectations of nurses, types of preventive and restorative care services in demand, distribution factors, quality of care, standards of care, geographic rural-urban needs, multi-disciplinary collaborative efforts, economic considerations, political factors influencing nursing care, cultural health norms, and management and organization models of nursing care services in different types of settings. Prediction models will be constructed and used on local, regional, and national bases, and will be tested for reliability and validity.

From the predictions of nurse-consumer ratios, it is anticipated that the number of students entering associate and baccalaureate degree nursing programs will be significantly smaller before 1980. There will be an oversupply of nurses, and especially of nonprofessional and technical nursing assistants. Nursing leaders must begin immediately *to regulate and monitor the number of nurses* so that our societal needs are met and our professional service goals, economic welfare, salaries, etc., are not compromised. Therefore, the admission of applicants into nursing programs will be a much more rigorous and selective process than it is today. We will also use selection indicators based upon research studies and a number of other indicators to predict the success of nurses in their future work. In addition, more thought will be given to nurses serving people in different geographic and cultural areas in this country and abroad.

Students from virtually every country in the world will be admitted to our nursing degree and continuing education programs. There will also be a marked increase in transcultural student exchange programs and this, in turn, will greatly enrich and expand learning opportunities for students and faculty alike. The determination of international admission requirements, program plans, and degree requirements will provide a great challenge to nursing administrators and faculty. Although nursing ethnocentrism with preference for our American nursing practices will still exist, nurse educators will gradually learn to understand and appreciate the health values and educational norms of different cultures, and in the process will learn much from them.

By 1980, the requirement for entrance at the first level of professional nursing practice in the United States will be the baccalaureate degree. However, by 1985, the requirement for entry at the first level of professional practice will be the master's degree. By 1990 the doctoral degree will be necessary for nurses who aspire to top leadership roles in nursing service and education. The apprenticeship system of nursing education will be a thing of the past and, in retrospect, will be viewed as a very primitive form of nursing education. Pockets of resistance to these trends will continue to exist among some nurses, but by the end of the century such anti-intellectual and anti-educational attitudes will have largely subsided. A perplexing problem will be what to do with the large number of associate degree nursing program graduates, as they will be in competition with professional nurses for the jobs they held in the past. Problems related to certification, recertification, licensure, and the diplomate status of nurses will be great. Serious problems related to certification of nurses, its cost, and its benefits will make nurse leaders wonder why certification was pursued because of the large numbers of practicing nurses with high levels of skills.

Baccalaureate and graduate degree programs will be more flexible than they are today and there will be many avenues to attain different educational goals. Audiovisual teaching aids, computer self-instruction models, and multidisciplinary educational unit instruction will be some of the modern ways of meeting the growing diverse interests and needs of future nursing students. Moreover, these students will be able to complete baccalaureate and graduate degree programs in less time than it takes today, and they will use more self- and group-pacing approaches, as predicted by the Carnegie Commission on Higher Education (Kerr, 1971). By 1985, nursing school faculties will be, as a rule, highly competent and well-prepared with the majority of their members holding doctoral degrees. This trend will revolutionize nursing education and help bring into focus nursing's contributions to higher education and to nursing service practices.

There will be a significant increase in the number, variety, and size of graduate programs by 1985 and in these aspects they will approximate current baccalaureate programs. The number of doctoral programs for nurses in the United States will mushroom, and this trend will continue until the close of this century (Leininger, 1976c). For example, there are presently twenty-four schools of nursing that plan to offer a doctoral degree in nursing (Leininger, 1976c, p. 207). The "nurse-scientist" programs that began in the early 1960s will be terminated by 1978, and this will initiate the new and important trend of preparing nurses in their *own* discipline rather than in a related one. As doctoral programs proliferate, major concerns about the quality of these programs, and especially about the quality of their faculties, will be expressed. There will be almost as many nurses desiring doctoral education as there are desiring baccalaureate education today. As a result of their doctoral preparation, a number of nurse-researchers, administrators, and educators will be employed in hospitals, health agencies, universities, and other such settings by the turn of the century. Some nurses who have doctoral degrees in nonnursing fields will be advised to pursue additional doctoral preparation in nursing fields in order to hold positions in university schools of nursing. There will be some major reconceptualizations of the types and purposes of nursing programs so that students will be better able to pursue combined subfield and multidisciplinary programs of study. Exchange programs, external degrees (per portfolio), multi-disciplinary studies, and many nontraditional types of nursing programs will be used more and more in the future.

With the advent of national health insurance in the United States, the demand for continuing education will increase with requests for both degree and nondegree courses. National health insurance will undoubtedly place many inactive nurses into practice in order to meet societal demands for health care. Continuing education will be the major means to reeducate or educate registered nurses who have been inactive for several years. Likewise, the demand for continuing educational programs for licensure, certification, and recertification will grow markedly in the future. Careful assessment of continuing education courses and credits assigned to the courses will be an ongoing problem for nursing educators.

Federal funds for nursing education programs and students will decrease in the near future. Nurses will compete vigorously with other health professionals for their share of the public health dollar. Private industries will move into the health educational arena in an attempt to contract for selected profit-making enterprises. These contract programs will pose problems for degree programs and institutions of higher education, but many will be linked with nurse licensure needs and continuing education programs.

Within the next decade, nursing education programs and faculty will be firmly established within institutions of higher learning and will be making some unique contributions to the academic community. Gradually, the achievement of nursing leaders who hold administrative and leadership positions in universities will be recognized and accepted. Women will be discovered to be highly competent, knowledgeable, and skilled educators and administrators, and eventually they will hold key administrative positions in universities and colleges.

NURSING RESEARCH TO ENSURE THE QUALITY OF NURSING PRACTICE AND EDUCATION

The future of nursing depends largely on its research. Nursing research will be essential for the generation of new knowledge, the refutation of outdated ideas, and the verification of existing practices. It will survive the struggles for research monies, the interprofessional challenges, and the limited administrative and federal support for research. By the turn of the century, the impact of nursing research findings on nursing practice and education in the United States will be evident. The importance of nurse scholars will begin to be recognized in spite of the anti-intellectualism of some nurses.

Nurse-researchers will not only present their research findings to nursing colleagues at national meetings, but they will also present their work to multidisciplinary health and behavioral science researchers. This will be a major step toward placing nurse-researchers firmly in university settings.

Nursing institutes and research centers will emerge inside and outside academic settings at home and abroad. Multidisciplinary research ventures will be stimulating but difficult for nurse-researchers until nursing's major domain, i.e., caring, is explicated. One of nursing's greatest needs is to explicate the behaviors and components that constitute caring. The study of caring is a research goal that is barely acknowledged today. Hospital and community field studies related to caring will need to be developed as well as other new research approaches to study communities.

I predict that the most significant development in nursing will be the growth of nursing research and its application to public health and nursing care problems. Nursing research in our scientifically oriented American culture will make a key difference in changing the image of nursing. It will modify client care, education, and general health care services. In addition, improved public education about nursing through mass communication will be essential to change the social reference, image, and status of nursing, and these changes will provide the bases for the nursing profession to move ahead in some extremely creative directions.

SUMMARY

Predicting and planning for nursing's future are very difficult but also very necessary tasks. The determination of nursing's future goals and priorities is critical and essential for nursing to remain a viable profession. To predict, guide, and shape the future of nursing, the largest health profession with more than 1 million members, is an overwhelming task and in order to be successful will require strong, intelligent, and creative leadership.

During this century, nursing has made some noteworthy achievements. However, the future looks even more exciting and promising provided that nurses plan for ways and means to shape new and strong directions. Without such thoughtful planning and predictions our future is most uncertain. Furthermore, one hopes that our three national nursing organizations will work together rather than compete with each other and duplicate their professional efforts. The organizational structures and purposes of these national organizations need to be reappraised and adapted to fit the needs of nursing today.

In the future, nursing will be much more complex, precise, and varied than it is today. Vigorous intellectual and professional leadership will continue to be needed in nursing, as well as creative thinkers and futuristic planners. There is yet much to be accomplished in determining the scientific and humanistic components of caring, the real essence of nursing, before we can hope to fulfill nursing's ultimate goal of providing care to many people. It is hoped that, by the year 2000, we will have explicated caring through rigorous study and documentation of different cultural groups. The future of nursing looks most promising, although there are tremendous challenges for us to meet and barriers for us to overcome in the health field.

BIBLIOGRAPHY

American Academy of Nursing: *Models for Health Care Delivery: Now and for the Future*, American Nurses Association, Kansas City, 1975.

Committee on Nursing Preparation and Utilization: "A New Nursing Model," Washington State Nurses Association, Seattle, Wash., October 1973, pp. 10–16.

Committee on Taxonomy: "Taxonomy of Nursing Practitioners," an unpublished working paper of the Committee on Taxonomy of the HEW, Analysis and Planning for Improved Distribution of Nursing Personnel and Services, 1976.

Eiseley, Loren: *The Unexpected Universe*, Harcourt Brace Jovanovich, New York, 1964.

Heneley, S. P., and J. R. Yates: *Futurism in Education*, McCutchen, New York, 1974.

Kerr, Clark: "Less Time, More Options," in Clark Kerr (ed.), *Higher Education for the Future: Reform or More of the Same*, Proceedings of the 20th SREB Legislative Work Conference, Atlanta, Georgia, Carnegie Corporation, New York, July 14–17, 1971, pp. 25–30.

Leininger, Madeleine: "Anthropological Issues Related to Community Mental Health Programs in the United States," *Community Mental Health Journal*, 7(1):50–62, March 1971.

———: "Health Care Delivery Systems for Tomorrow: Possibilities and Guidelines," in *Proceedings of Health of the Nation, 5*, University of Minnesota, Minneapolis, 1973*a*, pp. 24–31.

———: "An Open Health Care System Model," *Nursing Outlook*, 21(3):171–175, March 1973*b*.

———: "Political Systems of Health Science Centers," paper given at American Anthropological Association Meeting, New Mexico, 1974*a*.

———: "The Leadership Crisis in Nursing," *The Journal of Nursing Administration*, 4(2):28–34, March–April 1974*b*.

———: "Transcultural Nursing Presents Exciting Challenges," *The American Nurse*, 7(5):4, May 1975.

———: *Transcultural Nursing and Health Care: Theories and Practices*, Wiley, New York, 1976*a*.

———: "Transcultural Nursing: A Promising Subfield of Study for Nurse Educators and Practitioners," in Adina M. Reinhardt and Mildred D. Quinn (eds.), *Current Practice in Family Centered Community Nursing*, Mosby, St. Louis, 1976*b*.

———: "Doctoral Programs for Nurses: Trends, Questions and Projected Plans," *Nursing Research*, 25(3):201–211, May–June 1976*c*.

Santayana, George: *The Birth of Reason*, Columbia, New York, 1968.

Spicer, E. H. (ed.): *Human Problems in Technological Change*, Sage, New York, 1952.

EDITOR'S QUESTIONS FOR DISCUSSION

How might nursing be encouraged to plan for the future? How can leadership be developed in nursing? What factors within the profession may inhibit the development of leadership?

How may increased technology affect patient care? How is "rehumanization care" being provided today? What type of nurse may be best qualified to provide technological nursing care in the future? What measures might be developed to prevent the increased depersonalization of patient care? What are the implications of the marketing of nursing services for nursing and for patient care?

What evidence exists that the health care of tomorrow will be directed and regulated more by the government than by the patient? What effect(s) might national health insurance have on nursing education programs?

What are the implications for nursing of its increasing accountability in practice? What evidence is there that nursing may be preparing more specialists than generalists? What is the justification for the prediction that a master's degree will become a prerequisite for practice by 1985? What effect(s) might this have on the nursing profession and nursing practice? What will substitute for or replace the apprenticeship system of nursing education? What will be the effect(s) on practice and the profession if baccalaureate and graduate programs take less time to complete than they do today? What might be the *content* of doctoral programs in nursing? To what extent do you agree or disagree with the predictions that have been made? What evidence is there that the predictions may be accurate or inaccurate?

Chapter 39

The Nursing Profession: Vision of the Future

Rozella M. Schlotfeldt, R.N., Ph.D., D.Sc., L.H.D., F.A.A.N.
Professor, Frances Payne Bolton School of Nursing
Case Western Reserve University, Cleveland, Ohio

Rozella M. Schlotfeldt discusses the changing system of health care and the future definitions of nursing roles. Society's interest in health care is increasing, and Schlotfeldt focuses on the role of nursing in maintaining health and preventing illness. Unlike Christman and Leininger, she predicts the development of multiple community health centers. The nurse is designated as the health professional who will be responsible for primary patient contact. She will make initial health assessments, detect potential health problems, fulfill teaching and counseling roles, and be responsible for the health surveillance of persons of all ages. When problems occur, the nurse will refer the patient to a physician who will make a differential medical diagnosis and institute appropriate medical treatment. Accountability, peer review, self-evaluation, and research are needed to ensure superior nursing practices and the competency of nurses who provide comprehensive health care.

SOCIETY'S INTEREST IN HEALTH CARE

It is a strange paradox that while human beings have long professed that they value health, and while they proclaim that health is the bedrock on which social progress, personal attainment, and individual happiness are built, they have not, over the ages, consistently and actively sought health. Instead, they have primarily sought relief from their ills.

In primitive times, men implored their gods to send relief from their ills by asking them to exorcise the demons that had possessed them and to lift the curses that had befallen them. Subsequently, priest-physicians took responsibility for directing programs of healing that combined spiritual entreaties, the use of empirically tested potions and herbs, and physical therapies of several kinds. As man's knowledge increased, physicians became better and better educated and their methods of diagnosing and treating diseases of the body and mind became more and more sophisticated and specialized. Ordinary men came to regard medicine as practically a divine calling and viewed with awe the seemingly heroic acts that physicians performed. In the recent past, the eradication of dread diseases and the replacement of defective organs and limbs with artificial ones through the science of modern medicine have captured the imagination of laymen who marvel at such miracles; and yet, to health professionals, these so-called miracles have become routine practices. Indeed, physicians themselves often deplore the attention paid to such dramatic efforts to correct or cure maladies, in contrast to the lack of notice given to less glamorous endeavors designed to prevent disease and to promote health. A wise philosopher-physician recently commented on the relatively superior social value of the inexpensive contributions made by laymen who are successful in convincing their colleagues to quit smoking, in contrast to that of the remarkably costly contributions that are made by thoracic surgeons who remove cancerous lungs.

As added evidence to substantiate the allegation that man has not habitually sought health, one needs only to observe that most people in today's world eat too much and without proper consideration of diet; they exercise insufficiently and erratically; they use drugs of many kinds routinely, indiscriminately, and unwisely; and they take unnecessary risks that are dangerous to their lives and limbs. Many people respond eagerly to the passive consumerism that is promoted by the television industry. They accept without much question the notion fabricated by clever advertising agencies, that they suffer from illnesses, and they hasten to purchase popular, ineffective, and sometimes harmful remedies in order to cure these illnesses, or to relieve their trumped-up symptoms.

Without question, people have primarily sought the medical care and cure of their ills, and have often expected that they would be miraculously treated and restored, after having contracted maladies that could have been prevented in the first place. Why, then, is it likely that people can now be increasingly expected to change their time-worn behavior patterns, and to actively pursue health?

It is perhaps understandable that in our great society, where an abundance of all materials and services has generally been assumed to exist, perceived deficiencies in medical services, coupled with their high costs, have served as a strong force motivating people to actively seek health. There is little doubt that the high costs of sickness care, along with dissatisfaction with the lack of equity in its distribution, have led to numerous efforts to correct the imbalance between medical care and health care. The goal for the last half of the 1970s is to design and test new approaches to the delivery of care that will effectively promote health and prevent disease, as well as to bring about cures and to restore people to maximal levels of wellness. Well-educated nurses have major contributions to make in the attainment of this goal.

It is instructive, before we inquire into the characteristics of the new models proposed for the delivery of comprehensive health care, to point up the interrelationships that must exist between and among health care providers in order for us to have an efficient and effective health care delivery system. The focus and scope of the responsibilities of each of the health care providers must be agreed upon if that care system is to function properly as the sum of its parts, and the nature of the roles of the health care providers must be defined, with a view toward fulfilling the health needs of all people. Such decisions are best based upon conceptual analyses of the outcomes of the work of professionals who are primary functionaries in the system.

The term *health professional* encompasses a wide variety of persons—dentists, physicians, pharmacists, physical and diet therapists, sometimes social workers, and, of course, nurses. Each has a unique role to play and specific goals to attain in the delivery of health care.

The role of dentists is the advancement and use of dental science and technology with the long-range goal of eliminating the causes of dental pathologies, and with the immediate goal of correcting dental defects and pathologies and of promoting efficient mastication, optimal cosmetic effects, and good oral hygiene.

The medical profession is charged by society with responsibility for the diagnosis and treatment of all human diseases and disabilities, for the discovery of their causes, for the development and testing of effective cures, and for the means of controlling diseases the causes and cures of which are unknown. Of course, physicians are concerned with the general health of their patients and that of the nation at large. But the focus of medical practice, medical education, and medical research is on the discovery of existing pathologies and their causes, on the elimination or attenuation of their immediate effects, and on the provision of the means by which to minimize their harmful, long-range consequences.

Some professionals in the health care field are concerned with specific aspects of therapy. It is on them that sick people must rely for the exercise of judgment and the execution of skills necessary to bring about those positive outcomes that are the consequences of the effective use of particular types of treatments.

Pharmacists, for example, focus on the advancement and the use of knowledge of drugs and the dissemination of information about them with the intent of promoting their effective, efficient, and proper use in chemical therapies. Pharmacists function in a variety of settings and increasingly are providing drug information services to other health professionals, as well as to lay people. Such services include information about the proper use, misuse, overuse, and correct handling of medicaments. Pharmacists engage in the monitoring of drug utilization for the purpose of maximizing the positive effects of drug therapy and minimizing its negative ones.

Diet therapists use their knowledge of nutrition and the conditions related to it to enhance therapy programs through the proper and healthful use of foodstuffs. Their responsibility is limited to the surveillance of the patient's well-being solely as that responsibility pertains to the use of nutrients. Although concerned, of course, with the general well-being of patients, the dietitian's unique responsibility is diet therapy, not general health care.

The nature of social work brings professionals in that field into tangential contact with health professionals. The general focus of social workers is on the promotion of the greatest possible socialization of human beings. Since social and economic deprivations and unresolved life crises affect human beings' health, social adjustments, and productivity, social workers work quite frequently with health professionals. It is important that the focus of their work and their particular contributions to the health care system be understood.

The unique contribution of nurses to the health care system is the promotion of the optimal, general health of human beings, whether they are well, almost well, ill, injured, infirm, deprived, or dying. Nurses serve individuals, families, and communities, engaging in first contact and ambulatory care, in the care of persons who are acutely ill, and in the care of patients who require nursing services over protracted periods of time. The focus of their work is on the assessment of the health status and potentials of those they serve, and on the use of nursing strategies to promote their clients' optimal, general health. In addition, nursing's goal is to help people become maximally independent with regard to the successful execution of their own programs of therapy, and to encourage them to actively seek good health. Nurses are also expected to advance our knowledge of the ways and means man seeks health. Of course, nurses are concerned with pathologies and their prevention, and with medical therapies. But the focus of nursing practice, nursing education, and nursing research is on maximizing the health of human beings through the provision of scientifically sound, humanistic, nursing care.

Explicating the unique contribution and scope of responsibility of each of the several kinds of health professionals points up the complexity of any system of health care that is designed to meet the needs of all people. It points up the need for knowledgeably defining the roles of all health practitioners so that their talents and competencies are well and wisely utilized in providing those needed services. It points up the central, important, and indeed, *crucial* role of the nurse in any system of health care that is envisioned for the future. It points up the need for accountability on the part of each health professional to the society he or she serves. It points up the responsibility all health professionals have to work cooperatively, with one another and with other citizens, in designing a health care system that does in fact effectively and efficiently meet the needs of all people.

NEW MODELS OF HEALTH CARE

There is little question that the nationwide system by which health and medical services are currently delivered is about to undergo substantial change. Although previous attempts to develop a coordinated, national system of so-called health services have failed, each plan presented in the past offered at least a partial solution to the problem of the nation's health needs. The prospects are now high that a step-by-step campaign will be mounted to effect a health program that will enable each individual, by virtue of variously subsidized, prepaid insurance, to have access to care encompassing emergency services, dental services, periodic health assessment and surveillance, preventive services, diagnostic services, in-patient care during acute or episodic illnesses, and appropriate medical supervision, including home and institutional care, during chronic illnesses, protracted disabilities, and infirmities. Although the details of how to provide such a complete set of services must be worked out over time, it is possible to make fairly reliable predictions about the general characteristics of the health care system of the future. Within such predictions lies a vision of nursing's future.

First, the system will be characterized by the coordination of services on the community level, within regions, and nationally, and those services will be based on the needs of people for health and sickness care. Moreover, the services to be made available will be rationalized so that duplications will be minimized, gaps in services will be eliminated, and surveillance will assure that programs of care will be of uniformly high quality. Access to needed health care will be guaranteed to all citizens. Costs will be contained through monitoring of efficiency, through using the competencies of all practitioners wisely, through appropriate use of all available technologies, and through requir-

ing personal accountability on the part of each practitioner.

The allocation of responsibilities at national, regional, and community levels will assure the efficient collection of uniform data needed as indexes of the health of all of the nation's citizens. Such data will be used to identify needs for changes in the system and to monitor progress toward attaining agreed-upon goals. Although controversies may rage about the data bases needed, there is no question that information on the incidence of preventable diseases, disabilities, unnecessary and untimely deaths, and comparable, aggregate data on outcomes of health care and medical therapies will provide useful indexes of the nation's health status and of the value of the services delivered. The responsibility for surveillance over services will reside in community, regional, and national councils whose members will be both consumers and providers of health care.

Henceforth, health will increasingly be officially recognized as a national asset having claim on an appropriate, although as yet undetermined, proportion of the gross national product. Although some professionals, including nurses, will continue to offer their services on a private, or fee-for-service, basis, as is appropriate in our great democracy, it is instructive to look to the public and private systems of education to find a model that delineates the essential health care services provided through tax support in addition to those purchased through payment of additional, private funds.

A VISION OF NURSING'S FUTURE

In order to obtain a vision of nursing's future within the context of a coordinated health care system, it is useful to contemplate the services that will be made available at the community level, for these services will be representative of the practices of all health professionals. It should be noted that nurses, like all other health professionals, will be expected to serve along with lay people on community, regional, and national advisory panels, on governing councils, and on study commissions in order to insure the proper input of knowledge and experience into the design, execution, and evaluation of the health and medical care services to be provided.

Community health centers will be at the hub of the health and medical care system of the future. Each of these centers will serve a defined population within a specific geographic locale and each will provide a variety of services. Such services will encompass routine health surveillance, preventive services, and medical diagnoses and therapies for persons of all ages—at the center and in a variety of other settings; emergency care, acute care, long-term care, and rehabilitative services; residential and "at home" services for the aged and infirm, and institutional care for those whose mental or physical conditions require sustained help and supervision; and referral services of all kinds.

A network of services will be available locally, regionally, and nationally. A group of comprehensive, community health centers will be coordinated with a single, designated hospital offering highly sophisticated, specialty services of all kinds. Patients will be referred to those specialty hospitals for needed care and they will be returned to their community centers after receiving care that can be offered only by specialists in the several health professions. Each network of multiple community centers and their referral hospital will be joined with others like them to form regional health agencies; and those, in turn, will be interconnected to form a national system of health care services.

In the community health care network, services at intake or reception centers will encompass obtaining routine health histories and making health assessments of all people. Some of those evaluations will be carried out in schools, some at community health stations, some in the homes of people living in the community, some in work settings, and some in penal institutions. Health assessments are, of course, the responsibility of well-educated, competent nurses. Health education will be accomplished wherever health surveillance is provided and by means of local, regional, and national television networks as well. All modern technologies and teaching strategies will be employed with a view toward involving all citizens in the active pursuit of their own health and in their therapeutic regimens. Family planning and counseling services will be available at the community centers. Nurses will play those teaching and counseling roles. They will also be responsible for management of the health care and delivery of normal, pregnant women and for the health surveillance of persons of all ages.

Primary contact personnel will refer those persons who manifest signs of health problems to general physicians who will be responsible for making differential medical diagnoses and for instituting appropriate medical therapies. Nurses will be responsible for making such referrals.

Those persons who are judged at the reception center to need the additional services of nutritionists, pharmacists, social workers, the clergy, or lawyers will be appropriately referred; and it is anticipated that all of those services will be immediately available in the center. Nurses will perform that referral function. Those who need housekeeping, food, or child care services in order to maintain their independence at home, or to be gainfully employed, will similarly be referred by nurse-professionals at the reception center to personnel that can provide or arrange for such services. Some patients will be judged to need home health services. Such services will be provided by nurses working out of the community health centers. All reception or intake centers will be staffed on a 24-hour-a-day basis.

Emergency teams for each community health center will be available constantly, each serving a definitive geographic area and each having all needed transport and communication resources that can make maximum use of the most modern, appropriate technologies. Such teams will have immediate access to all needed diagnostic and therapeutic services. Nurses will serve on such emergency teams.

In the community hospitals, in-patients served will generally be those whose illnesses do not require the services of specialist physicians. They may, however, require the services of some specialist physicians on a consultant basis; and certainly the need for generalists and specialists in other health professions, including nursing, nutrition, pharmacy, physical therapy, and social work will be determined by the needs of the clientele.

It is anticipated that services for geriatric patients will henceforth be integral parts of the community health care centers, as will be care for mentally ill patients having behavioral problems that require ambulatory care and institutionalization. Such patients will thus have the attention they need from professionals, in contrast to the inadequate care they sometimes receive now. As it is expected that people will live longer in the future and this, in turn, will place increasing demands on the community health centers, long-range planning to meet these needs will be required. Similarly, long-range planning will be required to incorporate care for those who are mentally ill into the programs of the centers. It is for these reasons that a new health care system will be effected step by step, but with goals that are well defined. Surely professionals will need to retain some of the very fine services and resources now available, and to improve them, coordinate them, and add to them, as is appropriate, in order to attain the goal of having an efficient, effective, exemplary quality system of health and medical services available to all people in the immediate future.

Persons requiring the services of teams of specialists will henceforth, as now, be referred to specialty, primarily university, centers for such care. In those specialty hospitals, the complete range of health care services will be available. Some patients will, after treatment, be returned to their community centers for sustained care; others, whose conditions warrant it, will be treated over time in specialty hospitals.

Nurses of the future will, as they have in the past, play a key role in the delivery of health care. Henceforth, however, the well-prepared competent nurse professional will be recognized for the vital contributions she or he makes to the health and well-being of the nation. In turn, nurse professionals will, much more consistently than they have in the past, fulfill their obligations to the society they serve. Those obligations encompass the full range of practitioner responsibilities, and of professional responsibilities as well.

Working inside and outside of the community centers, the nurse will be the health professional primarily responsible for assessing the health status of people. Nurses will routinely obtain health histories and perform assessments of the physical, emotional, and social states of people who periodically or summarily present themselves, and provide care for those whose needs fall within the scope of nursing practice. They will refer to other health professionals those who need medical, legal, nutritional, or social services, or help from the clergy.

Nurses will continue to provide knowledgeable, competent services designed to assist sick, injured, and infirm persons retain or regain maximal levels of wellness during diagnostic and therapeutic regimens mandated by their physical and emotional impairments, whether these treatments are of short or long duration and whether the patients are treated in community or specialty hospitals. Those services will encompass compensatory, sustaining, comforting, guiding, and teaching functions for those whose physical or emotional states, or their inadequate knowledge, make them temporarily or permanently, partially or totally, dependent. In all circumstances, it will be the responsibility of nurses to act knowledgeably, competently, and judiciously to achieve the goal of helping persons to attain their highest possible levels of physical independence, social competence, and emotional well-being.

Included in the teaching and guiding responsibilities of nurses will be their helping patients to recognize and use their own strengths and assets, and to understand and accept whatever limitations are imposed on them by virtue of genetic inadequacies and the sequelae of diseases and injuries. Nurses, along with other health professionals, are expected to help patients become knowledgeable about and actively involved in the competent execution of their own programs of therapy.

It is in the care of chronically ill patients that nurses will have an especially challenging role to play, for the quality of life of those patients will be significantly enhanced through the knowledgeable ministrations of competent nurses. Such nurses will provide care to sustain patients and to prevent complicating and unnecessary maladies; they will monitor the health status of the patients and seek the consultation of physicians when their services are needed. In short, nurses will carry a large responsibility for maintaining the health status of patients who are chronically ill or disabled.

In addition to their referral, teaching and guidance, and direct care functions, nurse-professionals will play increasingly important roles as citizen-professionals. The advocacy role nurses will play must incorporate their judicious and skillful exercise of influence within social and political arenas. As citizens, professionals must not only demonstrate the social utility of their practices, but they must also interpret to other citizens in influential positions their need to act in ways to complement and enhance the services of professionals in order to improve the health of the nation.

The collective voice of nurse-professionals will be increasingly heard as they accurately identify the health hazards that exist in the environments in which people live, learn, work, and recreate. They also are, and will continue to be, in opportune positions to identify problems of child neglect and abuse, and deprivations, abandonment, and injustices suffered by persons who are old, infirm, and incompetent. They now understand and will continue to understand more about the dire consequences of the misuse and abuse of drugs. They now know and will continue to learn more about the consequences of poverty and deprivation, and of the exploitation of men by their fellow men. Their advocacy responsibilities as health professionals will surely lead them to the exercise

of proper social and political influence designed to promote programs and to enact legislation planned for the public good.

Self-evaluation and peer review as ways to ensure superior nursing practices and the competency of nurses must become more widely used than they are today. These are necessary safeguards through which the public can be assured of personal and group accountability on the part of all health professionals. Professional accountability encompasses responsibility to see that each health professional and each group of health practitioners demonstrates exemplary performance. It includes, in addition, active efforts on the part of health professionals to insure that all persons needing services actually receive them.

As part of their evaluative function, nurses must henceforth routinely and systematically identify situations where their knowledge base is inadequate to the task. Nurses, like other professionals, are responsible for the identification of what is not yet known as well as for the mastery of knowledge that has been discovered. The research function of nurses must continue to be significantly enhanced—for it is only through advancing nursing knowledge that the practices of health professionals can continue to be improved and society well-served.

Future generations of nurses must surpass the accomplishments of those of the present and the past in yet another way. Nurses of the future must work cooperatively with one another and with other health professionals. In turn, all health professionals must seek to know their respective roles and contributions to the total health care system, and must sustain and support one another in attaining the goals they all share. Health care of the future will only be effective and efficient if all practitioners demonstrate self-confidence, and respect for one another, for all those who are served, and for themselves. Nurses must increase their personal accountability and, by doing so, enhance their own self-confidence and self-respect.

Over a century ago Florence Nightingale set forth a vision of nursing's future. She envisioned nursing as a field of essential, scientific, humane and scholarly, as well as practical, work. She conceptualized nursing as work designed to keep people well, to help them avoid disease, and to restore them to their highest possible levels of health. She identified the need to discover knowledge that could be structured as the science of health. She knew that nursing would one day become a learned profession.

It is a timely coincidence that nursing's protracted and painful emergence as a full-fledged profession in the decade of the 1970s coincides with society's demands for improved and equitably distributed health care services. This co-incidence offers nurses the opportunity to create for themselves a future about which it may truly be said that nursing is the most exciting and potentially most rewarding of all of the health professions. That future rests with the young people who will be educated as nurses and with visionary teachers whose concept of nursing encompasses the fulfillment of the most demanding and, at the same time, most rewarding of all services—that of giving knowledgeable, humane, and comprehensive care designed to promote, sustain, and restore optimal health for all human beings.

EDITOR'S QUESTIONS FOR DISCUSSION

How can nursing diagnosis be applied and used in primary care? How does a nursing assessment of a patient differ from a medical one in terms of procedure and content? What are the responsibilities of a nurse in making a health assessment, providing referrals for treatment, and scheduling follow-up care? What should be the qualifications and educational preparation of nurses who are to be in primary care settings? How is the role of the nurse in primary care best communicated to the public and other professions? How will the role of the nurse in primary care be legitimated? What type of nurse will be attracted to the structure and organizational setting of a hospital versus those of ambulatory care centers?

Part Eight

Summary and Conclusions

In this summary chapter, the following topics, which correspond to the issues treated in this volume, are discussed: professionalization, nursing education, nursing research, nursing theory, nursing practice, interdisciplinary professional relationships, and the future of nursing. Observations are made about the current state of the profession from the perspective of the sociology of professions and occupations. More questions are raised and some possible answers are offered. These comments should be an example of the present search for meaning and definition of the professional role of nursing and should stimulate others to raise further questions and answers in the dialogue needed for the growth of the profession.

Chapter 40

Not Crystal Clear

Norma L. Chaska, R.N., Ph.D.
Research Associate, Mayo Clinic and Mayo Foundation
Rochester, Minnesota

The quest for meaning in a profession evokes many questions and stimulates the search for answers. This process also provides the members of the profession with an opportunity for self-examination. While searching for the right answers, nursing as a profession cannot afford to be without values. Society needs these values and patients expect them. In order to survive and grow, nursing needs different tested, proved values. Individuals within the profession need the behavioral guidance such values offer. Likewise, the process of asking questions can strengthen a profession as well as its members. Questions and uncertainty about the nature and future of a profession can provide the dynamics for that profession to move forward.

A static, crystal clear view of a profession provides logical explanations of society, the profession, and the professional, but such unchanging vision does not take into account the fact that we are constantly being influenced and indeed, changed, by our environment. On the other hand, however, professions have too often expected to derive their meaning and definition totally from external cultural, technologic, and economic forces. Nurses are beginning to realize that the meaning of nursing as a profession may be found within the profession and the person, not in the external environment. Nurses are defining their profession and their roles in this profession in terms of their internal strength. Nevertheless, nursing must be aware of external reality. Nurses

need to be in touch with, but not dominated by, their cultural, social, and economic environment and the environment of the health care system. Most importantly, they need to be in touch with others in the environment and with themselves.

Refusing to acknowledge diversity in society and in nursing will impede the growth of that profession. Acceptance of diversity is vital to the development of community, an essential attribute of a profession. Diversity of viewpoint within a profession provides a range of opinion from which answers can be selected and tested until the right ones are found. The best answer is seldom the most expedient one. To live with questions until the truth of answers has been tested by colleagues is often necessary.

Particularly for the caring professional, the final test of truth may be found in the positive response of the patient. Truth cannot be discovered in vacuum, by either an individual member of a profession or a profession itself. Thus the search for answers must be a responsible coordinated one. The professional who has no doubt about the correct answers must be patient with the testing process. Being patient does not mean being passive. Rather, one's being patient allows others to express their opinions and all answers to be tested.

Social and cultural forces such as the knowledge explosion, competition for health services, territorial disputes with medicine over the role of the nurse, the increasing knowledge of patients about health care and their rights, and the heightened concern with the quality of life make it imperative that each of the critical areas of nursing be examined in an overall analysis. This is essential for the growth of the profession and of the individual professional, who currently may feel alienated not only as a professional in society but also as an isolated member within the profession itself. If the profession as a whole is in a state of "mist," that is, confusion and change, individual members are undoubtedly experiencing similar feelings of uncertainty.

PROFESSIONALIZATION

A *profession* is usually envisioned as an abstract, broad category of occupational organization, whereas the term *professionalization* refers to the process by which occupations assume the attributes of a profession. Some of the structural characteristics that are necessary for the establishment of a profession have been mentioned in the section on professionalization. Perhaps the attributes most commonly cited are those designated by Greenwood (1957): the presence of systematic theory, formal and informal community sanction, a code of ethics, and a professional culture.

Most occupations striving to be recognized as distinct professions possess some or all of the above attributes to varying degrees. Perhaps another factor to consider is one indicated by Hall (1975, p. 75): the attitudinal orientations of the persons involved rather than the presence of structural characteristics may provide a different basis for professionalization. For example, the professional is usually characterized by a high level of personal involvement with his work, which is communicated to his clients by performance that indicates that he will always act in their best interest (Hall, 1975, p. 75). The professional actually has a well-developed sense of responsibility and obligation and is often thought of as one who would work for merely the intrinsic rewards

of his occupation (Hall, 1975, p. 75). Attitudinal consensus about professional behavior through close identification with one's professional colleagues and formal professional associations is usually considered to be the epitome of professionalism (Hall, 1975, p. 76).

If, indeed, the attitudes of members toward the profession are indicative of professionalism, there are important implications for the question of nursing's professionalism. The two types of commitment on the part of nurses to the nursing profession have been discussed in the section on professionalism (see the contribution by Yeaworth). These two types of nurses—those who regard nursing as a "job" and those who view it as a "career"—have always been present in nursing, and they represent two different degrees of involvement. Those who regard nursing as a job are more likely to be practicing it for the external rewards and are less likely to identify with the formal professional association. Those who regard nursing as a career presumably look for intrinsic satisfaction in their role performance and invest something of themselves in their formal professional associations. One cannot assume, however, that the part-time employee considers nursing as a job and that the full-time employee regards nursing as a career.

Many part-time nurses are the primary economic providers for their families; their part-time status does not necessarily imply any lack of commitment on their part to a career. Their common dilemma is that of the woman who combines family life with a career: which of the two roles receives priority varies with the situation. No single approach will resolve this dilemma for the nurse, the family, the profession, or the organization that is the employer. Whatever method is chosen to attempt to resolve the conflict, many part-time nurses remain committed to nursing as a career and are remarkably productive because their time of service is limited.

The problem of scheduling work hours for part-time employees is well known. One effective solution to this problem is to establish periodic exchanges between the part-time nurse and the employer to discuss what compromises can be made. If part-time nurses are not employed, a tremendous loss results. The profession loses the investment made in educating the person as well as the person-power, education, and experience of these nurses. The patient loses because of the decreased number of experienced nursing personnel. Unfortunately, some nurses who discontinue their careers for 2 or more years in order to raise their families discover that too many changes have occurred for them to return comfortably to practice. Nurses who drop out of the profession completely can no longer be afforded.

On the other hand, to believe that all full-time nurses are committed to their profession is unrealistic, as desirable as that state would be. The Women's Movement may have an increasing impact on the type of commitment a nurse might make to her profession. This influence should not be overestimated, however, because the Women's Movement has also opened doors to careers other than nursing for women.

It may be more realistic to explore the avenues by which the commitment a nurse makes to the profession may be increased. In their contributions to this volume, Jacox, Stein, and Monnig suggest that nursing students need teachers who can serve as role models, who are expert practitioners, and who are able to instill the important nursing values in their students. In addition, an increased study of the behavioral sciences should enable students to communicate more effectively with patients, and thus increase their personal commitment.

Monnig presents an interesting dilemma for nursing if one attempts to relate type of commitment to a basic educational program and degree of professionalism. A basic assumption in the literature is that the baccalaureate degree nurse is the professional nurse and the diploma graduate is the technical nurse. Yet, in Monnig's sample of nurses, the diploma graduate ranked higher than the baccalaureate degree nurse on all of the scales measuring professionalism, except on that of autonomy. Based on this finding, diploma nurses

may justly resent being excluded from the category of professional. How can such findings be explained?

Perhaps the answer lies in the scale itself. Hall's professionalism scale is a measure of *attitudinal* components. Generally, attitudes require time to develop and to be reinforced. Could the socialization process in the *practice* of nursing, which is longer for the diploma students than for the baccalaureate students, have reinforced professional attitudes by means of the role models of others who were significant as well as by means of the response of the patient? Furthermore, Hall's professionalism scale may not adequately reflect the impact of another variable, education, and the associated differences that are assumed to exist among professionals because of different educational backgrounds. Finally, it raises the question, Can the type of education cause a difference in the degree of professionalism one attains?

This question becomes even more legitimate when one reviews Monnig's finding that nurses with master's degrees had the least sense of calling to their profession according to that aspect of the professionalism scale. It would be important to know whether one's sense of calling is related to the type of commitment one makes to a profession. If it is, the implication might be that nurses with master's degrees are not necessarily more committed to nursing than nurses who have less education. Here is another reason to question whether professionalism and commitment are increased with education.

When students who are candidates for a master's degree discuss why they decided to enter graduate school, some will candidly admit that they "did not know what else to do." Others will explain that they did not feel adequately prepared to be *practitioners* in nursing after completing only a bachelor's program and that they hoped to acquire that ability from a master's program. If the student's expectations were high at the outset of the master's program, the graduate may still not feel adequately prepared at the end of the program. As a result, the master's program graduate nurse possibly displays less of a calling to the profession than do other nurses.

Whether a sense of calling is vitally important to professionalism, however, may be questioned. The skills that a professional with a master's degree has and uses may be more important to professionalism than a sense of calling. For example, how a clinical specialist applies her skills in order to assess a patient's condition most likely would be more important to the development of professionalism in nursing than whether or not the clinical specialist subjectively feels called to the profession. The whole issue of role performance, role deprivation, job satisfaction, and commitment of a graduate with a master's degree needs to be explored.

The question of values in nursing is an important one. For example, the issue of autonomy is becoming increasingly evident. In former times, a nurse was depicted as being passive and obedient. With the advent of the Women's Movement and with the change in values and mores that has come with the current generation, nurses are becoming more assertive. Stein's study shows that contemporary nursing students tend to be more self-directing and questioning. In our increasingly complex society, however, where the knowledge explosion and new technology have affected every profession, the plea for more autonomy is interpreted by some as demanding the right to be totally independent in role performance. Nurses need social control to define their roles as well as accountability to themselves and the patients they serve. This does not minimize the importance of collegial interdisciplinary and intradisciplinary relationships, which are definitely needed. No longer is it possible to make effective decisions about patient care via a hierarchical process. Rather, health care decisions are currently made through a collaborative process, and the skills and knowledge that nurses and physicians have to offer are recognized and utilized. Although every professional could not rightfully be called an expert, our complex society demands that appropriate disciplines and professions pool their resources and function as a health care team. A problem that will be explored later is the conflict between professions over territorial rights and boundaries in the care of patients as well as the necessity of the health care team having a designated "captain" in order to ensure the quality of patient care.

The finding by Braito that job dissatisfaction was unrelated to demands for increased control over who provides what type of patient care was particularly interesting in view of discussions in the nursing literature about the importance of striving for autonomy as a goal. The implications of the finding might be that the general nurse does not consider autonomy as an important issue, or at least that aspect of autonomy concerned with the right to control who provides what type of patient care.

This raises another question. How do we define and standardize the goals, criteria, and norms necessary for the nursing profession? Ideals for the profession are proposed by many nursing leaders, but these leaders may not be aware of the extent to which practicing nurses agree or disagree with what is posited for them as the ideal attribute or behavior for which to strive. Possibly, autonomy may be an example of a nursing ideal about which nurses have disparate views.

Another controversial issue is the importance of theory building in nursing. Some nurses would place nursing in the same category with other professions, according to Roth, that "have created a body of theory in order to justify their own existence" (1974). Hall explains that the emphasis on theory building may more likely be a result of the politics of higher learning than of the concrete demonstration of the importance of theory (1975, p. 78). As nursing strives to build a theory base for itself, it must be aware of the pitfall of developing theory for theory's sake; the utility of theory for nursing *practice* must be documented. The process of developing theory for nursing practice should be so innate to a nurse that she cannot perform a nursing action without reflecting on its underlying theory.

The development of nursing theory is perhaps considered to be a waste of time or an "ivory-tower" exercise by some staff nurses. This attitude may be due to the fact that nurses traditionally were socialized to perform certain tasks and functions. Emphasis was on the development of specific skills. Until the late 1950s, nurses were often assigned to patient care on the basis of their function—that is, the *treatment nurse*, the *medication nurse*, and so forth. Such an arbitrary system of role assignment is a typical example and outcome of the bureaucratic organizational structure of most hospitals. This functional method of assigning nurses to patient care presumably resulted in increased efficiency in the use of personnel and time. Emphasis was always on the outcome of patient care, i.e., in terms of whether or not all of the patients received their bath, treatment, and medications, and little thought was given to the theory underlying the nursing task or treatment for the patient. Even today many nurses, perceiving the quality of patient care to be excellent, may question the need for theory development. Likewise, organizations, such as hospitals, may question the usefulness of nursing theory and view it as an academic goal with little functional value and practical application to their bureaucratic structure.

These doubts about theory development need to be resolved. Perhaps the applicability of theory development to nursing may be understood through the example of another discipline, such as sociology. Some sociologists may view sociology as the study of the "taken-for-granted" behavior of everyday life and may contend, therefore, that sociology magnifies the obvious. Beyond this, a practical application of theory as derived from such a study may make theory development relevant to both nursing and sociology. Soares's study of the use of language in an intensive care unit examines such taken-for-granted behavior. We may assume that verbal interaction among the participants in an intensive care unit will be decreased because of the necessity, on the part of the staff, of performing many tech-

nological functions. What is important is that the results of such a study should reveal the effect on the patient of this lack of verbal communication. Such an examination of taken-for-granted behavior may therefore provide a basis for a change in nursing procedure. This study might also spur the development of a theory for the more effective communication of nurses with patients, particularly those in intensive care units.

Thus, the goal of developing theory in a profession is more than just a desire to ornament one's profession with recherché and irrelevant information. Through the study and analysis of nursing's taken-for-granted behavior—whether such behavior be of a communicative or treatment nature—the profession may identify what functions are uniquely nursing's. Furthermore, by understanding the theory underlying nursing actions or taken-for-granted behavior, the future actions of a professional or of a patient can be predicted, planned, or altered. Consequently, less time might be spent in adjusting nursing care plans or nursing actions, which were formerly based on the isolated responses of the patient. These predicted actions could become a basic framework on which a broader, more complete plan of care for a patient could be constructed. By developing theory that is applicable to nursing, the profession can gain control over what will be defined as uniquely nursing and in that sense can attain the type of autonomy that is desirable.

No single discipline concerned with patient care can claim a totally unique body of knowledge. Because the nature of man as a physical, social, and spiritual being is complex, the sharing of knowledge by disciplines is mandatory. Each discipline or profession has a particular perspective and applies its knowledge accordingly.

Many professions, according to Hall, dispute the existence of an inherent theoretical perspective or knowledge base (1975, p. 79). Many of the contributors in this volume present various aspects of nursing care that they believe should be claimed as the unique domain of nursing. For example, Murphy defines the mission of nursing as health maintenance and promotion. Her emphasis may be the result of nurses analyzing their taken-for-granted actions and determining what nursing really is. The social factors related to the health care needs of the patient are apparent. Murphy's emphasis may also be the result of isolating the inherent knowledge base of nursing and focusing on who should assume the responsibility of meeting the patient's needs. Moreover, it could be the result of nursing's struggle with the problem of autonomy in role performance, as well as the result of the prospective client's demand for services both as a person with multiple needs and as a member of a family unit, not just as a patient with an isolated health need to be met by individual experts.

Thus, many of the attributes of a profession can be demonstrated in nursing. To take the professional model too literally, however, would be an egregious error. Hall, in *Occupations and the Social Structure*, refers to Roth's article in an attempt to point out some of the negative aspects of using the model too literally as well as to clarify the positive use of the traditional professional model. Hall concludes that, in spite of its limitations, the more appropriate use of the professional model is as a basis of operations for occupations (1975, p. 80).

Perhaps the criteria for what constitutes professionalism or a profession are changing. Public acceptance has always been a critical factor in determining whether or not an occupation merited the title of "profession." The public is increasingly skeptical about professions. The inability of professions to enforce their own codes of ethics causes public disapproval. The meaning of the concepts of *service* and *rights* is debated by the patient. The respect previously enjoyed and expected by members of professions is presently being challenged. Today, more than ever before, a professional must be accountable for his or her behavior; the public demands it.

Nursing has an obligation to provide to the public the clearest possible definition of nursing and the clarification of the many roles in nursing. This volume represents a comprehensive attempt to accomplish that. Before nursing can progress as a profession, some basic conflicts and problems need to be identified.

Traditionally, there have been conflicting perspectives between nursing education and nursing practice. Differences have also existed among various nursing educational programs. Faculty members from different schools have not communicated with each other about their mutual problems and interests. The results have been duplication of efforts, inefficient planning, differing expectations of students, and students' unpredictable performance after graduation. All of this generates confusion for the practitioner when he or she first enters practice.

There is also discordance between those in nursing practice and those in nursing administration. Many nurses maintain that administrators neither know nor understand the problems encountered in practice. The universal complaint of nurses is about insufficient staffing, but the justification of this complaint is questionable.

Nursing administrators and nursing educators often may be at loggerheads. Administrators wish that educators were more knowledgable about the economics of providing services and educators desire the ideal clinical environment for students after graduation.

Another problem focuses on the nature of the community of nursing itself, which includes many members who have various degrees of educational preparation (for example, those with a master's degree, the licensed practical nurse, and the nurse assistant). The division of labor in nursing is such that many identify with nursing because of the nursing tasks they perform. All these tasks are essential to the overall nursing care of patients. Nevertheless, the diverse educational backgrounds of the various people involved in nursing care make it difficult for nursing to develop as a professional community. This great division of labor and the difficulties in maintaining a community are problems that may not exist in other professions.

The lack of a professional community in nursing is evident in the fact that the majority of nurses do not belong to their professional organization, the American Nurses Association. As long as the skills and tasks that lesser-prepared personnel perform are vital to nursing care, acceptance of these personnel is essential for the development of a professional community.

The challenge for nursing is to define the role and contribution of all nursing personnel in terms of the goals and desired professional development of nursing. The basic content of the labor force cannot be ignored while the further professionalization of nursing is promoted. Those who have advanced educational preparation for professional practice define the goals and establish the standards; concomitantly, the potential contribution of all those assisting with professional practice should be developed so that the goals, values, and ideals of the profession may be maintained as a community.

To meet these problems, nursing must have leaders who will confer with one another. The striving for professionalism is a process of continuous growth. To the extent that it is in the interest of the patient, nursing should strive to attain the attributes of a profession. This goal, however, should not be an end in itself. Nursing will be increasingly recognized as a profession to the extent that it develops the knowledge necessary to fulfill the needs of the patients it serves; monitors its membership in terms of qualifications, licensure, and credentials; defines mechanisms of accountability to the members of the profession and to the patient; and delineates and develops the role and functions of nursing.

NURSING EDUCATION

The issue of nursing educational programs continues to cause confusion and to arouse concern. Does education make a difference in nursing practice? Do nurses with advanced education offer higher quality care to the patient? Or do all nurses provide essentially the same quality of care? These questions have perplexed the nursing profession for years.

In attempting to address the issues, it is essential to recognize the increasing emphasis within the profession on the preparation of competent practitioners through nursing educational programs. If differences in nursing practice related to differing educational programs exist, it will become increasingly important to document such variations—for example, those reflected in the response of the patient. Nurse educators must define their criteria as to what constitutes competency in terms of the patient and in terms of the expectations of performance of nurses from each type of nursing program. Although time and experience are required before graduates will measure up to role performance expectations, potential differences in functioning should be apparent relatively soon after graduation. These differences, however, need to be verified. Nursing cannot afford, either professionally or economically, to tolerate ill-defined goals, lack of measurement of outcomes of educational programs, or duplication of services and efforts.

One problem that increases the confusion is the lack of a precise goal for the nursing profession. The expressed objective is to serve the patient, but the unstated goal may be to raise the status and level of professionalization of nursing. These are not necessarily conflicting goals. Presumably, professionalization will be increased by the placement of educational programs in a university environment. It cannot be assumed that placing nursing education in such a setting or increasing the number of years of education will enhance the quality of patient care without, at the same time, establishing specific documentation of nursing action and behavior.

For many years, there have been conflicts between nursing education and nursing practice, between the philosophy and perspective of nursing education in one school and those in another, between nursing education and nursing administration, and between nursing practice and nursing administration. These conflicts are being addressed, but more communication is needed among these groups before the problems can be solved.

Whereas formerly only those in nursing education and nursing administration could achieve status, recently the status associated with nursing practice has increased. This augmented status has improved the reciprocity between the nurse practitioner and both the nurse educator and the nurse administrator. Currently, the practitioner is defining her learning needs to educators and adamantly requesting assistance for performing nursing services.

The status of the nurse in practice may have increased because of clearer definitions of nursing and of the roles of the nurse. If nursing roles are defined as unique and valuable in health care delivery, the increased status of these roles may be anticipated. Status also may have been improved because of the development of new roles in nursing, such as the clinical specialist and the independent nurse practitioner. Increasing autonomy for nurses in these new roles also may have facilitated negotiations between the practitioners and the administrators.

The conflict between nursing administrators and nursing educators and practitioners is most often based on economic issues. Administrators tend to be pragmatic; thus their decisions about the staffing of nurses are based on the principle of using money where it will count most. This implies that the needs for quality patient care are identified and the available funds are distributed according to effective use. Administrators are not likely to hire a clinical specialist with a master's degree, particularly if they are unsure of her expertise, when they can hire two nurses with less education for the same salary. For the same reason, a graduate with an associate degree may be hired before a graduate with a baccalaureate degree. That the type of educational background of a nurse influences the quality of patient care has not been verified. To comprehend the economics of administration, nursing students preparing to be educators or practitioners should complete a course on the costs of health care delivery. This might prepare the practitioner for reality when she assumes her first position.

Educators should discuss with each other the objectives, similarities, and differences of their programs. Resources available to one school may not be available to another. In such instances, schools should not waste their energies and money attempting to duplicate scarce resources. Exchange programs in terms of faculty and resources should be developed to provide high quality nursing education.

Several factors that pertain to specific nursing programs must be examined. There is a growing consensus that the technical and professional aspects of nursing cannot be separated into two distinct programs. The technical aspects of care must be accomplished within the scope of nursing, and a professional manner is important in their performance. The baccalaureate degree nursing programs, however, should be distinct from the associate degree programs. For example, in preparing the nurse in an associate degree program, the value of providing experience in specialty areas of nursing, such as intensive care or dialysis units, is questionable. Such experiences seem more applicable to baccalaureate degree programs. On the other hand, in-depth experiences in general medical and surgical practice could be emphasized for the associate degree student, in order for her to function effectively and acquire the skills for practice that are expected but often are missing. If the goal of associate degree programs would be to develop the technical skills of patient care, the opportunity for this type of experience should be ample.

In the future, the type of skill development needed in hospitals may need to be oriented to the technology used. The type of care provided in hospitals of the future may conceivably require the skills of a bioengineer, with an extensive knowledge of physiology as well as engineering. Realistically speaking, associate degree programs could develop technologists who would be prepared to perform many complex technical functions. This does not imply that there would be less status for nurses performing this role. More appropriately, status should be ascribed to roles that are unique in nursing and that are indispensable for the total care of the patient. The technician will have an increasingly complex role in the future.

The role of the baccalaureate degree graduate may be broader, both in hospitals for crisis care and in health maintenance settings. With increased technology, more humanistic patient care will be needed. The behavioral sciences will need to be an important part of the curriculum of the baccalaureate degree nurse. She will need to be the health professional who integrates technological and humanistic patient care and who functions primarily to provide such holistic health care to the patient.

Each nursing program should have a unique area of focus, even though a common conceptual framework among nursing programs must exist. The holistic approach to man may provide such a common conceptual framework, with the focus in the associate degree program being on technology and the focus in the baccalaureate degree program being on human behavior. This does not imply that each program has exclusive domain over those aspects. The associate degree student needs a basic understanding of the behavioristic aspects of man, and the baccalaureate degree student needs to understand how to apply technology and engineering to patient care.

With the increasing emphasis in our society on health maintenance and prevention, hospitals may be utilized mainly for crisis care and complex surgical procedures. In that event, the baccalaureate degree nurse will be increasingly needed to integrate humanistic and technological patient care. She will be relied on to make nursing diagnoses and to plan and evaluate care. Although she may not be involved directly with technical equipment, she will need a knowledge of physics, engineering, and physiology to direct much of the care given by technologists.

Seemingly, the baccalaureate degree nurse will be in increasing demand in her role of providing health maintenance and preventing illness. Defining illness in a patient or maintaining his health involves behavioral responses. Hence, the study of behavior is becoming a primary focus in baccalaureate degree programs. It should be relatively easy for the baccalaureate degree nurse to make the transition from the hospital setting to outpatient clinics and offices. Her comprehensive educational preparation will also enable her to make initial health assessments of patients and to educate patients about existing or potential health problems.

There are also issues of concern that pertain to higher education programs. Undoubtedly, educational programs for the nursing profession should be provided in a university setting. This environment allows the student to have contact with many disciplines and enables a member of a profession to obtain a comprehensive appreciation for the needs and complexities of the clients they are to serve. Many believe that for nursing to achieve the status of a profession the education of nursing students must be based in the university. Contrary to this is the practice of certifying nurses in the new role of nurse practitioners via hospital-based programs, the educational standards of which may possibly be inferior to those set by the nursing profession. All education for nursing practice needs to be conducted in a college or university setting, not only to ensure similar education and practice standards and role preparation but also to guarantee a learning environment for the student and to certify the qualifications of the instructors of such programs. Nurse practitioner certificate programs in hospital settings may primarily emphasize apprenticeship learning and fail to use the theoretical knowledge and conceptual framework that would be included in a university-based master's degree program. Thus, it would seem prudent to confine the preparation of nurse practitioners to a university-based master's degree program and eliminate those programs based in the hospital.

Another issue is the one concerning doctoral programs for nurses. Three factors should be considered in planning doctoral programs: content of the program, resources in terms of faculty and facilities, and economics. In order to determine the content of doctoral programs, the need for specific programs has to be identified and objectives must be defined. Resources need to be studied and evaluated and economic realities must be taken into account. Keeping these three factors in mind, let us now raise a number of points for consideration. Would it not be advisable to consider the development of different types of doctoral programs in nursing to be located in various parts of the country? Four types of programs might be offered, with specialties in the following areas: research, practice, education, and administration. A sound program should be designed for each specialty. The decision about which specialty area a university would choose to develop would depend on the facilities that are available and on the ability of the university to attract the most competent and qualified teachers for its desired program. Such a plan would prevent program duplication as well as the development of weak doctoral programs in nursing and promote a more efficient and economic use of available facilities and personnel. One fact must be accepted—the lack of sufficiently qualified faculty, adequate facilities, and money will not permit the proliferation of doctoral nursing programs. The pooling of efforts and resources to develop excellent programs for each of the four specialties seems wise.

All doctoral programs should include content from each of the specialty areas, even though each program focuses on one specialty. The programs specializing in administration and education should require at least 2 years of experience in nursing practice as a prerequisite. Without this practical experience, the educator or administrator would not have the realistic awareness of the needs of the patient and the practitioner necessary to qualify as a leader of the profession, which is expected of the persons who complete these specialty programs. Nursing service administrators need to be prepared on a par with nursing educators in order to assume leadership roles in the profession. This does not imply that those special-

izing in nursing practice and research need not be prepared for leadership. The contrary is true; leadership is needed in all four nursing specialties. Traditionally, however, administrators and educators have been in positions of leadership. Obviously, one cannot understand the problems of nursing practice without experiencing practice. Those pursuing doctorates specializing in nursing practice or research must have considerable experience in the practice setting during the course of their studies. Research specialists cannot develop nursing theory for practice or test intervention strategies without being in practice. Moreover, nurses specializing in education should have substantial experience in nursing practice during their program in order to be able to serve as effective role models for their future students and to present a realistic view of nursing practice to them.

In addition, if nurses continue to obtain doctorates in disciplines other than nursing, the profession will be enriched. The diverse conceptual frameworks of such disciplines as sociology, psychology, anthropology, and biology should enable nurses to contribute to nursing from unique perspectives. It has been suggested that nurses who have received a Ph.D. degree should be encouraged to obtain a N.D. (doctor of nursing) degree. Although an additional doctorate in nursing may be helpful, particularly for potential leaders in the profession, it appears highly unlikely that this would become a trend. The high cost of higher education and the length of time required to complete such a program militate against such a trend developing.

The development of external degree programs in nursing should be mentioned. Although these programs vary in terms of content and requirements, one factor common to all of them has significance for nursing. These programs seemingly do not allow the student to experience the socialization process into nursing. If external degree programs are developed for nurses who have completed a basic educational program such as a diploma or associate degree program, there may be little concern about this factor. Most nurses who have completed a basic nursing program have gone through a socialization process. The concern would be for prospective nurses completing external degree programs who have had little opportunity to develop and understand the norms and values of the profession. (For example, such a prospective student may seek to obtain a degree in nursing while working full time and thus would have minimal contact with peers, a vital factor in the development of professional behavior.)

The present system of licensing in the nursing profession has been the subject of debate for years. If the proposed legislation is passed in New York, nursing will need to act to resolve the debate. Clearly, different types of licensing examinations should be required for different levels of practice. Although the issue of licensing has been thoroughly discussed in the literature, an alternative approach could be proposed.

Based on the suggestion of different types of licensing examinations for various levels of practice, examination and licensure for the associate degree graduate and the baccalaureate degree graduate obviously should be separate. The examination for the associate degree graduate should test the applicant for technical skills, and these graduates should be given the license that is equivalent to the present practical nurse license. The baccalaureate degree graduate should be tested for professional practice and should be given the license for registered nurses. In addition to the written examination, a demonstrated practice examination should be required of the candidates for all licenses. Such a requirement assumes that each person has a different level of skill development and abilities. Present diploma or associate degree graduates should be tested via challenge examinations plus demonstrated practice examinations before they receive a registered nurse license. The establishment of practice examinations as part of the licensing process would necessitate specific definitions of the various levels of practice expected for each type of license.

Up to this time, nursing has been the only profession not requiring a minimum of a bachelor's degree for practice. Advanced licensing perhaps should be required for nursing roles that are beyond the basic preparation. Additional licensing might be required for any nurse who has graduated from the minimum of a master's degree program and is functioning as an independent nurse practitioner, nurse practitioner, or clinical specialist. All three of these nursing roles demand great expertise in nursing practice, responsibility for the direction of nursing behavior of others, and more autonomy in role performance and decision making than other nursing roles. The patient and the profession need additional assurance of the qualifications and expertise of nurses in their roles. The licensing examination in this case likewise should be two-pronged; it should test the nurse's knowledge and ability in practice. Administrators cannot afford to pay a professional salary to someone who is not qualified. Reorganization of the licensing system in nursing is a necessity.

In addition to ensuring via licensing that nurses qualify for their positions, it is important to ensure the updating of nursing knowledge through continuing education. Continuing education cannot guarantee competency, however, unless some way to measure or evaluate the effect of such a program on nursing practice is incorporated in the program. The majority of the continuing education credits that a nurse may accumulate ideally should be in the area of her practice. The requirements perhaps need to be geared toward the specific needs of nurses. For example, nurse educators might be required to have a certain number of hours in nursing practice in addition to hours in methods in teaching. The value of legislating continuing education requirements is questionable, but the motivation of nurses to participate may increase if the effect on demonstrated practice is evaluated in the continuing education programs.

The issues of nursing educational programs and licensing are timely, and the profession should not ignore them. Nursing has sufficient documentation of past errors and present needs to plan and act effectively for the future. Nursing education is the foundation for the service the profession provides. Former conflicts between nursing education and nursing practice are diminishing. As increasing emphasis is placed on *practice* in educational programs, and methods such as simulation are utilized, less discrepancy should exist between the ideals projected in educational programs and the reality of actual service. The profession is now being challenged to identify and expand the knowledge unique to nursing.

NURSING RESEARCH

The primary task of nursing research is to develop theories that will serve as a guide for nursing practice. Unfortuntely, in the past, few of the studies completed have had relevance for nursing practice. This deficiency may have been caused by the fact that those performing research were not themselves involved in nursing practice. To conceptualize a research problem about nursing practice would be difficult without contact with or experience in nursing practice.

If the practice setting is not available to the persons in a research position, at least communication with those in that environment is essential. Collaboration between personnel in nursing research and nursing practice may facilitate the proposal of studying specific problems that have relevance for nursing practice. Such interaction may also enable those in nursing practice to understand the research process and accept the value of research.

Such an interrelationship should also generate more research about the physical needs of patients. Ironically, research in this area has been lacking even though the foremost goal of nursing education programs has been to prepare practitioners to care for the physical needs of the patient. Nurses should know which procedural techniques are more beneficial to the patient than others in giving physical care. For example, is the length of a patient's hospitalization and recovery affected by his frequency of ambulation? Does a patient relinquish the sick role sooner if he is given some responsibility for his care versus having

everything done for him? Is one method better than another in preventing and treating decubitus ulcers? What difference does it make in the monitoring of a patient and in his recovery if all patients are subject to routine procedures rather than to nursing care decisions based on individual patient needs? Whether nursing actually does make a difference to the patient's outcome needs to be documented. These are just some of the research questions that should be investigated. Nurses need to know why patients respond in particular ways to specific nursing actions.

The terms *nursing process* and *nursing diagnosis* are in vogue. The effects on patient care when these methods of approaching the patient are used should be explored. Are these terms merely jargon developed to give nursing the status of having its own special language, or are they references to meaningful behavior in nursing?

What is unique in the nursing role? Evaluation of nursing decisions and behavior is essential; such evaluation could result in goal development and effective planning of resources and utilization of personnel. What type of nursing personnel is most effective in caring for the needs of patients with a specific diagnosis? No new roles should be developed without evaluating the need for such roles as well as assessing the effectiveness of present roles. Is a clinical specialist who has a master's degree more effective in assessing the needs of patients and in directing other nursing personnel than a primary care nurse? How do patients evaluate their care from various types of nurses?

Research is needed in which the patient is viewed in terms of the family unit from which he comes and to which he will return. Illness will often affect the family unit and the family may in turn affect the response of a patient to his illness. Little is known about the follow-up of patients who have been cared for briefly on a nursing unit and are subsequently expected to comply with self-care directions at home. The teaching methods that are most effective in encouraging patients to care for themselves after they return home need to be determined. With the increase of outpatient care and clinics, emphasis on understanding the environment of the patient will be essential. If hospitals become settings primarily for acute crisis care, the needs of patients who require this type of care and treatment and the role requirements and functioning of nurses in this type of environment must be investigated extensively. To study the depersonalizing effect of increasing technology on patient care will be imperative, in order to prevent the alienation of the patient from the health care environment.

Some information is available about the attitudes and personality characteristics of nurses themselves and their perception of their roles. Further investigation is needed to identify problems in role performance and the needs of nurses as professional persons. What contributes to job satisfaction for a nurse?

It may also be helpful to explore further the effects on nursing of its being predominantly and traditionally a so-called woman's profession. How does combining roles such as that of a wife and mother with that of a nurse affect the profession as well as marriage and the family? What effects do the frequent moves of nurses from one hospital to another have on the profession and on the career development of the professional?

The questioning attitude needs to be encouraged as part of the education process in order for nurses in the practice setting to reflect automatically on their nursing behavior—what they are doing and why—and to have an appreciation for the measurement of outcome. Frequently, we devalue what we do not understand. Thus, nurses who have not internalized a value for the establishment of a rationale for nursing behavior may question the utility of research. The priority of most nurses is to accomplish certain nursing tasks. If it can be demonstrated that the manner in which tasks or functions are performed is critical to patient care, then research that determines the best approaches may be considered valuable.

Research is not an easy process. The dearth of research in nursing practice may be caused in part by how difficult it is to control the many interven-

ing variables in research studies. To prepare a study proposal is difficult in a practice setting. The research design may be limited because of the patient himself. For example, the patient's condition may change so rapidly that it may be difficult for him to remain in a study. This does not excuse the responsibility of nursing to develop research protocols but rather gives recognition to the fact that often great obstacles must be overcome to complete valid research. Research is a challenge. The rewards, however, lie in the knowledge that there is rhyme and reason in the behavior underlying patient care and that a particular nursing behavior may make a difference in the patient's outcome.

NURSING THEORY

To sell anyone a product for which they see no need is difficult. Unfortunately, this has been the situation in the last decade concerning the acceptance by many nurses in nursing practice of the need for theory development in nursing. To some practitioners the discussion about theory is evidence of the esoteric nature of those in education, who have long been the proponents of theory development to promote nursing as a profession. The practicing nurse may rationalize that she does not need anything that cannot be applied to practice. This attitude may be caused by the task-oriented nature of employment in organizations.

The source of the dilemma may be a lack of communication between those in nursing practice and those in nursing education. The meaning of nursing theory and the steps in theory development also may be grossly misunderstood. Furthermore, some nurses in practice may fail to recognize a conceptual theoretical framework underlying nursing behavior. Another contributing factor may be the failure of nurses to internalize a value or to question the why's and what's of their behavior. Consequently, some practicing nurses take their behavior for granted and function more by rote or routine than by reason.

Apparently, nurses in practice have not been

told that knowledge about the phenomena underlying their nursing actions is one of the first levels of theory development for determining the *use* of knowledge. Nurses are anxious to perform effectively in practice. To expend valuable energy on investigating the basic knowledge underlying practice may be interpreted by some practitioners as knowledge for its own sake and a waste of time.

Nursing educators and those in research who are attempting to define the knowledge base of nursing need to identify the relationship between the first and final levels of theory development. Unless practitioners are able to perceive theory as knowledge that eventually can be applied to nursing practice and service, it will be rejected as a value. At the same time, theory development must take place in the practice setting. The failure of academicians to make sufficient use of the practice setting as well as their failure to communicate with those in practice may have caused the unsystematic development of nursing theory.

Nurses would have difficulty developing situation-producing theory for practice without having first gone through the preliminary levels of theory development, as Menke suggests. It is not necessary, however, to wait until many theories have been developed at the lowest level before pursuing any one theory to the highest level of its development. That little theory has been developed at the level of situation-producing theory may have been caused by the fact that no one theory has been pursued to the practice level. Nursing has been groping unsystematically at the factor-isolating and factor-relating levels of theory development for too long.

Nursing can benefit from borrowing theory from other disciplines and applying it to nursing practice. For example, much of the theory of sociology can be applied to nursing, such as symbolic interaction theory and exchange theory. The use of symbolic interaction theory to explain behavior is evident in Soares's paper on verbal usage in the intensive care unit. Exchange theory in terms of understanding peers, social control, rewards, and punishment is applicable in nurse-

patient relationships. Functionalism is perhaps the theory traditionally underlying much of the behavior of nurses. This theory was evident in the tradition of assigning treatment nurses, medication nurses, and so forth, on a nursing unit in an attempt to organize patient care as a controlled system. The challenge is to apply the theory of another discipline to nursing as it is relevant to patient care.

Nursing needs to investigate specific nursing activities, not only to determine the underlying theory for each activity but also to be able to develop new theory for nursing practice. To define this underlying theory as unique to nursing is not necessary; in fact, to strive to do so may be a mistake. The nursing activity, however, may belong uniquely to nursing. Some nursing activities may not be based on theory borrowed or adapted from other disciplines, but this distinction may be difficult or unnecessary to determine.

The energy and time spent on defining theory that is unique to nursing and not borrowed or adapted from other disciplines may be more difficult for the practitioner to understand or accept. Those in practice may consider the search for nursing theory to substantiate their actions as totally irrelevant. To them, the significance of theory is doubtful because there has been no practical application of theory to effective nursing care. The nurse in practice may not be as concerned about nursing's attaining the status of a profession with a unique body of theoretical knowledge as are those in nursing education. The possibility of developing theory about nursing that is uniquely nursing theory, however, may lie in defining the activities and processes of nurses in practice, such as a *nursing diagnosis*.

A cultural lag exists between the documentation of theory by academicians and researchers and the acceptance of theory by nurses in practice. As the meaning and applications of such concepts as nursing diagnosis become understood, theoreticians and practitioners of patient care may realize their mutual contributions to improved patient care and may devise new ways to collaborate.

Thus, theory developed for the benefit of the patient will be considered relevant. It is not likely that a grand theory *about, of,* or *in* nursing will prove to be beneficial to nursing or will be advocated by the majority of those in the profession.

NURSING PRACTICE

In the last decade, the status associated with nursing practice has increased tremendously. One contributing factor has been that more nurses in practice have earned a master's degree in a clinical component. A possible outcome of obtaining higher education is that nurses have been able to identify practice problems via a conceptual, analytical framework and to implement plans to resolve them. Nurses with advanced education may also be better equipped to define the role of nursing. Peers on a nursing unit who have witnessed the use of skills by a clinical specialist, for example, may see the value of higher education.

From the point of view of education, the status associated with nursing practice has also improved because nurses who have earned a master's degree have returned to the practice setting. The level of educational preparation for nursing service administration has also increased. Slightly more than a decade ago, nursing administrators seldom had a master's degree. In effect, introducing higher education into the practice setting has resulted in increased status ascribed to nursing practice. Schools of nursing education have also promoted increased status for those in nursing practice. Approximately a decade ago, the trend developed to provide a master's degree program for specialization in clinical practice. Functional specialization, such as in administration or education, without minoring in a clinical component was frowned on. The emphasis on a master's degree for clinical practice did influence the status of nursing practice.

An interesting question remains. What was the impetus for this apparently sudden change in emphasis on the desirability of having master's degree programs in nursing? Were those in nursing education proposing that such a move might increase the quality and outcome of patient care? Was this attempt to introduce graduates with master's degrees into the practice setting aimed at reducing the gap between the theoretical world of education and the reality of patient care? Was this step primarily a maneuver to increase the status and the degree of professionalization of nursing that are assumed to be related to education? Perhaps the answer is a composite of all of these thoughts. It also may lie in the expressed need for expert patient care and in the awareness that the quality of patient care could be improved.

Whether all of the goals suggested in the above questions have been attained is yet to be documented, but undoubtedly the status formerly enjoyed by those in nursing education, and then by those in nursing administration, is now being experienced by those in nursing practice. This status is both achieved and ascribed—achieved from the perspective that the practitioner has earned an advanced degree and has demonstrated competence in her practice, and ascribed in that the status has been delegated by the profession to those who have attained a master's degree and returned to the practice setting. Increased status has not been limited to those with a master's degree for practice but has filtered down to improve the status of everyone involved in nursing practice.

In particular, expectations of the general nurse in practice may have changed because of her contact in practice with nurses who have had higher education. The staff nurse may have assimilated some of the values of the clinical specialist, for example. Values such as the use of judgment, autonomy, cognitive skills, and decision making may be a part of the desire to provide total, comprehensive, and individualized care for the patient. Because of her awareness of these values, the nurse in practice, whether in an organization setting or in private independent practice, may expect more interaction with a patient. Perhaps the increased interaction and direct involvement with patients allow more status to be ascribed to that nursing role. The patient is becoming more aware of his rights for quality service and may verbally reward those who provide it through direct patient care. Thus, the practicing nurse may have developed increased self-esteem and thus may regard her role as more important.

The increased status given to the nurse in practice, and specifically to the new role of the nurse practitioner and to those in joint and independent practice, may also be the result of the further division of labor in medicine. This function may apply especially to those who have primarily assumed a medical, rather than a nursing, orientation as nurse practitioners. Physicians have discovered the competency of nurses in performing certain tasks and consequently have delegated these responsibilities to nurses. The increasing demands on the physician's time and skills have facilitated a willingness to delegate these tasks. Concomitantly, medical practice laws have been changed to accommodate this process. This has had some unforeseen results on both those in medicine and those in nursing.

Some nurses, having experienced not only the challenge of decision making in planning some of the medical care of patients but also the heightened prestige and status of identifying closely with the medical model, desire further autonomy in offering medical care to patients. Members of the medical profession did not foresee this drive for autonomy that currently exists in some nurse practitioners. The outcome of this situation remains to be seen, but the blueprint apparently has been developed in the change in practice laws.* A norm might be established. To the extent that a nurse practitioner is functioning within the medical model and is applying medical skills in her practice, her domain legally will remain under the mandate of the physician. Nurses in such a role, however, are not using nursing skills but are assuming a defined medical role. ("By their works you shall know them!") Autonomy for nurses in patient care is not likely if that role is defined in

*As noted by Bullough in Chapter 30.

terms of medical behavior and within a medical model. If legislation is altered to permit nurses to perform medical tasks with greater autonomy, perhaps the legal definition of a new type of practice of medicine, not nursing, would be called for. This may account for the different approaches in the changes of the practice laws.

The combining of the medical and nursing models appears to present difficulties for many nurses. The mid-zone of role performance includes such activities as conducting an initial medical system assessment and examination of the patient, health teaching, counseling, and assessing total needs of the patient as a person and member of a family unit. In such practice settings, the distinction between the role of the physician and that of the nurse is minimal. Eventually, one role may receive primacy and the values associated with that role will be developed.

Admittedly, to decide what direction the role of the nursing practitioner should take is extremely difficult. Three schools of thought exist. The first is to develop the role of the nurse practitioner in primary care as a lower-level practitioner of medicine. The second is to combine medical activities, such as physical examinations, with nursing assessment and teaching. The third is to concentrate on the primary role and definition of nursing. To take a stance will require a crucial decision on the part of the nursing profession. Will the profession develop with a unique service to offer, or will it compromise and attempt to fill the need for increased medical services and to alleviate medical shortages? Nurses are capable of performing many of the initial tasks that a physician performs in making a medical diagnosis, such as assessing the preliminary medical needs of a patient, following up on the extent to which a patient has complied with medical treatment, teaching, investigating, and pursuing the social aspects of treatment. Beyond that, if nursing is to develop as a unique profession, nurses must concentrate on the unique role that nursing has to offer. Without this special effort on the part of nurses, nursing will be coopted as a profession.

There has been an apparent start, however, in the attempt to develop the unique role of nursing. The role of nurse practitioner allows for the development of an autonomy in nursing that is desirable for the profession. The contributions in the section on nursing practice focus specifically on nursing process, and the advent of nursing diagnoses provides distinct guidelines and directions for a method of developing nursing practice. The taken-for-granted activities of nursing are explicitly defined, and a prospective theoretical framework for nursing, which may assist those who are developing the role of nurse practitioner for nursing and not medicine, is presented. The nurse practitioner functioning predominantly as a nurse is just beginning to develop the potential of her role. With the development of any new role, gray areas about the domain of that role need to be discussed. This takes time and negotiation. To the extent that the gray areas of the nurse practitioner role are defined by the nursing profession as nursing and rationally can be understood as nursing, the role of the nurse practitioner may be accepted by both nursing and medicine as valuable and unique.

Perhaps the new, controversial nurse practitioner role has given the nursing profession the impetus to define nursing. The profession has been alarmed at the number of nursing dropouts—nurses who have entered medically oriented nurse practitioner programs and physician assistant programs. In effect, such nurses have been preempted by medicine. The nursing profession has been challenged to face the issues involved in defining nursing. What is presented in the section on nursing practice should greatly assist in defining nursing practice and the role of the nurse. It should apply not only to those in nursing practice in an organizational setting but also to those in ambulatory care and in joint or independent practice settings.

The unique role of nursing is similar in all of these settings; only the environment where it is applied varies. Some settings permit nurses more autonomous functioning than others, such as that of independent practice. Other specific nursing skills may need to be developed, depending on the setting. In our complex society, however, interdependency in role performance, and not only autonomy, is important. No one has the sufficient expertise in all areas necessary to provide the quality care that is needed today.

The growing impetus for nurses to deliver primary care presents many challenges to nursing. The nurse's role as a health teacher clearly will need further development. A viable definition of autonomy should be formulated. For example, the nurse in primary care may be autonomous in one area, such as in her methods of health teaching, but not autonomous in the total planning of care for patients. The primary care nurse should know when to consult other available resources. This decision-making skill is not likely to be developed in a basic baccalaureate degree program; its acquisition requires the experience of practice and perhaps advanced preparation in a clinical master's degree program. If fee-for-service or third-party reimbursement evolves for nursing services, nurses will need advanced preparation in order to measure up to the accountability that will be demanded of them.

If third-party reimbursement is further encouraged for nurses, nursing will have to define precisely the role of a specifically educated nurse both for the public and third-party payers. Expectations of service for various nursing roles will also need definition. However, nurses should be aware of the fact that third-party reimbursement could bring into play many bureaucratic procedures and regulations that might impede the type of individualized comprehensive care that they desire to give. Measurement of outcome in nursing care could become a legal requirement to justify third-party reimbursement. It is difficult enough to measure such subjective factors as interactions and quality of care without legislative considerations entering the process.

With the increase in technology and the knowledge explosion, the use of computers to direct nursing actions and predict patient needs is a real possibility and this, in turn, presents a danger to both nurses and patients alike. This danger lies in the potential negative effects of the increased use of such technology in nursing care, effects such as the dehumanization of the patient and the loss of the social meaning, relationship, and consequence of activity that Tomich defines as the essence of nursing. If social acts are programmed, the holistic approach of nursing to patient care will be endangered and if that approach is discarded, a role for nursing practice or the nursing profession will not exist.

INTERDISCIPLINARY PROFESSIONAL RELATIONSHIPS

The division of labor between medicine and nursing with respect to the social object (the patient) has increasingly become an area of confusion and conflict. At the basis of this conflict is the change in the culture of nursing itself. Although many interdisciplinary relationships are possible for nurses, the focus in this volume is on the nature of the relationship that exists between the physician and the nurse. Previous norms and values in role performance, such as the nurse acting obediently as the handmaiden of the physician, have been altered. Previously, the physician was regarded as the only professional expert in health care, and his specialized knowledge was the source of this authority. Nursing is developing its own specialized knowledge and defining the role of the nurse independently from, and interdependent with, that of medicine. This is being accomplished partly through negotiation with medicine. The interaction between medicine and nursing today is characterized by role bargaining and exchange. The conflict that has existed has not necessarily been a negative factor in the relationships between medicine and nursing. Conflict sets boundaries between groups and may strengthen group consciousness, thus establishing the identity of groups within the social system of health care. Nursing has been stimulated via the conflicts with medicine to identify its role and unique mission.

Interdependency is a check against the violation of agreements between nursing and medicine. The dialectics of stability and change, integration and conflict, and consensus and coercion historically have been a part of the physician-nurse relationship. With the emphasis on interdependency, more balance has been achieved in the power relationships between the two. To the extent that there is a balance between medicine and nursing in terms of each needing the other's services, power becomes less of a controlling factor.

The nature of the interdependence between nursing and medicine in terms of activities, use of resources, and client care needs further elaboration. A statement that clearly defines the established boundaries of medicine and nursing is needed. Extensive communication with physicians and among nurses is the essence of this social process. Communication is essential for nursing, not only for clarifying the incongruities in the nurse's self-concept and in her self-expectations but also for defining the concept and expectations others have of her. Once expectations are agreed on, defining the interdependency needed between nursing and medicine may be easier.

The existence of interdependent relationships may confuse the patient. Because the role of the nurse seems indefinite, the patient may not know what to expect from nurses in different role models. When the expressive aspects of the nursing role are combined with the instrumental aspects, as in the nurse practitioner role, the patient may be further confused. Standardization of nurse practitioner programs may facilitate expectations of that role for the patient.

In the process of defining nursing, the patient may feel "departmentalized" as he witnesses arbitration between nurses and physicians as they divide him up in relation to their role activities. There is hope, however. The care aspect of nursing is being scientifically defined in terms of process. In time, the patient should be able to differentiate nursing from medicine, as the nursing role assumes a consistent, defined pattern. Patients may recognize that pattern of care as their needs are met in a more consistent fashion. As nurses attempt to revise the conceptions that the public has of them, they will also be revising their conceptions of themselves and of their work. As they define their unique mission, nursing should gain in status, value, and prestige—not only among nurses but also in the view of physicians and the public.

Increasing the number of years of educational preparation is not necessarily what will increase the status of nursing in the eyes of the public and of members of the medical profession. Rather, the professional status of nursing may increase as a result of its providing a service that cannot be offered by another occupation. Nursing should capitalize on the opportunity to develop the service it has to offer since other avenues of status development are not available, for example, upward mobility is lacking in nursing.

Another aspect of the interdependency that exists between nursing and medicine is demonstrated in the legal process governing nursing practice. Not only is the collegial body the judge of professional competence but the licensing process acts as an evaluating mechanism as well. The tendency in some states to allow changes in nursing practice through laws governing medical practice may be contrary to the aims of the nursing profession. The licensing of nurse practitioners has been regulated by provisions in medical practice acts, which implies that the nurse is under the supervision of the physician. Such a trend may frustrate the development of true interdependent relationships with medicine.

The success of interdependent professional relationships depends upon the demonstration of competence and accountability by the nursing profession. Viable models for successful interdependent professional relationships between nurses and physicians exist. Medicine's and nursing's goal of being mutually supportive rather than being competitive and controlling is being realized.

FUTURE OF NURSING

The future of nursing may appear obscure and complex. Nevertheless, indications concerning the direction in which nursing as a profession is evolving have been presented. One thing is certain—continued change is inevitable. The predicted changes are based partly on the influence of the external environment on nursing and partly on factors within the health professions themselves.

That the government will have an increased role in health care delivery seems likely, if not specifically through a national health insurance program then through continued legislation for health care and health policy. Although patient involvement in health care delivery has been advocated, it is difficult for patients to be fully informed about the crucial issues in health care delivery. Input is needed from the patient, however; the patient may need to remind the health care experts that he is a holistic entity and more than merely a sum of parts to be treated by various specialists.

The patient's input to the health care process is apparently being promoted by the government. Attempts to establish grievance mechanisms for patients via legislation is an example of the government's acting as the patient's advocate. Such attempts may appear to be a means of safeguarding the rights of patients but, on the other hand, can represent an infringement on the health professions' autonomy and their rights to define the role of the health professional and the care to be provided by him. Grievances should be heard and acted upon, but when redress is legislated the superimposition of a generalized control on health care may result in the increased depersonalization of care. Whereas the public is aware that the government is continually being consulted to alleviate the escalating costs of care and to guarantee a certain amount of health care for all, it is not aware to the same degree about the implications of government intervention in the quality of care.

When the government intervenes in assisting with the economics of health care, the quality of health care will also be investigated, and that has future implications for the health professions. Specifically, it could mean that the government would define the role of the nurse and grant funds only to educational programs that develop certain nursing roles. Accountability to the government is certain to be demanded, both for quality and type of service provided.

One means of counteracting this type of control of nursing would be to develop the identity of nursing as a member of the health professions. The occupational consciousness of nursing will be raised as nursing continues to define its unique role, begins to document the service it provides, and evaluates the outcome of that service. As this is accomplished by nursing, nursing as a profession will become increasingly meaningful to its members. An external force such as the government may further unite the segmented interest groups of nursing (education, research, practice, and administration). A strong occupational consciousness increases a profession's potential political power. Nursing has not been actively involved in defining the policies of health care. As nursing continues to develop a role in health maintenance, the functions of this role will become increasingly relevant, and nursing may exert a more prestigious political influence.

The potential influence of the government may also be a catalyst to increase interdependent relationships between nursing and medicine. Obviously, medicine and nursing need the support and assistance of each other to provide the care needed and demanded by the patient. Some boundaries in patient care may always be arbitrary because of the acknowledged differences in abilities and competencies among individual professions as well as differences among the demands of certain settings, such as rural areas. To program precisely the roles of the physician and the nurse would probably limit the initiative and creativity of the professional, as well as fail to allow for the unforeseen factors that may crop up in providing care to human beings. Nursing and medicine are defining the crucial boundaries of their roles, and negotiation and exchange will continue in the future. Whereas in the past physicians often delegated tasks to nurses, at present nurses are negotiating with physicians for the right to perform tasks that are currently in the physician's domain but that in the future will be in the realm of nursing. The

mutual concern of both professions to provide the best possible health care to all will be the continued catalyst for improving relationships.

The reasons for health care will also inevitably change, partly because of an increasing desire to prevent serious illness that may result in devastating costs to the family but also because of increased knowledge about health maintenance. Presumably, with our increasingly complex and technologic society, health problems themselves may change. Suicide and mental illness may become more prevalent because of a person's alienation from himself and from others. These problems may be seen especially in patients in ambulatory care centers. Nurses need to be aware of the intervening social forces that influence the outcome of care, such as the effect the family has on encouraging health maintenance. They will need to identify the factors that impede expected healthy behavior and to take appropriate action to alleviate any conflict that may negatively affect the patient's recovery rate.

Hospitals may become centers for acute care and short-term stays for patients. Self-care or extended-care units may be further developed. The use of laser technology in surgical procedures may reduce the length of stay for patients in hospitals. Clinical specialists may be called upon more often to help meet unexpected complications in the nursing care of patients. Head nurses may be expected to provide more counseling and staff development as more nursing care is provided by technicians.

As the settings of health care change, the expectations and roles for members of the nursing profession and for others will need to be redefined. The nursing profession is obligated to accomplish this task, as it is the means by which it will demonstrate control over the work performance of its members and establish itself as an autonomous profession. Once there is consensus on what is expected of a nurse, the laws for nursing practice may more likely become standardized, and standards of practice may be defined for each nursing role.

Once expectations and standards of practice are

made explicit, educational requirements can be identified. Educational preparation should primarily focus on the qualifications necessary for a type of nursing practice rather than on increasing the professional status of nursing. Thus, it is critical that curricula and requirements be carefully planned and justified.

There is a growing consensus that a practice base is essential for nursing, whether one eventually specializes in education, research, administration, or practice. This agreement on the importance of practice may be the clue to the future of nursing. It is this identification of nursing's specific commitment to provide service and care to the patient that should enable the profession to retain a clear perspective for the future.

The problem of developing leadership for nursing remains. In the past, leadership in the profession has been left to chance. The process of gaining a position of influence in nursing is unsystematic. In part, such a position has been attained through the accumulation of educational credentials. Because practice has become increasingly important in nursing, it might be expected that future leaders will come from this area of the profession. The nursing practice base from which future leaders might develop is expected to be different from that of the past. Such future leaders will have an understanding of nursing theory and will be able to apply and develop it, draw on the significance of research findings for practice, and have a workable, realistic knowledge of economics in providing health care. Future leaders must have a comprehensive overview of nursing, and must not favor their own area of specialization. An eclectic theoretical and educational framework coupled with critical experience in nursing practice will provide the balance needed to enable effective planning for the future. Planning for change is the essence of leadership and the challenge that remains for nursing. Leadership development can be encouraged in the practice setting and in the education programs by establishing a climate conducive to raising questions and searching for the right answers. This volume has hopefully encouraged that type of climate. The exact nature of the future of nursing is not crystal clear, but the profession is a dynamic one and will continue to change and grow. Like the pilgrim who knows no certain path, the professional who is in the mist clears the path by going forward.

BIBLIOGRAPHY

Greenwood, Ernest: "Attributes of a Profession," *Social Work*, 2(3):45–55, July 1957.

Hall, Richard H.: *Occupations and the Social Structure*, 2d ed., Prentice-Hall, Englewood Cliffs, N.J., 1975.

Roth, Julius A.: "Professionalism: The Sociologist's Decoy," *Sociology of Work and Occupations*, 1:6–23, February 1974.

Index